Paediatrics Traumatology

Matías Sepúlveda O.
Editor

Paediatrics Traumatology

A Comprehensive Guide to Diagnosis and Management

Springer

Universidad Austral de Chile
Conocimiento y Naturaleza

Editor
Matías Sepúlveda O.
Instituto de Especialidades
Universidad Austral de Chile
Clínica Alemana Valdivia
Valdivia, XIV Los Ríos, Chile

ISBN 978-3-031-89484-8 ISBN 978-3-031-89482-4 (eBook)
https://doi.org/10.1007/978-3-031-89482-4

The original submitted manuscript has been translated into English. The translation was done using artificial intelligence. A subsequent revision was performed by the author(s) to further refine the work and to ensure that the translation is appropriate concerning content and scientific correctness. It may, however, read stylistically different from a conventional translation.
Translation from the Spanish language edition: "Traumatología Infantil" by Matías Sepúlveda O., © editor 2023. Published by National Society of Orthopedics and Traumatology in Chile (SCHOT). All Rights Reserved.

This Springer imprint is published by the registered company Springer Nature Switzerland AG
The registered company address is: Gewerbestrasse 11, 6330 Cham, Switzerland

Preface

This project has been developed with the support of "Funds for Scientific Publication 2021," from the Chilean Orthopedics and Traumatology Society, as a project of the Children's Orthopedics and Traumatology Committee. The book is a project included in the work plan of the directives for the years 2021 to 2023, with active participation of its members in each chapter.

Directive 2021
Pablo Schaufele M.
PRESIDENT
Catalina Larraín
VICE PRESIDENT
Matías Sepúlveda O.
SECRETARY

Directive 2022
Catalina Larraín
PRESIDENT
Matías Sepúlveda O.
VICE PRESIDENT
Alejandro Peña A.
SECRETARY

Directive 2023
Matías Sepúlveda O.
PRESIDENT
Alejandro Peña A.
VICE PRESIDENT
Cristian Artigas
SECRETARY

Valdivia, XIV Los Ríos, Chile

Matías Sepúlveda O.

Acknowledgment

The authors thank the Chilean Orthopedics and Traumatology Society for the support in carrying out this collaborative educational project, achieved with great effort.

For my part, I appreciate the time and work dedicated by each one of the authors of the different chapters of this book to achieve the task. This book is undoubtedly the result of committed teamwork, faithfuly representative the spirit of the Chilean Children Orthopedics and Traumatology Society (SCHOTI), committee of the Chilean Orthopedic and Traumatology Society (SCHOT).

The inspiration for this book comes from various conversations with Professor Lyhn Staheli, recently deceased, and Dalia Sepúlveda, my mentor. The idea of a book that simply guides the correct diagnosis of musculoskeletal pediatric trauma, presenting up-to-date treatment options available in our environment, is essential to improving access to adequate therapy and must be available to everyone.

The book is also a project developed by the team of the Faculty of Medicine of the Universidad Austral de Chile, seeking to be the primary bibliographic resource for the Annual Orthopedics and Traumatology Course. This course, held in Valdivia, Chile, and aimed at residents of the specialty of all the country, has been running continuously since 2010. Several of the book's chapter authors actively participate in the course as teachers.

Finally, I must thank my family. My parents for educating me and encouraging me to work daily for the ideals that I have. I thank my children for allowing me to dedicate the necessary time to this and other projects, and of course my wife, whose support makes these tasks possible. Also with a special mention to the drawings made by Estefanía, which support several chapters, another virtue in her.

Instituto de Especialidades
Universidad Austral de Chile
Clínica Alemana Valdivia
Valdivia, XIV Los Ríos, Chile

Matías Sepúlveda O.

Contents

Part I Generalities of Pediatric Trauma

1 Biology of Bone Repair in the Pediatric Patient 3
María Elena Pérez and Sergio Vial

2 Traumatic Injuries of the Growth Plate 15
Estefanía Birrer, Benjamín Cancino, and Julio de Pablos

3 Non-Accidental Injuries 35
Daniel Fodor and Carlos Saavedra

4 The Pediatric Patient with Multiple Injuries 47
Pedro Jorba and Nicolás Valdivia R.

5 Overuse Musculoskeletal Injuries in the Pediatric Patient 59
Claudia Alday and María Angélica Ibañez

6 Principles of Conservative Treatment in the Pediatric Patient 75
Erika Arana and Monica Foppiano

7 Principles of Surgical Treatment in the Pediatric Patient 89
Felipe Hodgson and Alexandre Arkader

8 Open Fractures in the Pediatric Population 109
Andres Ferreyra and Victoria Allende

Part II Upper Extremity Trauma

9 Clavicle Fracture 123
Martín D'Elía and Pablo Schaufele

10 Proximal Humerus Fracture 137
Juan Fuenzalida and Humberto Galleano

11 Humeral Shaft Fracture 147
Marco Morillo and Rodrigo Rivera

12 **Humeral Condyle Fractures** 159
Gino Martínez and Mauricio Silva

13 **Medial Epicondyle Fractures of the Humerus** 177
María Jesús Figueroa and Julio Toledo

14 **Supracondylar Fracture of the Distal Humerus** 191
Pía Franz, Unni Narayanan, and Matías Sepúlveda O.

15 **Radial Neck Fractures** 209
Theddy Slongo

16 **Monteggia Fracture-Dislocation** 233
Alejandro Baar and Jamil F. Soni

17 **Diaphyseal Fracture of the Radius and Ulna** 245
Cristian Artigas and Dalia Sepúlveda

18 **Distal Radius Fracture** 261
Juan Carlos Hernández and Verónica Vilches

19 **Fractures of the Phalanges of the Hands** 275
Jorge Gamboa

20 **Fingertip Injuries** 289
Macarena Morovic and Paulina de la Fuente

Part III Lower Extremity Trauma

21 **Pelvic Injuries in the Pediatric Patient** 305
Fernando Inostroza and Lenin Colmenares

22 **Hip Fractures in Children and Adolescents** 317
Laura Montes and Catalina Larraín

23 **Fracture of the Femoral Shaft** 331
Javier Besomi and Eric Gordon

24 **Distal Femur Fractures** 343
Claudio Meneses and Rodrigo Yáñez

25 **Tibial Eminence Fracture** 357
Florencia Espinoza, Daniel Green, and María Jesús Tuca

26 **Anterior Cruciate Ligament and Meniscal Injuries in Pediatric Patients** 373
Julio Javier Masquijo and I. Maximiliano Espinosa

27 **Fracture of the Anterior Tuberosity of the Tibia** 389
Gonzalo De la Fuente and Alejandro Gündel

28 **Proximal Tibia Fracture** 399
Astrid Medina and Daniel Pineda

29 Tibial Shaft Fracture 409
Hernán Guzmán and Constanza Ramírez

30 Ankle Fracture 425
Cristian Olmedo and Rodrigo Zuñiga

31 Transitional Ankle Fractures 439
Pablo Echenique and Pablo Wagner

32 Traumatic Injuries of the Pediatric Foot 451
Natalia Cifuentes and Consuelo Peirano

Index 473

Part I
Generalities of Pediatric Trauma

Chapter 1
Biology of Bone Repair in the Pediatric Patient

María Elena Pérez and Sergio Vial

1.1 Biology of Bone Repair in the Pediatric Patient

To understand the process of repair and remodeling of bone tissue after a fracture in pediatric patients, it is essential to know the structure of the organ called "bone," and the characteristics of the developing immature skeleton. Already from the seventeenth century, we find the works developed by Clopton Havers [1], who made the description of the bone canals that bear his name. The bone is composed of organic material (collagen and non-collagen proteins) and a mineral matrix (composed mostly of calcium and phosphorus). It is not an inert structure, but rather a living, complex tissue, with multiple constant functions, mainly through its three cell types: osteocyte, osteoblast, and osteoclast. The bone responds to external forces (load) and local and systemic signals (cytokines, growth factors, and different hormones: estrogens, androgens, parathyroid hormone, Vitamin D3, among others). In addition, it is in a constant communication with the cells of the immune and hematopoietic system.

1.2 Bone Tissue Structure

Bone tissue is a complex structure, with varied functions and biomechanical properties. Bone is a hard, resistant, and durable material, which can withstand high weight load and impact, and dynamically responds to mechanical challenges. It repairs and

---

M. E. Pérez (✉)
Clínica Universidad De La República, Montevideo, Uruguay

S. Vial
Clínica Santa María, Santiago, Chile

M. Sepúlveda O. (ed.), *Paediatrics Traumatology*,
https://doi.org/10.1007/978-3-031-89482-4_1

replaces itself throughout life and serves as a reservoir of ions (calcium, phosphorus) that are mobilized on demand from the body [2, 3].

Bone tissue is organized as a mosaic of connected units, whose base are the osteons that form the Haversian canals. These units freely lay as spongious trabecular bone or densely compact cortical bone. They adhere to each other by strong lines that have organic and non-organic components, which ensure the molecular union, maintaining its form during bone remodeling, while the bone is reabsorbed and forming new bone tissue. These "cellular teams," responsible for the alternation of the cycles of resorption and bone formation, are called Metabolic/Multicellular Bone Units (MBU), and are composed of osteocytes, osteoblasts, and osteoclasts. This physiological mechanism is what is known as "Bone turnover" (Fig. 1.1) [4, 5].

Both bone tissue and bone marrow are rich in undifferentiated pluripotential cells (called STEM cells), which can give rise to five cell strains: osteoblasts, chondroblasts, adipocytes, fibroblasts, and myoblasts. The generation of one or another cell type will depend on the activation of different genes. Among the recognized processes involved in differentiation towards the osteogenic lineage are those controlled by genes of the Hedgehog 3 family, Core transcription factors (Cbfa1 or Runx2), and bone morphogenetic proteins (BMPs). Collagen I and Osteopontin are expressed early in osteoprogenitor cells [6].

The Hedgehog pathway is essential in organogenesis and the modeling of embryonic structures, especially in the caudocephalic axis and the neural tube. Hedgehogs are a family of proteins that participate in the complex and intricate system of intercellular signaling. Its importance has also been determined in some tumors and in the maintenance and regulation of stem cells in some tissues. There are three genes from the Hedgehog family: Sonic Hedgehog (Shh), Indian Hedgehog (Ihh), and

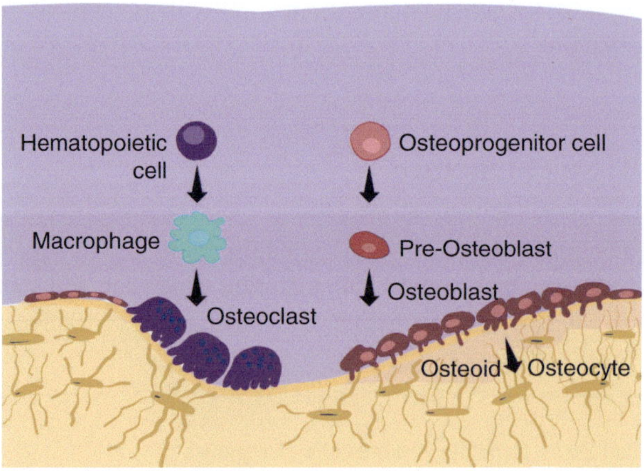

Fig. 1.1 Bone homeostasis is achieved through osteoclastic line activity (bone resorption) and osteoblastic line activity (secretion of hydroxyapatite and calcium, mineralization and osteocyte formation)

Desert Hedgehog (Dhh) which are homologous to the Hh gene of Drosophila (the "fruit fly") which was the first to be identified.

Shh plays a fundamental role in limb development, controlling the number and form of the fingers in all four limbs [9, 10].

Osteoclasts are large, multinucleated cells that develop from marrow hematopoietic stem cells, called Granulocyte and Macrophage Colony Forming Units (CFU-GM). The regulation of osteoclast formation is based on three key molecules: Osteoprotegerin (OPG), which is synthesized by osteoblasts and pre-osteoblasts; RANKL, which is a co-stimulating molecule of the pathway of cell activation of osteoclast precursors and of the transcription factors of the osteoclastogenic cascade; and RANK, which is the RANKL receptor found on the membrane of osteoclasts and pre-osteoclasts [11]. The osteoclast is the cell responsible for maintaining bone homeostasis; it performs osteocytic osteolysis to regulate calcemia, synthesizing and reabsorbing in a limited way certain components of the bone matrix. The active form of the osteoclasts is located in the Howship's lacunae, attached to the surface of the bone tissue that must be removed. They have a serrated edge with cytoplasmic projections by which they adhere to the edges of the cavity. It secretes protons and osteolytic enzymes (collagenases, gelatinases, cathepsins K, and matrix metalloproteinases [MMP-9]) to achieve the resorption of the mineralized surface of the bone (Fig. 1.2).

Osteoblasts are large cells, with a rough endoplasmic reticulum, that derive from pluripotent mesenchymal cells. They synthesize organic matrix or osteoid substance and present alkaline phosphatase and pyrophosphatase, which allow rapid mineralization. They produce matrix vesicles with accumulation of calcium and phosphate ions, direct the arrangement of the fibers of the extracellular matrix and mediate in the resorption performed by osteoclasts through the synthesis of specific cytokines.

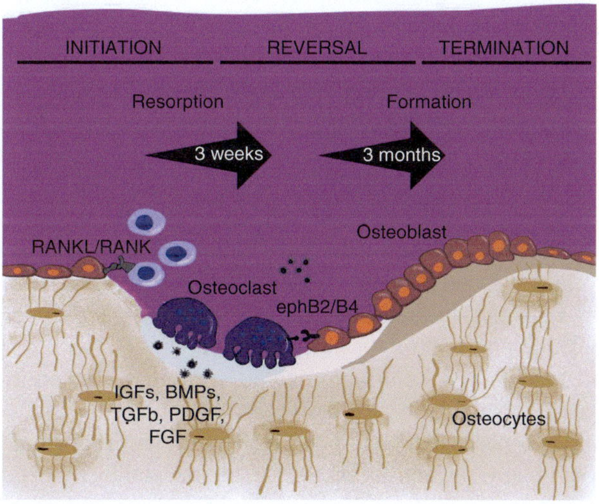

Fig. 1.2 Scheme of the three phases of the bone remodeling process

They also synthesize growth factors and type I Collagen, a fibrillar extracellular matrix protein, which determines the tensile strength of the bone. This type I collagen is not only in the bone, but also in ligaments, tendons, and skin. They also secrete Osteocalcin (OCN), a non-collagen protein that has a specific expression for bone, which has glutamic acids in its composition that leads to the formation of hydroxyapatite, inorganic component of the extracellular matrix.

The maturation stages of the osteoblast are: Immature Osteoblast or pre-osteoblast, Mature Osteoblast, Osteoid Osteocyte, Early Osteocyte, Mature Osteocyte, Differentiated Osteoblast. There is a "Master control gene" necessary for osteoblast differentiation called Runx2 transcription factor (Cbfa1, Osf2, Pebp2a1, or Am13). The absence of this factor (studied in mice) leads to no bone formation [2]. The transformation from Osteoblast to Osteocyte surrounded by bone matrix happens in 15% of the tissue. The rest remains on the surface of the newly formed bone tissue, constituting the flat cells of bone lining.

The osteocyte is the mature differentiation stage of the osteoblast, when it is surrounded by extracellular bone matrix in small tunnels called "canaliculi," that connect the entire length of the bone. The main function of the osteocyte is to distribute the direction and the amount of mechanical tension applied to the bone. Hence its location within the extracellular bone matrix, which supports the load of it. Its action is evident in elderly patients or patients under corticoid treatment, where the loss of osteocytes causes micro-damage that can lead to compression vertebral fractures. That's why it's so important to maintain the integrity of the "osteocytic network." Another important function of osteocytes is the regulation of mineral homeostasis, regulating the availability of calcium, especially under normal special conditions, such as lactation. It also regulates phosphate homeostasis.

The organic bone matrix [3, 12] is composed of collagen proteins (90%) and non-collagen proteins, proteoglycans, and lipids (10%). We also find plasmatic proteins, some with great affinity for the bone matrix, such as alpha2-HS glycoprotein (Fetuin A).

The most important collagen proteins are: a. Type I collagen, the most abundant protein in bone tissue, which is also present in ligaments, tendons, menisci, periosteum, and perichondrium, among others. It is a fibrillar collagen that contains a triple helix, which provides high tensile strength, important for bone and other tissues function. The coordinated expression of the COL1A1 and COL1A2 genes is essential to ensure the correct assembly of the different types of collagen chains; b. Type V collagen, which represents less than 5% of total collagen; and c. Type III collagen. In the collagen molecule, the Arg-Gly-Asp (RGD) sequence is identified, which interacts with the surface integrins of bone cells and contains the amino acids, hydroxylysine and hydroxyproline. This last amino acid is a specific marker of collagen phenotypes and its urinary excretion increases when the rate of bone resorption increases, as in Osteogenesis Imperfecta.

The non-collagen proteins in the bone tissue are: (a) interstitial proteoglycans (10% of non-collagen proteins), rich in Leucine, with four types described (Hyaluronan, Chondroitin Sulfate, Biglycan, and Decorin), and intervene in the initial phases of bone morphogenesis, and in the final stages of formation; (b) Fibromodulin and related small proteoglycans; (c) Thrombospondins; (d)

Osteonectin, the most abundant non-collagen protein in the mineralized bone matrix; (e) Alkaline Phosphatase, a glycoprotein that releases inorganic phosphate from phosphoric esters and is necessary for mineralization; (f) Osteocalcin; (g) Integrin-bound glycoproteins; (h) Bone sialoproteins; (i) Dental matrix phosphoproteins; (j) Osteopontin, phosphoprotein glycoprotein 1, which acts as a bone bridge between bone cells and hydroxyapatite; (k) Plasma proteins, Albumin, and alpha2-SH-glycoprotein; and (l) Growth factors, polypeptides that intervene in the differentiation, growth, and proliferation of cells.

The mineralized bone matrix represents 65% of the total bone weight. The main crystallized mineral of the body is Hydroxyapatite—$Ca_{10}(PO_4)6(OH)_2$—formed by calcium, phosphate, and carbonate (in a 10:6:1 ratio) and to a lesser extent magnesium, sodium, potassium, manganese, and fluorine.

The proteins of the organic matrix that have adhesive capacity, favor mineralization, while proteoglycans and pyrophosphate inhibit mineralization. The mineralization of the extracellular bone matrix occurs as the result of circulating systemic factors that regulate the homeostasis of mineral ions in blood, plasma fluids, and bone tissue along with local factors that act at the organic-inorganic interface [1, 3, 12].

1.3 Ossification Process

In modern vertebrates, the remnants of the exoskeleton (skull and rib cage), although have been fully integrated with those of the endoskeleton, are still formed differently during embryogenesis. These bones are generated by direct differentiation of mesenchymal cells into osteoblasts (Fig. 1.3) through what it's called "Intramembranous Ossification." On the other side, the bones derivatives of the

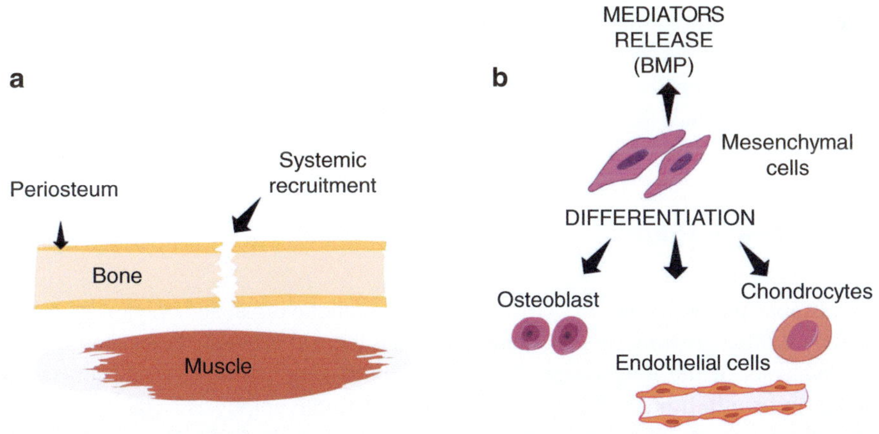

Fig. 1.3 (**a**) Origin of mesenchymal cells in the process of fracture healing. (**b**) Activity of mesenchymal cells at the fracture site

primitive endoskeleton first develop in cartilage molds, which are then replaced by bone through "Endochondral Ossification" [13].

1.3.1 Intramembranous Ossification

The genesis of the skeleton begins with the migration of mesenchymal cells to the sites of future bone formation, which occurs towards the end of the second month of gestation. These mesenchymal cells differentiate into mature osteoblasts, which produce an extracellular matrix, rich in collagen I. This differentiation occurs in some areas within the intramembranous bone, which is called "ossification centers." The beginning of this agglomeration is avascular, but then the differentiation of the osteoblasts and mineralization is closely related to the invasion of blood vessels. Therefore, the first bone formed in the human embryo is of an immature type, highly cellular, with disordered orientation of collagen fibers. At the time of birth, this bone is replaced by mature lamellar bone, with layers of collagen fibers oriented uniformly [14, 15].

1.3.2 Endochondral Ossification

This is a more complex process, triggered by the proliferation of chondrocytes in the center of the cartilaginous mold, giving a non-proliferative hypertrophic state that secretes a cartilage matrix with the presence of type II, IX, and XI collagen and proteoglycans. This initial condensation is performed in an avascular environment. The synchronous maturation and columnar organization of the chondrocytes result in a characteristic histological structure known as "growth plate" or physis. On the periphery of this condensation, the cells flatten and form a thin membrane called "perichondrium," which separates the cartilage from the surrounding mesenchyme. It has been established that these cells have a chondrogenic potential that aids radial growth by apposition. The thin layer that covers the newly formed bone is called periosteum and it supplies osteoblasts, which produce the bone matrix of the diaphysis [16].

1.4 Growth Plate

The physis, "physeal plate" or "growth plate," is a unique organ and only exists during the longitudinal growing stage of bone tissue. It is located between the metaphysis and the epiphysis of the long bones. Its function is to generate bone tissue, providing growth in length. It has different layers, which from the epiphysis to the metaphysis are: resting zone, proliferative zone, hypertrophic zone, and calcification zone [17, 18].

The small and relatively inactive cells are located in the reserve zone, near the secondary ossification center, while the proliferating chondrocytes are present in the adjacent proliferative zone. These cells undergo clonal expansion and align in columns, parallel to the direction of longitudinal growth. As the cells enter the hypertrophic zone, they stop proliferating and may undergo apoptosis [19].

The physeal plate is a mechanically weaker area than the rest of the osteoarticular complex, which is why it is a zone prone to injuries, referring to a lower resistance than the ligament tissue, usually damaged with sprains or dislocations in the adult. It is always important, if there is a direct or indirect traumatic history in the extremities and if in the clinic the pain is at the bone level, to rule out that it has a physeal injury and treat it accordingly [20–26].

1.5 Bone Repair

Bone tissue is one of the few in vertebrates that can repair with its own tissue, and not with connective tissue. Bone repair is divided into two types: primary (or direct) or secondary (or indirect). The first requires a stable fixation of the fracture lines, a situation created surgically by humans, so it is the least common to occur in pediatric patients [27].

Secondary repair is the most common process of bone tissue repair in pediatric patients (Fig. 1.4). It presents molecular and cellular patterns similar to bone formation in the embryonic skeleton, with the condensation of mesenchymal cells in endochondral ossification. This process consists of five stages [27, 28]:

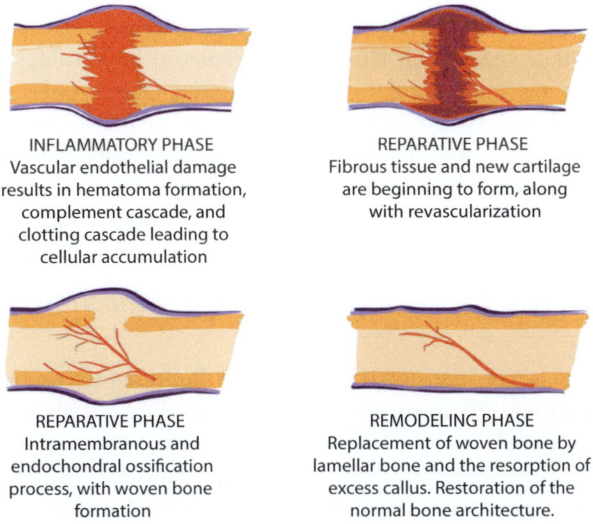

Fig. 1.4 Phases of secondary repair in bone tissue

1.5.1 Inflammatory Phase

It starts with the formation of the fracture hematoma, from the bone injury, periosteum, and adjacent soft tissues damage. Occurs immediately after the fracture, reaches its maximum at 48 h and disappears after 7 days. The Niche Cells surrounding the fracture line are activated. These regulate the response of the mesenchymal stem cells, promoting their differentiation, when they find damage in the bone tissue. Lymphocytes, polymorphonuclear cells, and macrophages are activated, which release cytokines to stimulate angiogenesis. The hematoma at the fracture site and under the periosteum prevents further bleeding and facilitates cell accumulation. The osteocytes near the fracture line die, resulting in bone necrosis, with hypoxia and pH decrease [4].

1.5.2 Reparative Phase with Intramembranous Ossification

It goes from the first days, until the second week after the fracture. A cartilaginous matrix appears in the fracture hematoma. The activity of the osteoblasts outside the bone tissue begins, forming the soft callus. The macrophages of the periosteum and endosteum are activated.

1.5.3 Reparative Phase with Chondrogenesis

Outside the bone callus, undifferentiated and mesenchymal cells form an avascular matrix of fibrous tissue, which will later be replaced by cartilaginous tissue [5]. Macrophages are recruited to remove necrotic tissue, and fibroblasts express extracellular matrix. These cells release growth factors and cytokines, mesenchymal stem cells are recruited from the bone marrow and the periosteum, which then differentiate into osteoprogenitor cells.

1.5.4 Reparative Phase (Endochondral Ossification)

After the second week, the newly formed cartilaginous tissue begins an endochondral ossification. Hypertrophic chondrocytes degrade glycosaminoglycans and osteoblasts initiate the calcification of the matrix. The periosteum provides intrinsic stability, helping to the calcification of the soft callus for greater stability. Capillaries of the bone tissue invade the calcified cartilage and the osteoblasts form bone tissue in the callus to connect the edges of the fracture. The periosteum thickens and the formation of the bone callus around the fracture line begins. The osteoprogenitor cells that are close to healthy bone tissue differentiate into osteoblasts, producing bone matrix, which later calcifies into bone. The cells that are further away, and consequently have less oxygen supply, differentiate into chondroblasts to form cartilage. At the same time, angiogenesis is induced so that this cartilaginous tissue ossifies endochondrally, when invaded by osteoclasts and osteoprogenitor cells. This whole process is similar to bone development in the embryonic period [5]. The endothelial cells of these new vessels interact with the osteoprogenitor cells to facilitate the differentiation of these into osteoblasts [4].

1.5.5 Remodeling Phase

The bony callus is replaced by lamellar bone following the mechanical loads to which it is exposed. Finally, a cortical bone and bone marrow similar to the prefracture are achieved.

Much less frequent is primary bone repair. Fractures in children are usually treated with relative stability methods, but occasionally there are cases that are managed with rigid fixation of the fracture [27]. The main characteristic of this type of repair is the absence of a bony callus. In this case, the edges of the fracture lines are in direct contact and without mobility. The BMUs (Bone Multicellular Units), which consist of osteoblasts, osteocytes, and osteoblasts, are activated. The osteoclasts from one edge reach the other, allowing the penetration of capillaries and thus new Haversian canals by bringing endothelial and osteoprogenitor cells.

1.6 Factors That Affect Bone Healing Process

The immobilization of the fracture is a critical factor for its proper repair. Excessive movement can delay the bone healing process, but absolute stability is also not always beneficial. Micromobility is required to achieve adequate repair in most of the cases. If there is a high mobility, a greater amount of cartilaginous callus will be produced due to a greater maturation of the chondrocytes in stage 4 of bone repair, and the formation of vascular bridges will also be altered. The micromovements of the fracture stimulate the proliferation of mesenchymal stem cells. Absolute stability, on the other hand, results in a weaker endosteum repair [6].

Multiple growth factors are expressed in different phases of bone repair, with different actions discovered until now: recruitment of mesenchymal stem cells from tissues adjacent to the fracture, proliferation of these and control their differentiation into chondrocytes and osteoblasts, invasion of blood vessels [6]. There are several growth factors involved in this process, but the main ones are Transforming Growth Factor beta (TGF-beta), Bone Morphogenetic Protein (BMP), Fibroblast

Growth Factor (FGF), Insulin-like Growth Factor (IGF), and Platelet-Derived Growth Factor (PDGF) [7].

Cell therapy can also stimulate bone repair. Osteoprogenitor cells, either in combination or not with mineral matrix and/or cytokines, could be applied to the bone defect and stimulate bone formation [8]. Current studies show that mesenchymal stem cells from bone marrow have great osteogenic potential and can be easily obtained from the iliac crest [29]. They can also be cultured in vitro to obtain a larger number of cells. Obviously, cell therapy would be an adjuvant for bone repair, with more important factors being the location of the fracture, patient age, condition of the soft tissues, vascularization of the area, and stability of the fracture.

1.6.1 Distraction Osteogenesis

Distraction osteogenesis has many similarities with bone repair. It consists of three phases [30]:

Latency phase: like the inflammatory phase of bone repair. Instead of a fracture, here it is an osteotomy that triggers the process. The inflammatory response releases cytokines, and mesenchymal stem cells are recruited and proliferate, which produce growth factors. The fracture hematoma appears.

Distraction phase: Here the space where the fracture hematoma formed is expanded, altering the expression of the growth factors, which increase in quantity and variety. The composition of collagen also changes, moving from a mixture of type I and II collagen, to predominance of type I. The calcification of the bone matrix begins. The Parathyroid Hormone (PTH) aids in the mineralization of the matrix along with the availability of Vitamin D and calcium. This phase is very similar to the intramembranous ossification phase of bone repair.

Consolidation phase: This phase is identical to the remodeling phase. At the end of bone distraction, the newly formed bone presents a central non-mineralized zone with tissue that begins its mineralization around it. There are peripheral zones with mineralized bone tissue that initiate the remodeling process. The presence of growth factors begins to decrease.

1.6.2 Use of Bone Grafts

The use of bone grafts in children is rare. In non-trauma situations, it is usually more used although considerably less than in adults. Complications from the donor site are the main reason to avoid its use. In the iliac crest, about 25% of patients have long-term pain, in addition to up to 15% with some degree of functional deficit. The larger the volume of graft taken, the higher the complication rate [31]. The supplementation of the autograft with allograft is as effective as the use of exclusive autograft. The bone autograft has Osteogenic properties (it stimulates the formation of bone tissue by its cells), Osteoinductive (it stimulates the differentiation of mesenchymal stem cells to Chondroblasts and Osteoblasts), and Osteoconductive (the process in which the recipient tissue orders the stimulation of mesenchymal stem cells, vascular development, and structure of the grafted tissue matrix). The allograft does not have Osteogenic properties although it does have Osteoconductive and Osteoinductive properties [32].

1.7 Final Message

A proper understanding of the processes of osteogenesis and bone repair is vital for planning the treatment of fractures. The choice of a treatment with external immobilization granting micromobility to the fracture site or favoring a reduction and osteosynthesis with primary or secondary bone repair is not random but based on solid foundations of bone biology.

In our usual practice, most of our treatments will be immobilization with plaster to induce secondary repair. It is this that we must fully understand, for its correct indication, placement of immobilizations, and the times of its use.

References

1. Trueta J. Osteogenesis. In: Trueta J, editor. The structure of the human body. Barcelona: Labor S.A; 1975. p. 3–14.
2. Jâhn K, Bonewald LF. Bone cell biology: Osteoclasts, osteoblasts, osteocytes. In: Glorieux FH, Pettifor JM, Juppner H, editors. Pediatric bone. Biology and diseases. Elsevier; 2012. p. 1–6.
3. Fernández-Tresguerres I, Gracia MAA, Pingarrón MC, Jerez LB. Physiological bases of bone regeneration I. Histology and physiology of bone tissue. Med Oral Patol Oral Cir Bucal. 2006;11:E47–51.
4. Salhotra A, Shah HN, Levi B, Longaker MT. Mechanisms of bone development and repair. Nat Rev Mol Cell Biol. 2020;21(11):696–711. https://doi.org/10.1038/s41580-020-00279-w.
5. Miclau T, Schneider R, Frank Eames B, Helms J. Common molecular mechanisms regulating fetal bone formation and adult fracture repair. In: Lieberman J, Friedlaender G, editors. Bone regeneration and repair. Humana Press; 2005. https://doi.org/10.1385/1-59259-863-3:045.
6. Kwong FN, Harris MB. Recent developments in the biology of fracture repair. J Am Acad Orthop Surg. 2008;16(11):619–25. https://doi.org/10.5435/00124635-200811000-00001.
7. Lieberman JR, Daluiski A, Einhorn TA. The role of growth factors in the repair of bone. Biology and clinical applications. J Bone Joint Surg Am. 2002;84(6):1032–44. https://doi.org/10.2106/00004623-200206000-00022.
8. Rosset P, Deschaseaux F, Layrolle P. Cell therapy for bone repair. Orthop Traumatol Surg Res. 2014;100(1 Suppl):S107–12. https://doi.org/10.1016/j.otsr.2013.11.010.
9. Azurmendi P. Regulation of organogenesis by the Hedgehog pathway [regulation of organogenesis by the hedgehog signaling pathway]. Medicine (B Aires). 2016;76(4):258–60.
10. Ros Lasierra M. The Hedgehog pathway: Embryogenesis and disease. In: Signaling networks and therapeutic strategies; 2009. SIBN 97884934430-9-2. p. 161–83.

11. Muñoz-Torres M, MdlH L-F, García DF. Advances in the knowledge of osteoclast biology: the osteo-protegerin-RANK ligand system. Clin Med (Barc). 2004;122(2):75–7.
12. McKee MD, Cole WG. Bone matrix and mineralization. In: Glorieux F, Pettifor J, Juppner H, editors. Pediatric bone. Biology and diseases. Elsevier; 2011. p. 9–48.
13. Gómez JG. The process of bone remodeling. Orthotips. 2008;4(3):170–6.
14. Berendsen AD, Olsen BR. Bone development. Bone. 2015;80:14–8. https://doi.org/10.1016/j.bone.2015.04.035.
15. Prenatal LF, Development B, In Glorieux F, Pettifor J, Juppner H. Pediatric bone. Biology and diseases. Elsevier; 2011. p. 39–48.
16. Fernández-Tresguerres I, Alobera MA, Canto M, Jerez LB. Physiological bases of bone regeneration II. The remodeling process. Med Oral Patol Oral Cir Bucal. 2006;11(2):E151–7.
17. Maes C, Kronenberg HM. Postnatal bone growth: growth plate biology, bone formation and remodeling. In Glorieux F, Pettifor J, Juppner H. Pediatric bone. Biology and diseases. Elsevier; 2011. p. 55–77.
18. Brian JM, Choi DH, Moore MM. The primary physis. Semin Musculoskelet Radiol. 2018;22(1):95–103.
19. Hosseinzadeh P, Milbrandt T. The normal and fractured physis: an anatomic and physiologic overview. J Pediatr Orthop B. 2016;25(4):385–92. https://doi.org/10.1097/BPB.0000000000000245.
20. Cepela DJ, Tartaglione JP, Dooley TP, Patel PN. Classifications In brief: Salter-Harris classification of pediatric physeal fractures. Clin Orthop Relat Res. 2016;474(11):2531–7. https://doi.org/10.1007/s11999-016-4891-3.
21. Woo SL, Ohland KJ, Weiss JA. Aging and sex-related changes in the biomechanical properties of the rabbit medial collateral ligament. Mech Ageing Dev. 1990;56(2):129–42. https://doi.org/10.1016/0047-6374(90)90004-y.
22. Woo SL, Orlando CA, Gomez MA, Frank CB, Akeson WH. Tensile properties of the medial collateral ligament as a function of age. J Orthop Res. 1986;4(2):133–41. https://doi.org/10.1002/jor.1100040201.
23. Martin RB, Burr DB. Skeletal tissue mechanics. Third Applied Chemistry International Edition, 6(11), 951–952. 1998.
24. Agashe V, Naik N. Biomechanics and biomaterials in orthopedics. In: Textbook of orthopedics and trauma, vol. 4; 2016. p. 725.
25. Martin RB, Burr DB, Sharkey NA, Fyhrie DP. Skeletal biology. In: Skeletal tissue mechanics; 2015. p. 35–93.
26. Bright RW, Burstein AH, Elmore SM. Epiphyseal-plate cartilage. A biomechanical and histological analysis of failure modes. J Bone Joint Surg Am. 1974;56(4):688–703.
27. Safeir C, Ho L, Doll B, Azari K, Hollinger J. Fracture repair. In: Lieberman J, Friedlaender G, editors. Bone regeneration and repair. Humana Press; 2005. https://doi.org/10.1385/1-59259-863-3:021.
28. Hing KA. Bone repair in the twenty-first century: biology, chemistry or engineering? Philos Trans A Math Phys Eng Sci. 1825;2004(362):2821–50. https://doi.org/10.1098/rsta.2004.1466.
29. Hernigou P, Mathieu G, Poignard A, Manicom O, Beaujean F, Rouard H. Percutaneous autologous bone-marrow grafting for nonunions. Surgical technique. J Bone Joint Surg Am. 2006;88(Suppl 1 Pt 2):322–7. https://doi.org/10.2106/JBJS.F.00203.
30. Hvid I, Horn J, Huhnstock S, Steen H. The biology of bone lengthening. J Child Orthop. 2016;10(6):487–92. https://doi.org/10.1007/s11832-016-0780-2.
31. Betz RR, Lavelle WF, Samdani AF. Bone grafting options in children. Spine (Phila Pa 1976). 2010;35(17):1648–54. https://doi.org/10.1097/BRS.0b013e3181ce8f4b.
32. Khan SN, Cammisa FP Jr, Sandhu HS, Diwan AD, Girardi FP, Lane JM. The biology of bone grafting. J Am Acad Orthop Surg. 2005;13(1):77–86.

Chapter 2
Traumatic Injuries of the Growth Plate

Estefanía Birrer, Benjamín Cancino, and Julio de Pablos

2.1 Traumatic Injuries of the Growth Plate

The word physis comes from Greek and translates as "grow," "sprout," or "the one that gives origin." It is also named "growth plate." Its primary function is the longitudinal growth of long bones, and therefore it can be considered an organ as such. The presence of this structure makes the real difference between the child skeleton and the adult skeleton, with its injuries being characteristic of childhood [1].

Physeal injuries have two special characteristics that we must keep in mind. The first is the severity of the sequelae that can remain, even after correct treatment. The second characteristic is its high frequency in pediatric age. According to Rang [2], they make up a third of the injuries in the child skeleton.

The physis is the "place of least resistance" (locus minoris resistentiae) of the skeletal tissue, given that the resistance of ligaments around it is greater, which is why injuries occur in this area more easily, although it is possible to find concomitant injuries in both structures.

E. Birrer (✉)
Hospital Base Valdivia, Clínica Alemana, Universidad Austral de Chile, Valdivia, Chile
e-mail: ebirrer@ortopediaytraumatologia.org

B. Cancino
Hospital Base Puerto Montt, Clínica Alemana Osorno, Osorno, Chile

J. de Pablos
Universidad de Navarra, Pamplona, Spain

M. Sepúlveda O. (ed.), *Paediatrics Traumatology*,
https://doi.org/10.1007/978-3-031-89482-4_2

2.2 Physeal Anatomy

The growth plate, or physis, develops from the cartilaginous model that remains between the primary (diaphyseal) and secondary (epiphyseal) ossification centers of the long bones. From there, it begins its organization in several layers, each with a specific function, which shape the final structure of the physis, until the end of the skeleton's growth, at which point it will disappear.

The physis is made up of cellular layers (Fig. 2.1), also called "zones" [1]:

Resting zone: Also called germinal zone or reserve zone (mesenchymal stem cells). It is located adjacent to the epiphyseal bone. This zone is made up of quiescent cartilaginous cells (chondrocytes), mainly producers of chondral matrix. It stores nutrients and has a close relationship with the epiphyseal vessels. Damage to this area will be related to long-term growth sequelae.

Proliferative zone: Characterized by a high rate of mitosis of the cells and scarce chondral matrix. Injury to this layer can lead to local growth cessation. Involved in longitudinal growth, like the columnar and hypertrophic zones.

Hypertrophic zone: Called the zone of cellular columns. The chondrocytes maintain a "stack of coins" arrangement and increase their size (ten times their original size), prior to degenerating and undergoing apoptosis, coinciding with vascular invasion. This produces three areas: maturation, degeneration, and transient calcification. It is the zone where there is the highest metabolic activity. In this zone, extracellular matrix is produced.

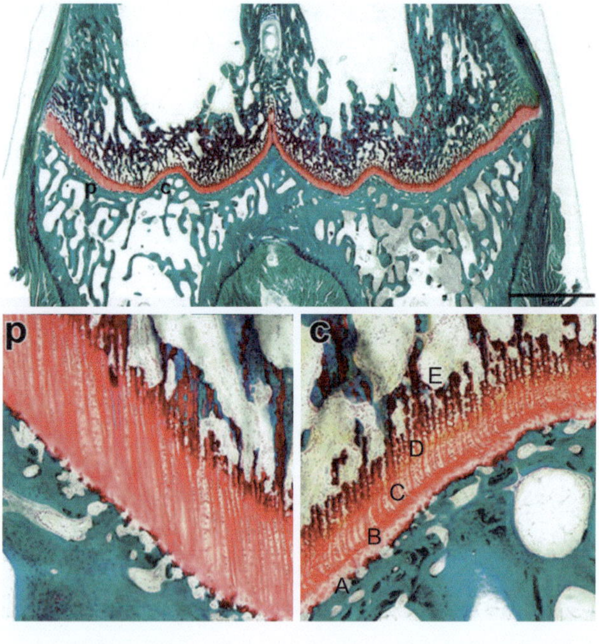

Fig. 2.1 Bright field images of histological section stained with Safranin (SOFG), from the left metatarsus of a sheep (*p* periphery, *c* central), with the zones of the growth plate: (**a**) resting zone, (**b**) proliferative; (**c**) columnar; (**d**) hypertrophic; (**e**) temporary calcification

Ossification zone: Also called "primary spongy." It is the zone adjacent to the metaphysis. From the metaphysis, blood vessels invade the residual cells after the apoptosis of the chondrocytes, and the process of ossification of the physis (endochondral ossification) begins. When this ossification process slows down or stops, there is an accumulation of chondrocytes that results in a generalized widening of the physeal line. Rickets is a good example of this phenomenon.

The mechanically weakest point of the physis is the junction of the ossification zone with the hypertrophic zone, where most of the traumatic epiphyseal detachments occur.

The physis is surrounded by a fibrocartilaginous structure called the "perichondral complex" [3]. It is composed of Ranvier's ossification groove, which, through appositional growth, produces an increase in bone diameter, and LaCroix's perichondral ring, which provides circumferential mechanical resistance to the growth cartilage. This resistance seems to decrease during puberty, which partly explains the greater predisposition to traumatic physis failure during this period of development. The Ranvier zone is also responsible for the latitudinal growth (increase in thickness) of the metaphyseal bone.

The physis has different growth capacities depending on age, being greater in physiological outbreaks, such as puberty, and its location. The growth cartilages with the greatest contribution in length are those located around the knee (distal femur and proximal tibia), and in the proximal humerus (Fig. 2.2).

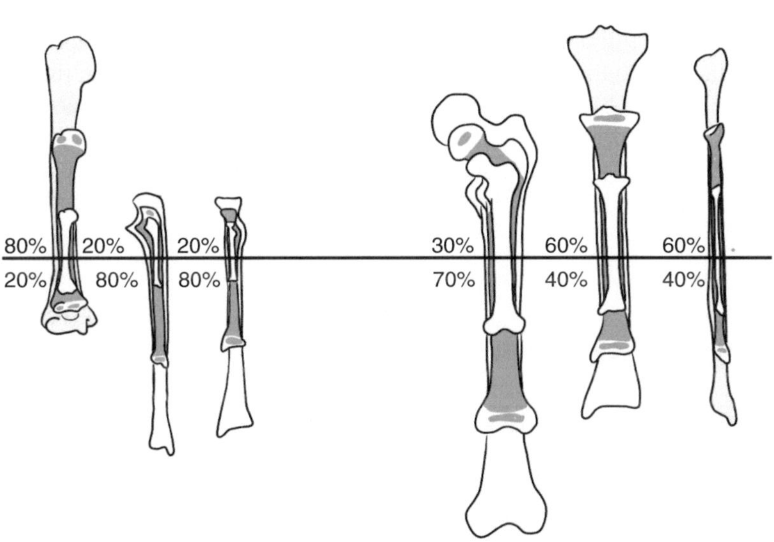

Fig. 2.2 Contribution in percentage of each physis to longitudinal growth, in the long bones of the extremities

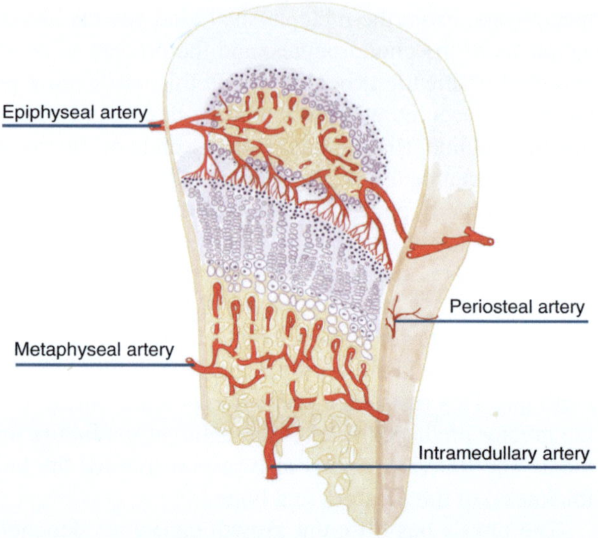

Fig. 2.3 Scheme of physeal vascularization

The growth cartilage is irrigated by epiphyseal vessels, metaphyseal in the center and perichondral on its periphery (Fig. 2.3). The epiphyseal vessels are directly related to the germinal layer of the physis, and their alteration can cause cessation or slowing of growth dependent on that physis. The metaphyseal vessels are fundamental in the process of endochondral ossification on the metaphyseal side of the physis, so their interruption will cause the cessation of this function. In the early years of life, the epiphyseal and metaphyseal vessels cross the physis, and communicate with each other, but over time these connections disappear, leaving the hypertrophic zone relatively avascular, particularly in older children [4].

2.3 Growth Regulation

The longitudinal growth of the bone is governed by a complex network of endocrine signals, generated by growth hormone, Insulin-like Growth Factor I (IGF-I), glucocorticoids, thyroid hormone, estrogens, androgens, vitamin D, and leptin [5]. The growth hormone seems to act directly, producing an increase in chondrocyte proliferation, and indirectly, stimulating the local production of IGF-I, which in turn stimulates the differentiation and hypertrophy of chondrocytes. The increase during puberty of growth hormone and testosterone levels on the one hand stimulate growth, but on the other hand decrease the mechanical resistance of the physis cartilage, favoring the production of epiphyseal detachments, traumatic or not, at this time of life [2].

The effects of mechanical conditions on skeletal growth were already observed by Jacques Delpech in the nineteenth century and embodied in the Hueter-Volkmann law. It states that growth is inhibited by compression forces and stimulated by distraction forces. Compression produces a decrease in chondrocyte proliferation, while distraction forces cause the opposite effect [6].

The growth cartilage also undergoes changes in its structure and function in relation to other factors, whose mechanisms we do not know, but which seem evident. This is the case with malnutrition, which is often associated with the appearance of physis bone bridges and multiple bone deformities. Also, other socioeconomic factors, such as environmental pollution, are associated with alterations in skeletal development.

Finally, it is important to note the sensitivity of the physis to problems that generate some type of stressful situation in the pediatric patient, such as infections or severe trauma. In these situations, it is common to see temporary growth stops, which are radiologically manifested as metaphyseal condensation lines (growth stop lines or "Park-Harris" lines), which move away from the physis, once normal growth is reestablished (Fig. 2.4). Despite their evidence in X-rays, their clinical repercussion is generally unimportant.

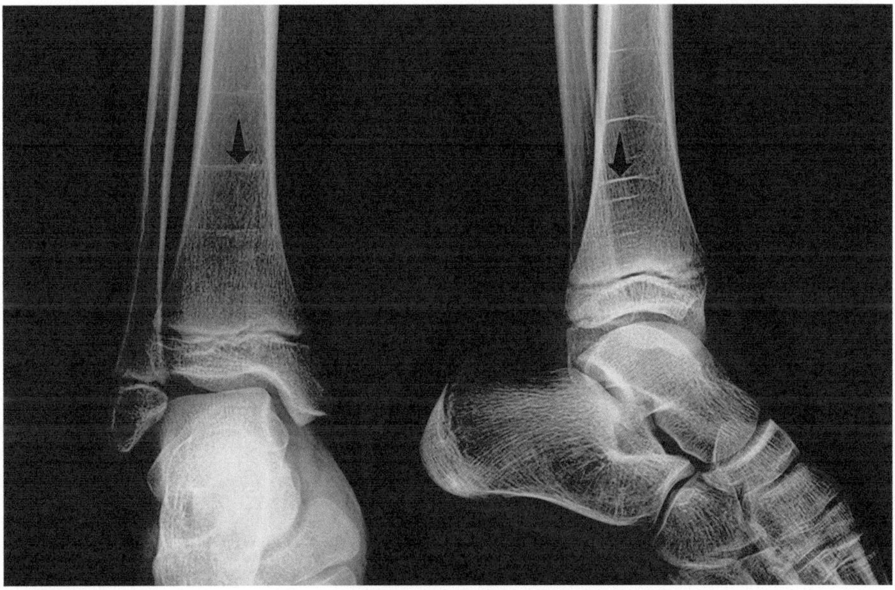

Fig. 2.4 Anteroposterior and lateral radiographs of the right ankle of a 10-year-old girl, with Park-Harris lines (arrows), parallel to the physis, indicating symmetrical growth

2.4 Physeal Trauma

Histologically, we can find two basic types of traumatic physeal failure. One is the metaphyseal-epiphyseal separation, which typically is located between the hypertrophic and ossification layers of the physis. The other is the longitudinal physeal fracture, transphyseal, which is reported more associated with the formation of post-traumatic physeal bridges, probably due to producing a communication between the metaphyseal and epiphyseal circulation, or due to the interruption of the epiphyseal and/or metaphyseal irrigation. This is common to see in completely articular epiphyses, for example in the proximal femoral epiphysis [7, 8].

The widening of the physeal line, which is very often seen 2 to 3 weeks after a fracture type physeal separation, is due more to an accumulation of degenerative cells due to temporary interruption of endochondral ossification, than to a possible physeal stimulus [9]. Once this endochondral ossification is restored, the thickness of the physis tends to normalize.

2.5 Diagnosis

Physeal trauma should be studied with conventional radiographs of the affected segment, in two planes (Fig. 2.5). If there is doubt in the diagnosis, oblique projections can be requested (e.g., in humeral condyle fractures). Stress radiographs are not recommended because they cause pain to the patient.

Magnetic resonance imaging (MRI) has proven to be a very useful examination as it allows the detection of the fracture, determine its morphology, assist in therapeutic decision-making, locate and plan the surgical treatment of bone bridges, and even guide the prognosis, even in minimal injuries (Fig. 2.6). Its main disadvantage is the high sensitivity, with the risk of false positives.

Computed Axial Tomography (CT-scan) allows a better understanding of the fracture features in articular injuries (Fig. 2.7) and is associated with better results after treatment [10, 11].

Other exams, such as bone scintigraphy or ultrasound, are of more limited value.

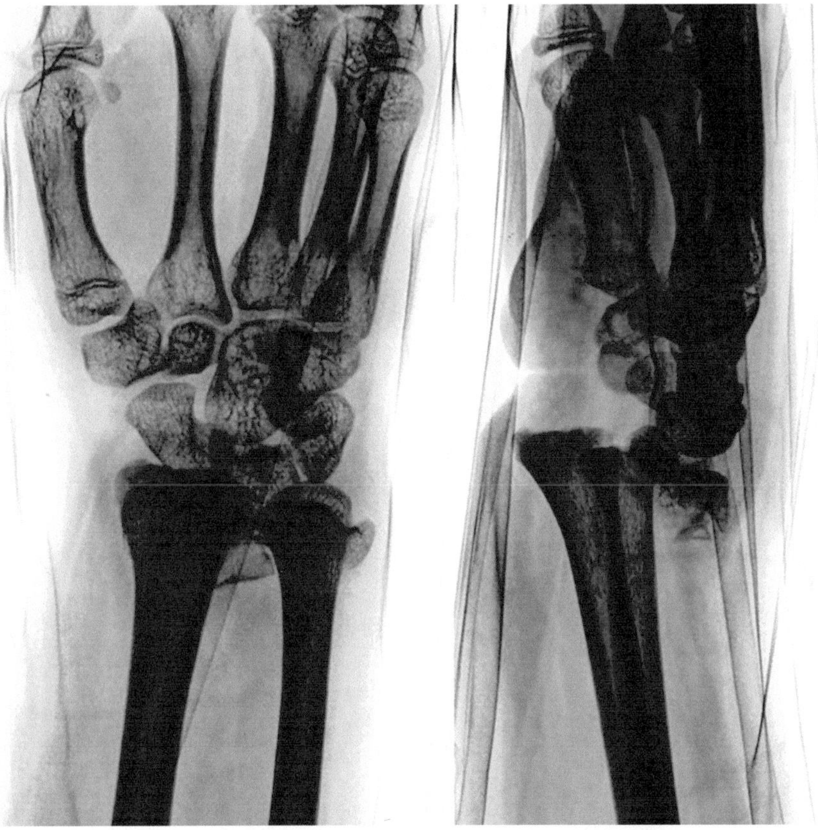

Fig. 2.5 Anteroposterior and lateral wrist x-ray of the wrist of a 12 years-old girl, with a Salter and Harris type II fracture, with a fragment of Thurston Holland dorsal metaphyseal

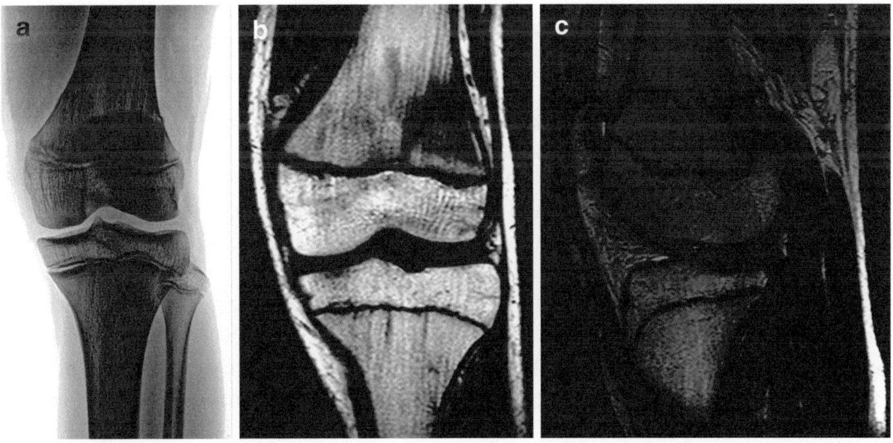

Fig. 2.6 Anteroposterior radiograph of the left knee of a 14-years-old boy, with a Salter and Harris II distal femur fracture, not evidente (**a**). Magnetic resonance imaging in coronal sequence T1 (**b**) and sagittal plane T2 sequence (**c**) confirm the injury

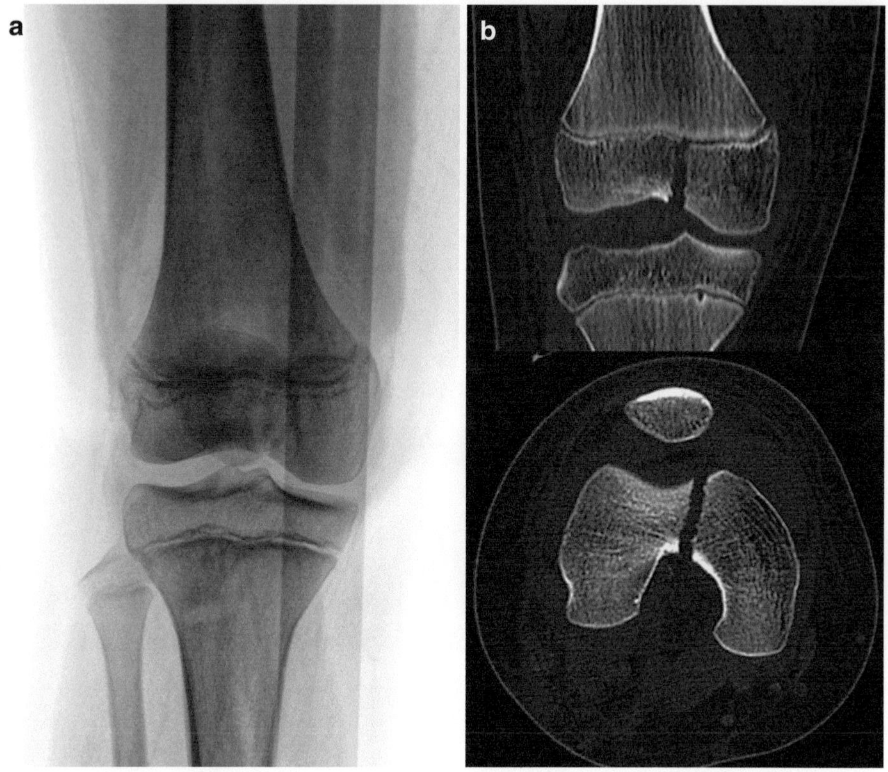

Fig. 2.7 Anteroposterior radiograph (**a**) and coronal and axial sections of CT-scan (**b**) of the right knee of an 11-year-old girl. The displaced Salter and Harris type III fracture can be seen

2.6 Classification

In 1863, prior to the era of X-rays, Foucher reported the first classification of physeal fractures in the book *De la Divulsion des Epiphyses*. Years later, Poland makes the greatest contribution to this topic, writing the classification extracted from numerous clinical cases and preparations, making illustrations of this classification, being the pillar for the twentieth century. At that time, this type of injury was widely studied and classified. Bergenfeldt [1], Aitken [2], and Brashear [9] made their own classifications, but the dissemination of these was not as successful because some of them were not originally written in English [1, 9].

Robert Salter and W. Robert Harris, from Canada, describe their classification of 1963 with five types of injuries (Fig. 2.8). It includes the four types previously described by Poland, adding a type without acute radiographic correlation (Type V). This classification is still the most popular, used, and taught around the world [12].

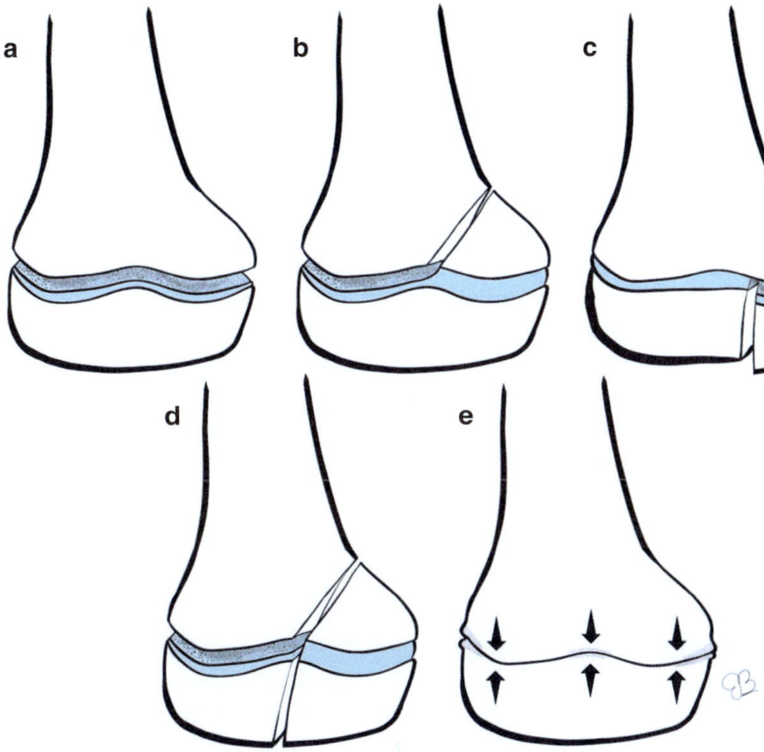

Fig. 2.8 Salter and Harris classification scheme. (**a**) type I; (**b**) type II; (**c**) type III; (**d**) type IV; (**e**) type V

2.6.1 Salter and Harris (SH) Classification

2.6.1.1 Type I

It consists of a complete epiphyseal-metaphyseal separation. Its prognosis is generally good. In proximal femoral epiphyseal detachments, avascular necrosis of the epiphysis may occur, due to its completely intra-articular location and its vascular anatomy.

2.6.1.2 Type II

This is the most common type of physeal fractures. The fracture pattern is very similar to type I, but after running along most of the physis, it enters the metaphysis, leaving a small metaphyseal fragment ("Thurston Holland" Fragment). Its reduction is usually easy to obtain, as the intact periosteum and the metaphyseal fragment act as a hinge, preventing overcorrection. The prognosis is almost always excellent and the vascular supply to the epiphysis is usually not affected.

2.6.1.3 Type III

In these fractures, part of the fracture line is also a pure physeal separation, as in type I, but at a certain point an inflection occurs and crosses the physis and the epiphysis to reach the articular surface. These are much rarer fractures and have a more reserved prognosis, for two fundamental reasons. Firstly, it is an intra-articular fracture, which can potentially cause an incongruity of the articular surface if it is not anatomically reduced. Secondly, there is a communication of the epiphyseal and metaphyseal circulation that can lead to the appearance of premature partial closures of the growth cartilage (bone bridges). For these reasons, its anatomical reduction is fundamental.

2.6.1.4 Type IV

In this type, the fracture line begins on the articular surface and crosses the epiphysis, the physis, and the metaphysis, constituting a kind of combination between type II and III fractures. Type IV fractures are intra-articular, and due to the trace, there is a communication of the metaphyseal circulation with the epiphyseal. This can lead to articular incongruity and/or premature partial cessations of physeal growth. Like type III, they require an anatomical reduction.

2.6.1.5 Type V

This is a physeal trauma by compression. This would cause a physeal crushing and consequently a communication of the epiphyseal and metaphyseal circulations. This fact confers a particularly poor prognosis, with the appearance of a premature physeal closure, occupying the entirety or a large part of the affected physis. The diagnosis is retrospective, when a premature physeal closure is observed in a bone that has previously suffered trauma.

There is debate on some points about this classification. Regarding its prognostic value, a significant percentage of type I and II injuries, especially around the knee, produce growth disorders due to premature physeal closure, not conditioning the good prognosis associated with these types.

Another limitation is that some physeal fractures cannot be included in the classification. Peterson [1, 13] proposed a classification adding two types (Fig. 2.9).

Finally, type V fractures, by compression, are still controversial, as some authors defend their existence [9], while others, on the contrary, do not admit it precisely, due to the lack of evidence that a fracture has occurred [14, 15].

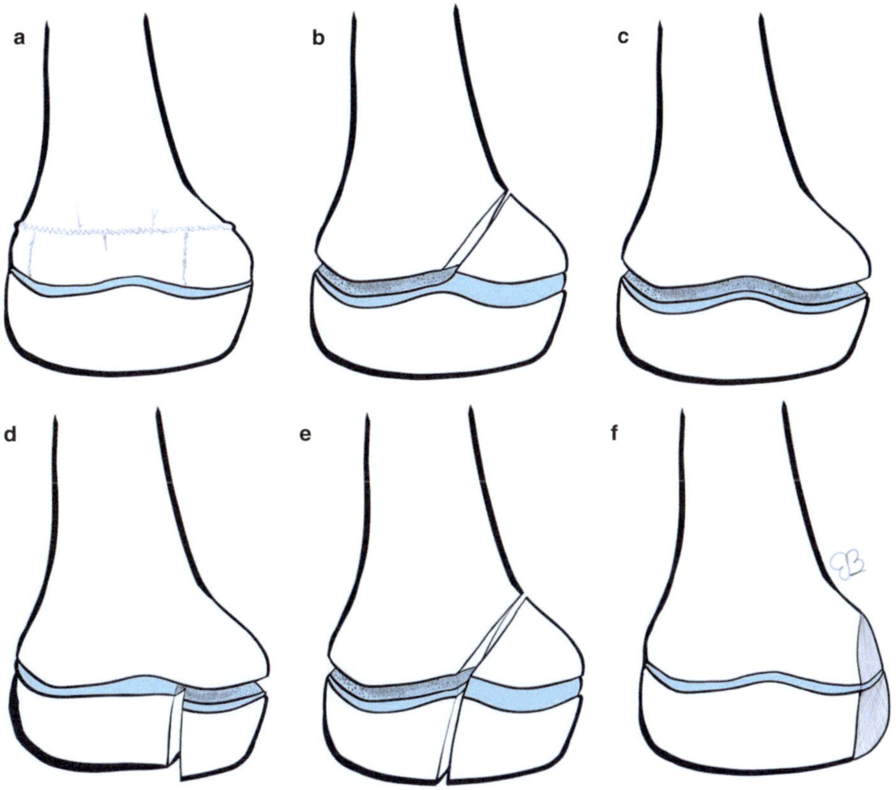

Fig. 2.9 Peterson classification scheme. (**a**) transverse fracture metaphyseal extending to the physis; (**b**) metaphyseal fracture continuing transverse in the physis, with a metaphyseal fragment attached to the epiphysis by physis segment undamaged; (**c**) physeal fracture with complete separation of the metaphysis from the epiphysis; (**d**) epiphyseal fracture that continues transverse in the physis; (**e**) fracture that crosses metaphysis, epiphysis and physis; (**f**) loss of physeal fragment

There are other special types of traumatic physeal injuries: overload (stress) fractures due to the repeated application of sub-maximal force, slow epiphysiolysis, typically the result of joint imbalance, and physeal fractures in adults, for example, at the level of the clavicle in its proximal third, which can be confused with a sternoclavicular dislocation.

2.7 Incidence

Physeal fractures represent 15–30% of all pediatric fractures [8, 16, 17]. These fractures are more common in adolescence than at earlier ages, as in the latter the epiphysis is more cartilaginous and acts as a buffer for a significant amount of force that is transmitted to the metaphysis.

Boys are affected twice as often as girls. This is explained because their physes remain open until an older age, and due to the greater sports participation of males. Despite this, the overall incidence of epiphyseal injury peaks at 12 years old, both in boys and girls, and the average age is 10.3 years old in boys and 8.9 years old in girls [17]. Regardless of the site, the distal physis of each bone is more frequently affected than the proximal one, with the distal radial physis being the most common site of involvement, followed by the physis of the phalanges and distal tibia [18, 19].

Traumatic injury to the physis can cause growth disturbances, and this is mainly due to damage to the germinative cells, loss of vascular supply, infection, or formation of bone bridges between the epiphysis and metaphysis. The rate of permanent growth plate damage, resulting in significant growth disturbance, ranges between 1% and 10% of physeal fractures [20].

Kawamamoto [17], found that Salter-Harris type I injuries accounted for 28.6% of physeal injuries, type II 60.9%, type III 6.8%, and type IV 3.7%. Type V cases were not identified in this study. The main cause of physeal injuries were accidents during sports practice (37.0%), compared to other causes, such as falling (17.2%) or traffic accidents (1.7%). Most cases were treated conservatively. However, in load-bearing limb injuries and in the elbow, there was a trend towards surgical resolution. Salter-Harris type I (80.0%) and type II (72.3%) injuries were mainly treated conservatively.

2.8 Mechanism of Injury

Most of these injuries occur during the accelerated growth period of the child, when the physis is weakest. Active children are most likely to suffer physeal-related injuries, as the ligaments and joint capsules surrounding the growth cartilage tend to be much stronger and stable. Therefore, the ligaments and capsules can withstand greater external loads on the joint, in relation to the physis itself.

Physeal fractures tend to occur between the hypertrophic and ossification zones; however, they can cross several zones depending on the type of injury or the external force applied (e.g., shear forces, versus compression, versus tension).

2.9 Treatment

A physeal injury represents a unique therapeutic challenge, as the sequelae could cause future growth alterations. These growth alterations could manifest as differences in limb length or angular deformities. Of all physeal fractures, growth alterations are observed in 1–10% of cases [19].

Physeal injuries heal faster than pure bone injuries. Generally, a physeal fracture would heal in 3–4 weeks. In the case of an injury to a large undulating physis, such as a distal femur physeal fracture, the fracture plane would cross several zones of

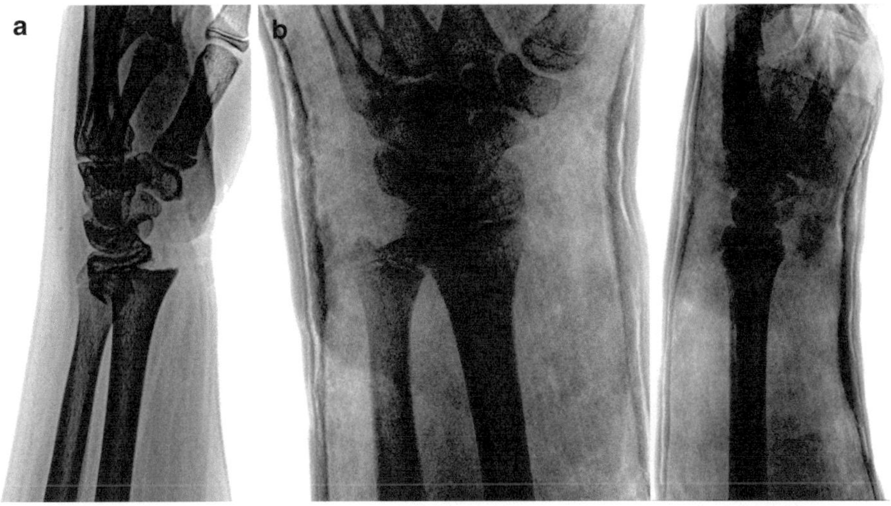

Fig. 2.10 Fracture of the left distal radius, in a 12-year-old boy, with a Salter and Harris II type fracture (**a**). A closed and stable reduction was performed, with stabilization in a 3-point molded plaster (**b**)

the physis. Likewise, intra-articular physeal fractures, such as Salter-Harris type III and IV fractures would cross several or all zones of the physis. Such injuries have a worse prognosis, as the chances of bone formation along the physis increase when multiple zones are injured, with the consequent determination of physeal bridges.

According to the Salter-Harris classification, a safe closed reduction is possible as treatment without significant problems in most type I injuries, except in the displaced proximal femur. Closed reduction is also safe in most type II injuries, the most commonly seen fracture type (Fig. 2.10). Open reduction with internal fixation may be necessary in some areas, such as the distal femur, where the risk of growth alteration is higher [20].

Salter-Harris type III and type IV injuries are intra-articular fractures. Growth disturbances, joint stiffness, and non-union can be observed. Open reduction and internal fixation are often preferred to restore the anatomy of the joint and growth plate and to avoid such complications (Fig. 2.11).

The following principles are recommended for treating physeal injuries in pediatric patients, with some modifications depending on the location of the injury and the age [19]:

- The displaced physeal fracture should be reduced with sustained traction and gentle manipulation. Avoid forced reduction maneuvers, repeated reduction attempts, or the insertion of instruments into the physis to manipulate the fracture fragments, as this could cause an iatrogenic physeal injury. Open reduction is better than multiple closed reduction attempts.
- For an extra-articular physeal fracture (Salter-Harris type I and II), late reduction, beyond 5–7 days after the injury occurred, should be avoided. This is due to

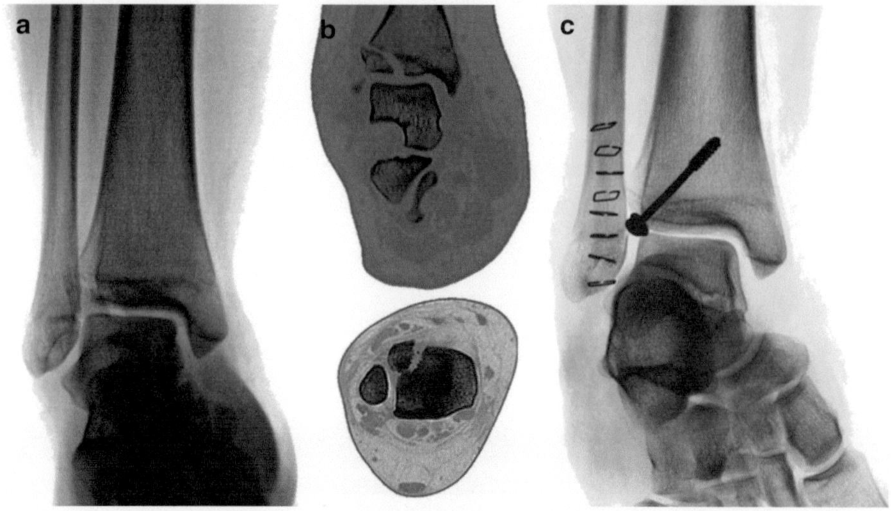

Fig. 2.11 Anteroposterior radiograph (**a**) and coronal and axial sections of computed tomography (**b**) of the right ankle of a 13-year-old girl, with a Salter and Harris type III fracture (Tillaux Juvenile). It was treated by open reduction and stabilization with cannulated screw (**c**), transphyseal due proximity to the end of growth and state of closure of the physis

the high risk of causing an iatrogenic physeal injury, and the resulting growth arrest. Instead, it is better to allow the fracture to heal and remodel. The treatment of a malunion is safer than that of growth arrest in a young patient [21].

- Displaced intra-articular physeal fractures (Salter-Harris III and IV) should be anatomically reduced and stabilized by internal fixation, regardless of their time of presentation. The congruence of the articular surface is of utmost importance. There are several methods to assess the accuracy of the articular surface reduction for Salter-Harris type III and IV physeal fractures. These include direct visualization, fluoroscopy, arthrography, or arthroscopic evaluation.
- The implants used for internal fixation should be installed respecting the physis. Kirschner wires and screws should ideally be parallel to the physis when the fracture geometry allows it. If an implant is placed through the physis (transphyseal), compression should be avoided (Fig. 2.12).
- If more than 2 years of growth remain, a transphyseal implant should be removed once the fracture has consolidated.
- For an exposed or crushed physeal injury, an anticipatory Langenskiold procedure can be performed. This consists of the use of free fat graft to cover the physis, helping to prevent growth arrest [22, 23].
- Growth arrest lines ("Park-Harris" lines) are transverse lines seen in the metaphysis. Their orientation and relationship with the physis are used to assess growth and its alterations, ideally being parallel to it [24, 25].
- For a displaced physeal fracture, the patient should be monitored for growth disturbances for at least 1 year, or until the patient reaches skeletal maturity. For

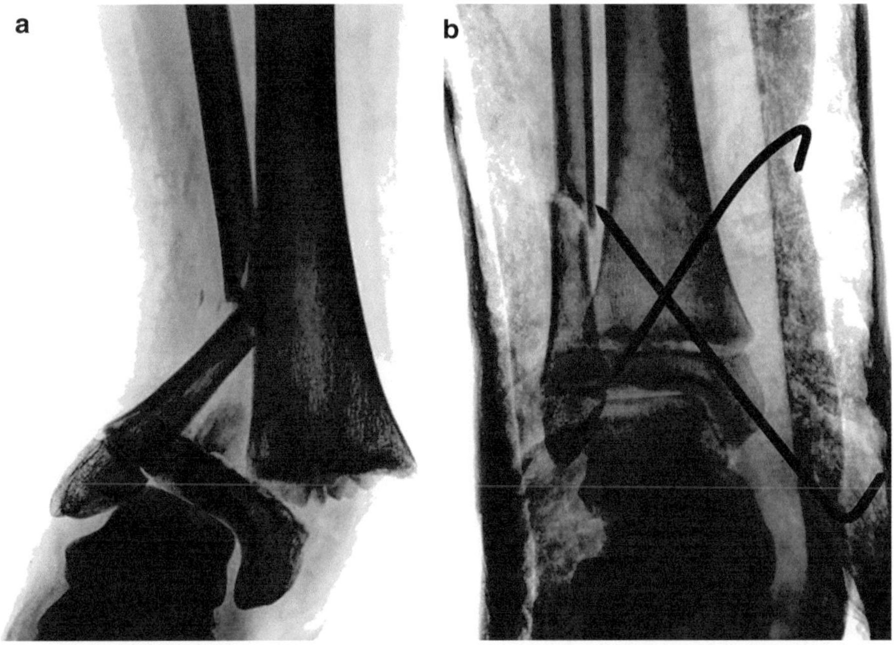

Fig. 2.12 Anteroposterior radiograph of the right ankle of a 12-year-old boy, where a Salter and Harris type II fracture of the distal tibia is observed, associated to fibula fracture (**a**). Closed reduction and stabilization are performed with smooth, transphyseal Kirschner wires, avoiding compression (**b**)

a non-displaced physeal fracture, there is no need for serial radiographs. Instead, the family should be advised about the low potential for growth arrest and follow-up if symptoms are noticed or deformities are evident, especially in distal femur injuries.

– Performing a transphyseal drilling has been shown to have a significantly higher risk in the formation of physeal bridges [26].

2.10 Complications

The most catastrophic complication is the formation of bone bridges across the physis. Once the physeal bridge is formed, it is mandatory to perform a thorough imaging study to define the size and location (Fig. 2.13). A small fibrous bridge can resolve spontaneously [27].

Although the specific mechanism through which different etiological agents cause premature physeal closure is poorly understood, it seems clear that, in the case of physeal fractures, the contact between the epiphyseal and metaphyseal tissues, and the subsequent ossification that occurs, particularly in transphyseal

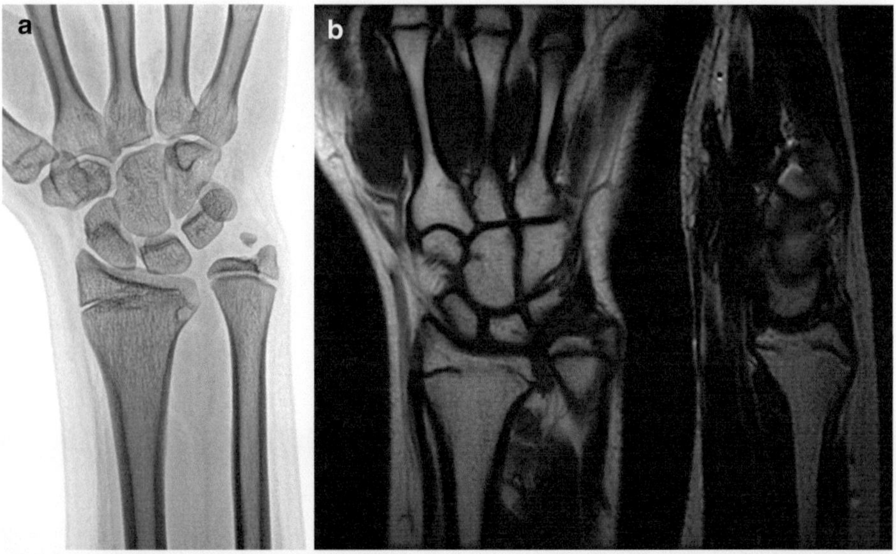

Fig. 2.13 Anteroposterior x-ray of the left wrist of a 14-years-old girl, with a post-traumatic bone bridge and the consequent growth disturbance (**a**). Magnetic resonance imaging in coronal and sagittal planes in T1 sequence (**b**) demonstrate the structure of the bone bridge

fractures (Salter-Harris types III, IV, and V) are the most likely causes of post-traumatic premature physeal closure. However, post-traumatic premature physeal closure can also be a consequence of non-transphyseal fractures (Salter-Harris types I and II), as unlikely as it may seem from a conceptual standpoint [28].

An interruption of blood flow (ischemia), in or around the physis, may be due to a microembolism, which causes very localized damage, or massive epiphyseal ischemia, with reduction of blood supply to the germinal layer of the physis, as may be the case in patients with intracapsular fractures of the femoral neck. In addition, post-traumatic premature physeal closure has been seen after some high-energy diaphyseal fractures, in growth cartilages located at a distance from the fracture. Although there could be an ischemic element involved, the actual mechanism of the injury is not yet fully understood.

Physeal closure can also be iatrogenic. Several animal studies have shown a correlation between transphyseal fixation with Kirschner wires and growth disorders [28, 29]. Boyden and Peterson [30] observed that premature physeal closure was potentially related to the size of the wires, their location within the physis, the obliquity with respect to the physis, the use of threaded wires, and the longer duration of wire retention in the physis. Therefore, transphyseal Kirschner wires should be used judiciously, in fractures where they are truly necessary. However, it is not recommended to avoid their use arbitrarily, as in unstable fractures, the risk of loss of reduction is significantly higher in patients who were not fixed [31]. It is advisable to avoid the use of multiple wires, multiple insertion attempts, use of large size wires, intrafocal, and permanent [19].

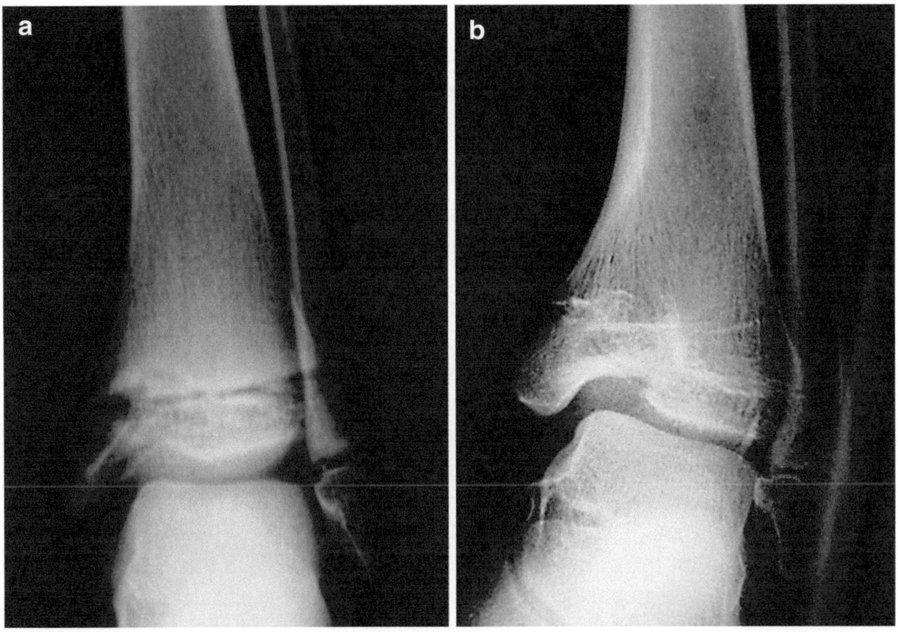

Fig. 2.14 Anteroposterior x-ray of the left ankle of a 7-years-old girl (**a**), with a Salter and Harris 3 fracture of the distal tibia. It is observed on an x-ray at 10-years-old, the formation of a post-traumatic bone bridge and a varus deviation of the ankle (**b**)

These growth alterations, secondary to post-traumatic premature physeal closure, could manifest as a difference in limb length or angular deformities (Fig. 2.14). Of all physeal fractures, growth arrest or alterations are observed in 1–10% of cases. This corresponds to 70% of all post-traumatic premature physeal closures that we can observe in our clinical practice [28].

We can classify a premature physeal closure as follows:

- Complete physeal closure, where we will see a difference in length of the affected segment in relation to the contralateral, but there may be minimal angular changes.
- Partial physeal closure, with predominance of angular alterations. These can be subclassified according to the location of the bar in the physis, to predict its behavior: Central, with length difference, Peripheral, with angular alteration, and Linear, with complete closure.

2.11 Final Message

The physis, or growth cartilage, is the structure that makes the difference between the child and the adult. We can consider it as an organ in its own, as it is a set of cells and tissues that fulfills the primary function of the infant skeleton, which is the longitudinal growth of the long bones.

Its great potential for remodeling in response to traumatic injuries, and the ability for angular reorientation are not unlimited and we must know their limits, as well as recognize the physes with greater activity.

Injury to the resting and proliferative layers can lead to local cessation of growth. The weakest area is the junction between the hypertrophic layer and the ossification layer, where most post-traumatic epiphyseal detachments occur.

The most common etiology of physeal injuries is trauma, but we must not forget injuries from burns, ischemia, electricity, among others. Injuries range from a simple metaphyseal-epiphyseal separation, less severe, to transphyseal injuries with a worse prognosis due to the potential production of physeal bone bridges.

The physiological reparative response to damage is immediate, for this reason, physeal injuries should be managed in a timely manner, knowing that a week after the trauma, a reduction could be more harmful than beneficial.

When the injury destroys the entire thickness of the physis or, simply when a transphyseal vascular communication occurs, it can generate ossification between the epiphysis and metaphysis (physeal closure, physeal arrest, or definitive physeodesis) that will alter the growth of the rest of that physis. Whether the bone bridge has a greater or lesser impact on the growth of a bone segment depends mainly on the patient's age (the younger, the greater) and on the activity of the physis where it assists (the more active, the greater). Thus, for example, physeal injuries around the knee, especially in younger patients, are some of the ones that will leave the greatest sequelae in the long term (Fig. 2.15).

Permanent traumatic damage to the physis can cause a bar. Taking into account the area where it is located, it could generate angular deformities, as well as length differences. Both injuries will leave permanent sequelae with loss of function and disability in "adult life."

The care of the physis is the task of the doctor and above all of the Pediatric Orthopedist.

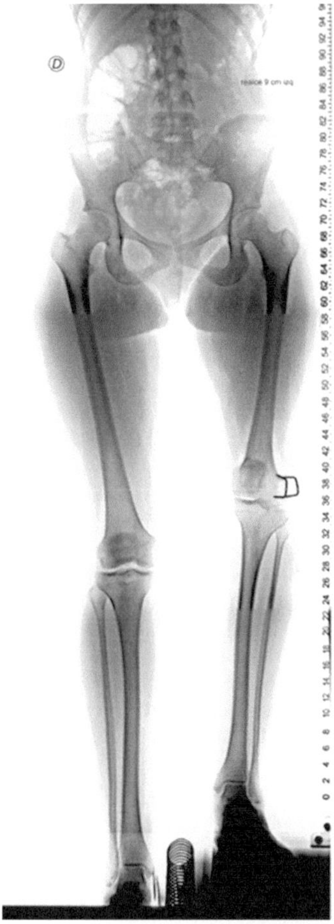

Fig. 2.15 Standing lower extremities AP x-ray of the lower extremities of a 20-year-old girl with a traumatic injury to the distal physis of the left femur, with angular deformity and shortening

References

1. Peterson HA. Epiphyseal growth plate fractures. Springer; 2007. ISBN 978-3-540-33801-7
2. Rang M. Injuries of the epiphysis, growth plate and Perichondrial ring. In: Rang M, editor. Children's fractures. Philadelphia: JB Lippincott; 1974. p. 7–17.
3. Chung SM, Batterman SC, Brighton CT. Shear strength of the human femoral capital epiphyseal plate. J Bone Joint Surg Am. 1976;58(1):94–103.
4. Trueta J, Amato VP. The vascular contribution to osteogenesis. III. Changes in the growth cartilage caused by experimentally induced ischemia. J Bone Joint Surg Br. 1960;42-B:571–87. https://doi.org/10.1302/0301-620X.42B3.571.
5. Nilsson O, Marino R, De Luca F, Phillip M, Baron J. Endocrine regulation of the growth plate. Horm Res. 2005;64(4):157–65. https://doi.org/10.1159/000088791.
6. Apte SS, Kenwright J. Physeal distraction and cell proliferation in the growth plate. J Bone Joint Surg Br. 1994;76(5):837–43.
7. Lee MA, Nissen TP, Otsuka NY. Utilization of a murine model to investigate the molecular process of transphyseal bone formation. J Pediatr Orthop. 2000;20(6):802–6. https://doi.org/10.1097/00004694-200011000-00021.
8. Wattenbarger JM, Gruber HE, Phieffer LS. Physeal fractures, part I: histologic features of bone, cartilage, and bar formation in a small animal model. J Pediatr Orthop. 2002;22(6):703–9.

9. Hefti F. Basic principles: growth. In: Hefti F, editor. Pediatric orthopaedics in practice. Berlin and Heidelberg: Germany, Springer Medizin Verlag; 2007. p. 41–8.
10. Olgun ZD, Maestre S. Management of pediatric ankle fractures. Curr Rev Musculoskelet Med. 2018;11(3):475–84. https://doi.org/10.1007/s12178-018-9510-3.
11. Kim JR, Song KH, Song KJ, Lee HS. Treatment outcomes of triplane and Tillaux fractures of the ankle in adolescence. Clin Orthop Surg. 2010;2(1):34–8. https://doi.org/10.4055/cios.2010.2.1.34.
12. Salter RB, Harris WR. Injuries involving the epiphyseal plate. J Bone Surg. 1963;45-A:587–622.
13. Peterson HA. Physeal fractures: part 3. Classification. J Pediatr Orthop. 1994;14(4):439–48. https://doi.org/10.1097/01241398-199407000-00004.
14. Keret D, Mendez AA, Harcke HT, MacEwen GD. Type V physeal injury: a case report. J Pediatr Orthop. 1990;10:545–8.
15. Peterson HA, Burkhart SS. Compression injury of the epiphyseal growth plate: fact or fiction? J Pediatr Orthop. 1981;1(4):377–84. https://doi.org/10.1097/01241398-198112000-00004.
16. Mann DC, Rajmaira S. Distribution of physeal and nonphyseal fractures in 2,650 long-bone fractures in children aged 0-16 years. J Pediatr Orthop. 1990;10(6):713–6. https://doi.org/10.1097/01241398-199011000-00002.
17. Kawamoto K, Kim WC, Tsuchida Y, et al. Incidence of physeal injuries in Japanese children. J Pediatr Orthop B. 2006;15(2):126–30. https://doi.org/10.1097/01.bpb.0000191874.69258.0b.
18. Duart J, de Pablos J. Pediatric orthopedics for residents. Spanish Society of Pediatric Orthopedics; 2019.
19. Singh V, Garg V, Parikh SN. Management of physeal fractures: a review article. Indian J Orthop. 2021;55(3):525–38. Published 2021 Jan 13. https://doi.org/10.1007/s43465-020-00338-6.
20. Ömeroglu H. Basic principles of fracture treatment in children. Eklem Hastalik Cerrahisi. 2018;29(1):52–7. https://doi.org/10.5606/ehc.2018.58165.
21. Parikh SN, Wells L, Mehlman CT, Scherl SA. Management of fractures in adolescents. Instr Course Lect. 2011;60:397–411.
22. Foster BK, John B, Hasler C. Free fat interpositional graft in acute physeal injuries: the anticipatory Langenskiöld procedure. J Pediatr Orthop. 2000;20(3):282–5.
23. Langenskiöld A. The possibilities of eliminating premature partial closure of an epiphyseal plate caused by trauma or disease. Acta Orthop Scand. 1967;38(1–4):267–79. https://doi.org/10.3109/17453676708989640.
24. Lee TM, Mehlman CT. Hyphenated history: Park-Harris growth arrest lines. Am J Orthop (Belle Mead NJ). 2003;32(8):408–11.
25. Ogden JA. Growth slowdown and arrest lines. J Pediatr Orthop. 1984;4(4):409–15. https://doi.org/10.1097/01241398-198408000-00003.
26. Gruber HE, Ashraf N, Cox MD, Ingram JA, Templin M, Wattenbarger JM. Experimental induction of physeal injuries by fracture, drill, and ablation techniques: analyses of immunohistochemical findings. J Pediatr Orthop. 2019;39(9):479–86. https://doi.org/10.1097/BPO.0000000000001093.
27. Jaramillo D, Hoffer FA. Cartilaginous epiphysis and growth plate: normal and abnormal MR imaging findings. AJR Am J Roentgenol. 1992;158(5):1105–10. https://doi.org/10.2214/ajr.158.5.1566676.
28. de Pablos J, Arenas-Miquelez A, Arbeloa-Gutierrez L. Update on premature physeal closure. Diagnosis and treatment. Curr Opin Pediatr. 2021;33(1):79–89. https://doi.org/10.1097/MOP.0000000000000990.
29. Escott BG, Kelley SP. Management of traumatic physeal growth arrest. Orthop Trauma. 2012;26(3):200–11.
30. Boyden EM, Peterson HA. Partial premature closure of the distal radial physis associated with Kirschner wire fixation. Orthopedics. 1991;14(5):585–8. https://doi.org/10.3928/0147-7447-19910501-13.
31. Sengab A, Krijnen P, Schipper IB. Displaced distal radius fractures in children, cast alone vs additional K-wire fixation: a meta-analysis. Eur J Trauma Emerg Surg. 2019;45(6):1003–11. https://doi.org/10.1007/s00068-018-1011-y.

Chapter 3
Non-Accidental Injuries

Daniel Fodor and Carlos Saavedra

3.1 Non-Accidental Injuries

There are different definitions of Child Abuse, a concept currently replaced in the medical literature as Non-Accidental Injuries (NAI). The Chilean Law N°19.324 [1] on domestic violence defines it as the "result of an action or omission that causes damage to the physical or psychic health of minors." UNICEF [2] understands it as children and adolescents up to 18 years old who "occasionally or habitually suffer acts of physical, sexual or emotional violence, whether in the family group or in social institutions." However, the most complete and specific definition is given by the World Health Organization (WHO) defining it as the abuses and neglect suffered by minors under 18 years old and includes all types of physical or psychological abuse, sexual abuse, neglect, negligence, and commercial or other exploitation that cause or may cause harm to the health, development, or dignity of the child. The term "Child Abuse" has been widely used, a concept currently replaced in the medical literature as NAI [3–6].

The global prevalence of NAI varies according to the definition of the diagnosis used, as broader definitions provide higher prevalence rates. There is also inconsistency in the reporting of cases in the global literature due to underdiagnosis. It is estimated that between 2% and 10% of children who are treated in emergency services present NAI, estimating that 20% of fractures due to NAI in children under 3 years old are not diagnosed [4].

D. Fodor (✉)
Servicio De Salud Araucanía Sur, Clínica Mayor Redsalud, Temuco, Chile

C. Saavedra
Universidad de Chile, Santiago, Chile

M. Sepúlveda O. (ed.), *Paediatrics Traumatology*,
https://doi.org/10.1007/978-3-031-89482-4_3

3.2 Introduction

Musculoskeletal injuries are presented as the first cause for consultation in up to a third of patients with NAI, and 1 out of every 8 children of 18 months old or younger with a fracture, is a result of NAI. The most frequent forms of presentation are bruises, and fractures in second place. It should be considered that between 25% and 50% of patients present recurrence of NAI, and of these, 5–10% can be fatal [5].

We should always consider that an NAI is present at all levels in society, without distinction of educational level, socioeconomic status, race, or religion [6]. In addition, there are some risk factors described in the literature [7, 8]. Child risk factors are considered to be an unplanned or unwanted pregnancy, a preterm newborn, with chronic diseases or with special needs. The risk factors of the parents or caregivers are harmful alcohol or substance use, and a negative perception of a child's behavior. Environmental risk factors are also described, such as social isolation, poverty, or unemployment.

There is a myth that it is easy to recognize an NAI. However, we know that most injuries in the pediatric population are not the result of an NAI. In fact, most injuries in children do not even require medical attention. To further complicate the diagnosis, there are injuries with unusual patterns that are also the result of accidental injuries, as children are involved at younger ages in dangerous games. Finally, it is common for there to be no witnesses to the accident, or for the victims not to want to speak out of fear of retaliation, or simply because of their limited communication skills if they are in the preverbal stage of their development. It should also be noted that there may be a possibility on the part of the medical staff not to want to raise the diagnosis of NAI, due to the associated situations and loss of trust. For all these considerations, to propose or diagnose an NAI (Non-Accidental Injury) is one of the most difficult responsibilities in the practice of medicine with children. However, we must know that early identification can stop the abuse; therefore, we must take it as an opportunity for mandatory intervention in medical practice.

3.3 Diagnosis

To achieve the diagnosis of an NAI, the objective of the anamnesis should be to collect the information in a detailed, but not accusatory, manner in order to recognize a potential NAI. It is not the objective of this to identify a particular aggressor. In the face of suspicion, a basic radiological study should be carried out (first focused on the injury for which consultation is sought), and refer or complement its action with other specialist, for the complete evaluation, investigation, and treatment of the patient [9, 10]. Broad questions, an initial spontaneous account from the patient without interruptions, and subsequently questions from the doctor about the event:

time, witnesses, patient's behavior before, during, and after the accident. The patient's and his family's history should be taken into consideration, recording those focused on the differential diagnosis of NAI: musculoskeletal diseases (e.g., osteogenesis imperfecta), metabolic bone diseases, coagulation disorders [11].

There are some anamnestic elements that suggest NAI and that should be an alert: vague or null explanation regarding a serious injury, explicit denial of trauma in a patient with an evident injury, changes in the story, or witnesses who give different versions of an event, an explanation that is inconsistent with the pattern, severity of the injury, age or with the patient's physical abilities (e.g., in children using orthoses or wheelchairs), unexplained delay in seeking medical attention, aggressive or evasive companion. In younger, or preverbal, children, changes in behavior should be investigated. It is suggestive of NAI that different witnesses give different versions (unlike the fact that several witnesses give a single version).

NAI can range from minor injuries to those that pose a life-threatening risk or are fatal. They can be reported by the patient himself, by a caregiver (e.g., teachers), or by a witness to the events. As with any injured child, the priority will be to stabilize their medical condition.

We must remember that rarely an injury is pathognomonic of NAI, so it is essential to consider together the clinical history, the complete physical examination, and the analysis of the complementary tests [12, 13].

It is recommended to perform a systematized or protocolized physical examination, always accompanied by another medical service provider. We must always observe the behavior of the patient and his caregivers and be attentive to suspicious injuries. In case of finding them, it is advisable to keep a photographic record or a body diagram of them, in order to document the findings. If injuries not mentioned in the account are found during the physical examination, the appropriate thing is to ask about the mechanism of injury. In the case that any is a relevant injury for treatment, ask about whether the patient has received it adequately.

Signs of neglect in the form of abandonment should also be sought: malnutrition (use height and weight charts according to age), numerous dental cavities, untreated diaper rash. Physical abuse and neglect can be concomitant.

In the segmental physical examination, we must look for injuries in skin, mouth (frenulum injuries in infants), head (traumatic alopecia), rib cage (fractures), neurological alterations (suggestive of trauma), and extremities (careful inspection and palpation). Sentinel injuries [14] are defined as those injuries that, being medically of lesser severity, are recognized by doctors or relatives before the diagnosis of NAI. They are infrequent in accidental injuries, but common in NAI: they are present in 25% of abused children. Although "bruises" are common soft tissue injuries in childhood, they are also the most frequent manifestation of NAI. Despite this, they are not considered by the treating physician as sentinel injuries in half of the severe and fatal cases of NAI. Characteristic injuries predictive of NAI (Sensitivity of 97%–Specificity of 84%) are "bruises" on the trunk, ears, or neck in children up to 4 years old or any "bruise" in children under 4 months old [15–17] (Fig. 3.1).

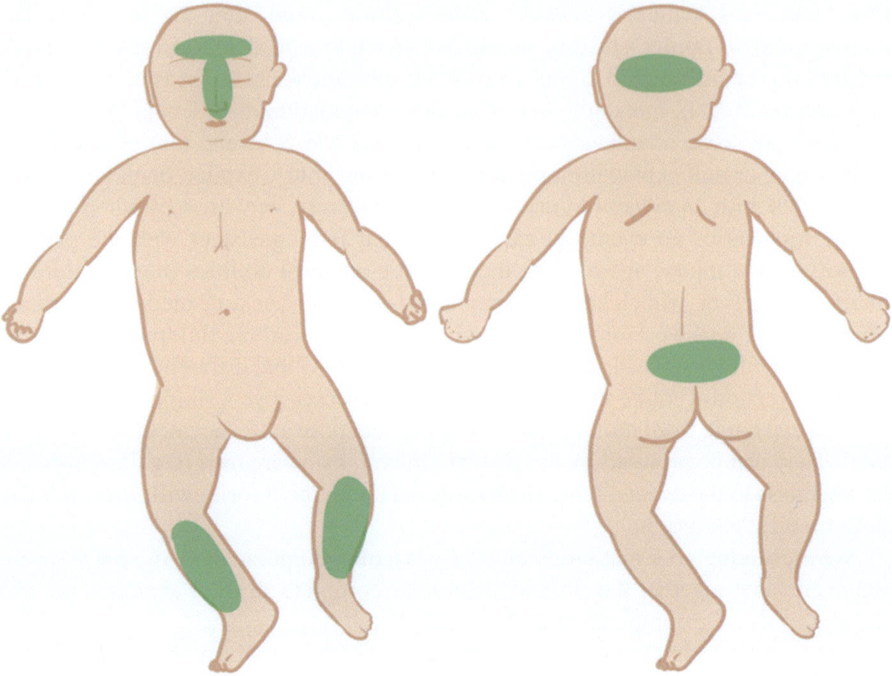

Fig. 3.1 Typical sites of accidental injury: bony prominences in the lower limbs such as knees, tibias, but also head and forehead

Petechiae are present in 22% of patients with NAI, while only in 2% of accidental injuries. The pattern and location of accidental bruises directly correlates with the degree of the patient's independent mobility (Fig. 3.2). Remember: "if it doesn't walk, it doesn't get injured!."

Other important soft tissue injuries to consider [18] are: Clusters of injuries, which present in a typical defensive mode (Fig. 3.3); Human bites, highly suggestive of non-accidental mechanism; Burns, which are not typical injuries of NAI; however, this mechanism should be suspected if they are severe, if they have an immersion pattern (demarcation line that involves genitals, buttocks, and lower limbs in a symmetrical way); imprint of the element used to cause the damage (Fig. 3.4).

Also associated with NAI are soft tissue injuries in non-ambulatory children, in multiple systems, at different stages of evolution, with imprint of objects, in typical locations, without clear mechanism and concomitant with other types of abuse.

Do not forget that these children may present injuries in other systems different from the musculoskeletal, so in the face of suspicion, the presence of sexual abuse, thoracoabdominal injuries and cranial injuries should be explored as a team. Also, do not forget the differential diagnoses (Osteogenesis imperfecta, nutritional deficiencies—vitamin C, vitamin D, copper) [11].

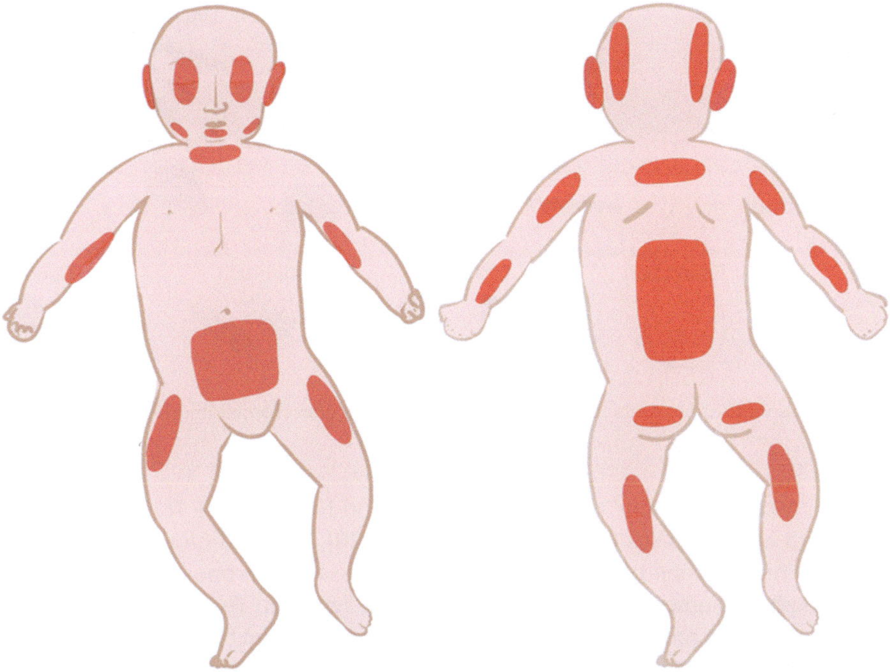

Fig. 3.2 Frequent sites of non-accidental injuries

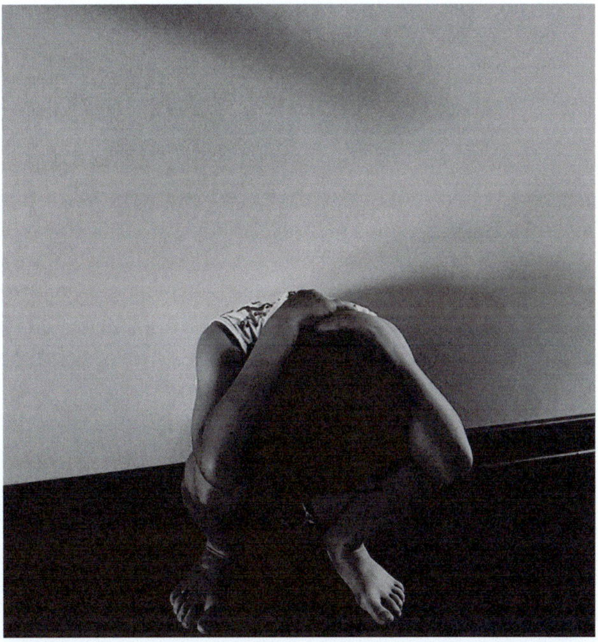

Fig. 3.3 Typical defense position, in which injuries are found on the outer side of the forearms, the outer side of the knees, and the back of the head

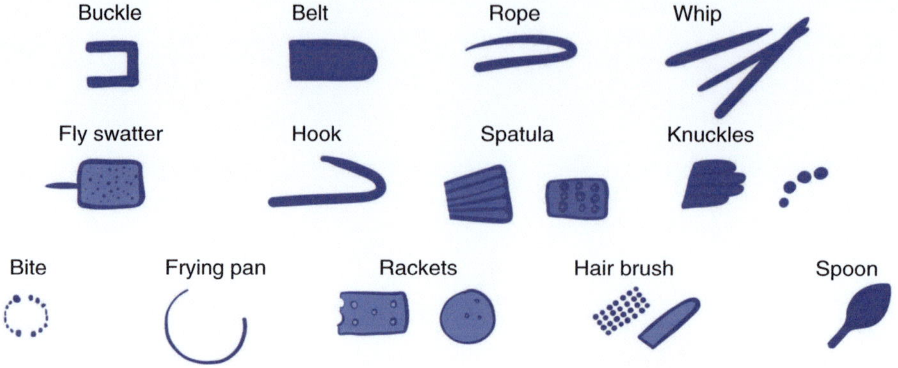

Fig. 3.4 Imprints of elements that can be seen in cases of non-accidental injuries

The "Skeletal Survey" is the standard method for detecting fractures in children with other injuries suspected of NAI [19, 20]. This radiological evaluation includes radiographs of the appendicular skeleton (Anteroposterior projection radiograph of humerus, forearm, hand, femur, legs and foot) and of the axial skeleton: (Chest radiograph in anteroposterior projection, lateral and rib cage, anteroposterior pelvis, lateral lumbosacral spine, lateral cervical spine, anteroposterior and lateral skull). An analysis of 700 of these exams found 11% of unreported fractures, half of which were NAI. Repeating the "Skeletal Survey" 2–3 weeks after the first attention allows to detect 25% of additional fractures to those observed at the beginning [21].

The "Skeletal Survey" should be regularly requested for every child under 2 years old, with evident injuries from NAI, every child under 2 years old, with injuries suggestive of NAI, patients with unexplained intracranial injuries and siblings of a patient who has suffered NAI.

Highly suggestive findings of NAI in the radiological evaluation [21] are femur fracture in children under 1 year old, humerus fracture in children under 3 years old, scapula fracture, sternum or spinous process fracture, and fractures in different phases of consolidation. These last ones are present in 70% of NAI cases in children under 1 year old, and in 50% of all patients with NAI (Fig. 3.5).

Rib fractures occur by an anteroposterior-lateral compression mechanism (Fig. 3.6). Metaphyseal corner fractures in femur and tibia are the result of a traction mechanism and rotation, where a complete fracture feature is generated in the metaphyseal spongy bone, and a thick peripheral bone fragment that includes physis, periosteum, and bone (Fig. 3.7) [22].

Multiple fractures, especially if they are bilateral, finger fractures in non-ambulatory individuals, and epiphyseal separation by traction mechanism that

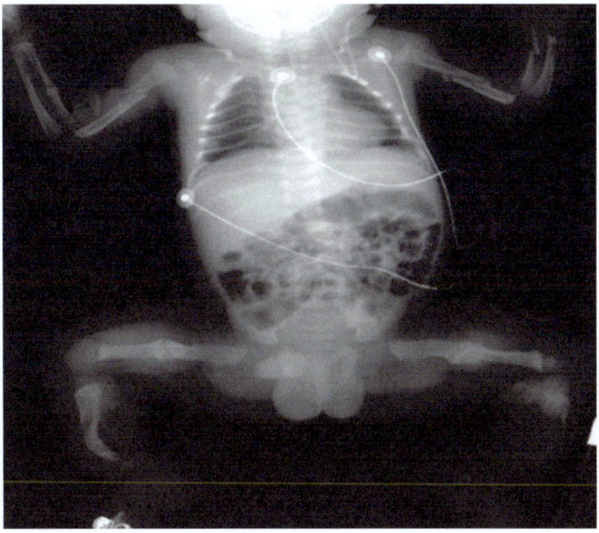

Fig. 3.5 Fractures in different stages of evolution. (Photo courtesy of Gerardo Aguilar, Mexico)

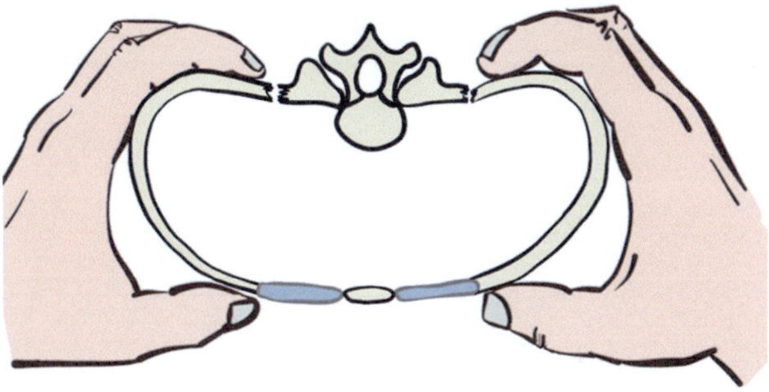

Fig. 3.6 Mechanism of rib fractures associated with non-accidental injuries due to chest compression

produces a listhesis of the distal humerus physis (Fig. 3.8) are moderately specific findings in radiological evaluation. This fracture can be difficult to diagnose, especially in very small patients. It can also occur in the context of birth trauma. It can be confused with an elbow dislocation, especially if the capitellum is not ossified. Ultrasound can be useful as a complementary examination.

Therefore, we must suspect NAI in the presence of a fracture in non-ambulatory children, in diaphyseal fractures of the humerus in the femur in preschoolers, in unusual and highly specific fractures (metaphyseal corner, sternum, scapula, spinous processes), rib fractures, associated with soft tissue injury or other systems, multiple fractures or in different phases of consolidation and accident history that does not explain the fracture.

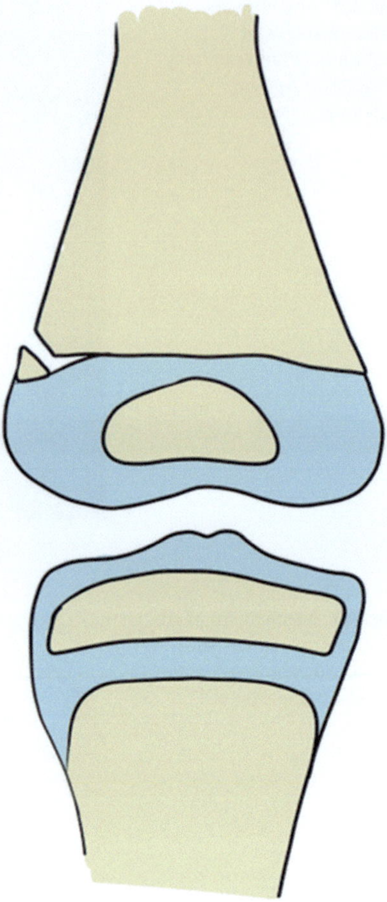

Fig. 3.7 Diagram of a metaphyseal corner fracture, associated with non-accidental injuries due traction

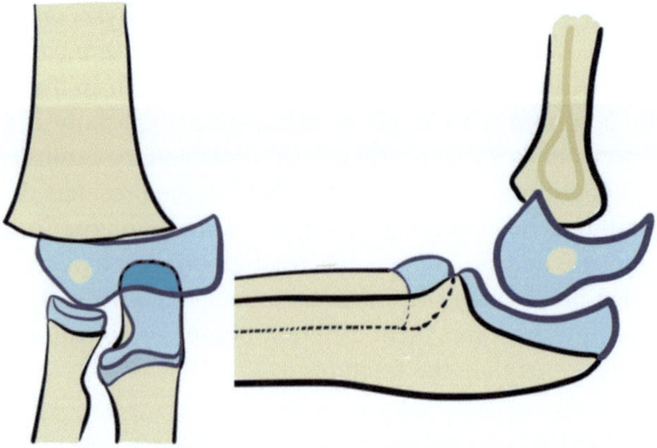

Fig. 3.8 Epiphyseal separation: a traction mechanism that produces a physiolisthesis of the distal humerus

3.4 Treatment

The role of the trauma surgeon in suspected NAI cases varies according to the severity of the case, the specialist's own training, and local legislation. In cases that present a biomedical risk of serious functional sequelae or death (0.25% of cases [23]), our primary duty is to make efforts in relation to the rescue of our patient. However, the vast majority of NAI cases do not present with severe biomedical risk injuries immediately [23]; therefore, our management should have other characteristics in a suspicious case.

Sink [24] in his work presents an optimal role, which includes a proper medical history, a thorough physical examination, obtaining adequate radiographs, and notification to auxiliary agencies, depending on the country.

The suggestive elements of NAI in the anamnesis and the requirements to request the skeletal imaging study have already been mentioned, highlighting the importance of the physical examination in the first attention. It is demonstrated in suspected NAI cases, 1 out of every 5 cases receives suboptimal treatment [25], with which patients with fractures due to NAI run the risk of delay in diagnosis and repetition of the abuse pattern.

Regarding notification to social services, in the face of a suspicion of NAI we must activate a first response, which consists of "health actions aimed at interrupting abuse, establishing safe conditions and protection for the affected child or adolescent" [26].

Secondly, the first response will also facilitate the criminal prosecution and the sanction of those responsible. In Chilean legislation, this is defined as "the legal act that consists of making a possible crime known to the corresponding authority." To report, it is enough to suspect a situation of abuse, since its verification or not is the function of the Public Ministry and not of the reporting doctor. The deadline to make the complaint is "twenty-four hours following the moment they became aware of the fact" [27]. Complaints can be made Police, Public Ministry, or Guarantee Family Courts.

The suggestion of these authors is that in case of suspicion or certainty of NAI, the patient should be hospitalized, regardless of the biomedical severity of the condition, to be evaluated by the multidisciplinary team of each center in charge of managing these cases (Fig. 3.9) [28].

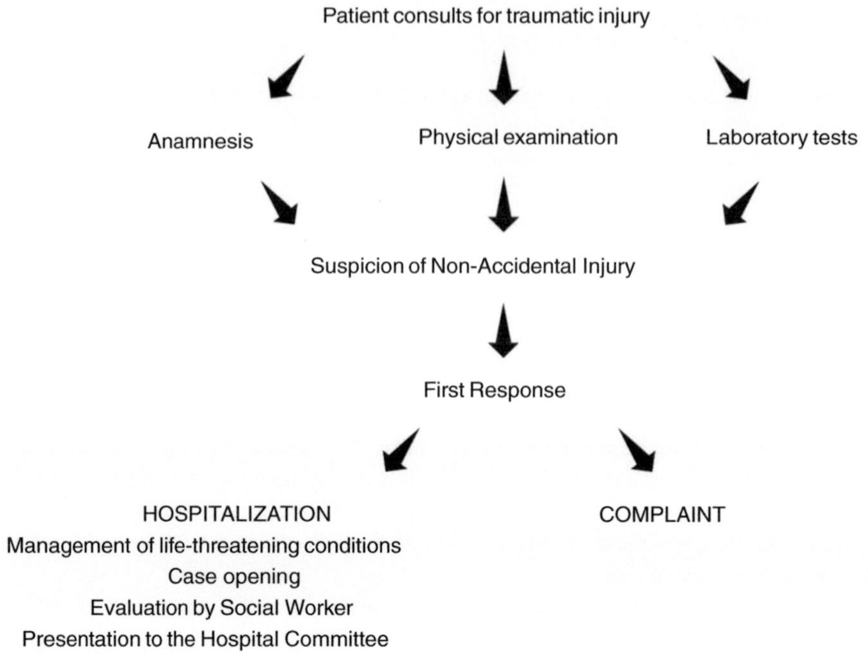

Fig. 3.9 Proposed flowchart for suspected or detected non-accidental injury

3.5 Final Message

As with any medical diagnosis, the proper management of the pathology begins with paying attention to the details during clinical practice. Non-accidental injuries are not an isolated entity, but correspond to a clinically verifiable event within a timeline of abuse. A high index of suspicion must be maintained and local protocols and interdisciplinary teams involved in the management of these patients must be known.

References

1. Ministry of Justice, Republic of Chile. Law N° 19.324. Official Gazette of the Republic of Chile, August 19, 1994. http://bcn.cl/2qc3q. Accessed 12 June 2022.
2. UNICEF. 4th Study Child Abuse in Chile comparative analysis 1994–2000–2006–2012. Santiago, Chile: UNICEF; 2012. Available at: https://www.unicef.org/chile/media/1306/file/4to_estudio_de:maltrato_infantil_en_chile.pdf. Accessed 12 June 2022
3. Teeuw AH, Derkx BH, Koster WA, van Rijn RR. Educational paper: Detection of child abuse and neglect at the emergency room. Eur J Pediatr. 2012;171(6):877–85. https://doi.org/10.1007/s00431-011-1551-1.

4. McMahon P, Grossman W, Gaffney M, Stanitski C. Soft-tissue injury as an indication of child abuse. J Bone Joint Surg Am. 1995;77(8):1179–83. https://doi.org/10.2106/00004623-199508000-00006.
5. Jayakumar P, Barry M, Ramachandran M. Orthopaedic aspects of paediatric non-accidental injury. J Bone Joint Surg Br. 2010;92(2):189–95. https://doi.org/10.1302/0301-620X.92B2.22923.
6. Kocher MS, Kasser JR. Orthopaedic aspects of child abuse. J Am Acad Orthop Surg. 2000;8(1):10–20. https://doi.org/10.5435/00124635-200001000-00002.
7. Austin AE, Lesak AM, Shanahan ME. Risk and protective factors for child maltreatment: A review. Curr Epidemiol Rep. 2020;7(4):334–42. https://doi.org/10.1007/s40471-020-00252-3.
8. Sivasundaram L, Trivedi NN, Gatta J, Ning AY, Kim CY, Mistovich RJ. Demographics and risk factors for non-accidental orthopedic trauma. Clin Pediatr (Phila). 2019;58(6):618–26. https://doi.org/10.1177/0009922819829045.
9. United Nations Children's Fund. Hidden in plain sight: A statistical analysis of violence against children. New York, UNICEF; September 2014. https://www.unicef.org/publications/index_74865.html. Accessed 12 June 2022
10. Loder RT, Feinberg JR. Orthopaedic injuries in children with nonaccidental trauma: demographics and incidence from the 2000 kids' inpatient database [published correction appears in J Pediatr Orthop. 2008 Sep;28(6):699]. J Pediatr Orthop. 2007;27(4):421–6. https://doi.org/10.1097/01.bpb.0000271328.79481.07.
11. Wood JN, Christian CW, Adams CM, Rubin DM. Skeletal surveys in infants with isolated skull fractures. Pediatrics. 2009;123(2):e247–52. https://doi.org/10.1542/peds.2008-2467.
12. Christian CW. Committee on child abuse and neglect, American Academy of Pediatrics. The evaluation of suspected child physical abuse [published correction appears in Pediatrics. 2015 Sep;136(3):583]. Pediatrics. 2015;135(5):e1337–54. https://doi.org/10.1542/peds.2015-0356.
13. Sheets LK, Leach ME, Koszewski IJ, Lessmeier AM, Nugent M, Simpson P. Sentinel injuries in infants evaluated for child physical abuse. Pediatrics. 2013;131(4):701–7. https://doi.org/10.1542/peds.2012-2780.
14. Wood JN, Fakeye O, Mondestin V, et al. Prevalence of abuse among young children with femur fractures: a systematic review. BMC Pediatr. 2014;14:169. https://doi.org/10.1186/1471-2431-14-169.
15. Expert Panel on Pediatric Imaging, Wootton-Gorges SL, Soares BP, et al. ACR appropriateness Criteria® suspected physical abuse-child. J Am Coll Radiol. 2017;14(5S):S338–49. https://doi.org/10.1016/j.jacr.2017.01.036.
16. Onyon C, Rabb L, Debelle G. Non-accidental injury and bone fragility disorders: the need for a multidisciplinary perspective. Child Abuse Review. 2009;18:346–53. https://doi.org/10.1002/car.1086.
17. Carpenter RF. The prevalence and distribution of bruising in babies. Arch Dis Child. 1999;80(4):363–6. https://doi.org/10.1136/adc.80.4.363.
18. Maguire S, Mann M. Systematic reviews of bruising in relation to child abuse-what have we learnt: an overview of review updates. Evid Based Child Health. 2013;8(2):255–63. https://doi.org/10.1002/ebch.1909.
19. Kemp AM, Dunstan F, Harrison S, et al. Patterns of skeletal fractures in child abuse: systematic review. BMJ. 2008;337:a1518. Published 2008 Oct 2. https://doi.org/10.1136/bmj.a1518.
20. Flaherty EG, Perez-Rossello JM, Levine MA, et al. Evaluating children with fractures for child physical abuse. Pediatrics. 2014;133(2):e477–89. https://doi.org/10.1542/peds.2013-3793.
21. Harper NS, Eddleman S, Lindberg DM, ExSTRA Investigators. The utility of follow-up skeletal surveys in child abuse. Pediatrics. 2013;131(3):e672–8. https://doi.org/10.1542/peds.2012-2608.
22. Sugar NF, Taylor JA, Feldman KW. Bruises in infants and toddlers: those who don't cruise rarely bruise. Puget Sound Pediatric Research Network. Arch Pediatr Adolesc Med. 1999;153(4):399–403. https://doi.org/10.1001/archpedi.153.4.399.

23. Pierce MC, Kaczor K, Aldridge S, O'Flynn J, Lorenz DJ. Bruising characteristics discriminating physical child abuse from accidental trauma [published correction appears in Pediatrics. 2010 Apr;125(4):861]. Pediatrics. 2010;125(1):67–74. https://doi.org/10.1542/peds.2008-3632.
24. Sink EL, Hyman JE, Matheny T, Georgopoulos G, Kleinman P. Child abuse: the role of the orthopaedic surgeon in nonaccidental trauma. Clin Orthop Relat Res. 2011;469(3):790–7. https://doi.org/10.1007/s11999-010-1610-3.
25. Ravichandiran N, Schuh S, Bejuk M, et al. Delayed identification of pediatric abuse-related fractures. Pediatrics. 2010;125(1):60–6. https://doi.org/10.1542/peds.2008-3794.
26. U.S. Department of Health and Human Services AfCaF. Administration on Children, Youth and Families, Children's Bureau. Child Maltreatment. 2017; https://www.acf.hhs.gov/sites/default/files/cb/cm2017.pdf. Accessed 29 March 2019
27. Ministry of Health, Government of Chile. CLINICAL GUIDE: Detection and first response to children and adolescents victims of abuse by relatives or caregivers. Santiago de Chile: Editorial Valente Limited; 2013. https://www.minsal.cl/sites/default/files/files/Guia_maltrato_Valente26dic2013.pdf. Accessed 12 June 2022
28. Ministry of Justice, Republic of Chile. Article 175 of the Criminal Procedure Code. Official Gazette of the Republic of Chile; 2000. http://bcn.cl/2f7dm. Accessed 12 June 2022

Chapter 4
The Pediatric Patient with Multiple Injuries

Pedro Jorba and Nicolás Valdivia R.

4.1 The Pediatric Patient with Multiple Injuries

Intentional injuries, unintentional injuries, and homicide cause more deaths in those over 1 year old up to 18 years old, than all other causes of death combined [1]. According to the latest reports from the World Health Organization, injuries caused by traffic accidents are the leading cause of mortality in the population aged 5 to 29 years old [2].

According to the latest update of the ATLS (Advanced Trauma Life Support), trauma-related injuries are the most common cause of mortality and disability in the United States in children over 1 year old, with approximately 10,000 deaths per year [3]. During 2016, there were 20,360 deaths in children and adolescents. More than 60% of these deaths were secondary to trauma injuries. Motor vehicle accidents were the leading cause of death in children under 19 years old, representing 20% of all deaths, gunshot injuries accounted for 15%, followed by deaths from suffocation and suicide [4].

4.2 Introduction

Given the alarming numbers during the beginning of 2000, the implementation of new regulations regarding accident prevention and stricter laws in the United States, mortality from accidental trauma decreased by 29% between the years 2000 and

P. Jorba
Legaria Children's Hospital, Ciudad de México, Mexico

N. Valdivia R. (✉)
Hospital Víctor Ríos Ruiz, Los Ángeles, Clínica Andes Salud, Clínica Sur, Concepción, Chile

M. Sepúlveda O. (ed.), *Paediatrics Traumatology*,
https://doi.org/10.1007/978-3-031-89482-4_4

2009, that is, from 15.5 to 11.0 per 100,000 individuals. During 2009 there were 9143 deaths of children due to accidental causes [5]. This is why it is of vital importance to implement governmental policies in each country, with regulations about the correct use of child-adapted safety systems (with their proper mode of use) inside vehicles, in addition to strict laws and penalties that help raise awareness of the consequences of not complying with them.

Regarding the distribution by gender, boys are twice as likely to suffer a trauma injury compared to girls, and there is evidence that a higher percentage of injuries in boys may require hospitalization for their management [6].

In our country, accidental trauma injuries correspond to the third cause of death among 0 to 19 year old, after perinatal pathology and congenital malformations, representing, in 2014, 20.5% of the recorded deaths, with a mortality rate of 12.5 x 100,000 inhabitants [7].

4.3 Causes of Death

The most frequent causal agent of death from trauma in pediatric patients is cranial trauma (associated or not with other injuries), which is more frequent in infants. This is followed by thoracic trauma, usually associated with other injuries, and in third place abdominal trauma, which in 90% of cases is closed, and in 85% is exclusively non-surgical management [7].

When we talk about a patient with multiple injuries, penetrating trauma is much rarer in children compared to adults, and as they approach adolescence, the trend is for this type of injury to be similar to adults. Closed trauma secondary to vehicular accidents, falls from height or abuse is more associated with pediatric patients than adults.

Fractures are quite common in polytrauma patients and significantly contribute to their morbidity, but they are rarely the direct cause of mortality. Almost two-thirds of these patients have fractures of the limbs. Within this group, fractures of the long bones, mainly femur fractures, are associated in 22% of cases. It is common to find fractures of long bones in both the upper and lower limbs ipsilaterally in vehicular accidents.

4.4 Special Characteristics of the Pediatric Polytrauma Patient

The anatomical conditions of the pediatric skeleton and those related to high-energy trauma are classically described. Children under 6 years old have a head size that is considerably larger/heavier in proportion to the rest of the body, which makes them more prone to cervical injuries, cranial trauma. It is important to keep this in mind when immobilizing and transporting (see below).

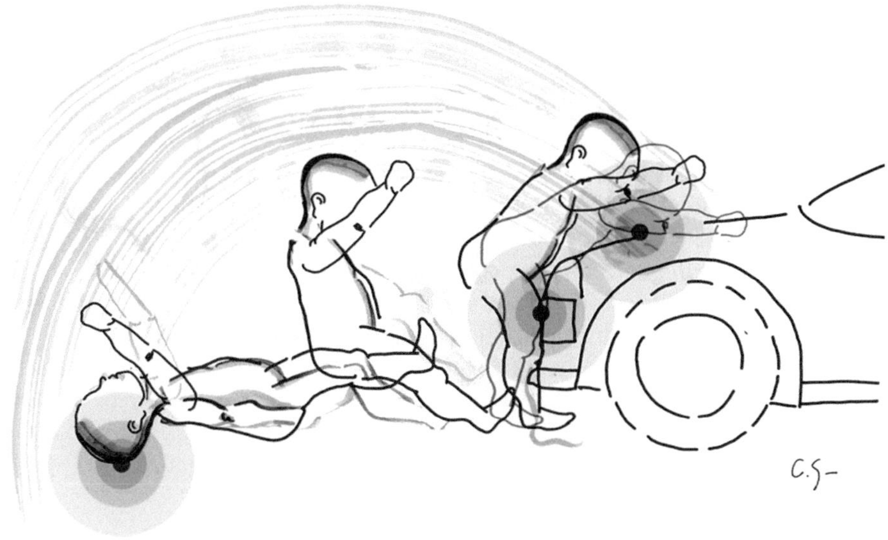

Fig. 4.1 Wadell's triad. The car hits the minor's thigh, then the torso hits the hood, and finally the skull hits the ground

In preadolescents and minors who are hit by a car, we must keep in mind the Waddell triad, which consists of the child initially being hit in the thigh by the vehicle's bumper (causing a femur fracture), followed by trauma around the chest or abdomen on the hood, and finally the head region when hitting the ground (Fig. 4.1).

4.5 Systemic Response of the Pediatric Polytrauma Patient

In a polytrauma patient, the injury of multiple organs and systems triggers an inflammatory cascade, resulting in increased endothelial permeability, interstitial edema, intravascular occlusion, microvascular ischemia, and eventually failure of the affected organ or multiple organs. In general, the pattern of multiple organ failure in the pediatric patient is pathophysiologically distinct from that of the adult.

The timing of multiple organ failure in children and adults is different. In children, its onset is practically immediate, affecting almost all organs simultaneously after trauma, unlike adults, where it occurs between 48 and 72 h after trauma, with initial pulmonary involvement. We must emphasize that lung injuries in children are six times less frequent than in adults [8].

The physiological response to pediatric trauma is characterized by being more buffered at the systemic level, but with a much more intense response at the level of the injured tissue, which favors tissue repair at the local level, generating less systemic damage. This could tip the balance towards early definitive management in surgical fractures.

In the management of the adult polytrauma patient, there is evidence that tips the balance towards the concept of "Damage Control Orthopedic Surgery," meaning that definitive fracture management is performed in a deferred manner and only temporary stabilization of these is performed, as it would reduce the risk of multiple organ failure, a lower systemic inflammatory response, and less risk of respiratory distress. In the pediatric patient, there is no evidence that this is the case. In fact, the emergence of the concept "Early Total Care" (ETC) would allow for early and definitive treatment of fractures. Few studies are focused on the most appropriate time for stabilization and definitive fixation in pediatric patients, so it is very difficult to reach a consensus. In 2019, a study was published where 5512 trauma victims were analyzed, including 316 children, and the use of conservative management, "Damage Control" and "Early Total Care" was recorded. It is noteworthy that the use of external fixator increased with age, most children immediately received ETC and that when comparing these patients with the adult group there were no differences in mortality, complications such as sepsis and multiple organ failure [9].

4.6 Evaluation and Treatment

The treatment of a polytrauma patient can be divided into two parts: pre-hospital, where the first vital support care and transfer are received, and the management in the emergency service, once the patient has been transferred.

It is of crucial importance that the patient must be transferred appropriately to the referral center, that is, securely immobilized, with a proper airway and oxygen support, depending on the patient's requirements and the degree of consciousness impairment (Glasgow Scale). In addition, two caliber venous routes must be kept permeable (intraosseous route as an alternative), and adequate physical measures to prevent hypothermia.

Cervical spine injury should always be assumed in a polytraumatized patient until proven otherwise. The immobilization of the cervical spine should be done through a collar suitable for the child's size, and using a pediatric spinal board. This is because, in children under 8 to 9 years old, the head is disproportionately larger than the trunk and to leave the cervical spine in a neutral position and the airway clear there are two alternatives: a spinal board with a hole at the head level, or with a raise (sheets or blankets) under the body [10] (Fig. 4.2).

Once the patient is received in the emergency service, they must be quickly admitted to the resuscitation room, and evaluated by a team, which is usually led by a pediatrician or a pediatric surgeon. One of them will be the person responsible for indicating the resuscitation and/or stabilization maneuvers of the patient.

While the doctor in charge of resuscitation evaluates the patient, the trauma surgeon simultaneously (without interfering in resuscitation/stabilization maneuvers) must perform a first evaluation, looking for musculoskeletal injuries that could affect the patient hemodynamically or neurologically (pelvis fractures, multiple long bones, spinal column), and temporarily immobilize them to reduce their

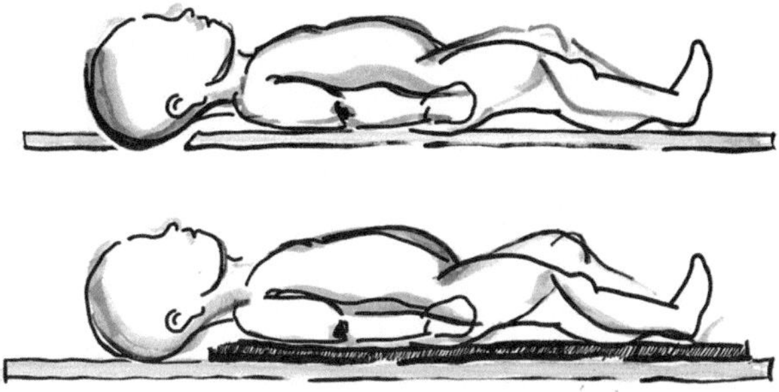

Fig. 4.2 Adequate transport position for a polytraumatized pediatric patient, avoiding cervical flexion and maintaining a clear airway

bleeding. The use of pneumatic splints or with side bars and soft part traction systems for lower limbs allow to align and quickly stabilize a bone segment, reducing bleeding, and acting with a significant analgesic effect. We must remember that a femur fracture in an adult can lose 1000 to 1500 cc of blood or approximately 30% of the volemia. Despite this, children rarely require a transfusion when they have isolated femur fractures, but when associated with other injuries the possibility of transfusion increases to 39% [11].

Pelvis fractures are usually due to high-energy closed traumas, such as car accidents or falls from height, so a high suspicion must be held in these cases. The integrity and stability of the pelvic ring must be carefully evaluated. Pelvis fractures are an indicator of severity when present, which should make suspect associated injuries such as traumatic brain injury and intra-abdominal, with a higher risk of bleeding [12]. Like femur fractures, these fractures when isolated (without concomitant injuries) do not present a higher risk of hemodynamic compromise, unlike adults [10].

Once the patient is uncovered, a new evaluation is performed, where the trauma surgeon must look for injuries in the musculoskeletal apparatus more carefully than at the beginning. Areas with wounds, indurated, edematous or deformed, with hypoperfusion distal to some limb (pallor, absence or decrease of pulses, slow capillary refill) and/or signs of compartment syndrome, must be identified and described in detail.

Most young children who are victims of polytrauma who enter the emergency service without consciousness impairment, do so very scared, crying or with psychomotor agitation. It is not uncommon to see them brought by ambulance personnel without the company of a known person or family member. These conditions make the patient's evaluation very difficult (especially small children). It is important to try to be calm, in order to soothe the child and obtain any information about the accident (mechanism of trauma, areas of pain, etc.), which will allow us to approach a more precise diagnosis.

Any patient who does not move or refuses to move a limb is a sign indicative of a fracture until proven otherwise.

An evaluation of the spine should be performed while keeping the cervical spine immobilized, moving the patient as a block without removing the spinal board.

Look for skin injuries suggestive of trauma, palpate and look for painful points or deformity along the spine.

A detailed neurological examination checking for sensory or motor deficits will allow us to identify possible injuries early and alert the resuscitation team when moving the patient, transferring to another unit (imaging, operating room, etc.), and guide when taking imaging tests during the diagnostic process.

4.7 Imaging Diagnosis

Diagnostic imaging studies are a crucial complement to the careful physical examination in the evaluation of the polytraumatized child. Although there are a large number of imaging techniques available, the time constraints in an emergency situation force us to choose and efficiently use imaging studies. For this reason, sensitivity is usually prioritized over specificity, with the goal of preventing significant injuries from going unnoticed.

The American College of Surgeons, through the recommendations of Advanced Trauma Life Support (ATLS), recommends performing, at least, three radiographs in the polytraumatized patient: lateral projection of cervical spine, anteroposterior projection of chest, and anteroposterior projection of the pelvis. Although there is no specific recommendation for the pediatric patient, this same recommendation has been usually extended to them although there is not the same evidence support as in adults.

Khan [13] reports a series of 176 pediatric patients polytraumatized to whom the standard trauma series was performed. None of the patients presented clinically or radiographically identifiable cervical injuries. Regarding the chest, 100% of the patients in whom a radiographic injury was identified also presented clinical suggestive data. The pelvis projection reported a bone injury in 6.25% of the patients, of which only 18% (2 out of 11) did not have positive clinical data for the segment. These findings together suggest that the trauma panel is of limited utility in conscious children with normal physical examination.

The use of Whole-Body Computed Tomography (WBCT) has been shown to be able to decrease mortality in adult polytraumatized patients. However, in pediatric patients the increased risk of cancer derived from radiation forces us to be more selective when indicating CT studies. Frellesen [14] correlated clinical variables with WBCT findings in 100 pediatric patients, finding that no clinical variable by itself was able to predict an abnormal imaging study, with the exception of the Glasgow coma scale, which was able to predict an abnormal brain CT with a score of 13 or less. It is likely that it is preferable to perform CT on specific body segments, according to clinical findings.

Whole-body Magnetic Resonance Imaging has been suggested as a radiation-free alternative for pediatric patients, with high sensitivity to detect injuries.

However, the significantly longer time required for the study limits its use to patients who are hemodynamically stable, which reduces its utility in the clinical situation. Further studies are needed to define the precise indications of this imaging modality [15].

4.8 Scores in Pediatric Polytrauma

For decades, different scoring systems have been developed for trauma patients. These scores have proven to be useful in facilitating the triage of these patients, defining the severity of injuries, and allowing to predict the need for surgical treatments. The very definition of what is a polytrauma is linked to the rating of the most used tool, the Injury Severity Score (ISS), considering that it exists when it is greater than or equal to 16. However, there is still controversy about this, and the search for an ideal definition continues [16]. Brown [17] proposes taking an ISS score greater than or equal to 25 as indicative of polytrauma in children, after analyzing mortality patterns and differences with the adult patient.

Despite the demonstrated utility of the ISS, and its widespread use in the world, there is concern that it may not be the best option in children, so specific scores have been designed for pediatric patients. The most used is the Pediatric Trauma Score (PTS), which values the size of the child, as well as the state of his airway (Table 4.1). The PTS has a rating range of 6 to 12, and the lowest scores strongly correlate with a poor outcome, finding a linear relationship between the score and mortality, being the latter 100% when it is equal to or less than 0, and 9% when the score is equal to or greater than 8 [3].

Interestingly, the PTS has not been able to demonstrate a clear superiority over the ISS in predicting the need for surgery, or the risk of mortality. None of the available scores has the ability to predict the severity of the head injury [18], so the combined use of both scores is probably the best option for the management of pediatric patients. In view of the profound physiological differences between children and adults, we must continue searching for better and more accurate tools for the evaluation of polytrauma in the pediatric patient.

Table 4.1 Score for obtaining the Pediatric Trauma Score (PTS)

+1	+2	+3	
WEIGHT	>20 kg	10–20 kg	<10 kg
AIRWAY	Patent	Maintainable	Not maintainable
PAS	>90 mmHg	50–90 mmHg	<50 mmHg
CNS	Awake	Obtunded	Comatose
FRACTURE	None	Closed	Multiple, closed or open
WOUND	None	Minor	Major, penetrating, burns

PAS systolic blood pressure, *CNS* Central nervous system

4.9 Associated Injuries

In the pediatric polytrauma patient, Traumatic Brain Injury (TBI) is one of the most common injuries, being present in 17% of cases, and is the leading cause of death and permanent disability. As mentioned, TBI is more common in children due to the anatomical factors that predispose them. In children, up to 80% of patients will develop increased intracranial pressure, which is the main cause of secondary brain injury. When this increase is caused by intracranial hematomas, timely drainage can allow a full recovery; when it is caused by diffuse cerebral edema without occupational injuries, the prognosis is worse, despite the performance of decompressive craniotomies [19]. Early multidisciplinary management is crucial to seek the best outcomes in these potentially devastating injuries.

Thoracic trauma occurs in 8–62% of pediatric polytrauma patients. When accompanied by TBI or abdominal trauma, the mortality rate is up to 25%. Compared to adults, sternal and rib injuries are uncommon, and when they do occur, they may indicate severe cardiopulmonary injuries. Pulmonary contusions are the most frequently presented thoracic injuries and require timely management to avoid developing secondary complications that can be associated with significant morbidity and mortality. Cardiac contusions, although rare, should always be considered as the possible cause of shock without apparent etiology. Elevated troponin levels in polytrauma children are associated with a longer stay in intensive care unit (ICU), and a higher mortality, secondary to pulmonary and/or myocardial contusions, so it can be useful as a prognostic indicator [20].

Abdominal injuries are reported in approximately a quarter of polytrauma patients. Due to the greater physiological reserve of children, the hemodynamic repercussions of an abdominal bleeding usually delay their appearance until there is a significant volume loss. Due to their relative larger size in the infant abdomen, splenic and hepatic injuries are the most common. When there is hemodynamic stability, conservative management may be appropriate, but the threshold for deciding surgical exploration should be low. Two-stage management for severe liver injuries, with perihepatic packing and subsequent definitive repair allows avoiding large hepatic resections.

Once the initial surgical management of the polytrauma child has concluded, monitoring and medical management should continue in a Pediatric Intensive Care Unit, specialized, with a multidisciplinary team. Management in a Pediatric ICU optimizes the possibilities of survival and functional recovery [21].

4.10 Treatment of Orthopedic Injuries

Once the polytrauma pediatric patient has been initially addressed and the objectives of resuscitation have been met, musculoskeletal injuries should be treated as part of the secondary evaluation. Orthopedic management should focus on the management of severe open fractures, as well as early stabilization of other fractures.

In closed long bones fractures, it is advisable to avoid the use of large splints or casts for prolonged periods, particularly if the patient requires management in an Intensive Care Unit (ICU). Immobilization devices hinder nursing care, limit bed mobilization and carry a non-insignificant risk of causing pressure skin ulcers, particularly in patients with altered consciousness.

Early use of temporary external fixation devices has multiple advantages in the management of the polytraumatized pediatric patient. They can be applied quickly, without hindering the performance of urgent surgeries on other body segments, and significantly simplify the subsequent management of the patient, reducing pain and the risk of complications secondary to the instability of fractures. It is critical to consider at the time of installing the external fixator, the type of definitive fixation that will eventually be performed, to avoid interfering with potential approaches. Always consider the possibility that it may never be possible to perform another definitive fixation on time, either due to deterioration in the patient's medical condition or for any other factor beyond the control of the orthopedic surgeon. For this reason, it is always advisable to seek the best possible reduction when applying external fixation.

The definitive management of closed fractures of long bones is usually the same as would be chosen in a similar isolated fracture, and, as previously mentioned, in general, definitive osteosynthesis is sought as soon as the patient's conditions allow it, as the benefits of Damage Control Surgery in pediatric patients have not been documented so far.

Open fractures in pediatric patients are usually the result of high-energy trauma and are most commonly classified with the Gustilo-Anderson classification. Despite the fact that there is no specific classification for children, the management principles used in adults generally apply in pediatric patients, although one should always be more conservative in children, particularly when deciding between early amputation or trying to salvage a severely injured limb.

In open fractures of the tibia, the evolution in children tends to be favorable, unlike what happens in adult patients. Several studies have shown that primary fixation with titanium elastic nails, even in type II or IIIA Gustilo-Anderson injuries, is safe and gives results comparable to the use of initial external fixation with deferred osteosynthesis [22, 23]. In open fractures of the femoral shaft or forearm, in which the soft tissue cover is superior to that of the tibia, definitive osteosynthesis with titanium elastic nails can also be used early.

4.11 Final Message

Trauma injuries are the leading cause of death in children and adolescents from the age of 1 year old. In this age group, the most common cause of death is traumatic brain injury, followed by chest trauma. Although skeletal system injuries almost never cause death, they can lead to permanent disability.

Unlike in adults, in children and adolescents the metabolic response to polytrauma begins immediately and is more marked at the tissue level than systemic. This makes it feasible to perform total early treatment in most cases, instead of damage control. In the case of open fractures, likewise, definitive osteosynthesis can be chosen from the beginning, when the state of the soft tissue coverage allows it. These two factors make the evolution and results of orthopedic injuries in polytraumatized children superior to those of adults, with less risk of complications.

References

1. Committee on Pediatric Emergency Medicine, Council on Injury; Violence, and Poison Prevention, Section on Critical Care, Section on Orthopaedics, Section on Surgery, Section on Transport Medicine, Pediatric Trauma Society, and Society of Trauma Nurses Pediatric Committee. Management of pediatric trauma. Pediatrics. 2016;138(2):e20161569. https://doi.org/10.1542/peds.2016-1569.
2. World Health Organization. Children: new threats to health. November 19, 2020. Accessed 29 April 2022. https://www.who.int/news-room/fact-sheets/detail/children-new-threats-to-health
3. Galvagno SM Jr, Nahmias JT, Young DA. Advanced Trauma Life Support® update 2019: management and applications for adults and special populations. Anesthesiol Clin. 2019;37(1):13–32. https://doi.org/10.1016/j.anclin.2018.09.009.
4. Cunningham RM, Walton MA, Carter PM. The major causes of death in children and adolescents in the United States. N Engl J Med. 2018;379(25):2468–75. https://doi.org/10.1056/NEJMsr1804754.
5. Abzug JM, Kozin SH, Zlotolow DA. The pediatric upper extremity. New York, NY: Springer; 2015. https://doi.org/10.1007/978-1-4614-8515-5.
6. Borse N, Sleet DA. CDC childhood injury report. Patterns of unintentional injuries among 0- to 19-year olds in the United States, 2000–2006. 2009;32(2):189. https://doi.org/10.1097/01.fch.0000347986.44810.59.
7. Wegner AA. Damage control resuscitation in pediatric severe trauma. Rev Chil Pediatr. 2018;89(1):118–27. https://doi.org/10.4067/S0370-41062018000100118.
8. Pandya NK, Upasani VV, Kulkarni VA. The pediatric polytrauma patient: current concepts. J Am Acad Orthop Surg. 2013;21(3):170–9. https://doi.org/10.5435/JAAOS-21-03-170.
9. Horst K, Andruszkow H, Weber CD, et al. Surgical treatment strategies in pediatric trauma patients: ETC vs. DCO-an analysis of 316 pediatric trauma patients from the TraumaRegister DGU®. Eur J Trauma Emerg Surg. 2019;45(5):801–8. https://doi.org/10.1007/s00068-019-01092-7.
10. Loubani E, Bartley D, Forward K. Orthopedic injuries in pediatric trauma. Curr Pediatr Rev. 2018;14(1):52–8. https://doi.org/10.2174/1573396313666170911140044.
11. Compton E, Andras LM, Murgai RR, Skaggs DL, Illingworth KD. Isolated femoral shaft fractures in children rarely require a blood transfusion. Injury. 2020;51(3):642–6. https://doi.org/10.1016/j.injury.2020.01.005.
12. Spiguel L, Glynn L, Liu D, Statter M. Pediatric pelvic fractures: a marker for injury severity. Am Surg. 2006;72(6):481–4.
13. Alam Khan T, Jamil Khattak Y, Awais M, et al. Utility of complete trauma series radiographs in alert pediatric patients presenting to Emergency Department of a Tertiary Care Hospital. Eur J Trauma Emerg Surg. 2015;41(3):279–85. https://doi.org/10.1007/s00068-014-0413-8.
14. Frellesen C, Klein D, Tischendorf P, et al. Indication of whole body computed tomography in pediatric polytrauma patients-diagnostic potential of the Glasgow coma scale, the mechanism

of injury and clinical examination. Eur J Radiol. 2018;105:32–40. https://doi.org/10.1016/j.ejrad.2018.05.022.
15. Ludwig J, Heumann P, Gümbel D, et al. Full-body MR imaging: a retrospective study on a novel diagnostic approach for children sustaining high-energy trauma. Eur J Trauma Emerg Surg. 2022;48(3):2165–72. https://doi.org/10.1007/s00068-021-01736-7.
16. Rau CS, Wu SC, Kuo PJ, et al. Polytrauma defined by the new berlin definition: a validation test based on propensity-score matching approach. Int J Environ Res Public Health. 2017;14(9):1045. Published 2017 Sep 11. https://doi.org/10.3390/ijerph14091045.
17. Brown JB, Gestring ML, Leeper CM, et al. The value of the injury severity score in pediatric trauma: time for a new definition of severe injury? J Trauma Acute Care Surg. 2017;82(6):995–1001. https://doi.org/10.1097/TA.0000000000001440.
18. Wendling-Keim DS, Hefele A, Muensterer O, Lehner M. Trauma scores and their prognostic value for the outcome following pediatric polytrauma. Front Pediatr. 2021;9:721585. Published 2021 Sep 3. https://doi.org/10.3389/fped.2021.721585.
19. Figaji AA. Anatomical and physiological differences between children and adults relevant to traumatic brain injury and the implications for clinical assessment and care. Front Neurol. 2017;8:685. Published 2017 Dec 14. https://doi.org/10.3389/fneur.2017.00685.
20. Braun CK, Schaffer A, Weber B, Huber-Lang M, Kalbitz M, Preßmar J. The prognostic value of troponin in pediatric polytrauma. Front Pediatr. 2019;7:477. Published 2019 Nov 20. https://doi.org/10.3389/fped.2019.00477.
21. Naqvi G, Johansson G, Yip G, Rehm A, Carrothers A, Stöhr K. Mechanisms, patterns and outcomes of paediatric polytrauma in a UK major trauma Centre. Ann R Coll Surg Engl. 2017;99(1):39–45. https://doi.org/10.1308/rcsann.2016.0222.
22. Pandya NK. Flexible intramedullary nailing of unstable and/or open tibia shaft fractures in the pediatric population. J Pediatr Orthop. 2016;36(Suppl 1):S19–23. https://doi.org/10.1097/BPO.0000000000000754.
23. Hong P, Rai S, Tang X, Liu R, Li J. External fixation versus elastic stable intramedullary nailing in the treatment of open tibial shaft fractures in children. J Orthop Surg Res. 2021;16(1):528. Published 2021 Aug 25. https://doi.org/10.1186/s13018-021-02679-w.

Chapter 5
Overuse Musculoskeletal Injuries in the Pediatric Patient

Claudia Alday and María Angélica Ibañez

5.1 Overuse Musculoskeletal Injuries in the Pediatric Patient

A child's physical activity is a set of actions, both daily, recreational and formal sports. Recently, the practice of competitive sports has increased in the pediatric population, which, despite its benefits, implies a risk of morbidity associated with specialization and intensive training. Understanding overtraining pathology, its risk factors, and clinical characteristics contributes to an early diagnosis and early treatment of these injuries, avoiding significant sequelae. Additionally, it allows implementing preventive practices to avoid future injuries.

On the other hand, over the past decades, we have witnessed an increase in competitive and recreational sports activities in the pediatric and adolescent population, which, while generating countless physical, psychological, and mental benefits for this age group, brings with it the risk of morbidity associated with sports specialization and intensive athletic training. Terms such as burnout, overtraining, and overuse injuries, conditions that were previously thought to only occur in elite athletes, have become more common [1]. This phenomenon has led to an increase in musculoskeletal system injuries, which have particularities that must be considered when treating and preventing [2].

Musculoskeletal system injuries can occur acutely or subacutely, the former being associated with trauma at a certain moment, where a structure fails due to the mechanical load exerted, while the latter occur progressively when a structure is subjected to repetitive loads without it having enough time to repair the damage [3, 4]. We will call these latter overuse injuries or excessive use injuries.

C. Alday
Hospital Hernán Henríquez Aravena, Universidad de la Frontera, Temuco, Chile

M. A. Ibañez (✉)
Universidad Católica de Chile, Santiago, Chile
e-mail: maibanez@ucchristus.cl

M. Sepúlveda O. (ed.), *Paediatrics Traumatology*,
https://doi.org/10.1007/978-3-031-89482-4_5

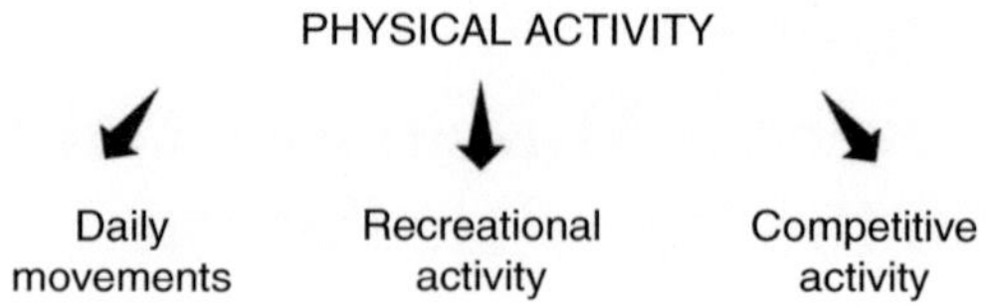

Fig. 5.1 Activities to consider when determining the physical activity performed by the patient

Compared to acute traumatic sports injuries, there is little literature on the epidemiology of overuse injuries in the pediatric population. A possible reason for this is the difficulty for the inexperienced pediatric athlete to identify and recognize overuse injuries, due to their presentation and clinical characteristics. These types of injuries can have an insidious onset, with fluctuating symptoms depending on the current level of activity of the athlete, and may not result in loss of sports activity time, misinterpreting vague symptoms as fatigue or decreased performance. It is also less likely that children will seek care, possibly continuing activities despite pain, due to the chronic nature of these injuries and the increasing pressures from families, coaches, or teammates [5].

This chapter will focus on the possible risk factors for overuse injuries in the immature skeleton. In addition, we will show some of the most common overuse injuries observed in the clinical setting, their diagnosis, treatment, and ways of prevention.

5.2 Introduction

Analyzing a child's physical activity is not simply a matter of adding up the number of hours they dedicate each week to organized sports, but also the amount of recreational activities, both inside and outside of school (Fig. 5.1). We must consider that there is a general decrease these days in such daily activity, which is replaced by sedentary activities, such as working on the computer or playing video games. This leads to a lower level of basic physical fitness in children who start a sport, increasing their risk of injury [2, 6].

5.3 Anatomical Considerations

Among the characteristics of the growing musculoskeletal system, there are special mechanical and functional conditions, which differentiate it from those of the adult (Table 5.1).

Pediatric patients have a higher risk of suffering injuries due to overuse because of their immature skeletal system. The elasticity of soft structures, associated with the relative fragility that cartilaginous and bone structures have, determine that the

Table 5.1 Differences in the developing locomotor system of the pediatric patient and that of the adult patient

Bone	Different areas than in adults: epiphysis, physis, metaphysis, diaphysis, and apophysis
	Greater flexibility
	Secure consolidation
	Capacity for remodeling
	Cartilaginous epiphysis and apophysis
	Cartilaginous osteotendinous union
Others components	More elastic ligaments and tendons
	Muscles of variable mass and elasticity
	Varied body proportions

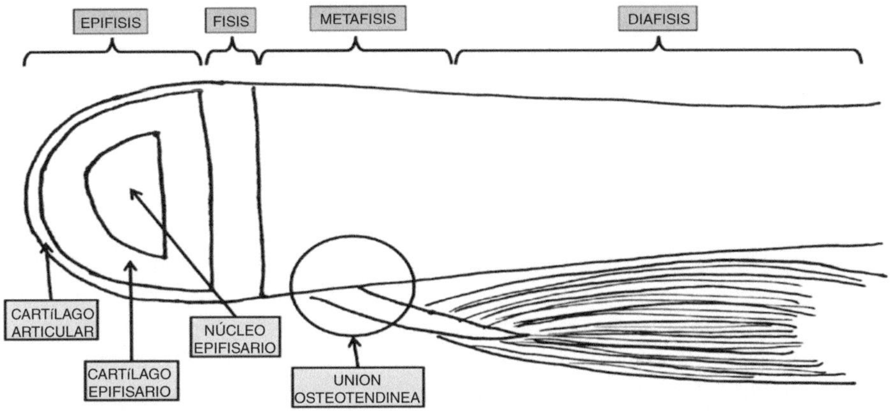

Fig. 5.2 Risk zones for injury in pediatric patients

injury patterns are variable depending on the child's age. Specifically, areas such as the physis-epiphyseal unions, apophyses, or osteotendinous unions are exclusive areas of children and places at risk of injury due to stress (Fig. 5.2).

5.4 Pathophysiology

Overuse injuries are usually related to repetitive physiological stress, sub-maximum, and the load of the musculoskeletal system, without the body having enough time to recover. This results in a tissue adaptation. Although such adaptation can be beneficial, it can also result in a harmful tissue injury when ongoing stress factors are combined with inadequate rest [1].

Generally, repetitive strain injuries occur at the junction points, where multidirectional mechanical forces are transmitted to tissues of different consistencies and tensile resistances. The injury patterns depend on the specific mechanism

Table 5.2 Risk factors for musculoskeletal injuries due to overuse

Extrinsic factors	Early specialization
	Incorrect training technique
	High training volume and intensity
	Year-round sports participation
	Repetitive motion sport
	Inadequate equipment
	Pressure from parents and coaches
Intrinsic factors	Skeletal immaturity
	Accelerated growth
	Anatomical factors
	Level of cognitive development
	Flexibility
	Age
	Sex
	Body mass index (BMI)
	Previous injuries

associated with the sport performed, as well as the maturity of the skeleton. In the young athlete, the weakest part of the musculoskeletal system is the junction of the growth plate cartilage with the adjacent ossified bone tissue, at the base of the epiphyses and apophyses. With maturity, the sites of tendinous insertion become the weakest structure. The most common stress injuries in pediatric age are stress fractures, traction apophysitis, and repetitive physeal injuries [7].

Although there is a lack of research regarding specific injuries or treatments for pathology caused by overuse in children, recent literature has tended to identify risk factors (Table 5.2), both intrinsic and extrinsic [1, 8, 9].

5.5 Classification

The most commonly used term to define these injuries is "osteochondrosis," which corresponds to an alteration of endochondral ossification, including osteogenesis and chondrogenesis, in subjects without initial growth disorder. Osteochondrosis can be epiphyseal, physeal, or apophyseal, depending on the affected site. While there is no consensus on the etiology of osteochondrosis, multiple vascular, traumatic, or combined factors seem to be involved (Fig. 5.3) [2].

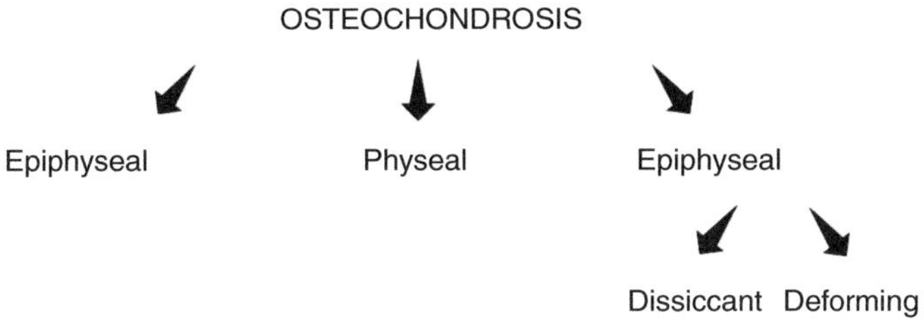

Fig. 5.3 Described types of osteochondrosis

Fig. 5.4 Evolutionary stages of a musculoskeletal injury due to overuse

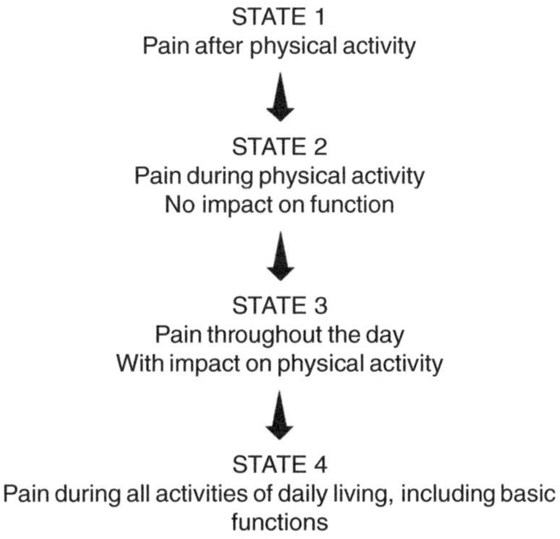

5.6 Treatment

When evaluating a pediatric athlete, a complete medical history and physical examination are essential [1].

In the medical history, mechanical pain is the main sign of overuse injuries. It significantly limits or prevents participation in sport or daily activities [2, 8]. Regarding pain, it is important to find the precise location, determine when it was first noticed in the affected area, when it began to affect performance, the intensity of the symptom and the actions that trigger it. Pain allows injuries to be divided into four stages according to their evolution (Fig. 5.4).

In addition, it is important to obtain information about present risk factors:

- Sports in which the patient participates and the degree of commitment in them (schedules, number of clubs or leagues).
- Training errors.
- Recent introduction of some new technique or training method.
- Rest days from activity each week.
- Time off from activity during the last 6–12 months.

- Type of equipment being used and when it was last replaced.
- Previous injuries and how they were treated (or not).
- Determination of pubertal, menstrual, and growth curve status.
- Child's motivation.
- Parents' expectations.
- Existence of any nutritional or sleep disorder.

The physical examination should try to locate the injured tissue as accurately as possible, always recommending to compare both limbs. Carefully palpating the painful area is essential. Alignment, flexibility, joint laxity, and muscle tone should be evaluated. Observe the patient to detect muscle and/or tendon stiffness. It should be considered that hyperlaxity can also be a source of pain. The physical examination should address the joints above and below the area in question, as referred pain can be part of the underlying clinical picture. Evaluation of dynamic and static stabilizers and anatomical reference points within the area. A neuromuscular examination is also pertinent, which includes perfusion, sensation, and motor function of the affected area.

Many overuse injuries can be diagnosed and initially treated without the need for diagnosis with complementary exams, but these should be requested in the case of unilateral commitment or unusual pain, such as nocturnal or inflammatory pain and those injuries that do not respond to initial treatment.

Radiographic studies can be considered to support or refute the history and components of the physical examination. Comparative views of the contralateral side can be useful when anatomical variants are unclear, either as the origin of the pathology or as a normal variant in maturation. In these cases, it is important to carefully evaluate the need for additional images, including ultrasound, bone scintigraphy, magnetic resonance imaging (MRI), or computed tomography (CT), for cases that require very specific data for diagnosis and treatment.

5.7 Most Frequent Overuse Injuries

5.7.1 Upper Limb Injuries

Overuse injuries of the upper limbs are less frequent than those of the lower limbs. The overhead athlete, such as the swimmer, the baseball pitcher, the tennis player, as well as athletes who bear a lot of weight on the upper limbs, such as gymnasts, may seek medical attention for these types of injuries.

With weight-bearing activities of the upper limbs, the distribution of forces through the wrist can equate to almost double the body weight. These compression and shear forces are transferred through the distal physis and can exceed the limit of what the growing body is capable of withstanding, especially in the context of inadequate rest. This can lead to alterations in the physis structure (Fig. 5.5).

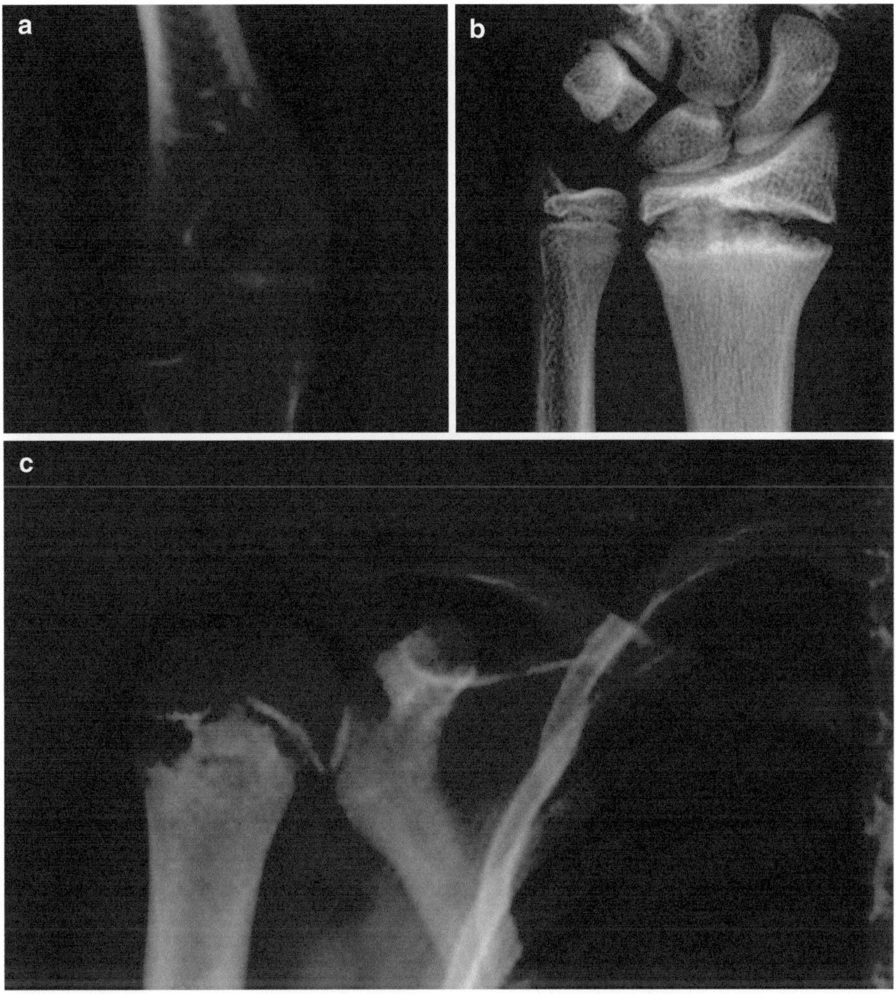

Fig. 5.5 Radiographs of upper extremity overuse injuries, with characteristic findings. (**a**) Little League elbow; (**b**) Gymnast's wrist; (**c**) Little League shoulder

Table 5.3 summarizes the most frequent overuse injuries of the upper limb and their affected segment.

5.7.2 Lower Limb Injuries

Young athletes are vulnerable to apophysitis of the lower limbs during times of rapid growth and development. The three areas of the lower limb most frequently affected are the calcaneus (Sever), the tibial tubercle (Osgood Schlatter) (Fig. 5.6),

Table 5.3 Most common upper extremity overuse injuries

Injury	Sport	Location	Mechanism	Findings	Imaging	Treatment
Minor league shoulder	Baseball, tennis, volleyball, swimming	Proximal physis of humerus	Rotational torque when throwing	Pain and fatigue when throwing.	Normal or physeal widening. MRI with physeal closure.	Rest for 6 weeks. Gradual return. Risk correction.
Minor league elbow	Baseball	Medial epicondyle of humerus	Valgus tension	Pain with flexion and instability in valgus	Normal or widening of apophysis medial epicondyle	Rest 4–6 weeks. Physiotherapy, correct risk factor.
Osteochondrosis Capitelum Dissecans	Basketball, baseball, gymnastics	Lateral capitellum	Microtraumatic vascular insufficiency due to valgus	Pain and limitation of mobility, with joint blockage	MRI with fragmentary lesion and chondral damage of capitellum	Stable, rest. Unstable, surgical treatment.
Gymnast's wrist	Gymnastics	Distal physis of radius	Weight bearing with EE.SS.	Epicritic pain in physis.	Physeal widening	Rest, muscle strengthening, physiotherapy

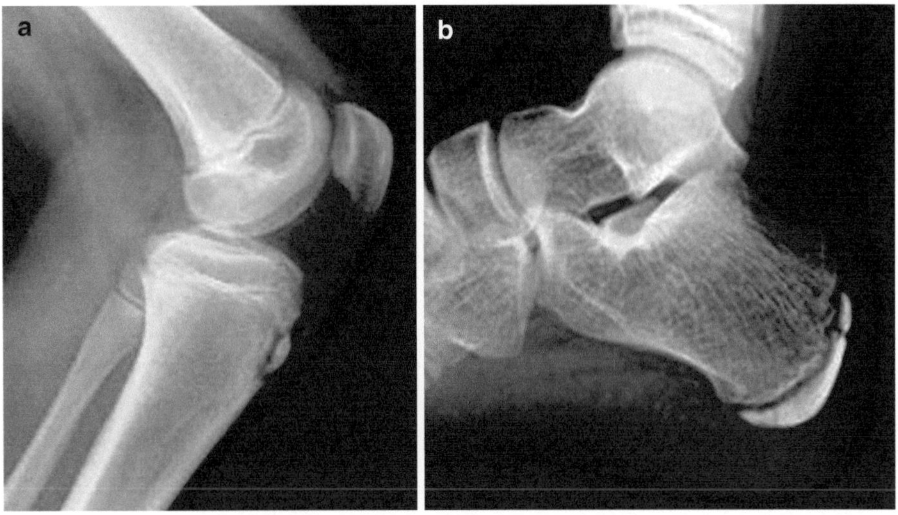

Fig. 5.6 Radiographs of lower extremity overuse injuries, with characteristic findings. (**a**) Osgood Schlater; (**b**) Sever's disease

and the inferior pole of the patella (Sinding Larsen). In general, they are self-limiting in nature and present clinically with fluctuations in symptomatology. A description of each of these areas is described in more detail in Table 5.4.

5.7.3 Pelvic Injuries

The pelvis of a young athlete presents multiple open apophyses that are prone to injuries, both acute and from overuse. The tendon, muscle, and ossified bone are much more resistant than the partially cartilaginous apophysis, in dynamic development.

There are seven large muscle insertion sites in the pelvis, and these are generally the most common areas of involvement, both for tendinitis and for apophysitis. This is related to skeletal age and the state of ossification of the patient. Having knowledge of the anatomy of the area helps to complete an appropriate examination (Table 5.5).

Once an apophyseal pelvic injury is diagnosed, rest, the removal of repetitive forces through the injured area, and occasionally, a period of weight unloading, are necessary for healing. Without proper care and rest, these apophyseal areas can widen, and even progress to acute and sudden avulsion injuries.

Table 5.4 Most frequent injuries due to overuse of the lower extremity

Injury	Sport	Location	Mechanism	Findings	Imaging	Treatment
Calcaneal apophysitis (sever)	Athletics, gymnastics	Calcaneal process, insertion of Achilles	Traction of Achilles and impact on heel	Thalagia, 8–10 years	Normal or fragmentation of second nucleus of calcaneus	Relative rest, soft heel pad, stretching
ATT apophysitis (Osgood Schlatter)	Football, soccer, basketball, volleyball,	Insertion of patellar tendon in ATT	Microtrauma due to traction	Pain in ATT, increase in volumen	Normal or fragmentation of TAT. Calcification patellar tendon.	Rest and muscle strengthening. Local cold and NSAIDs.
Lower pole apophysitis of patella (Sinding Larsen Johanson)	Running	Lower pole of patella	Repetitive traction patellar tendón	Pain in the lower pole of the patella and inflammation	Fragmentation of the lower pole of the patella	Rest and muscle strengthening. Local cold and NSAIDs.
Base apophysitis fifth metatarsal (iselin)	Running, jumping	Insertion of the short peroneal tendon	Traction of the short peroneal at the base of the fifth metatarsal	Pain and increase in volume at the base of the fifth metatarsal	Sclerosis and fragmentation parallel to the physis of the fifth metatarsal	Rest, NSAIDs. Removable boot for 4 weeks.

Table 5.5 Processes around the pelvis and associated musculature

Iliac crest	Origin of tensor fascia lata, insertion of internal and external oblique muscles, and transverse abdominis muscle
Anterior upper iliac spine	Insertion of sartorius muscle
Anterior lower iliac spine	Origin of rectus femoris muscle
Ischiatic tuberosity	Origin of hamstrings
Pubis	Origin of adductors and gracilis muscle
Greater trochanter	Insertion of gluteus maximus and medius muscle, piriformis, and hip rotators
Less trochanter	Insertion of iliopsoas muscle

5.7.4 *Spine Injuries*

Back pain in athletes is a warning sign, especially in those who perform repetitive hyperextension of the spine. Of the adolescent athletes seeking attention for their lower back pain, about 50% of them will have spondylolysis. The incidence of spondylolysis in adolescents is in the range of 8–15%. Athletes at high risk of such injuries include gymnasts, divers, wrestlers, weightlifters, throwing athletes, and even rowers [1, 5].

Spondylolysis is a fracture of the pars interarticularis of the vertebral arch and can be unilateral or bilateral. The pars portion of the bone is the weakest point of the neural arch, and with repetitive stress and mechanical load through hyperextension maneuvers, the bone elements fatigue similarly to the mechanism of a stress fracture. With bilateral pars fractures, there is the possibility of an anterior slippage of the vertebrae resulting in spondylolisthesis.

The examination is characterized by focal lower back pain and to the extension of the lumbar spine. Initial radiographs may be negative, which does not rule out spondylolysis, and advanced imaging, such as CT, MRI, or bone scintigraphy, may be necessary.

Treatment consists of cessation of activities for a few weeks, to move on to a later period of physiotherapy, aimed at muscle strengthening. The use of orthopedic devices is controversial.

5.7.5 *Stress Fractures*

Stress fractures occur from repetitive loads on a bone that does not manage to repair itself in the time between trainings. They are relatively infrequent in children, so they can represent a challenge in diagnosis. Their frequency is higher as the child approaches skeletal maturity.

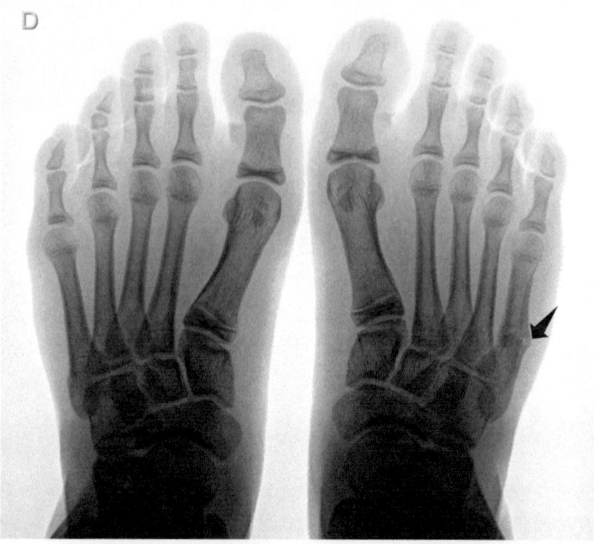

Fig. 5.7 Stress fracture of the left fifth metatarsal (Arrow)

The most frequent location is in the lower limbs. It is common in the proximal tibia and in the metatarsals in runner patients (Fig. 5.7). In athletes who use the upper limbs, these and the lumbar spine can be compromised.

It manifests as long-standing pain, generally in relation to physical activity. It should be studied with radiographs, which will show a periosteal reaction if it is an advanced process, which can be complemented with bone scintigraphy and magnetic resonance imaging.

The treatment consists in rest from sports from the activity that caused the injury, being tolerable only activities without impact.

5.8 Treatment Options

It is important that we understand the basal problem to better comprehend why these injuries occur. Curative treatment should not mean suspending all sports activities until the child stops growing, but should be adapted case by case. Preventive treatment should continue because the main goal is that the children can resume their favorite physical activities, as quickly and completely as possible [8].

If the injury is considered from overuse, either from an inadequate rest and/or due to modifiable risk factors, testing a conservative management with rest and activity modification is almost always the first-line therapy. The removal of stress from the growth plate and/or growing apophysis often allows for adequate healing. Once pain levels improve, physiotherapy can be initiated and factors such as flexibility and balance can be improved.

5.9 Prevention

Most injuries in children occur in unstructured activities, so they cannot be modified by institutional sports prevention policies, but they can be addressed through good education to the population [10].

However, despite the scarce information for pediatric sports practice, there are recommendations aimed at the athlete, in order to decrease the risk of overuse injuries [8–12]:

- Weekly rest, 1–2 days.
- 2–3 months of rest per year from specific sports training, to transition to a more free recreational game [13].
- Specialization in a sport should be delayed until late puberty [14–16].
- The use of protective elements for contact sports or with risk of falls is recommended. These are helmet, dental protectors, wristbands, shin guards, gloves, as appropriate to the sport. Such protections must be of the right size and quality.
- Specific equipment, of the best possible quality, of the right size and meet the technical characteristics of that particular sport.
- Programs for the prevention of specific injuries [15, 16]. In children, these programs have more difficulties to be implemented, but it is recommended in each sport to look for those that have been shown to lower the incidence of injuries [16–20].
- Healthy lifestyle habits: sleep, adequate rest, healthy eating, and no use of alcohol and drugs [16].

Finally, it is expected that scientific guidelines will be developed that generate specific prevention policies for children and adolescents in sport, as there are for brain concussions, which are very developed [17].

5.10 Final Message

Overuse injuries in children are common, especially in athletes during rapid growth period. The increasingly competitive nature of youth sports, early specialization, and year-round participation, with inadequate rest periods, seem to contribute to the increase in the prevalence of this type of injury in the pediatric population.

The management of these pathologies is not only medical; it must also involve the patient, the family and the coach, making them aware of these risk factors, which is fundamental to help prevent these injuries.

Early diagnosis, and appropriate treatment, help the athlete return to play in a timely manner and avoid long-term sequelae.

5.11 Authors' Recommendations

- Pain in children during sport should not be considered normal, but may be a warning sign.
- Accurate diagnosis is made by knowing the technical gestures of the sport performed, in addition to a directed anamnesis and exhaustive physical examination.
- The suspicion of an overuse injury may require a modification or decrease in activity, a review of technical elements or training methods.
- It is very important to identify and control the anxiety of parents, teachers, and the patient during the process.
- The support of the health team is essential for the child to be able to return to their normal activities.

References

1. Magrini D, Dahab KS. Musculoskeletal overuse injuries in the pediatric population. Curr Sports Med Rep. 2016;15(6):392–9. https://doi.org/10.1249/JSR.0000000000000303.
2. Launay F. Sports-related overuse injuries in children. Orthop Traumatol Surg Res. 2015;101 (1 Suppl):S139–47. https://doi.org/10.1016/j.otsr.2014.06.030.
3. Hyman M. The most expensive game in town. The rising cost of youth sports and the toll on today's families. Boston, MA: Beacon Press; 2012.
4. Luke A, Lazaro RM, Bergeron MF, et al. Sports-related injuries in youth athletes: is overscheduling a risk factor? Clin J Sport Med. 2011;21(4):307–14. https://doi.org/10.1097/JSM.0b013e3182218f71.
5. Wu M, Fallon R, Heyworth BE. Overuse injuries in the pediatric population. Sports Med Arthrosc Rev. 2016;24(4):150–8. https://doi.org/10.1097/JSA.0000000000000129.
6. Valovich McLeod TC, Decoster LC, Loud KJ, et al. National Athletic Trainers' Association position statement: prevention of pediatric overuse injuries. J Athl Train. 2011;46(2):206–20. https://doi.org/10.4085/1062-6050-46.2.206.
7. Bedoya MA, Jaramillo D, Chauvin NA. Overuse injuries in children. Top Magn Reson Imaging. 2015;24(2):67–81. https://doi.org/10.1097/RMR.0000000000000048.
8. DiFiori JP. Evaluation of overuse injuries in children and adolescents. Curr Sports Med Rep. 2010;9(6):372–8. https://doi.org/10.1249/JSR.0b013e3181fdba58.
9. DiFiori JP, Benjamin HJ, Brenner JS, et al. Overuse injuries and burnout in youth sports: a position statement from the American Medical Society for Sports Medicine. Br J Sports Med. 2014;48(4):287–8. https://doi.org/10.1136/bjsports-2013-093299.
10. Nauta J, Martin-Diener E, Martin BW, van Mechelen W, Verhagen E. Injury risk during different physical activity behaviours in children: a systematic review with bias assessment. Sports Med. 2015;45(3):327–36. https://doi.org/10.1007/s40279-014-0289-0.
11. Ridenour R, Hennrikus W. Overuse injuries in pediatric athletes. Adv Pediatr. 2020;67:171–82. https://doi.org/10.1016/j.yapd.2020.04.001.
12. Trentacosta N. Pediatric sports injuries. Pediatr Clin N Am. 2020;67(1):205–25. https://doi.org/10.1016/j.pcl.2019.09.013.
13. Sporting Goods Manufacturers Association Research/Sports Marketing Surveys USA. U.S. trends in team sports report. Jupiter, FL, 2011. Updated May 2011.
14. van Reijen M, Vriend I, van Mechelen W, Finch CF, Verhagen EA. Compliance with sport injury prevention interventions in randomised controlled trials: a systematic review. Sports Med. 2016;46(8):1125–39. https://doi.org/10.1007/s40279-016-0470-8.

15. Carder SL, Giusti NE, Vopat LM, et al. The concept of sport sampling versus sport specialization: preventing youth athlete injury: a systematic review and meta-analysis. Am J Sports Med. 2020;48(11):2850–7. https://doi.org/10.1177/0363546519899380.
16. Gao B, Dwivedi S, Milewski MD, Cruz AI Jr. Lack of sleep and sports injuries in adolescents: a systematic review and meta-analysis. J Pediatr Orthop. 2019;39(5):e324–33. https://doi.org/10.1097/BPO.0000000000001306.
17. Göpfert A, Van Hove M, Emond A, Mytton J. Prevención de lesiones deportivas en niños en la escuela: una revisión sistemática de las políticas. BMJ Open Sport Exerc Med. 2018;4(1):e000346. Publicado el 4 de junio de 2018. https://doi.org/10.1136/bmjsem-2018-000346.
18. Mugele H, Plummer A, Steffen K, Stoll J, Mayer F, Müller J. Programas de prevención de lesiones generales versus específicos para deportes en atletas: Una revisión sistemática sobre el efecto en las tasas de lesiones. PLoS One. 2018;13(10):e0205635. Publicado el 19 de octubre de 2018. https://doi.org/10.1371/journal.pone.0205635.
19. Falk B, Dotan R. Harefuah. 2019;158(8):515–9.
20. Brown T, Moran M. Lesiones relacionadas con el deporte pediátrico. Clin Pediatr (Phila). 2019;58(2):199–212. https://doi.org/10.1177/0009922818810879.

Chapter 6
Principles of Conservative Treatment in the Pediatric Patient

Erika Arana and Monica Foppiano

6.1 Principles of Conservative Treatment in the Pediatric Patient

Musculoskeletal trauma in children is a common pathology. One in four injuries secondary to trauma will be accompanied by a fracture. The increasing participation of minors in sports activities and the rise in obesity in the child population have led to an upward trend in traumatic injuries. In addition, in recent years there have been a greater number of high-energy injuries due to car accidents [1].

The particular characteristics of the immature skeleton, the wide variability of the age range, and the presence of growth cartilages make the management of these injuries a challenge. The goal should be to achieve an optimal result, with the least amount of necessary actions, and to avoid iatrogenic actions that generate progresive sequelae. To achieve this, in most cases, conservative treatment will be the choice, guiding the reparative response in children and adolescents. However, there are complex cases, such as open fractures, with associated neurovascular injuries, polytrauma, or lesions in pathological bone, which will require more aggressive treatment and usually surgical procedures [1].

E. Arana
Hospital Civil de Guadalajara, Fray Antonio Alcalde, Guadalajara, Jalisco, Mexico

M. Foppiano (✉)
Hospital Hernán Henríquez Aravena, Universidad de la Frontera, Temuco, Chile

M. Sepúlveda O. (ed.), *Paediatrics Traumatology*,
https://doi.org/10.1007/978-3-031-89482-4_6

6.1.1 Characteristics of Pediatric Bone Tissue

A child is not a small-sized adult. There are several characteristics of their skeletal tissue that differentiate them. The bone has a higher amount of water, cortical porosity, and a higher percentage of cartilaginous component, which allows a great capacity to absorb the energy of trauma, so we observe special, incomplete fractures, which are only seen in children. In addition, there is greater elasticity of the joints, with a low incidence of sprains [2].

On the other hand, the presence of the physis, or growth plate, which allows the longitudinal growth of the bone, can manifest with specific fractures of childhood. Although it allows a large amount of bone remodeling after a fracture, if damage to this structure occurs, with sufficient remaining growth, there is the possibility of significant sequelae, such as alteration of axes or limb length discrepancy. Also, this structure, together with the presence of the ossification centers that appear during growth, can make radiographic interpretation difficult for personnel not accustomed to managing pediatric patients [1].

It should be noted that the force of a trauma in a child impacts on a smaller body surface, with less fatty and elastic connective tissue, being able to penetrate and impact internal organs, which in polytraumatized patients can be lethal, even without the appearance of bone lesions. We must also consider that in children, blood loss and body heat loss are proportionally greater [2].

Finally, the pediatric periosteum is a more vascularized, thick and resistant tissue than that of the adult. It helps to provide stability, reducing the complexity and displacement of the fracture fragments. Along with the fracture hematoma, it contributes to the rapid formation of a bone callus, promoting that the fracture heals faster than in adults. Once bone healing is achieved, the growing bone can remodel some of the residual angular deformities, possibly even remaining without signs of having had an injury [3]. The younger the patient, the greater the potential for remodeling. An adolescent who is close to skeletal maturity will have less remodeling capacity due to limited remaining growth [2].

Due to these characteristics, we can say that most of the fractures in the pediatric patient can be treated non-surgically, by maintaining alignment and protecting the injury with the use of immobilization or a well-molded cast, having few chances of joint stiffness, delay in consolidation and non-union.

6.1.2 Bone Repair Process

Bone repair is divided into three phases. These are: inflammatory phase, reparative phase, and remodeling phase [4].

The inflammatory phase occurs acutely, after the loss of integrity of the bone structures, with the formation of the fracture hematoma. This hematoma contains fibrin, which is replaced by a collagen structure, which serves as a matrix for bone tissue. In addition, proteins are produced and signal cascades are generated that stimulate cell differentiation for the formation of new bone. In the reparative phase, the initial bone callus is produced, with the formation of endochondral (endosteal) and intramembranous (periosteal) bone. This occurs in the first 2–3 months of the reparative process, providing the initial stabilization. Finally, the remodeling phase occurs, which can last months or years, where the provisional callus is replaced by new bone, in a more structured form, that can withstand normal physical activity (Fig. 6.1) [5].

In children, bone remodeling can restore the alignment of fractures that initially consolidated with small malunion, allowing that, in many cases, anatomical reduction is less essential than in adults. This remodeling also depends on muscle action, joint reaction forces, and physiological body weight load. Remodeling, in most cases, can correct translation, angulation, and shortening; however, it is important to consider that rotational remodeling is almost nonexistent [5].

The most important factors that determine the potential for remodeling are: (a) skeletal age, which is proportional to the potential for remaining growth, greater in children under 8 years; (b) the proximity of the fracture to the physis; (c) the specific growth potential of the nearby physis, with greater remodeling around the knee, in the proximal humerus or in the distal forearm; (d) the orientation of the deformity, given that in the plane of movement the joint axis, remodeling will be greater; (e) the degree of deformity to be remodeled; and (f) the affected segment, with better remodeling described in the lower limb, apparently due to being subject to greater mechanical load. The thick and active periosteum in children also contributes to remodeling due to the presence of osteoclasts and appositional growth that shapes the bone callus [5].

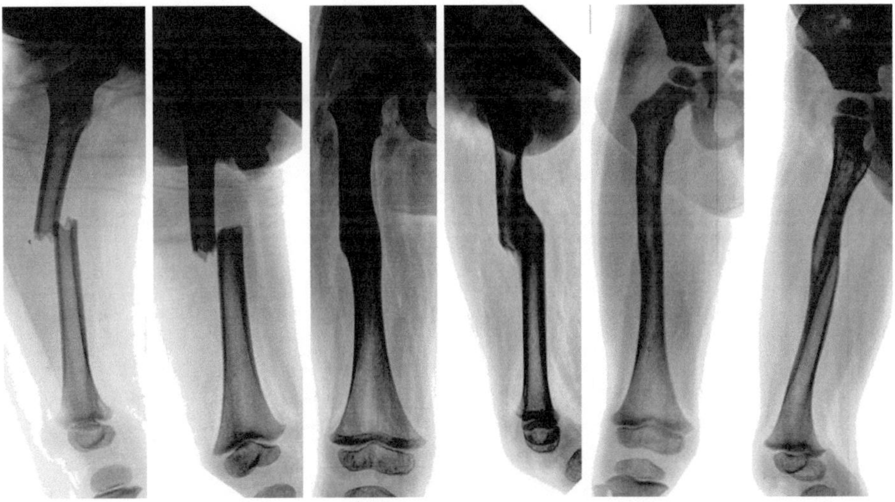

Fig. 6.1 Bone repair process in a femur fracture in a 2-year-old child treated conservatively

Bone remodeling will be different according to the location of the fracture in the bone segment. The metaphysis is an area of active remodeling, adjacent to the physis, due to its great vascularization and osteogenic potential, it facilitates fracture repair . On the other hand, the diaphysis is an area with latent osteogenesis, where the production of bone tissue is a balance between subperiosteal intramembranous ossification, on the surface, and endosteal bone resorption, in the medullary canal. In addition, in the diaphysis, the bone is rigid and compact (cortical bone), relatively avascular. For these reasons, there is less potential for remodeling in this area, so fractures can take longer to heal and remodel [4]. In the diaphysis, remodeling is guided by Wolf's law, which describes that the stimulation of bone formation is produced on the concave side of the angulation, by compression forces, while on the convex side, under tension, bone resorption occurs. Approximately 20% of the remodeling potential of a fracture would occur in this area (Fig. 6.2) [6].

Longitudinal growth, provided by the physis, is responsible for approximately 75% of the remodeling of a posttraumatic angular deformity. This is through asymmetric growth of it, until achieving perpendicularity with the axial axis of the bone, following the law of Hueter-Volkmann. After this, the symmetric growth of the growth cartilage is restarted (Fig. 6.3) [5].

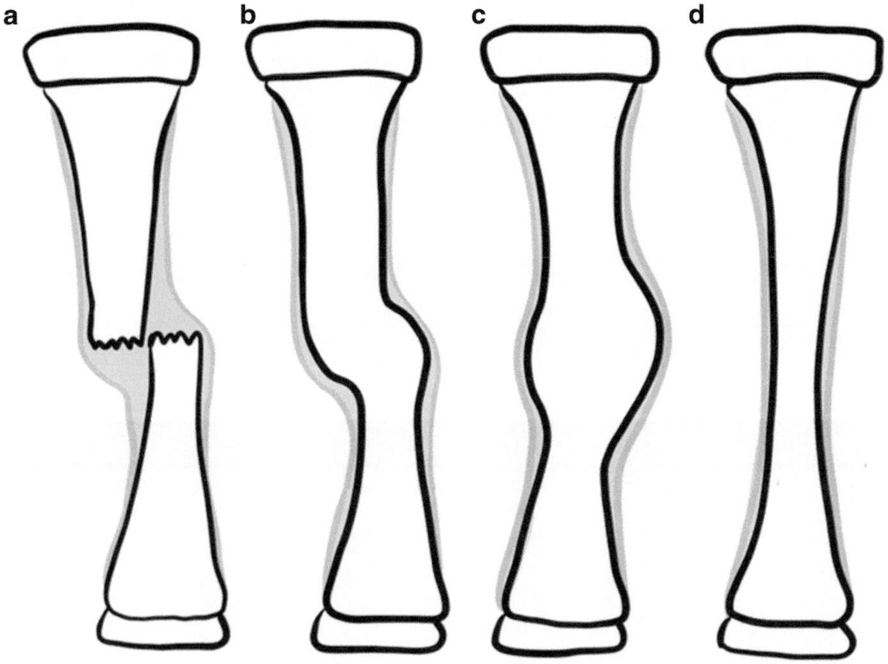

Fig. 6.2 Diagram of the diaphyseal remodeling process of long bones. (**a**) fracture with subperiosteal hematoma; (**b**) initial bone callus; (**c**) prominent bone callus on the concave side; (**d**) recovery of normal anatomy

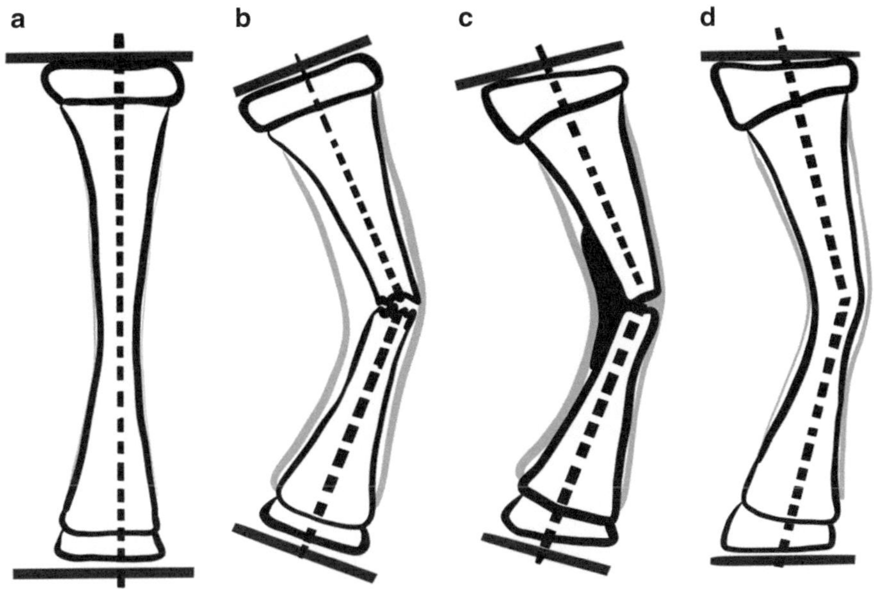

Fig. 6.3 Diagram of the contribution of the physis to the remodeling process of long bones. (**a**) normal axis; (**b**) loss of axis due to fracture; (**c**) asymmetric physeal growth, greater on the concave side, seeking to correct the axis; (**d**) corrected articular axis, and subsequent symmetric growth

"Overgrowth" of a bone segment can also occur during the healing process of a fracture. This situation mainly occurs in the diaphysis of the femur, with an average of 9.2 mm (6.9–11 mm), and in the tibia of 5.7 mm, (4–6 mm) [4]. This greater growth could be due to an increase in blood flow in areas adjacent to growth areas, which can last up to 3 years after injury.

6.1.3 Diagnosis

The diagnosis of a fracture requires a complete anamnesis of the traumatic incident, considering the type of accident, mechanism, and previous treatment received. Physical examination must be complete, looking for increased volume, pain, functional alterations, deformation of the segment, bruising, loss of axes, abnormal mobility, and bone crepitus. The concordance of the event with the injuries found is important. If not, or in non-ambulatory small children, non-accidental injury must be ruled out [7].

A simple radiograph is the first pillar of diagnostic support, being in most cases sufficient to guide the treatment. At least two projections of the area should be obtained and include adjacent joints (Fig. 6.4).

On some occasions, it will be useful to obtain oblique or contralateral projections, and indirect signs of fracture should always be sought (Fig. 6.5).

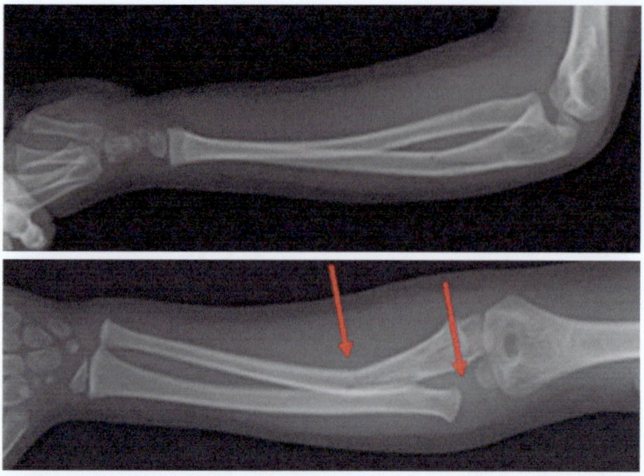

Fig. 6.4 Forearm fracture associated with proximal radius dislocation (Monteggia fracture-dislocation), revealing the importance of including adjacent joints in the radiological study

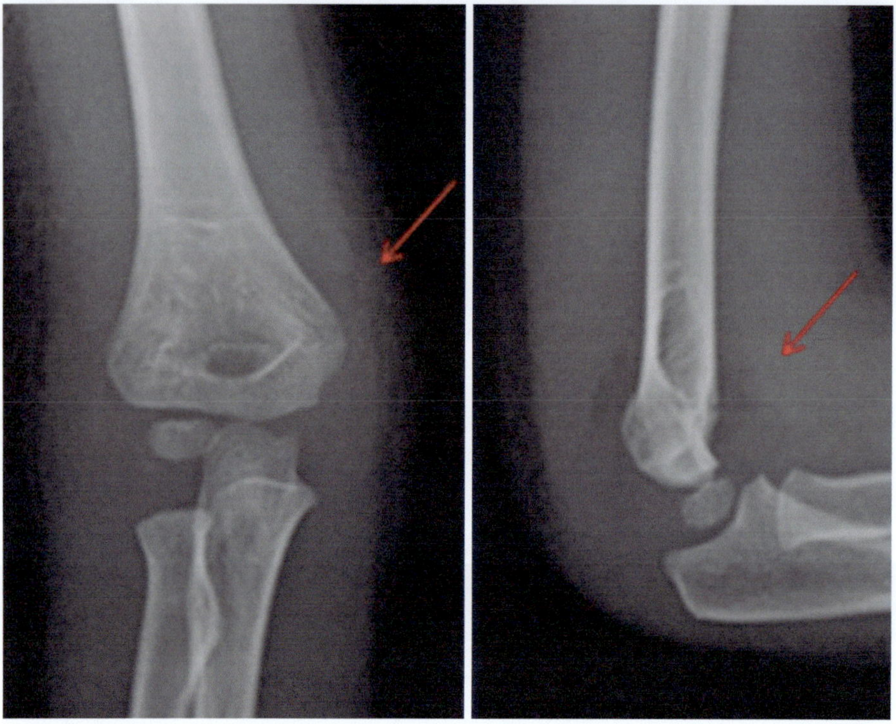

Fig. 6.5 Supracondylar fracture of the distal humerus, showing the anterior fat pad sign (arrow) that guides the diagnosis

Ultrasound is a complementary examination that has the advantage of being non-expensive and very useful in cartilaginous injuries not visible on radiographs. Its main disadvantage is that it requires an operator experienced in pediatric bone pathology [7].

In more complex cases, the use of ct scan (CT) is useful. This examination is quick to perform and provides excellent visualization of bone lesions. In addition, it allows a three-dimensional analysis, very useful when deciding the treatment of some injuries. It has the disadvantage of higher associated radiation. Magnetic resonance imaging (MRI), although it does not irradiate, is more expensive, not always accessible, and requires sedation or anesthesia in small children due to its duration [7].

6.1.4 Indications for Conservative Treatment

For the treatment of fractures in children, it is essential to understand the general principles of bone remodeling, but it is also important to know the variations and limits of acceptance of residual angulation for fractures in different bones and at certain ages. This will help us make appropriate decisions for the treatment of fractures in children [6].

Clavicle fractures are the most common of the long bone fractures in pediatric patients. They are frequently seen in the emergency departments of hospitals, and comprise up to 10–15% of all pediatric fractures. They allow a wide margin of deformity, and for this reason, in most cases, the ideal treatment is non-surgical. However, there are some parameters, which, when combined, it is preferable to choose surgical treatment to avoid complications. Among these parameters are the degree of displacement (lack of contact between the fragments), male patient, and being a teenager (between 13 and 15 years of age) [8]. For the femur, tibia, proximal and diaphyseal humerus, and the radius diaphysis, we can guide ourselves, according to the age and deviation in the sagittal and coronal planes [5] (Table 6.1). Greater deformity ranges will not be fully corrected by the remodeling process.

According to this, most fractures in children can be successfully treated with non-surgical methods. However, it has limitations for its use in children with multiple traumas, open fractures, fractures in pathological bone, associated vascular injuries, those with a history of initial non-surgical treatment failure and in fractures where there will be poor results, such as femoral neck fractures, some physeal fractures, displaced supracondylar fractures of the distal humerus, fractures of the femur, tibia and forearm diaphysis in older children or adolescents, and in unstable fractures of the pelvis and acetabulum [1].

Table 6.1 Tolerable residual deformity ranges by segment for conservative treatment of fractures in pediatric patients

Proximal humerus		
Age	Displacement	
<5 years	<70° angulation/complete displacement	
5–12 years	40°–70° angulation	
>12 years	<40° angulation/50% apposition	
Humeral shaft		
Displacement	Angulation	
Varus	20–30°	
Anterior apex	20°	
Radius shaft		
Age	Angulation	Rotation
<9 years	15°	45°
>9 years	10°	30°
Femur shaft		
Age	Varus/valgus	Sagital
<2 years	30°	30°
2–5 years	15°	20°
6–10 years	10°	15°
>10 years	5°	10°
Tibia shaft		
Deformity	<8 years	>8 years
Varus	10°	5°
Valgus	5°	5°
<Posterior	5°	0°
<Anterior	10°	5°
Rotation	5°	5°
Shortening	10 mm	5 mm

6.1.5 *Options for Conservative Treatment*

It is necessary to remember that to perform a non-surgical treatment of a fracture in a pediatric patient, we must consider the three basic principles of it: fracture reduction, immobilization to maintain the proper position (retention), and finally recover the function of the affected segment [9].

The fracture reduction must be adequate, considering the limits of the remodeling of the bone to treat [10]. If it is necessary to perform maneuvers to achieve this, in most cases they are carried out by the reverse mechanism that produced the fracture.

Immobilization should always neutralize muscular forces to avoid displacements, so its optimum installation is fundamental. The application of a cast should aim to prevent the loss of reduction. To achive this, it must be properly molded, imitating the shape of the limb and not excessive padding. However, at the initial moment of the injury, and according to the mechanism of injury, the use of splints or bivalve circular casts is recommended, in order to avoid an increase in the intra-compartmental pressure secondary to the edema that will occur.

Special care must be taken to protect bone prominences and the edges of the cast to avoid wounds from rubbing, pressure areas, and even ulcers. It is essential to instruct patients and their caregivers of the cares of the cast and alarm signs [11] (ulcers on the edges of the cast, presence of purulent material, broken cast, excessive pain or increased analgesia requirements, excessive bad smell, change in coloration, or delay in capillary filling).

If the fracture is not displaced or has an acceptable deformity, the purpose of the cast is to maintain that alignment while achieving bone healing. If the fracture has an unacceptable alignment, it must be reduced to achieve suitable alignment in all planes [12], to accomplish this it will be essential to analyze the fracture to know how the forces that caused it acted. Once we determine the mechanism, we can perform the manipulation maneuvers, resembling the forces that caused it, but in reverse. We must also take into account how muscular forces act, which can displace the reduction of the bone in treatment, to neutralize them. To perform a closed reduction, it is essential that the patient is sedated or anesthetized to avoid pain and facilitate maneuvers through muscle relaxation [13]. Depending on the special characteristics that each patient may have, regional blocks can be performed, or even hematoma infiltration, to be able to manipulate the fracture without pain.

In general, cast is the most used material to maintain the reduction of a fracture. The best material to use in the immobilization should be moldable, with the ability to maintain the desired shape (Moldability). Currently, there are different types of materials, more sophisticated, lighter, and easier to remove. In a study conducted by Aronsson [14], where they compared three types of materials to assess their molding capacity (plaster of Paris, fiberglass, and semi-flexible bandage), the "plaster of Paris" turned out to be more moldable than fiberglass and the semi-flexible bandage, therefore, in those cases where we require precision to mold and maintain the reduction, it is the preferred material. In cases where precision in molding is not required, fiberglass and semi-flexible fibers are the choice, for being lighter, water-resistant, and having a wide range of colors, which can be more friendly for pediatric patients [14].

In those cases susceptible to non-surgical management and in which a closed reduction is not achieved, we can perform maneuvers aided with the use of a percutaneous Kirschner wires [15], which is then removed, followed by the usual immobilization (Fig. 6.6).

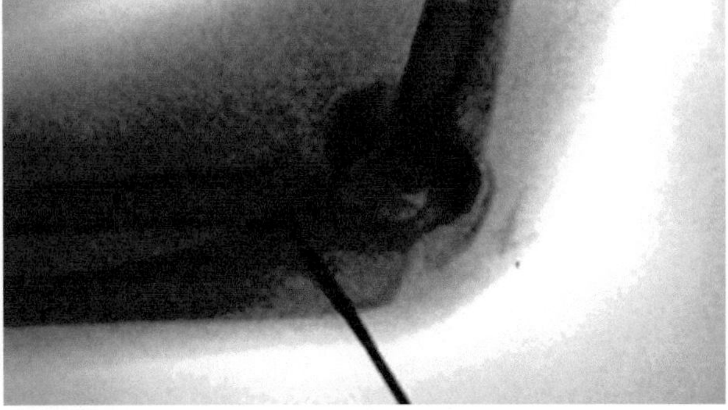

Fig. 6.6 Reduction of a radial neck fracture with the assistance of a percutaneous Kirschner wire, as a lever arm

6.1.6 Complications

Performing non-surgical treatment to resolve a fracture does not exempt us from complications [2, 16]. It is common to see skin lesions (erythema, skin irritation, pressure points, ulcers) that appear due to the installation of inappropriate or poorly molded casts (Fig. 6.7).

Superficial skin infections can occur due to moisture and skin alterations. Thermal injuries can also occur due to the heat generated during the setting of the plaster. This is related to the use of hot water to inmerse the bandages (>50 °C) and/or a thicker plaster, which concentrates the heat [10]. In a study conducted by Sawyer [11], it is reported that, over a period of 5 years, there were 168 unplanned visits to a hospital emergency room, all related to plaster problems. Of these, 29% were related to wet plasters, 23% with tight plasters, and 13% with loose plasters. Wet and dirty plasters can favor skin maceration, and even promote the appearance of necrotizing fasciitis and toxic shock syndrome.

It is also very common for patients to introduce all kinds of objects inside the plaster (Fig. 6.8). This can cause pressure points and skin infection. Any object inside the plaster can cause problems, so it is essential to remove ornaments or jewelry prior to its installation (Fig. 6.9).

Another complication is the loss of fracture reduction, which can condition us to the need of a new procedure, either closed or open reduction, and/or use of fixation [17].

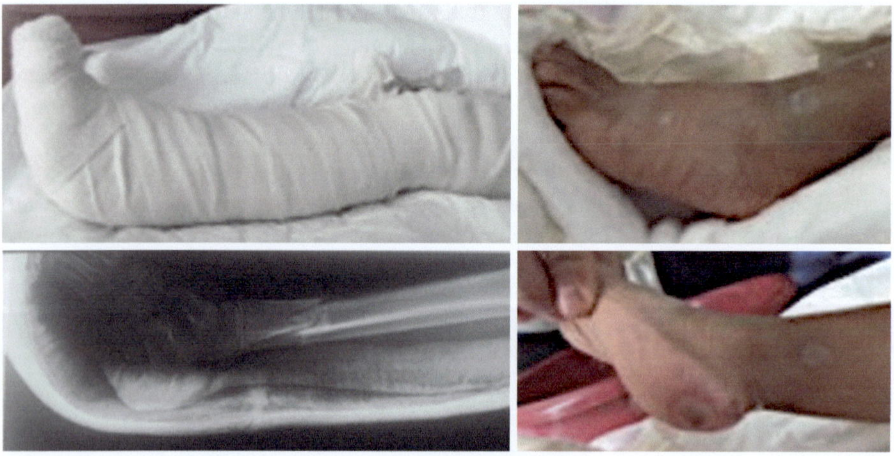

Fig. 6.7 Poorly molded plaster valve, showing an inadequate pressure zone. Upon removal, badly positioned and scarring in the pressure zone are evident

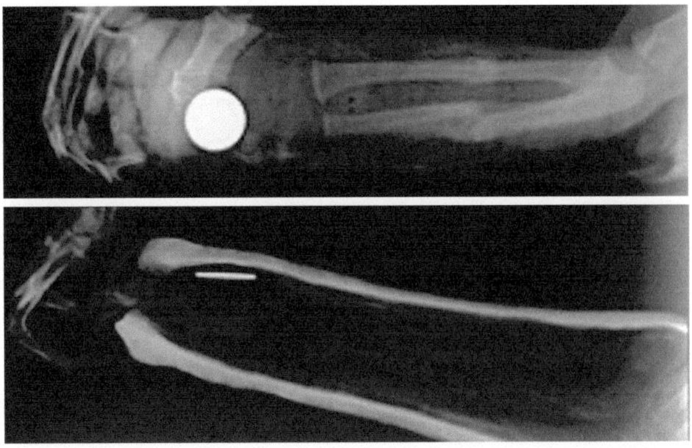

Fig. 6.8 X-ray of a forearm immobilized in a cast, showing the presence of a metallic foreign body inside it

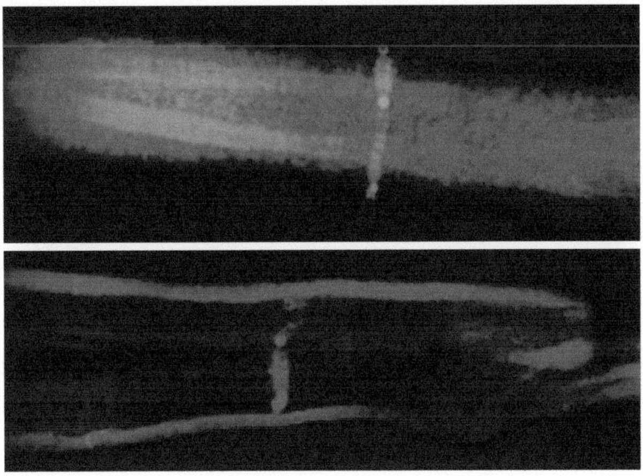

Fig. 6.9 X-ray before and after the installation of the short-arm cast, with the presence in both of the patient's bracelet, not removed at the time of the installation of the cast

6.1.7 Final Message

The great potential for remodeling in children allows accepting deformities within certain ranges that will improve over time. This remodeling, together with the biological and mechanical characteristics of growing bone, makes it feasible that the vast majority of fractures in pediatric patients can be treated non-surgically. Thus, most displacement in translation completely remodels in children under 10 years [5]. However, we must take into account that the remodeling of rotational displacement practically does not occur.

6.1.8 Authors' Recommendations

It is always important to achieve an aligned axis, stabilize it with adequate immobilization, and close follow up on patients to detect possible loss of reduction. The use of bivalve casts or splints is recommended in acute cases to avoid complications due to edema. The best material for immobilization will depend on the fracture to be treated [18].

Remember the phrase "Crooked casts, for straight bones" (Monnier's Maxim). For example, placing a long boot in equinus to avoid recurvatum of a leg fracture; or a forearm cast with the wrist in slight flexion and cubitalization to maintain the alignment of a distal radius fracture displaced dorsally. We also use the phrase "Fingers for reduction, palms for containment" (Carrasco's Maxim), referring to using the fingers for the Blount maneuver and then the palms to leave the cast molded, not compressive.

The molding of the cast should aim to have 3-points of contact to avoid displacement of the fracture. Always think about the location of your assistant, in favor of the necessary molding of the cast and in a comfortable position. It is important to do this with a relaxed and calm patient, ideally with fluoroscopic assistance. If a simple closed reduction cannot be achieved, the use of K wires can help us with the reduction, limiting traumatic maneuvers that can cause problems.

The placement of splints or circular casts should be carried out under the best possible conditions, that is, patient and orthopedist comfortable, facilitate handling acting in favor of gravity. For example, if a short plaster splint is placed for a foot or ankle fracture, the patient in prone position facilitates work in favor of gravity and not against it, as when we place that same patient in supine position. In a tibia fracture that we intend to immobilize with a long leg cast, ideally the patient should sit at the edge of the table, with knee flexion at 90°, and the applier sitting at the height of the knee for the placement of the cast and molding on the leg.

Remember that the pediatric patient is not a small-sized adult; it requires delicacy, tact, and kindness to achieve tranquility, both for him and his caregivers, for a successful treatment.

References

1. Ömeroglu H. Basic principles of fracture treatment in children. Eklem Hastalik Cerrahisi. 2018;29(1):52–7. https://doi.org/10.5606/ehc.2018.58165.
2. Jevsevar DS, Shea KG, Murray JN, Sevarino KS. AAOS clinical practice guideline on the treatment of pediatric diaphyseal femur fractures. J Am Acad Orthop Surg. 2015;23(12):e101. https://doi.org/10.5435/JAAOS-D-15-00523.
3. Lindaman LM. Bone healing in children. Clin Podiatr Med Surg. 2001;18(1):97–108.
4. Stilli S, Magnani M, Lampasi M, Antonioli D, Bettuzzi C, Donzelli O. Remodelling and overgrowth after conservative treatment for femoral and tibial shaft fractures in children. Chir Organi Mov. 2008;91(1):13–9. https://doi.org/10.1007/s12306-007-0003-6.
5. Naik P. Remodelling in children's fractures and limits of acceptability. Indian J Orthop. 2021;55(3):549–59. Published 2021 Mar 10. https://doi.org/10.1007/s43465-020-00320-2.
6. Wilkins KE. Principles of fracture remodeling in children. Injury. 2005;36(Suppl 1):A3–A11. https://doi.org/10.1016/j.injury.2004.12.007.
7. Kraus R, Wessel L. The treatment of upper limb fractures in children and adolescents. Dtsch Arztebl Int. 2010;107(51–52):903–10. https://doi.org/10.3238/arztebl.2010.0903.

8. Strauss BJ, Carey TP, Seabrook JA, Lim R. Pediatric clavicular fractures: assessment of fracture patterns and predictors of complicated outcome. J Emerg Med. 2012;43(1):29–35. https://doi.org/10.1016/j.jemermed.2011.06.132.
9. Herman MJ, McCarthy JJ. The principles of pediatric fracture and trauma care. In: Weinstein SL, Flynn JM, editors. Lovell and Winter's pediatric orthopaedics. 7th ed. Philadelphia: Wolters Kluwer; 2014. p. 1661–93.
10. Halanski M, Nemeth BA, Noonan KJ. Cast and splint immobilization, remodeling and special issues of children's fractures. In: Rockwood and Wilkins' fractures in children. 8th ed. Wolters Kluwer Health; 2015. p. 57–94.
11. Sawyer JR, Ivie CB, Huff AL, et al. Emergency room visits by pediatric fracture patients treated with cast immobilization. J Pediatr Orthop. 2010;30(3):248–52. https://doi.org/10.1097/BPO.0b013e3181d213bc.
12. Hubbard EW, Riccio AI. Pediatric orthopedic trauma: an evidence-based approach. Orthop Clin North Am. 2018;49(2):195–210. https://doi.org/10.1016/j.ocl.2017.11.008.
13. Mora F, Espíndola J, Mejía L, López A, Isunza A, Hernández S, Antonio C. Remodeling of displaced fractures of the distal metaphysis of the forearm in children. Rev Esp Méd Quir. 2012;17(3):186–90.
14. Daines SB, Aronsson DD, Beynnon BD, Sturnick DR, Lisle JW, Naud S. What is the best material for molding casts in children? J Pediatr Orthop. 2014;34(7):743–8. https://doi.org/10.1097/BPO.0000000000000178.
15. Laaksonen T, Puhakka J, Stenroos A, Kosola J, Ahonen M, Nietosvaara Y. Cast immobilization in bayonet position versus reduction and pin fixation of overriding distal metaphyseal radius fractures in children under ten years of age: a case control study. J Child Orthop. 2021;15(1):63–9. https://doi.org/10.1302/1863-2548.15.200171.
16. Pace JL. Pediatric and adolescent forearm fractures: current controversies and treatment recommendations. J Am Acad Orthop Surg. 2016;24(11):780–8. https://doi.org/10.5435/JAAOS-D-15-00151.
17. Kosuge D, Barry M. Changing trends in the management of children's fractures. Bone Joint J. 2015;97-B(4):442–8. https://doi.org/10.1302/0301-620X.97B4.34723.
18. Ömeroglu H, Cassiano NM. Tendency towards operative treatment is increasing in children's fractures: results obtained from patient databases, causes, impact of evidence-based medicine. EFORT Open Rev. 2020;5(6):347–53. Published 2020 Jun 1. https://doi.org/10.1302/2058-5241.5.200012.

Chapter 7
Principles of Surgical Treatment in the Pediatric Patient

Felipe Hodgson and Alexandre Arkader

7.1 Principles of Surgical Treatment in the Pediatric Patient

Over the past few decades, the treatment of fractures in children and adolescents has become increasingly invasive, and the variety of osteosynthesis materials on the market have led the pediatric trauma surgeon, especially the younger ones, to apply more frequently surgical treatments for pediatric fractures, unlike what happened half a century ago, when most of the fractures in patients under 18 years of age were resolved non-surgically. It is important to clarify that, in some types of fractures, the results obtained in the middle of the last century were not entirely good, but thanks to advances in fracture fixation methods, mainly in the forearm, elbow, and femur, the results have improved substantially in terms of better bone healing, in addition to reintegrating patients into their activities much more quickly [1].

7.2 Introduction

We must consider that the child's bone presents a series of peculiarities in its structure and physiology compared to the adult one, and during a fracture, characteristic reactions of immature skeletal tissue are generated.

Children and adolescents have high elasticity, with the child's bone being more plastic and less fragile than the adult's; it also has a thick periosteum, which gives it

F. Hodgson (✉)
Universidad Católica de Chile, Hospital Dr. Sótero del Río, Santiago, Chile
e-mail: fahodgso@uc.cl

A. Arkader
University of Pennsylvania, Philadelphia, PA, USA
e-mail: arkadera@chop.edu

M. Sepúlveda O. (ed.), *Paediatrics Traumatology*,
https://doi.org/10.1007/978-3-031-89482-4_7

more resistance. Because of these characteristics, incomplete fractures, such as greenstick type fracture, are very common. If the doctor is not used to distinguishing them, some of these may go unnoticed. Likewise, the fractures' locations differ in children compared to adults. The most important difference lies in the fact that the bone is still developing and fractures can affect the growth plate, representing up to 20% of total fractures. All the above determines the great difference in the approach and management of patients between the general trauma surgeon and the pediatric orthopedic surgeon.

When asking the question of when and why we should perform an osteosynthesis in children and adolescents, the most logical answer should be objective and relatively standardized, but usually each surgeon approaches the treatment based on their own experience. Age is the most important parameter that should be taken in consideration when we treat a fracture in pediatric patients because, as mentioned previously, the bone remodeling power decreases over time. It is not the same to have a forearm angulation in a 3-year-old child as in a 14-year-old adolescent; in the first, in a few months the deformity will be able to correct completely, but in the second the correction will not be perfect.

Another important factor in relation to treatment with or without osteosynthesis is the location of the fractures since those that occur near the growth plate and those where the angulation is in the movement direction of the nearest joint have more opportunity to correct. Likewise, fractures angled in other directions will have less remodeling capacity. When the fracture compromises the growth plate, it is very important to reduce it urgently and maintain that reduction stable, to void further damage of the physis. Most of the time immobilization with a cast for as long as necessary will be sufficient, and in others the use of some osteosynthesis material (usually Kirschner wires to reduce the risk of physeal damage) is required.

There are other factors that we should also consider in the decision for invasive surgery, such as the injury mechanism, with high-energy injuries often requiring the use of osteosynthesis. In turn, patients with associated injuries or multiple fractures, especially in patients in intensive care, are another factor that we should consider in favor of osteosynthesis [2].

Many changes have occurred in the fixation of fractures in children and adolescents in recent years, mainly due to scientific advances in the fields of biomechanics and in the biology of consolidation, in addition to understanding the important differences of children and their growth.

There are not many publications on the pathophysiology of fracture healing in children where some osteosynthesis material is used. Téot described, in 1987, how the consolidation of fractures occurs in children where flexible intramedullary nails were used, conducting studies of biological aspects, such as the preservation of the periosteum and the fracture hematoma. He highlighted the fundamental role of the conservation of the periosteum and the importance of medullary vascularization. In addition, he revealed the role of bone morphogenetic proteins (BMP), osteoblast-osteoclast interactions, the contribution of ischemia and hypoxia, and the phenomenon of electrical induction [3].

Over the past decades, the internal fixation of diaphyseal fractures has evolved enormously under the auspices of the AO Foundation. The concept of rigid anatomical fixation has transformed into a more biology-friendly design, resulting in locked plates. The desire to maintain the mechanical environment through muscle balance and bone vascularization led to the idea of a minimally invasive surgery. Stem cell-based therapies and osteoinductive factors are now used clinically. Since children rarely have alterations in bone healing, the world of pediatric orthopedics is a spectator of these developments, for now. However, without true pediatric studies on bone healing, we can only extrapolate recent scientific findings to children.

Regarding fracture fixation, the following points are already well known to favor healing in a biological context: maintain the periosteum intact, do not alter the fracture hematoma, some flexibility during fixation (some biomechanical stress is essential for proper bone healing) and development of percutaneous surgery [4].

7.3 Role of Fixation

It is important to underline that this period of the life is characterized by growth, a process that is driven by two specific structures: the growth plate (or physis) and the periosteum, which is a true ally of the pediatric orthopedic surgeon. Each of these structures can present its own problems and challenges during the fracture fixation. Although growth corrects many cases of defective consolidation, it is a mistake to believe that it solves everything. Rotational deformities or in the opposite direction to the movement of the adjacent joint have less chance of remodeling.

We must always remember that conservative (non-surgical) treatment leads, in most cases, to a faster and more reliable bone healing than open fracture fixation. Fixation is only indicated if the fracture's healing process does not have sufficient remodeling capacity or is altered by other factors. The indications will mainly depend on the child's age and the location of the fracture. Exceptions to this rule are polytraumatized children, refractures, displaced intra-articular fractures, association with severe head trauma, pathological bone fractures or those determined by underlying diseases such as neurological deterioration, bone fragility, or displaced physeal fractures. Something more debatable, especially in children, is the fixation of fractures in high-performance athletes for an early return to their activities [5].

The following rules of bone remodeling guide indications for the fixation of a fracture. A defective union will usually remodel adequately if the child is young enough (less than 10 years of age in males and 8 in females), and if the defective union is close to an active metaphysis, with a high growth potential (near the knee, far from the elbow). In addition, if the main plane of the deformity corresponds to the main movement of the closest joint, it will have a greater capacity for remodeling (high tolerance in the wrist to volar-dorsal angulations, and little or no tolerance for varus-valgus displacement in the ankle).

Something more debatable is the correction of rotational alterations since it is a deformity with less potential to correct itself. Historically, it was explained that rotational alterations do not remodel; however, their location and the compensation capacity of neighboring joints will determine future function. Because of this, we must be careful with supracondylar fractures in the elbow, the fixation of the middle diaphysis of the humerus, the femur, and fractures of metacarpals or phalanges.

All these factors help to explain the high success for the conservative or non-surgical treatment of wrist or proximal humerus fractures and a large number of surgical indications for fractures at the elbow and in the ankle level.

7.4 Preserve the Periosteum at all Costs

The fixation of diaphyseal fractures in children for a long time were perform with "adult" implants, which consisted of quite long plates. However, these plates had various complications, such as the need for large surgical approaches, the risk of hemorrhage and infection, and overgrowth related to the need to remove the periosteum. Advocates of this method, which is used less frequently in pediatric trauma, believe that better control over rotation is achieved, and that the patient and surgeon are subject to less radiation. Two successive events broke these beliefs: the arrival of flexible intramedullary fixation and the development of locked plates. Also, advances in fluoroscopy and radiological protection have been fundamental in reducing the risks of radiation exposure.

7.5 Elastic Intramedullary Nailing

The technique of flexible intramedullary nailing, developed in 1980 by surgeons from Nancy, France, has been perfected. This technique is also known as elastic stable intramedullary nailing (ESIN). It is now universally used since intraoperative images were available. Currently, this is the standard treatment for diaphyseal fractures in long bones of the pediatric population and is governed by the biological criteria described above (the hematoma and its growth factors are preserved). The periosteum, outside of the damage related to the fracture, is not destroyed. The flexibility of the construct allows the necessary micromovements to stimulate the periosteum and ensure healing. The nails do not completely fill the medullary canal, so they do not alter the callus in the endosteum. The stability of the construction is assured in the three planes: frontal, sagittal, and rotational (Fig. 7.1) [6].

With the nails molded in opposite directions, three-point support ensure balance and stabilize the fracture each time a deforming load is placed on the bone. Rotational movements are controlled by the medullary anchoring of the curved tips. The technique was initially developed for the fixation of the femur, which due to its characteristic circumferential endomedullary tubular canal allows its adequate anchoring. Other areas, such as the triangular endomedullary canal of the tibia, may

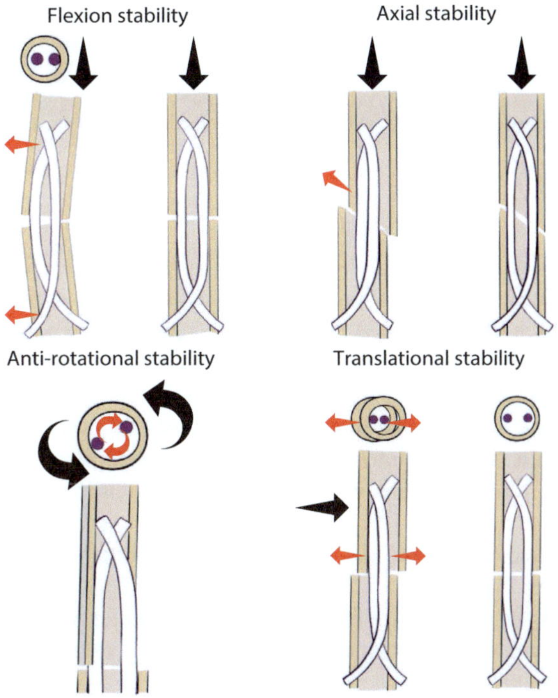

Fig. 7.1 Stability of elastic intramedullary nailing in all planes of motion. Under deforming forces (black arrow), the restoring force of the nail shape (red arrow) maintains the reduction in relative stability as long as a symmetrical configuration is achieved

present less stability, requiring protection with plaster or external orthoses. Ender's nails were the basis for the design/nails, which can be molded.

The usual surgical technique for the insertion of flexible intramedullary nails in long bones includes the use of a radiolucent table, the patient under general anesthesia and fluoroscopic control. Nails of a diameter corresponding to 30–40% of the medullary canal at the isthmus, or twice the thickness of the bone cortex, are used. The fracture is reduced by manipulation and traction, checked under fluoroscopic in anteroposterior and lateral projections. The insertion point is determined 1–2 cm proximally from the physis. For femur and tibia, two incisions are made, one medial and one lateral, 1 cm from the point of insertion. Two holes are made, one on each side of the bone, using the starter punch at a 45° angle to the longitudinal axis of the diaphysis, taking care not to perforate the opposite cortical bone.

Before introducing the nails, it is advisable to bend their distal end at a 30° angle. The rest of the nail will be curved in a "C" shape, up to three times the diameter of the canal. The nail is mounted on a T-handle and is inserted perpendicularly into the previously made hole. The nail is oriented in the opposite direction of the physis and is advanced manually to the fracture site with rotational movements, and in the same way the next nail.

Once the appropriate reduction under fluoroscopy is verified, one of the nails is introduced, and then the second, until it is close to the opposite physis. The nails are cut once the position is defined, protruding 5 mm from their insertion point to facilitate extraction. The use of end-caps is an alternative for unstable fractures; for example, in comminuted, spiral and long oblique fractures, in order to avoid further impaction. (Fig. 7.2) [7].

7.5.1 Choice of Materials

The nails are available in titanium or stainless steel. Both have the same type of curvature and similar instrumentation. Titanium is more elastic than stainless steel, which makes more suitable for increasing micromovement in the construct and stimulating the periosteum. Stainless steel nails are more rigid. The stiffness of a stainless steel nail of a given diameter is the same as that of a titanium nail 0.5 mm larger in diameter. As a result, a larger diameter titanium nail is needed to achieve the same stiffness as a stainless steel nail, but the medullary canal may not be large enough to use it (remember that 70–80% occupancy of the medullary canal diameter is required). Since both types of materials suffer similar amounts of friction-related corrosion, the choice of material depends on the desired degree of stiffness. In general terms, titanium can be used in small patients, when a greater degree of elasticity is allowed. Stainless steel is indispensable in larger patients and adolescents who still have open growth cartilages, and in whom stability is essential. It is important to consider that titanium nails have greater osteointegration, so their removal, especially in the forearm, can be more difficult. The final decision comes down to biomechanics, surgeon's preference, and financial considerations (titanium may be more expensive).

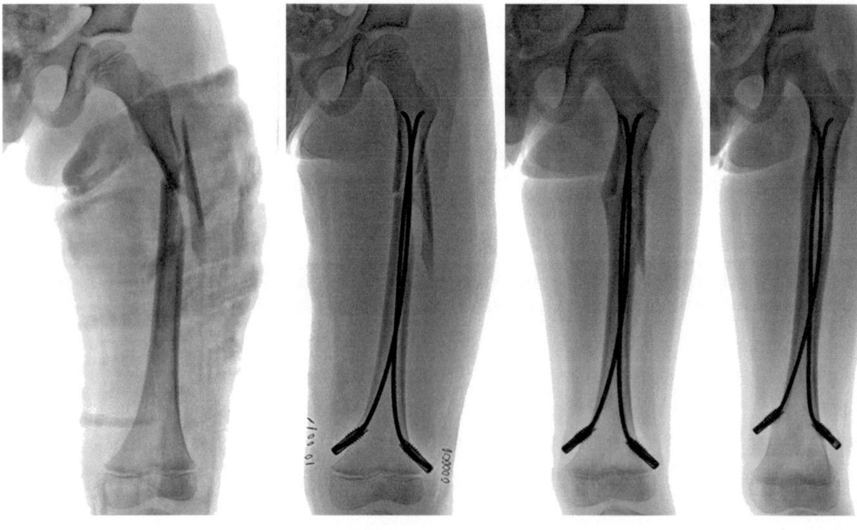

Fig. 7.2 Femur fracture in a 6-year-old child, stabilized with elastic nails and with support of a end caps. Postoperative control (without the need for plaster cast), 3 months and 1 year postoperatively

7.5.2 Diameter of the Intramedullary Nail

Several methods have been described to guide the size selection for the femur: endomedullary canal diameter × 0.4; (endomedullary canal diameter/2) − 1; according to age (3 mm for patients <7 years old; 3.5 mm for 7–10 years old; 4 mm for >10 years old). In the tibia, 3–4 mm wide nails are used, and in the forearm, 2–2.5 mm. These dimensions are more complicated to measure in digitized radiographs with reduced image sizes, which can lead to errors. The nail should be as long as possible, considering the insertion point as distal as possible in relation to the fracture site and also far enough from the LaCroix perichondral ring. The intramedullary end must be anchored enough in the cancellous bone to preserve the biomechanics of the construct. The nails are manually bent until they are symmetrical and the curve is located over the fracture site. We must be especially careful not to cross both nails to maintain three-point support.

7.5.3 Main Indications for Elastic Intramedullary Nails

This method was first used in the femur. Retrograde ascending nailing is preferred, except in cases of fractures of the distal end of the femur. If greater stability is needed in distal fractures, epiphyseal anchoring with individual paths for each nail is allowed. The minimum age is defined by the limits of diaphyseal remodeling, with a more reduced capacity after 5 years old. From this age, standard fixation of these fractures should be considered. Exceptions are polytraumatized patients, fractures in pathological bone or those with associated conditions (neurological, congenital), or significant fracture instability that is not adequately controlled with conservative treatment (spica cast). This construct may not be rigid enough in adolescents. The need for greater stability and the risks of fracture impaction, especially when the fracture is comminuted, has led to two additional improvements: the use of end-caps that are screwed into the distal end of the nails or at the proximal end of the tibial nail. This technique avoids the impaction of the fracture site or the sinking of the nail with active muscle contraction in addition to the development of special rigid nails for adolescents, with trochanteric insertion.

The upper limit for indications of flexible intramedullary nails is determined by skeletal maturity and the patient's weight. Studies have determined that the maximum weight for their use is 49 kg in the femur [8]. Traditional rigid nails (with or without locking) and their entry points are dangerous at this age due to the risk of femoral head necrosis or pseudoarthrosis of the femoral neck. Tibial fractures are rarely treated with flexible nails, most of these fractures are treated non-surgical. In adolescents, the technique is limited by the possibility of nailing, ideally when the anterior tuberosity of the tibia is completely fused, due to the risk of genu recurvatum.

The proximal humerus has a high capacity for remodeling, so indications for surgical fixation are infrequent. In diaphyseal fractures of the humerus, especially in adolescents, it may be a good indication as an alternative to the usual treatment with functional braces or cast. It is reserved for fractures in pathological bone or fractures with intra-articular extension that require hybrid fixation methods. Intramedullary nailing in this location has a risk of skin-related complications. Nailing is used very limitedly for supracondylar fractures of the humerus, a demanding but effective technique. One advantage is that it is not necessary to immobilize the elbow.

Stable intramedullary nailing fixation in the forearm (Fig. 7.3) is indicated in open fractures, unstable fractures, unacceptable angular deformities, new displacements, in irreducible fractures due to soft tissue interposition, in refractures and when accompanied by multiple traumas. Since the ulna and the diaphyseal radius have a low remodeling capacity, closed reduction must provide a good alignment, and at least 2–3 months of immobilization are required. This explains why the installation of elastic nails is widely used in children over 8–10 years old. In these cases, only one nail is placed in each bone; the interosseous membrane unites the forearm bones. If fluoroscopy is not available or reduction is difficult, a small incision can be made over the fracture site to help insert the nails. The nails should be left in place for at least 6 months before being removed. On some occasions, it may be necessary only the fixation of one of the forearm bones or hybrid constructs may be useful, such as a plate to the distal radius and an elastic nail to the ulna.

Complications are rare if certain technical rules are followed. In 2001, Lascombes reported a surgical revision rate of 4% and a sequelae rate of 0.1%. Skin problems occur in 14% of cases, mainly with humerus or tibia fractures, but also in the femur if the nails are inserted distally. Less than 1 cm of limb length discrepancy has been

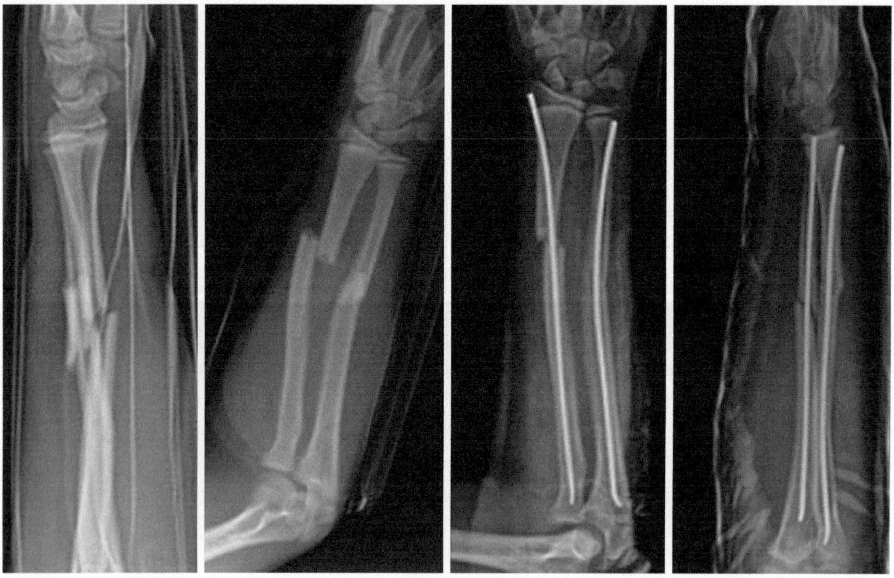

Fig. 7.3 Forearm fracture in an 11-year-old girl, closed reduction and fixation with flexible intramedullary nails was performed

found in isolated femur fractures. Refractures are common in the forearm if the material is not left in place for at least 6 months. Other complications are due to technical errors. The most common technical errors are: incorrect choice of nail size; nails that are too short; nails inserted in the wrong direction; nail orientation; inaccurate assessment of the patient's age or size, especially with adolescents; failure to achieve a double arc and having the nails crossed several times ("corkscrew" effect). The problems encountered during surgery are often due to patient-related issues or a lack of reduction before starting nail insertion. The surgeon should not rely on the curved tip to achieve fracture reduction, as its true purpose is to guide the nail. The reduction should be performed on the traction table or by external maneuvers. In some cases, such as 15% of forearm fractures, an incision is made in the skin over the fracture site to achieve proper reduction. Late consolidation and pseudoarthrosis are rare, but can occur due to an infection, an open reduction of the fracture, and especially a technical error.

The material can be removed approximately 6 months after insertion, once the fracture callus shows signs of an intramedullary canal in order to avoid refractures.

7.6 Locked Compression Plate (LCP)

Currently, the standard fixation of diaphyseal fractures are flexible intramedullary nails, however, for the fixation of some fractures in the diaphysis, long and rigid plates have been used. Compression at the fracture site has been a secondary problem and the disadvantages of these plates are soft tissue injuries, large scars, and aggressive periosteal extraction that cause excessive lengthening. Supplementary immobilization induces muscle atrophy, as occurs in adults. The arrival of locked plates has generated a significant advance from a biological point of view and has also changed the way postoperative care is performed. These plates are equivalent to using an external fixator, internally. The construction is short and rigid, while allowing the rest of the shaft to remain flexible. The plate is not attached to the bone, so the periosteum can heal, immobilization is not necessary, and there is less postoperative pain. In addition, this type of plate is indicated when there is poor bone quality due to other pathologies. Rehabilitation can be started quickly and weight-bearing is allowed almost immediately. These advantages are fundamental in cases of neurological diseases and can be considered as an alternative to fixation with intramedullary nails.

In general, short and straight plates are used, with four to six holes (equal to having a screw in eight cortical surfaces) in the femur, tibia, or humerus, to maintain rotation. The other indications for fixation with this type of plates are mainly in the hip. The enormous range of available implants includes multiple variants of blade-plates, with more screw. Each surgical team has its preferred materials, but many of these systems still require the use of immobilization after surgery. Blade-plates have the disadvantage of being more difficult to correctly place, so they are usually used more in osteotomies than in acute fractures. The concept of locking screws has led

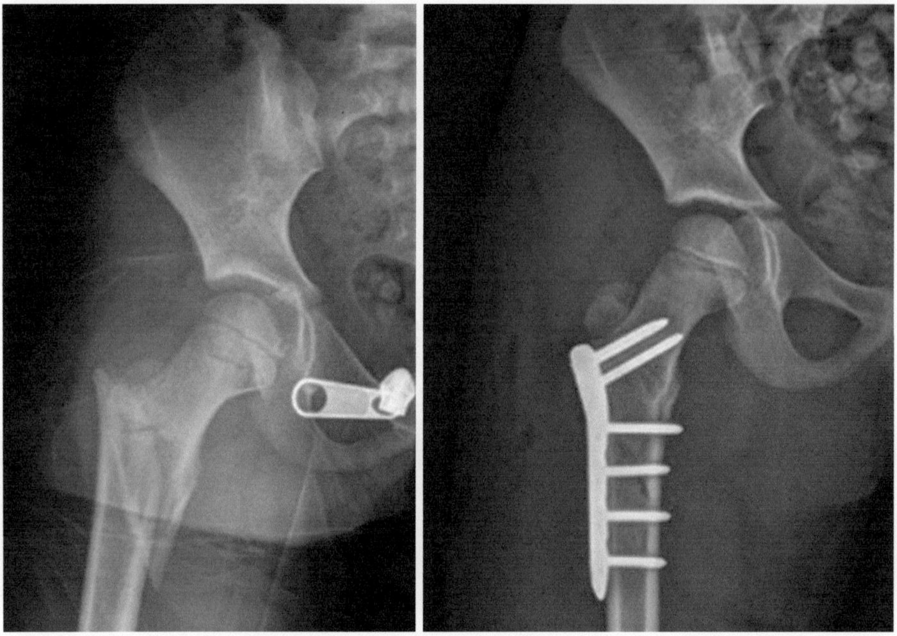

Fig. 7.4 Displaced hip fracture in a 6-year-old girl, treated with open reduction and pediatric hip locking plate fixation

to the development of specific pediatric hip plates for each age group, used for stabilization in proximal femur fractures (Fig. 7.4). As mentioned earlier, their main advantages are early mobilization and weightbearing. The triangulation of the proximal locking screws in the femoral neck ensures that the screws do not come out.

7.7 External Fixation (EF)

External fixation is indispensable in the initial treatment of closed or open fractures with severe soft tissue injury. The choice of fixator is based on the place to be installed, the surgeon's preferences and training, and economic limitations. The pros and cons of each type (ring, unilateral or combination) must be well understood, and the surgeon must be familiar with the specific implantation techniques for each one. Circular fixators are mainly used in distal segments, while that straight monolaterals in diaphyseal segments. Modular fixators have multiple uses, but often require a variety of accessory pieces. In trauma, initial use is limited to closed fractures, or open fractures with severe soft tissue injury (Fig. 7.5), revisions, treatment of delay in bone healing, infections although some surgeons have maintained their use in some closed fractures of the femur as a definitive treatment. It also offers the possibility of gradual axial correction, through various alignment modifications or by

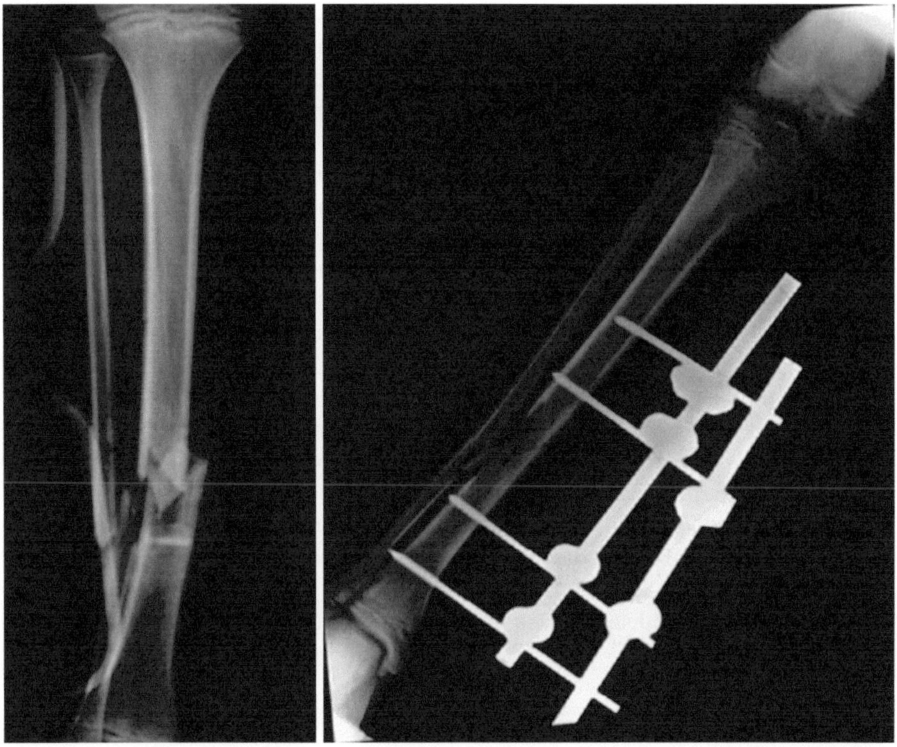

Fig. 7.5 Adolescent with an open fracture of the right leg. Initial stabilization was performed with a modular external fixator

asymmetric distraction, to reduce the risk of compartment syndrome. In some cases, it can be used as a help to achieve an adequate reduction of a fracture, and at that moment perform the definitive osteosynthesis with intramedullary nails or other devices. External fixators would also be useful in tropical climates where casts are not well tolerated. The ability to weightbearing stimulates the fracture callus formation almost immediately and reduces the risk of thromboembolism in older patients. Its disadvantages are related to the discomfort of the device and its unaesthetic appearance. It also requires special care of the screws and wires to reduce the risk of infection. Ideally, external fixation should be considered as an initial treatment in order to convert to internal osteosynthesis methods as soon as the conditions allow it.

7.8 Fractures Due to Bone Fragility

We have already insisted on the systematic fixation in polytraumatized patients, regardless of age, which goes against the usual rules surrounding pediatric trauma cases. In addition, some pathologies associated with bone fragility that benefit from fracture fixation are described, as patients with osteogenesis imperfecta in whom fixation has two objectives to treat the fracture and prevent recurrence. The chosen fixation ideally should allow for growth and endomedullary devices are preferred (Fig. 7.6). Fassier-Duval type telescopic nails are the most used; however, the material must be changed as the child grows.

In patients with neurological diseases, conservative treatments should be performed with care, as the dominant symptom is spasticity or hypertonia. Prolonged immobilization increases the risk of pressure ulcers, tendon contractions, muscle contractions, and rapid muscle atrophy. The immobilization period should be as short as possible, and rehabilitation should start as soon as the pain disappears. Fixation with intramedullary nails is more indicated, which requires a shorter immobilization period in patients who do not walk. Locked plates can also be used depending on the type of fracture.

In patients with tumors, intramedullary nails allow to protect benign lytic bone lesions (simple bone cyst, aneurysmal bone cyst, fibrous dysplasia). It is compatible with current treatments that include filling with bone graft, bone marrow injection, alcohol, and corticosteroids. Depending on the patient's age, an "adult" type fixation device will be used, such as locked nails, cephalo-medullary nails, and others, for permanent lesions. In the femur, there are currently pediatric nails with trochanteric lateral entry to reduce the risk of avascular necrosis of the femoral head, with smaller nail diameters.

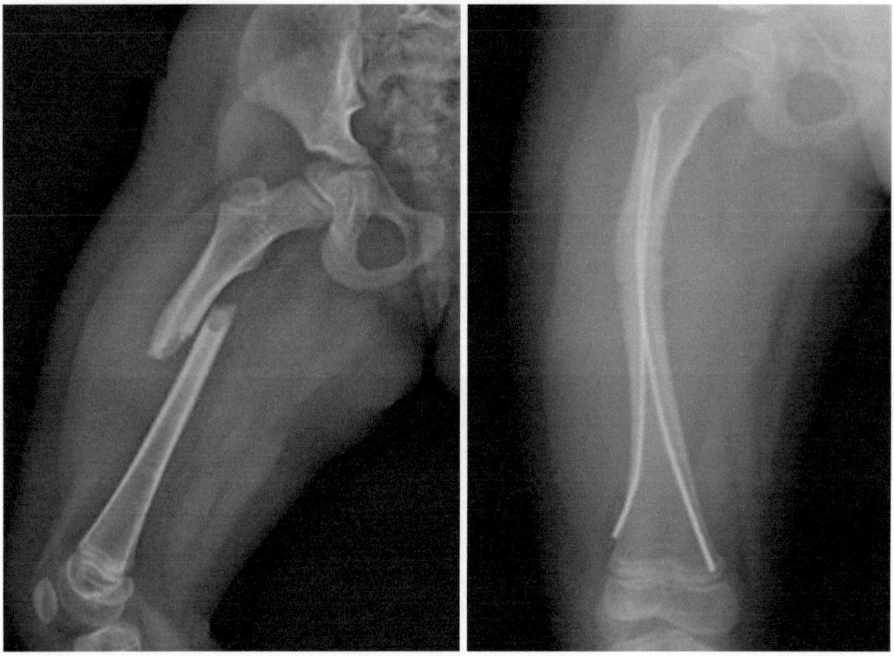

Fig. 7.6 Displaced femur fracture in a 7-year-old girl with osteogenesis imperfecta. Closed reduction was performed with a flexible intramedullary nail

7.9 Considerations with the Physis

The injury that affects the articular surface, requires an anatomical reduction, which is synonymous with surgery and fixation. The main complication of these injuries is the premature closure of the physis, but it is also possible to observe epiphyseal necrosis or pseudoarthrosis. Although the appearance of complications depends on the type of fracture, the time before the reduction and the quality of the reduction, surgical treatment is a significant source of risk factors in relation to the type of material and the surgical approach used. An extensive open approach, especially in the elbow and hip, can induce devascularization of the fragment, especially if the electrocoagulator is used excessively.

Altered olecranon growth has also been described after tension band osteosynthesis with wires. These complications have been reduced through the development of minimally invasive percutaneous surgery and anatomical specific implants.

We must avoid physeal injury when use osteosynthesis materials. This damage can be by direct compression or related to an alteration of cartilage activity. A study carried out on the distal femur of rabbits showed that the amount and duration of the applied compression are the main factors affecting the activity of the physis. The initial compression provided by a fixation device and the time before removing the material should be considered. Conversely, this reduced growth can be induced on purpose when epiphysiodesis is desired (fixation with screws, staples, figure-eight plates) or intentional fusion of the femoral epiphysis, choosing an implant of greater diameter, size, and volume [9].

It has been demonstrated in rabbits that Kirschner wires should have a diameter less than 2 mm to avoid altering growth. If we extrapolate these findings to the size of various physes in pediatric patients, 1.8 mm is the maximum diameter that can be used in a medial malleolus, for example. Based on the requirements described above, we must remember that the use of plate fixation in the physis area is practically prohibited because it eliminates the periosteum from the perichondral area and induces physis compression, and the formation of bone bridges. The options for this type of fractures are external fixation, especially Ilizarov type circular external fixation, which makes it possible not to cross the physis, and offers the option of using olive Kirschner wires to compact the fragments. The downside is that it can induce compression and the use of an external fixator in an emergency situation is complex, with a construct volume that can be bothersome.

Flexible intramedullary nails meet the established requirements. They are useful and effective in epiphyseal fractures without joint involvement, such as radial neck fractures. A nail, preferably made of stainless steel for greater rigidity and ease of removal, should be inserted retrogradely through the distal end of the radius (Fig. 7.7).

Kirschner wires are an osteosynthesis material extensively used by pediatric surgeons in the fixation of epiphyseal-metaphyseal fractures. As mentioned above, the diameter of the Kirschner wire ideally should not exceed 2 mm because practically no compression is induced. However, the diameter will depend on the size of the patient, the affected physis, the number of wires installed, in addition to the energy involved in the injury. It is a stable construct option, but not strong. It should

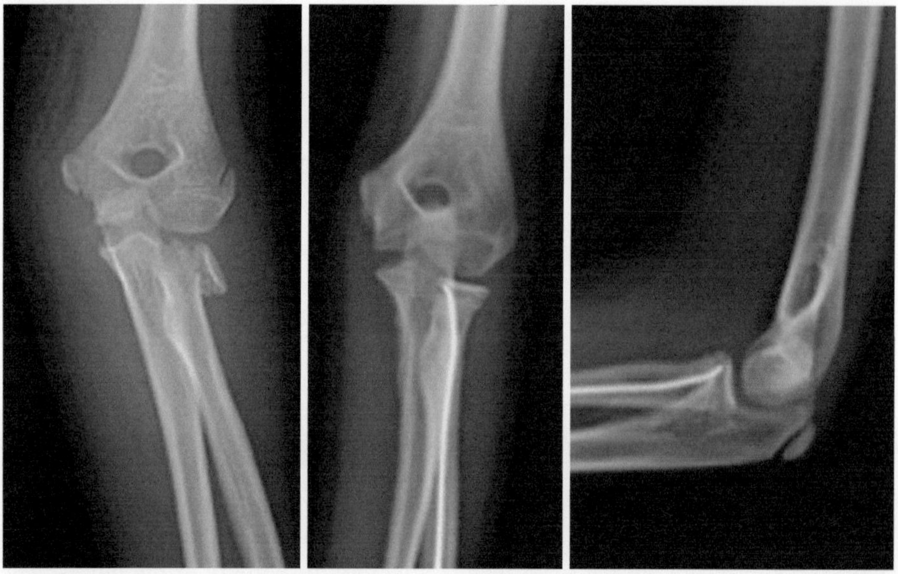

Fig. 7.7 Displaced radial neck fracture in a 12-year-old girl. Closed reduction with a flexible intramedullary nail was performed

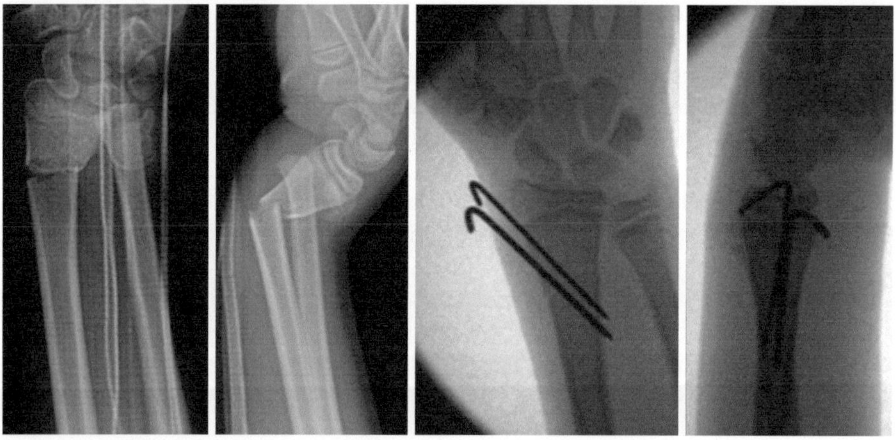

Fig. 7.8 Distal forearm fracture in a 14-year-old male. Closed reduction and ostesynthesis with Kirschner wires was performed, protected with plaster cast

always be accompanied by a cast protection, until consolidation is achieved (Figs. 7.8 and 7.9).

Kirschner wires are usually inserted percutaneously and left exposed through the skin, to be removed between the third and fourth week, once consolidation has progressed. Let's remember that prolonged immobilization of a joint in children does not produce stiffness as in adults. Without this additional immobilization, the construct may suffer secondary displacement.

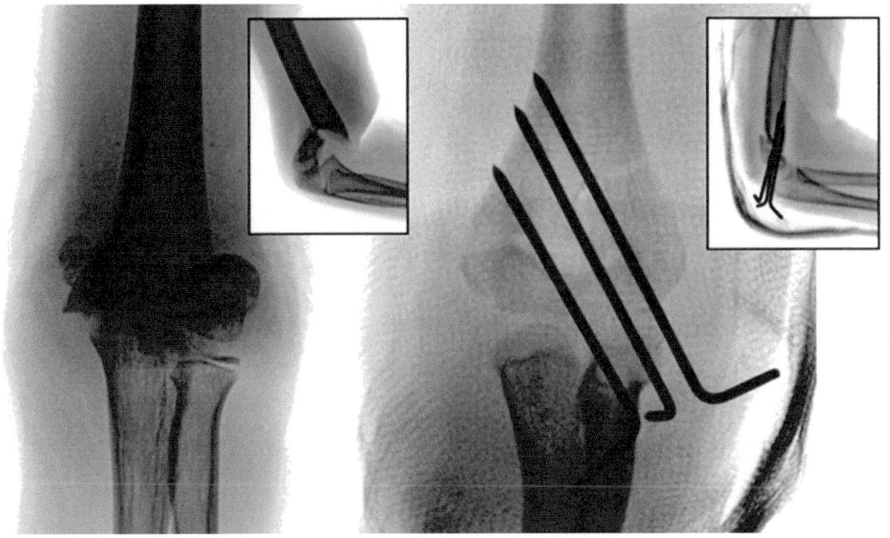

Fig. 7.9 Supracondylar humerus fracture in a 8-year-old girl. Treated with closed reduction and percutaneous Kirschner wires from lateral

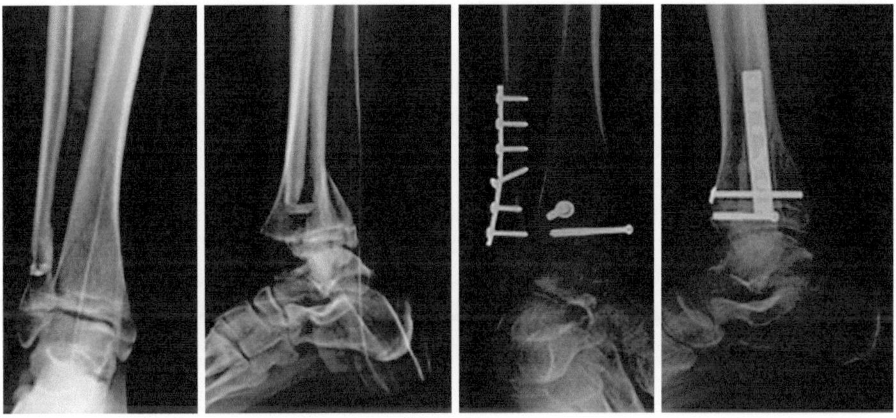

Fig. 7.10 Triplanar ankle fracture in a 12-year-old girl. Open reduction and fixation with screws and a plate to the fibula was performed

7.10 Screws

Screw fixation is used when compression of two fragments is required and ideally does not cross the physis. The development of cannulated screws of various diameters has led to increased use of percutaneous fixation. The main indications for small diameter screws are ankle (Fig. 7.10) and medial epicondyle fractures (Fig. 7.11).

Larger diameter screws are used for fractures of larger epiphyses, such as distal femur, femoral neck fractures and, by extension, in slipped capital femoral epiphysis.

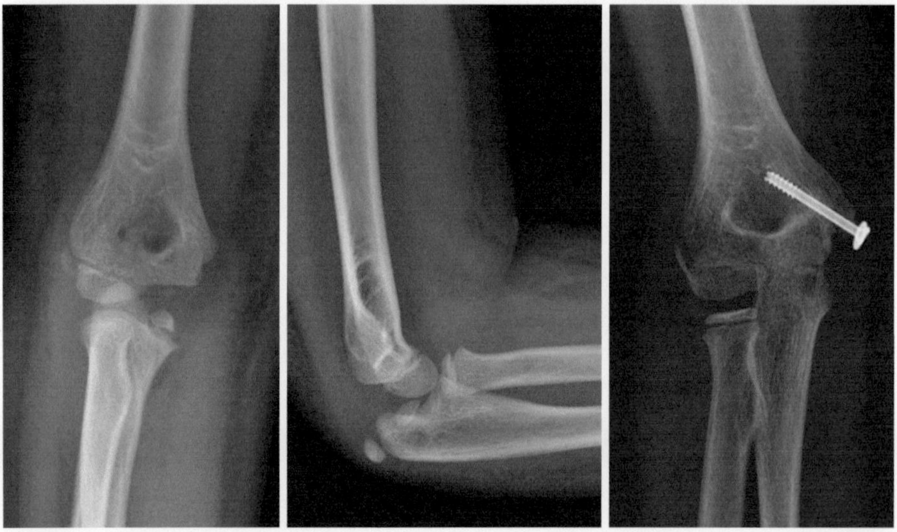

Fig. 7.11 Displaced intra-articular epitrochlea fracture after elbow dislocation in a 9-year-old girl. Open reduction and fixation with a cannulated screw were performed

7.11 Other Osteosynthesis Options

Fixing fractures does not always require metallic devices. Bone fragments can also be stabilized by other means. The absorbable sutures are useful for stabilizing some small fragments or treating epiphyseal or apophyseal avulsions. The development of titanium anchors with large caliber absorbable sutures has expanded indications in children. Apart from tendon transfers, these techniques can be very useful in medial epicondyle fractures, tibial spine fractures with a loop at the base of the anterior cruciate ligament (Fig. 7.12) and ankle sprains with bone avulsion (talofibular ligament). Absorbable pins can also be used during the fixation of certain fractures.

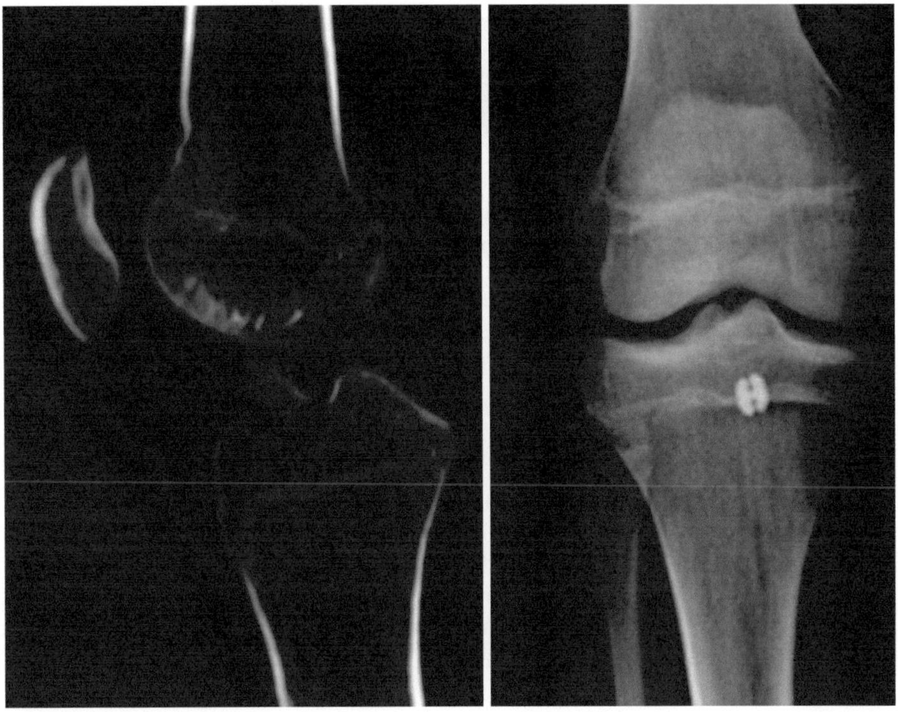

Fig. 7.12 Displaced tibial spine fracture in a 14-year-old boy. Arthroscopic reduction and suture fixation through bone tunnels was performed

7.12 Removal of Osteosynthesis

Fractures in skeletally immature patients often require only conservative treatment; however, certain injuries require surgical intervention and the use of osteosynthesis material. Using these devices can lead to the need for secondary procedures to remove them. The indications in pediatrics for the extraction of this osteosynthesis material are varied, and there are few evidence-based guidelines for clinical decision-making.

It has been repeatedly shown that osteosynthesis material serves as a possible nest for infection. Boulos' review found that *S. aureus* was the most common infectious organism (32%), followed by MRSA (15%) and other gram negatives. This is important to keep in mind when prescribing antibiotics to patients with infected osteosynthesis material before identification [10].

In Boulos' study, they also observed that the cause of removal was 30% due to infection, 25% due to symptomatic osteosynthesis material, 13% due to pain, and 5% due to pseudoarthrosis. Other authors have observed that the main reasons for the extraction of intramedullary nails in the femur and forearm include the prominence or discomfort of the nail end. Of forearm fractures treated with plates in pediatric patients, about 20% choose to remove the implant due to irritation. It has been described that patients with osteosynthesis material in the foot and ankle experience more pain, associated with the resumption of weightbearing in activities, and patients have significantly less pain after elective removal of the implant. In those procedures where the main indication for removal was pain, they could not identify an obvious cause. This emphasizes the need for further research in order to reduce unnecessary surgeries and their associated costs.

In addition to infection and symptomatic osteosynthesis material, surgeons may recommend implant removal to avoid future complications; this includes difficulty in removing implants later in life, peri-implant fracture due to stress, migration of osteosynthesis material with growth, metal allergy and possible carcinogenesis due to corrosion of metallic elements. However, implant removal is not without risks and can result in possible postoperative complications such as refracture, infection, hematoma, wound dehiscence, blood loss, and prolonged operative time. In a survey of pediatric orthopedic surgeons, many believed that implants should be preserved due to the aforementioned complications and concerns related to anesthesia. One study found for patients undergoing implant removal in the USA, the average hospital charge after implant removal for any cause was $36,349, and $21,040 if we exclude infectious causes of extraction. This is not an insignificant amount and can cause financial stress for both patients and hospitals, especially if the implant removal is not performed for symptomatic reasons.

There is scarce evidence-based literature and practical guidelines keep the topic of debate between the need for implant removal, versus its retention after fracture consolidation. However, the complication rates of implant removal in elective, non-symptomatic patients, suggest that material removal should be performed only for clinical indications or valid reasons.

7.13 Final Message

Most fractures in pediatric patients should be treated non-surgically, but some require fixation with different devices to achieve adequate bone healing. This fixation may seem easy or simple to some surgeons, associated with the knowledge that growth corrects many defects. However, it has been shown that this apparent simplicity hides certain complications, so learning should never stop.

Although we have a better understanding of bone biomechanics, it is essential to understand its biology so as not to compromise bone consolidation and not to damage structures such as growth cartilage or the periosteum.

In case of using fixation, we recommend flexible intramedullary nails for diaphyseal fractures, and as an alternative we have the use of locked plates. In fractures that compromise the epiphyseal or metaphyseal region, it may be necessary to stabilize with Kirschner wires associated with cast immobilization, and on some occasions, we can use screws or intramedullary nails. The use of external fixation is reserved for the stabilization of fractures with extensive soft tissue involvement.

New developments for the treatment of fractures in children should combine our knowledge of mechanics with advances in tissue engineering and materials.

References

1. Ömerolu H, Cassiano Neves M. Tendency towards operative treatment is increasing in children's fractures: results obtained from patient databases, causes, impact of evidence-based medicine. EFORT Open Rev. 2020;5(6):347–53. Published 2020 Jun 1. https://doi.org/10.1302/2058-5241.5.200012.
2. Juanto M, Fernández E, Ramacciotti A, et al. Osteosynthesis in pediatrics. When and why? Ortho-tips. 2015;11(1):7–14.
3. de Billy B, Gindraux F, Langlais J. Osteotomy and fracture fixation in children and teenagers. Orthop Traumatol Surg Res. 2014;100(1 Suppl):S139–48. https://doi.org/10.1016/j.otsr.2013.11.006.
4. Ömerolu H. Basic principles of fracture treatment in children. Eklem Hastalik Cerrahisi. 2018;29(1):52–7. https://doi.org/10.5606/ehc.2018.58165.
5. Beaty JH, Kasser JR. Rockwood-Wilkins. Fractures in children. 5th ed. Marban, Madrid: Lippincott Williams & Wilkins; 2003.
6. Métaizeau J-P. L'embrochage centro-médullaire élastique stable (ECMES). Rev Chir Orthop Reparatrice Appar Mot. 2006;92(4):409–11., ISSN 0035-1040. https://doi.org/10.1016/S0035-f1040(06)75791-9.
7. Dietz HG, Schmittenbecher P, Slongo T, Wilkins K. Elastic stable intramedullary nailing (ESIN) in children. 1st ed. New York: Thieme; 2006.
8. Donovan RL, Harries L, Whitehouse MR. Flexible nails have a significantly increased risk of complications compared with plating techniques when treating diaphyseal femoral fractures in children aged 5-12: a systematic review. Injury. 2020;51(12):2763–70. https://doi.org/10.1016/j.injury.2020.09.024.
9. Mäkelä EA, Vainionpää S, Vihtonen K, Mero M, Rokkanen P. The effect of trauma to the lower femoral epiphyseal plate. An experimental study in rabbits. J Bone Joint Surg Br. 1988;70(2):187–91. https://doi.org/10.1302/0301-620X.70B2.3346285.
10. Boulos A, DeFroda SF, Kleiner JE, Thomas N, Gil JA, Cruz AI Jr. Inpatient orthopaedic hardware removal in children: a cross-sectional study. J Clin Orthop Trauma. 2017;8(3):270–5. https://doi.org/10.1016/j.jcot.2017.06.020.

Chapter 8
Open Fractures in the Pediatric Population

Andres Ferreyra and Victoria Allende

8.1 Open Fractures in the Pediatric Population

Open fractures are those in which the soft tissues and skin are disrupted, and the bone has been exposed to the environment. Open fractures are rare in the pediatric population, with an incidence rate between 0.7% and 2% of all pediatric fractures, usually affecting the fingertips during exploratory activities (Fig. 8.1). More complex injuries are the result of high-energy trauma, such as motor vehicle accidents or falls from heights.

High-level evidence articles on open fractures in the pediatric population are scarce. Many treatment recommendations are extrapolated from adult's literature [1–5].

There are several differences between adults and children regarding bone physiology. Children's periosteum is a thick tissue, active, and highly vascularized. It allows less fracture displacement and promotes faster fracture healing. High remodeling potential is another characteristic of the children's bone tissue (Fig. 8.2).

A unique aspect of the pediatric long bones is the presence of an open physis, which, when involved in a fracture pattern, can lead to growth disturbances.

A. Ferreyra (✉) · V. Allende
Sanatorio Allende, Cordoba, Argentina

M. Sepúlveda O. (ed.), *Paediatrics Traumatology*,
https://doi.org/10.1007/978-3-031-89482-4_8

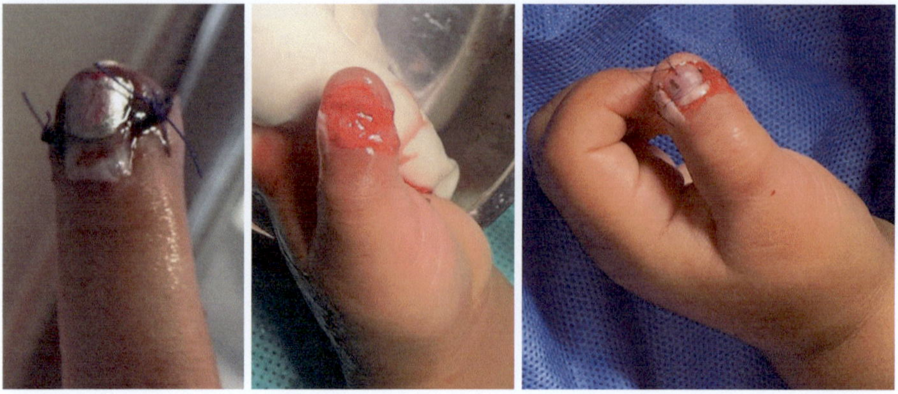

Fig. 8.1 Fingertip injury, with exposed phalanx fracture, nail disinsertion and damage to the nail bed, which required surgical debridment, nail bed repair and temporary replacement of the nail with sterile plastic

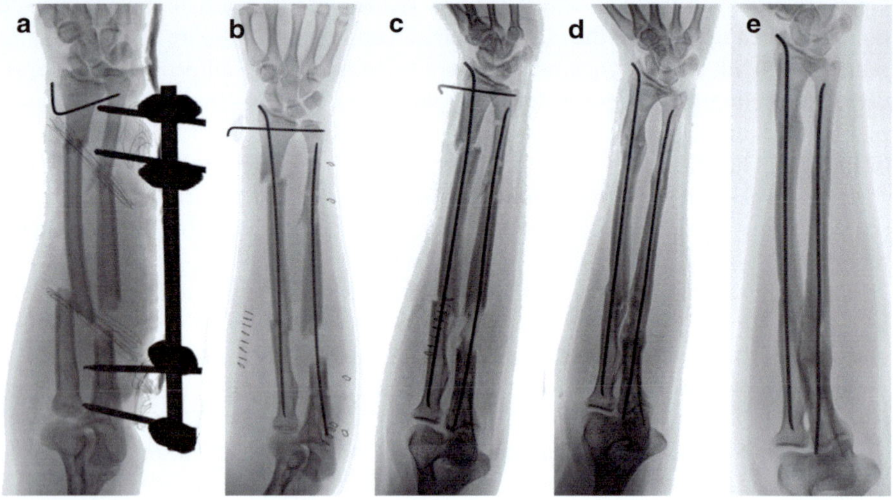

Fig. 8.2 Exposed forearm fracture in a 13-year-old boy, initially stabilized with an external fixator after wound debridement (**a**). In the second stage, periosteal repair was performed at the site of the bone defect (arrow), and stabilization was achieved with elastic nails (**b**). Initial bone formation is visible at 4 weeks after surgery (**c**), with solid bone at 4 months (**d**), and complete bone healing at 9 months (**e**)

8.2 Goals of Treatment

The primary goals of treatment are to prevent infection of the wound and fracture site, while allowing for soft tissue healing, fracture union, and ultimately restore the limb to its previous function [2].

8.3 Classification

The Gustilo and Anderson (GA) classification is widely accepted for defining the severity of open fractures. It is based on the wound size, the extent of soft tissue damage, and the fracture characteristics [1, 2, 6, 7]:

- Type I: Clean wound with a size less than 1 cm, simple fracture pattern, minimal soft tissue injury, and minimal contamination.
- Type II: Wound larger than 1 cm, moderate soft tissue crushing. Associated with transverse or oblique fractures. Skin grafts or flaps are generally unnecessary.
- Type IIIA: Adequate soft tissue coverage despite extensive soft tissue injury.
- Type IIIB: Extensive soft tissue injury with bony exposure, usually associated with severe contamination. Requires soft tissue coverage, such as skin grafts or flaps.
- Type IIIC: Any type of open fracture associated with arterial injury that requires surgical repair.

8.4 Treatment

An open fracture must be considered an orthopedic emergency due to the contamination increases the risk of infection, osteomyelitis, malunion, nonunion, and long-term disability [9].

Initial emergency management includes the administration of prophylactic antibiotic, coverage of the wound with sterile dressings, appropriate splinting of the segment, and tetanus toxoid administration, all carried out while currently stabilizing the patient.

Prompt antibiotic administration is crucial to minimize the risk of infection associated with open fractures and should be initiated as soon as possible [4, 9]. Infection rates are similar for patients in whom surgical debridement was performed within the first 6 h after injury, and those treated between 6 and 24 h after injury, provided that antibiotics are administered promptly [8].

8.5 Antibiotic Prophylaxis

For Type I and II Open Fractures, current evidence supports the use of first-generation cephalosporins against Gram-positive organisms. For Type III open fractures, aminoglycosides (e.g., gentamicin) are generally added to extend coverage. Although there is no clear consensus on prophylaxis against Gram-negative bacteria in Type III Open Fractures, evidence supports the use of this combination [4, 9].

The optimal duration of antibiotic prophylaxis remains controversial [4]. A 1-day course of antibiotics has a similar efficacy than a 5-day course, but studies exclude pediatric patients [10]. In general, the recommendation is 24–48 h of perioperative administration of antibiotics. Penicillin or one of its derivatives should be added for prophylaxis against anaerobic and Clostridium species prophylaxis, especially when dealing with soil-contaminated wounds or vascular injuries [9].

8.6 Debridement and Irrigation

There is consensus in the literature regarding the treatment of Type I Open Fractures on pediatric patients, with primary irrigation and superficial wound debridement in the emergency department [3, 9].

In contrast, Gustilo-Anderson Type II and III Open Fractures often require more extensive debridement (Fig. 8.3a, b), even as initial debridement should be more conservative in the pediatric population. Bone fragments with doubtful viability and scarce soft tissue attachments should be preserved because they may contribute on the fracture healing process [9, 11].

Traditionally, irrigation with saline solution has been recommended. The commonly accepted volumes are 3 liters for type I, 6 liters for type II, and 9 liters for type III injuries [5].

Singh [11], in a systematic review and meta-analysis of 1093 pediatric Open Fractures, reported a reduced risk of osteomyelitis, wound infection, and nonunion with nonoperative treatment across all Gustilo-Anderson types. They stated that, for grade III fractures, operative management did not reduce the risk of osteomyelitis or wound infection.

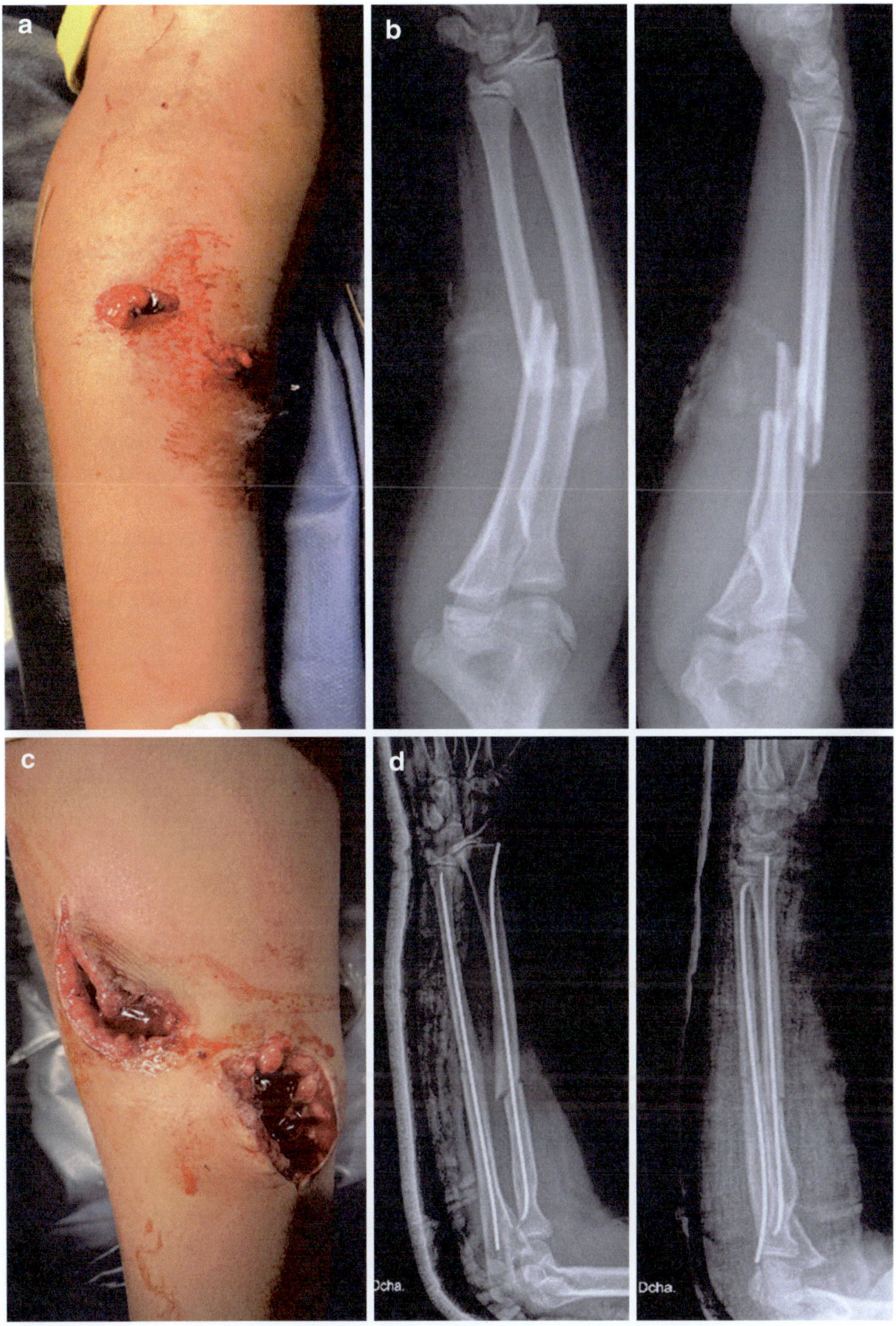

Fig. 8.3 12-year-old male who sustained a Gustilo Anderson type II open fracture of the forearm (**a**), following a fall from a horse. Initial AP and lateral X-rays of the forearm shows a displace fracture of the radius and ulna at the same level (**b**). (**c**) Soft tissue injury on the palmar aspect of the forearm was surgically enlarged for proper irrigation and debridement. (**d**) Postoperative radiographs following surgical debridement and internal fixation with elastic nails

8.7 Fracture Stabilization

Once the patient is stable, imaging studies such as X-rays, CT scans, or ultrasound are performed to guide treatment planning.

Fracture stabilization facilitates soft tissue management and should be considered simultaneously during surgical planning [1, 2]. While "damage control" orthopedics is well studied in adult literature, there is limited literature in pediatric patients [2]. External fixation provides safe and quick stabilization of fractures in clinically unstable patients and can even be performed in the intensive care unit (ICU) (Fig. 8.4).

This option is usually chosen for cases involving segmental bone loss, bone transport or significant soft tissue damage (Fig. 8.5). Care should be taken to reduce as close as anatomical as possible during the external fixator application since in some cases this will be the first and definitive treatment (Fig. 8.6).

Casts and splints could be suitable for some type I or II fractures with minimal soft tissue involvement but are generally inadequate for unstable type II and most type III injuries [2].

Distal forearm fractures can be managed with percutaneous K-wire pinning and a short-arm cast. Elastic endomedullary nailing provides sufficient stability for diaphyseal forearm fractures, allowing easy soft tissue dressing. These elastic endomedullary nails are also recommended for most open tibial (Fig. 8.7a, b) and

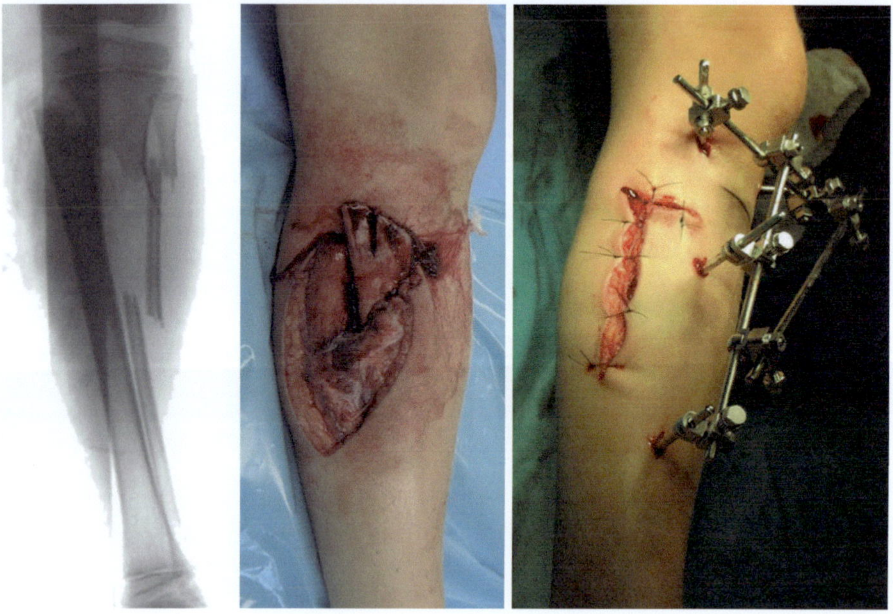

Fig. 8.4 Open fracture of the right leg in a 7-year-old girl. Surgical debridement and temporary partial wound closure, in addition to stabilization with an external fixator, were used for damage control surgery

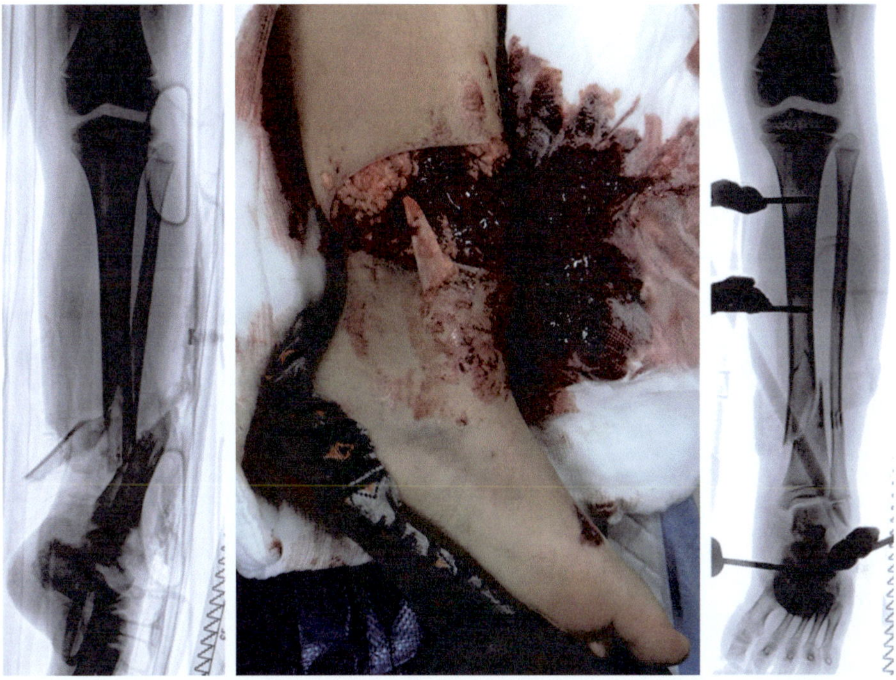

Fig. 8.5 Left leg open fracture in a 10-year-old boy, with significant soft tissue involvement. Surgical debridement and external fixation was performed, to allow adequate soft tissue management

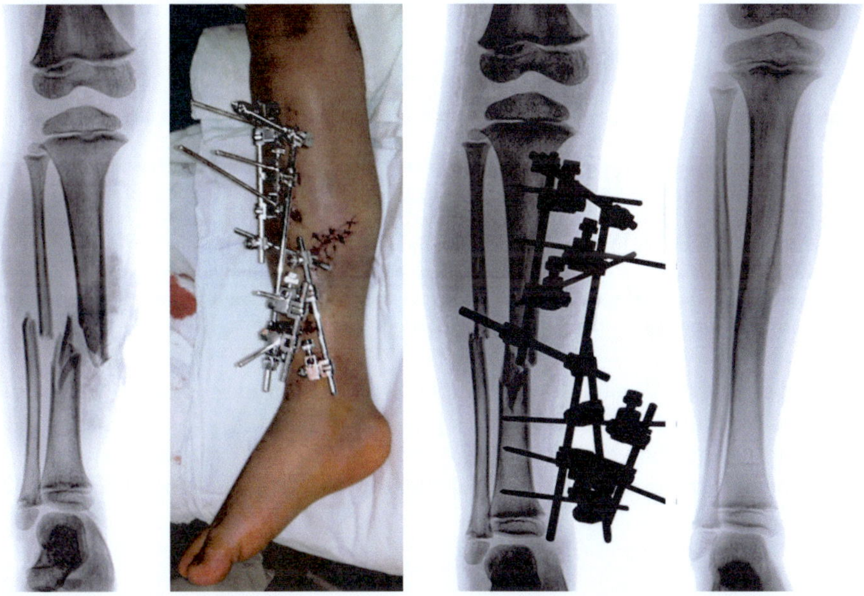

Fig. 8.6 Open fracture of the right leg of a 5-year-old boy. External fixation after appropriate surgical cleaning was the definitive stabilization of the fracture, without the need for other treatments

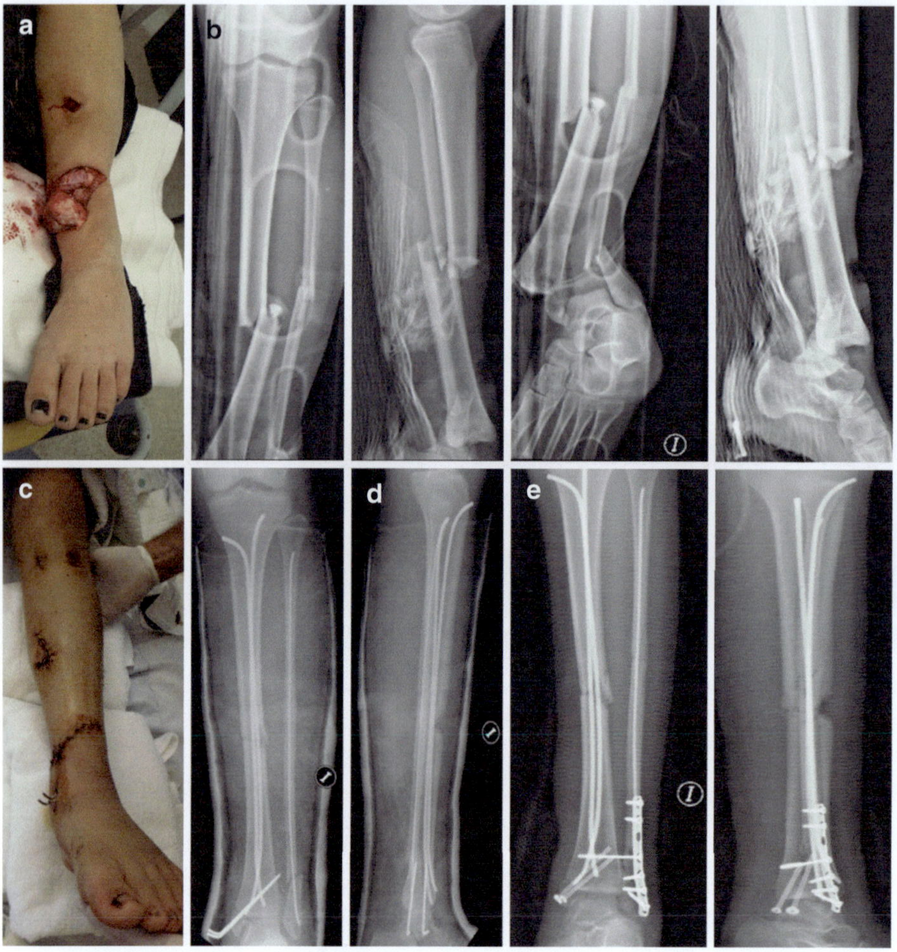

Fig. 8.7 (**a**) A 14 years-old girl, involved in a motor vehicle accident sustained a Gustilo Anderson type IIIA open fracture of the left leg, along with an ankle fracture-dislocation. (**a**) Significant soft tissue damage, with exposure of the tibial plafond. (**b**) X-rays of the fracture in both bones of the lower leg. (**c**) Closure of the skin following initial treatment, which included irrigation, debridement, and fixation with an elastic intramedullary nail. (**d**) Post-initial surgery X-rays show good alignment of the shaft but unacceptable fixation of the joint. (**e**) X-rays following open reduction and internal fixation of the ankle fracture-dislocation

femoral fractures. Wound care is simpler with this fixation method and is better tolerated by patients and their families [2].

For intra-articular open fractures, open reduction and internal fixation are the recommended treatments, with special attention to avoid damaging the physis [2].

8.8 Amputation

Open fractures that do not heal in adults, often heal satisfactorily in children. For this reason, efforts should be made to preserve the injured extremity in kids for most cases [2].

Wound management associated with Gustilo Type IIIB open fractures in children often requires muscle flaps, skin grafts or, in rare cases, amputation. These injuries presentat with a broad spectrum of severity, ranging from easily treatable to barely salvageable. The most used score is the Mangled Extremity Severity Score (MESS). MESS includes four factors: (1) the force of injury, (2) presence or absence of shock, (3) ischemia to the limb, and (4) age of the patient. A score of six points or less suggests that the limb should be salvaged, while a score of 7 or more is indication for amputation [12]. The utility of this scoring system, or any other scoring system, is further questioned given the major advances that have been made in the management of severely mangled extremities, including increased use of tourniquets, numerous new hemostatic agents, advanced tissue transfer techniques, novel vascular interventions, use of external fixators, advances in reconstructive microsurgery and bone loss management, such as induced membrane technique [12–15]. Lower extremity injury severity scoring systems should not be used as an absolute indication for early amputation in children. Using them as a strict indication would have recommended amputation in several limbs that were finally reconstructed [15]. The decision to amputate must be made on a case-by-case basis [12].

The vacuum-assisted closure (VAC) device is an alternative and effective method for providing an occlusive dressing for management of soft tissue defects, and has allowed wound closure without the need of a flap for defect coverage [16]. This method can also be used in conjunction with external fixation device for fracture stabilization.

8.9 Complications

Timing of antibiotic administration is a crucial factor in preventing infections in open fractures. As infections are the primary complication to avoid, antibiotic administration as soon as possible after injury is considered best practice [4].

Compartmental syndrome should be suspected in cases of high-energy trauma affecting the forearm or the leg and clinical status should be assessed periodically in these patients. The "3 A's" (increasing Analgesic requirement, Anxiety, and Agitation) are usefull indicators for diagnosing of compartment syndrome in the pediatric population. When suspected, open fasciotomy of all affected compartments should be performed urgently, and the wounds should be left open.

8.10 Final Message

Due to the scarcity of data regarding Open Fractures in the pediatric population, most recommendations are based on adult studies. Most treatment protocols recommend prompt intravenous antibiotic prophylaxis before operative intervention to decrease the infection rates. Initial management should include sterile dressing moistened with normal saline, and temporary fracture stabilization [5], if definitive fixation is not an option.

References

1. Weinstein SL, Flynn JM, editors. Lovell and Winter's pediatric orthopaedics. 7th ed. Lippincott Williams & Wilkins; 2014.
2. Flynn JM, Skaggs DL, Waters PM, editors. Rockwood and Wilkins' fractures in children. 8th ed. Wolters Kluwer Health; 2015.
3. Godfrey J, Choi PD, Shabtai L, Nossov SB, Williams A, Lindberg AW, Silva S, Caird MS, Schur MD, Arkader A. Management of pediatric type I open fractures in the emergency department or operating room: a multicenter perspective. J Pediatr Orthop. 2019;39(7):372–6. https://doi.org/10.1097/BPO.0000000000000972.
4. Pace JL, Kocher MS, Skaggs DL. Evidence-based review: management of open pediatric fractures. J Pediatr Orthop. 2012;32(Suppl 2):S123–7. https://doi.org/10.1097/BPO.0b013e318259f326.
5. Bhandari M. Evidence-based orthopedics. Chief editor: Blackwell Publishing Ltd 2012.
6. Gustilo RB, Anderson JT. Prevention of infection in the treatment of one thousand and twenty-five open fractures of long bones: retrospective and prospective analyses. J Bone Joint Surg Am. 1976;58(4):453–8.
7. Gustilo RB, Mendoza RM, Williams DN. Problems in the management of type III (severe) open fractures: a new classification of type III open fractures. J Trauma. 1984;24(8):742–6. https://doi.org/10.1097/00005373-198408000-00009.
8. Skaggs DL, Friend L, Alman B, Chambers HG, Schmitz M, Leake B, Kay RM, Flynn JM. The effect of surgical delay on acute infection following 554 open fractures in children. J Bone Joint Surg Am. 2005;87(1):8–12. https://doi.org/10.2106/JBJS.C.01561.
9. Aulisa AG, Marsiolo M, Basiglini L, Aletto C, Giordano M, Falciglia F. Management of open pediatric fractures: proposal of a new multidisciplinary algorithm. J Clin Med. 2023;12(19):6378. https://doi.org/10.3390/jcm12196378.
10. Dellinger EP, Caplan ES, Weaver LD, Wertz MJ, Droppert BM, Hoyt N, Brumback R, Burgess A, Poka A, Benirschke SK, et al. Duration of preventive antibiotic administration for open extremity fractures. Arch Surg. 1988;123(3):333–9. https://doi.org/10.1001/archsurg.1988.01400270067010.
11. Singh A, Bierrum W, Wormald J, Eastwood DM. Non-operative versus operative management of open fractures in the paediatric population: a systematic review and meta-analysis of the adverse outcomes. Injury. 2020;51(7):1477–88. https://doi.org/10.1016/j.injury.2020.03.055.
12. Venkatadass K, Grandhi TSP, Rajasekaran S. Use of ganga hospital open injury severity scoring for determination of salvage versus amputation in open type IIIB injuries of lower limbs in children-an analysis of 52 type IIIB open fractures. Injury. 2017;48(11):2509–14. https://doi.org/10.1016/j.injury.2017.09.010.
13. Loja MN, Sammann A, DuBose J, Li CS, Liu Y, Savage S, Scalea T, Holcomb JB, Rasmussen TE, Knudson MM, AAST PROOVIT Study Group. The mangled extremity score and

amputation: time for a revision. J Trauma Acute Care Surg. 2017;82(3):518–23. https://doi.org/10.1097/TA.0000000000001339.
14. Stein AM, Badina A, Pannier S, Saghbini E, Fitoussi F. Improvements in pediatric bone loss reconstruction with the induced membrane technique. J Pediatr Orthop. 2024;44:e748. https://doi.org/10.1097/BPO.0000000000002736.
15. Stewart DA, Coombs CJ, Graham HK. Application of lower extremity injury severity scores in children. J Child Orthop. 2012;6(5):427–31. https://doi.org/10.1007/s11832-012-0439-6.
16. Mayers A, Dunleavy ML, Chau MM, Hennrikus W. The vacuum-assisted closure device increases value in the treatment of Gustilo grade IIIb open tibia fractures in children. Cureus. 2020;12(9):e10194. https://doi.org/10.7759/cureus.10194.

Part II
Upper Extremity Trauma

Chapter 9
Clavicle Fracture

Martín D'Elía and Pablo Schaufele

9.1 Clavicle Fracture

Clavicle fracture is one of the three most common fractures presented during childhood, so the knowledge of its epidemiology, injury mechanism, treatment, and possible complications is of vital importance for the trauma surgeon, and even for the non-specialist doctor. Its most frequent location is in the diaphyseal segment, being in more than 95% of conservative treatment. In this chapter, we will address both classic and modern concepts, for its diagnosis and treatment.

9.2 Epidemiology

Clavicle fractures represent 8–15% of the general fractures in pediatric patients, which makes them one of the most common fractures in pediatric age. 63% occur in males and, if we only consider patients over 10 years old, this percentage increases to 77%. It is in this last age group where 30% of these injuries are concentrated [1].

M. D'Elía
Hospital de Niños Víctor J Vilela, Universidad Nacional de Rosario, Rosario, Argentina

P. Schaufele (✉)
Universidad de Concepción, Hospital Clínico Guillermo Grant Benavente, Concepción, Chile

M. Sepúlveda O. (ed.), *Paediatrics Traumatology*,
https://doi.org/10.1007/978-3-031-89482-4_9

9.3 Mechanism of Injury

In 85% of cases, the mechanism of injury is a fall on the shoulder or a direct blow. This is usually the result of a fall from the bed in infants and preschoolers, who begin to explore the environment or simply enjoy playing. In schoolchildren and adolescents, it is associated with injuries during sports practice, such as football and rugby, for example. In younger infants, who do not start walking, it is important to consider a non-accidental injury in the absence of an evident accidental traumatic mechanism.

According to the mechanism or energy of the trauma that causes the fracture, we can divide them into: (1) low energy (falls at ground level), (2) medium energy (direct blow in sports activity, fall on bicycle or skateboard); and (3) high energy (serious sports accident during the practice of football, hockey, skiing, snowboarding, all-terrain vehicle, motocross, and motor vehicle collision injuries). There are also fractures that occur during the birth process, where, due to a dystocic presentation or fetal macrosomia, they occur accidentally and/or directed by the medical team, to facilitate birth.

9.4 Anatomy

Morphologically, the clavicle is a long bone in the shape of an "S", with a medial epiphysis that leans forward, and a lateral epiphysis towards the back. Because the middle third of the clavicle is thin and devoid of muscular or ligamentous stabilizers, the fracture of this portion of the clavicle is the most common. Its muscular insertions, and therefore, the main forces that displace the fragments of the clavicle fracture, are the sternocleidomastoid in the medial fragment, which elevates it, and the weight of the body along with the pectoralis major muscle in the distal fragment, which make it descend (Fig. 9.1).

Functionally, the clavicle connects the axial skeleton with the thoracic limb, helps to support the weight of the upper limb, in addition to protecting neurovascular structures. It mainly participates in three axes of movement: (1) scapular antepulsion and retropulsion, (2) scapular elevation and descent, and (3) scapular rotation and rocking.

The clavicle is the first bone to start its ossification, at 5 weeks in utero [12]. Its medial physis contributes 80% of the growth of the clavicle, and its closure occurs between the ages of 23 and 25. According to the studies of Smekal and McGraw [2], at 10 years of age, the clavicle will have reached 80% of its total length. After this age, and until the closure of the physis, it will only change by 20% [3]. This would support the idea of the need for anatomical reduction in adolescent patients. However, recent studies affirm that between the ages of 12 and 25, the clavicle grows by 34% in males and 26% in females, which accounts for the remaining growth and remodeling in the final stage of skeletal development [4]. For this

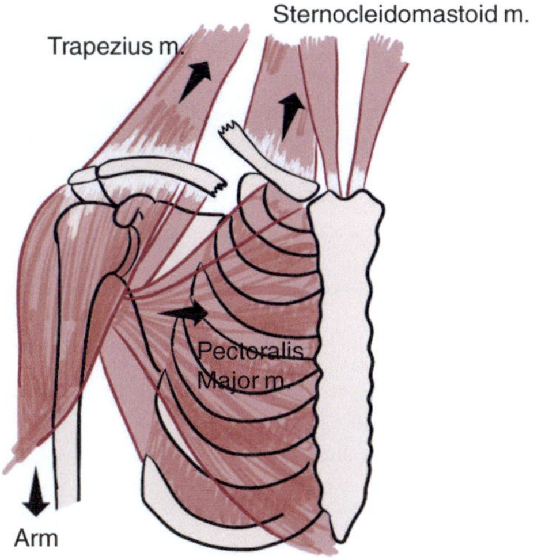

Fig. 9.1 Diagram showing the muscular forces that generate displacement of a middle third clavicle fracture

reason, management in adolescents remains in discussion, especially due to the good functional results of non-surgical management.

9.5 Diagnosis

The clinical scenario that accompanies this fracture is different between newborns and the rest of the patients. Newborns may present irritability due to pain, a very nonspecific symptom, but indicative of some alteration. In these patients, the Moro reflex is generally incomplete, even possibly absent, especially if the fracture is accompanied by a brachial plexus injury. This problem can be found in up to 10% of clavicle fractures at this age. It is for this reason that a neurological examination is vital in the newborn with this fracture. Given their scarce symptomatology, only about 11% are detected in the first neonatal evaluation, and only 50% have the diagnosis described at the time of hospital discharge. The remaining 50% are diagnosed around 2 weeks after the fracture, in the presence of the prominent bone callus (Fig. 9.2).

In older patients, localized pain is the cardinal sign, and increases when making shoulder movements or palpating the fractured area. There is an increase in volume mainly due to the deformity, due to the fracture hematoma, or due to the bone callus when the diagnosis is late. Patients may also present cervical tilt or head turns towards the fracture as a way to antalgically relax the sternocleidomastoid muscle. Bruising in the area is a late presentation and can be significant (Fig. 9.3).

Finally, bone crepitus, described in the literature, causes pain, so it is not advisable to look for it.

An important sign to evaluate in the presence of a proximal clavicle fracture with posterior displacement is difficulty swallowing or ventilating, and these are

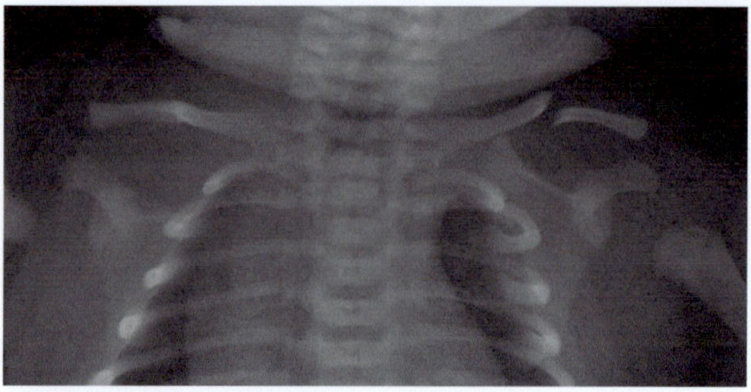

Fig. 9.2 Clavicle fracture in the middle third, 1 week old, in a newborn patient

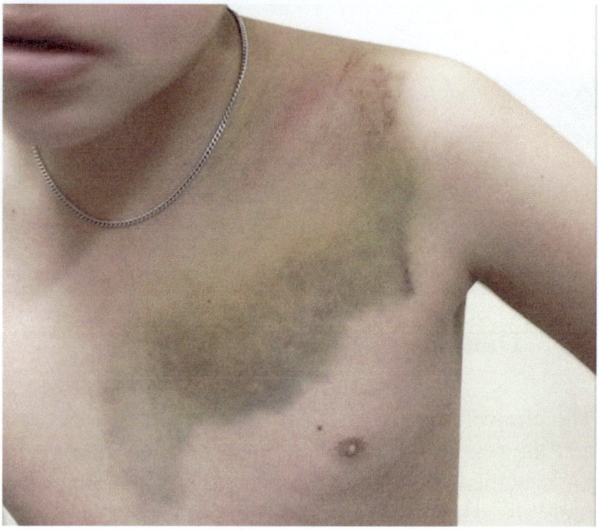

Fig. 9.3 Bruising 1 week after fracture of the left clavicle

indicators of the need for emergency resolution, with the support of a specialist thoracic medical team.

In relation to the diagnosis with images, usually the anteroposterior radiograph is sufficient to make it. However, other projections can provide details such as the cephalic projection, where the arm is placed in internal rotation and the X-ray beam is directed perpendicular to the coronal plane of the body.

The use of the apical lordotic projection is also described, with the patient in supine or standing position and the beam in a cephalic direction of 30°, at 1 m of distance; and the scapular axial projection, which is obtained with the patient standing or prone, with the anterior margin of the affected side rotated 30° to 45° towards the beam.

For fractures of the distal third, a weight-bearing radiograph (5 kg) in comparative anteroposterior projection can contribute to the diagnosis and management decision.

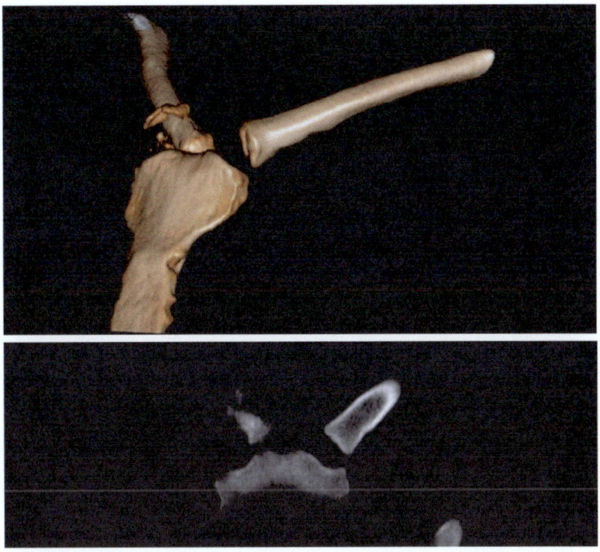

Fig. 9.4 CT scan of a 13-year-old girl with a clavicle fracture in the proximal third, Salter Harris type 2, with no evidence of ossification in the proximal epiphysis of the clavicle

For proximal clavicle fractures, the "serendipity" projection provides us with information in relation to the displacement of the clavicle. It is performed supine, a projection centered on the sternum, with a cephalic angulation of 40°. However, computed tomography (CT) is more useful and should be requested in every patient with this fracture (Fig. 9.4).

Finally, the use of ultrasound is an excellent option for the diagnosis in neonate patients, where ossification is scarce.

9.6 Classification

The most commonly used classification for these injuries is that of Allman (1967), who divides them into three types, numbering them according to the frequency of their presentation (Fig. 9.5). Thus, type 1, which corresponds to the fracture of the middle third, has a frequency of up to 85% in the original publication, but in our reality it is around 90%. Type 2 of this classification corresponds to the fracture of the distal third and would reach between 12% and 28%. Finally, the Type 3 fracture corresponds to the fracture of the proximal third, and its frequency would be between 3% and 6%.

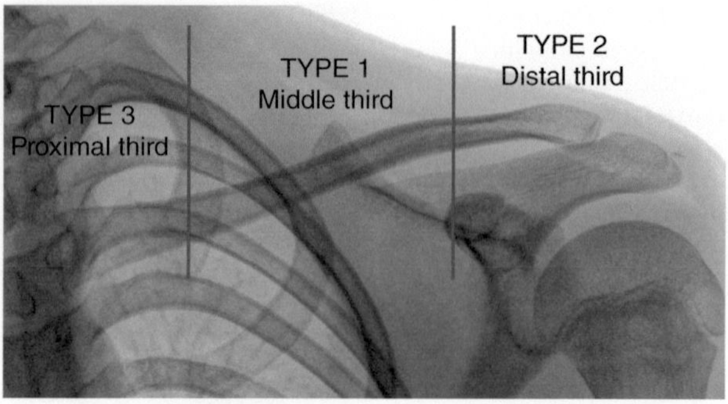

Fig. 9.5 Classification of clavicle fractures according to Allman

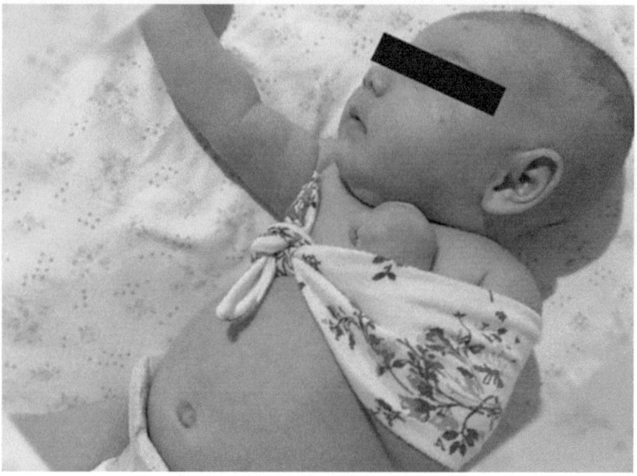

Fig. 9.6 Immobilization of the left arm in a newborn with a left clavicle fracture

9.7 Treatment

To define the treatment to be performed for these injuries, patients must be grouped by ages.

In the group of newborns, the Allman Type 1 fracture is even more frequent, close to 96% of the cases, so the treatment is non-surgically. Immobilization of the affected limb is indicated, attaching it to the chest, either with a simple adhesive cloth over the clothes or by securing it with a safety pin from the sleeve of the clothes to the chest area of it, for 7–10 days (Fig. 9.6).

In preschool, school-age, and preadolescent patients, with a Type 1 fracture, management is by immobilization with a sling for 3–4 weeks. In more restless children, a shoulder immobilizer sling can be used to ensure adherence (Fig. 9.7).

Other management alternatives described are the "figure eight" bandage or ring bandage, but they have fallen into disrepute due to presenting neurovascular complications, due to tension at the axillary level, and as there are no differences in the final result with the use of the sling.

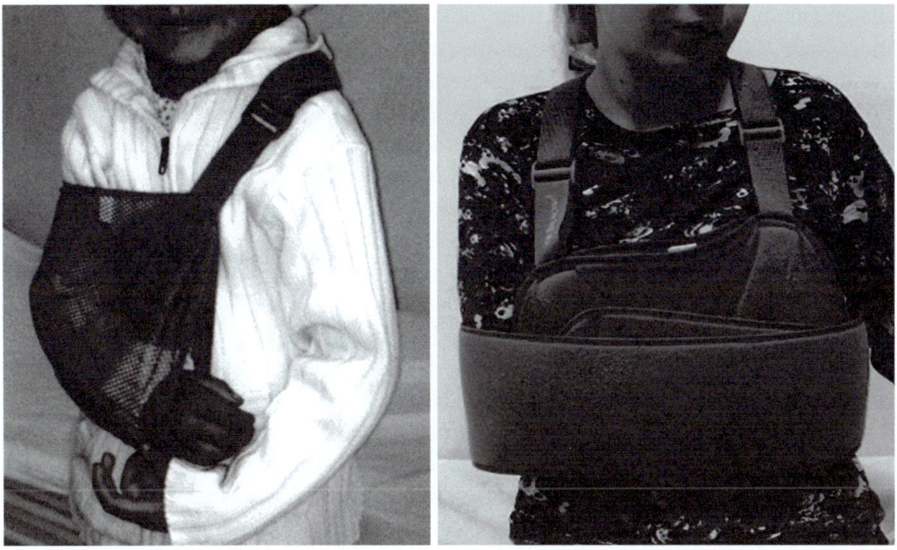

Fig. 9.7 Alternatives for the treatment of clavicle fractures. Simple sling and shoulder immobilization

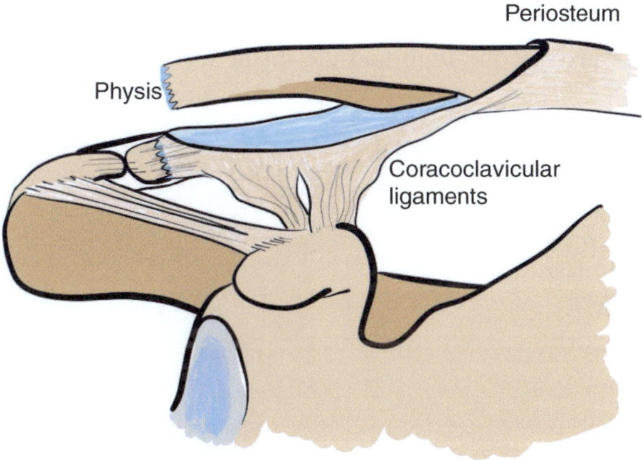

Fig. 9.8 Diagram showing the presence of periosteum with attached coracoclavicular ligaments in an Allman Type 2 fracture

In this same age group, for the management of Type 2 fractures, of the distal third, it must be taken into account that in them the thick and vascularized periosteum of the clavicle tears in the upper area, remaining attached to it the coracoclavicular ligaments below (Fig. 9.8).

In addition, these fractures are mostly metaphyseal or transphyseal, so, in the absence of radiological ossification of the distal epiphysis of the clavicle, they can be confused with an acromioclavicular disjunction, which is extremely rare in children under 18 years old. Therefore, before adolescence, these fractures are intrinsically stable, and their displacement usually does not reach 100%, which is why their management is conservative, similar to Type 1. However, in cases where there is more than 100% displacement when measuring the coracoclavicular distance comparatively from both shoulders, in a Zanca projection (supine position, AP projection centered on the acromioclavicular joint with a cephalic angulation of 10°), or the fracture is unstable, displaced posteriorly, or with risk of exposure, surgical treatment of them is recommended. This is carried out through an open reduction, closure of the torn periosteum, and fixation with a Kirschner wire (1 or 2), material that is left outside the skin at its lateral end, and is removed after 3 weeks (Fig. 9.9).

Another treatment alternative is closed reduction and percutaneous fixation with a Kirschner wire, or the use of a fixation system with sutures and a button, which keeps the clavicle in position while tissue healing occurs (Fig. 9.10).

For the management of Type 3 fractures or of the proximal third, it is essential to remember that most of these are Salter and Harris Type I or II fractures, since the epiphysis is fixed to the sternum through the sternoclavicular ligaments, so the force is dissipated through the weakest structure, which is the growth cartilage. Given its location, there is the possibility of damage to the neighboring thoracic structures, so it is advisable to perform a CT-scan for its evaluation, especially if surgical treatment is indicated.

If the fracture is very displaced anteriorly, it is recommended perform a longitudinal traction of the upper limb, while direct pressure is applied to the distal fragment of the clavicle, in a gentle manner. If, on the other hand, the displacement is posterior, it is suggested to have a thoracic surgeon at the time of performing the reduction, as their help may be required. The reduction is performed by traction on the axis of the limb and the distal segment of the clavicle with a Backhaus type

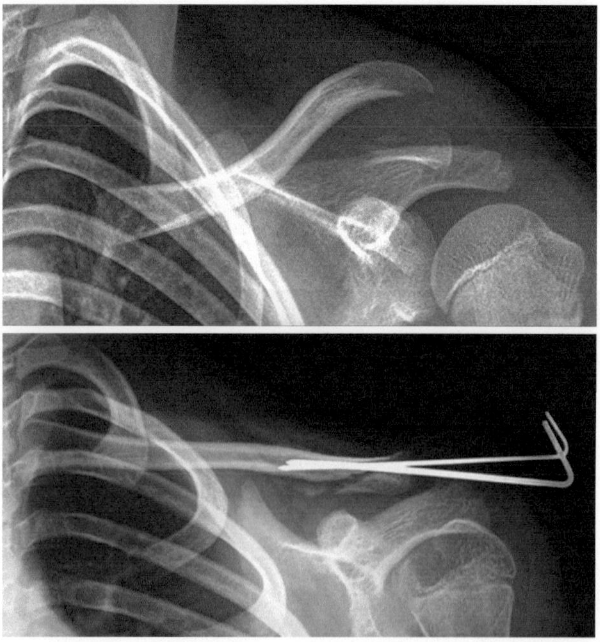

Fig. 9.9 Allman 2 clavicle fracture, treated with open reduction, periosteal repair, and stabilization with percutaneous Kirschner wires

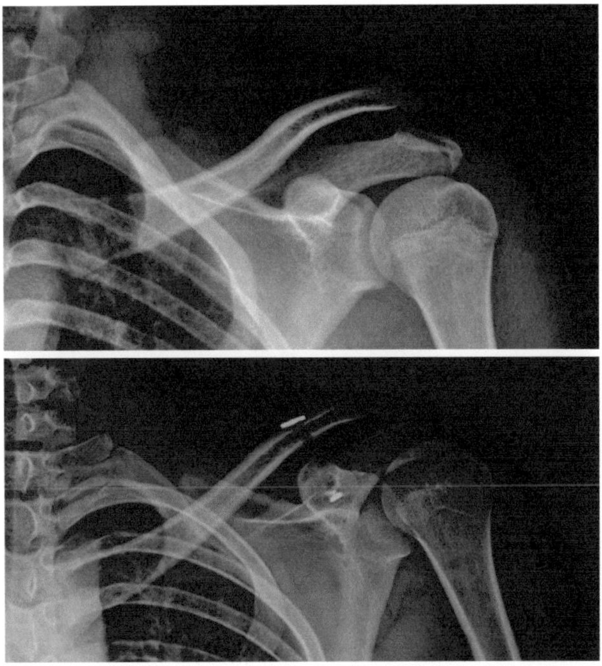

Fig. 9.10 Allman type 3 fracture, reduced with button and suture

clamp. After obtaining the reduction of this fracture, they are usually stable, so the limb is immobilized with a shoulder immobilizer sling for 3–4 weeks. If the reduction is not stable, transosseous sutures can be placed.

Traditionally, clavicle fractures in postpubertal adolescents have been treated conservatively [3, 5]. Surgical treatment was reserved for patients in the context of polytrauma, open injuries, skin compromise, or neurovascular injury, but the degree of displacement or shortening were not considered as reference. However, recent studies in adults report high rates of nonunion and biomechanical deterioration after non-surgical treatment of displaced and shortened fractures [2], which has been extrapolated to this age group. Cases with 20 mm or more of displacement would fall into the range of surgical option. However, studies by Schulz and Baeet [6] have suggested that even fractures with more than 15–20 mm of shortening are not associated with functional limitations in adolescents treated conservatively. Moreover, new research suggests that traditional measurement techniques may overestimate the actual displacement of the fracture, not taking into account their oblique nature. For this reason, the caudo-apical projection is recommended, with an X-ray tilt of between 20° and 40°, to perform an adequate evaluation and therapeutic decision. In addition, it should be considered that adolescent patients differ from adults in terms of remaining growth, remodeling potential and activity level. Therefore, any functional deterioration can be severe and have lasting consequences for the adolescent patient [3, 7], so all these biological factors, as well as aesthetic requirements, should be included in an informed treatment decision (Fig. 9.11).

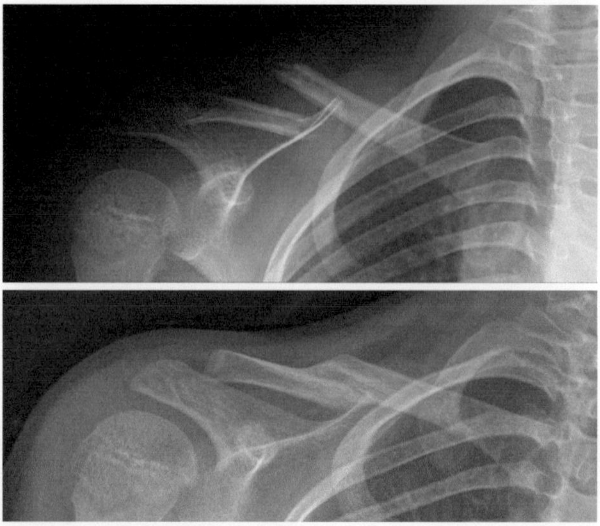

Fig. 9.11 13-year-old patient with displaced Allman type 1 fracture, treated conservatively. Favorable evolution can be seen after 3 months

McGraw [2] digitally analyzed chest radiographs of 961 individuals between birth and 18 year old, mapping the clavicular growth patterns. Constant growth of the clavicle for both sexes was demonstrated, from birth to 12 years old, at a rate of 8.4 mm per year. In addition, it was found that in girls the clavicle grew 2.6 mm per year after 12 years old, while in boys the annual growth was 5.4 mm after that age. In general, the clavicle reached 80% of its length at 9 years in girls, and at 12 years in boys. However, other recent publications show that the average growth of the clavicle significantly increases between the ages of 12 and 25, in both men and women. In these articles, for men the increase from 16 to 25 years described is 17.5 mm, which represents 10.6% of the total length of the clavicle. In women, the increase described from 14 to 25 years was 7.7 mm, which represents 5.2% of the total length of the clavicle. We then find that from skeletal maturity, until the closure of the secondary ossification center, growth was 17.5 mm in males (10.6% of the total length of the clavicle) and of 7.7 mm in females (5.2% of the total length of the clavicle) [5].

Understanding this potential for growth in length of the clavicle influences management decisions [5] and should be considered in the evaluation, along with the tolerable limits of fracture fragments displacement (shortening greater than 20 mm or angulation greater than 30°, risk of bone exposure due to prominence of the fracture fragments), taking into account the patient's functional requirement in their daily activities.

If a non-surgical treatment is decided, the use of a sling is recommended, which can be supported with a shoulder immobilizer for pain management. There is consistent evidence that the conservative treatment of isolated closed fractures of the clavicle shaft in adolescents is successful, with a low rate of complications, high rate of return to previous activity level and a high rate of union. The evidence is inconclusive to define which of the immobilization options is better, so one of the greatest comfort for the patient is recommended [2].

The indications for surgical treatment of the clavicle, despite there being no absolute consensus in the literature, are: skin damage above the fragments, angulation greater than 30° of the fragments, significant bone comminution, and shortening greater than 20 mm.

The option of surgical treatment should also be discussed in patients who perform high-demand activities with the upper limb, such as high-performance athletes who perform movements above the shoulder level, where functional alterations in their activity are described if the bone structures are not repaired anatomically.

For surgical treatment, the fracture can be fixed with a plate with screws, or with an intramedullary nail, preferably elastic endomedullary nails.

Fixation with endomedullary nails is a procedure that is recommended for wedge fractures, fragmented and angled in the middle area of the clavicle. For the other patterns, stabilization with plate and screws is preferred. The goal of treatment with endomedullary nail for this type of fractures is to achieve the anatomical reduction and then the internal splint effect with the intramedullary fixation. The shape of the nail maintaining that of the bone achieves the anatomical alignment. Shortening is avoided by the bone contact of the fragments. If the use of Kirschner wire for this method is decided, the limited size option, its limited flexibility to replicate the "S" shape of the clavicle and the high rate of complications described in the literature should be taken into consideration [8].

It is recommended to use the insertion by medial approach, or retrograde, in which through a medial anterior incision, 2 cm from the sternoclavicular joint, the perforation of the clavicle in its medial third is performed, inserting the nail from medial to lateral. This nail usually has a diameter of 2–3 mm. Special care must be taken in the narrowing of the medullary canal by the thinning of the clavicle in its lateral third, being able to perform the opening of the canal with a drill, and avoid perforating the lateral cortex. The reduction can be performed with reduction forceps percutaneously or through minimal incisions [9]. This configuration of the fixation presents a higher probability of skin irritation, so an adequate measurement must be taken prior to performing the procedure and a good impaction at the nail entry. The probability of major complications is very low (Fig. 9.12).

For the use of a plate with screws, the subclavicular approach is recommended to achieve good soft tissue coverage for the implant. During the surgical approach, the supraclavicular sensory branches must be identified and avoided from being

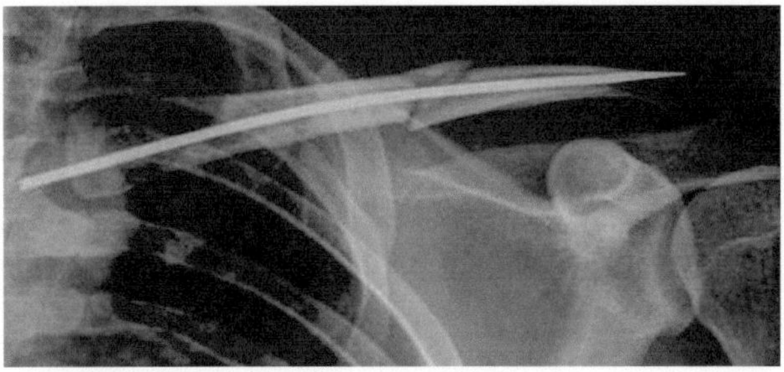

Fig. 9.12 Fixation of Allman 1 clavicle fracture with intramedullary nail, from medial to lateral

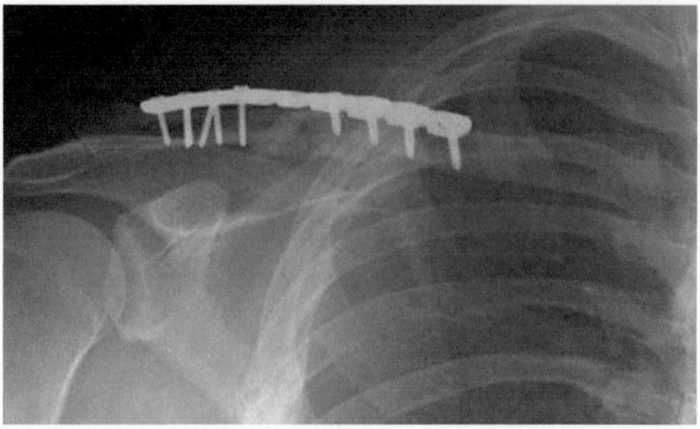

Fig. 9.13 Allman Type 1 clavicle fracture in a 14-year-old adolescent, treated with osteosynthesis plate with screws

damaged. It is suggested to always stay in a subperiosteal plane, so that this layer of tissue acts as protection for the neighboring neurovascular structures. The placement of the plate on the anterosuperior edge of the clavicle would have biomechanical advantages over the superior position, which would have greater secondary discomfort, usually requiring a second surgery for the removal of the implant (Fig. 9.13). Currently, there are anatomically contoured implants, with locked screws, with biomechanical advantages in comminuted fractures. It is recommended to use interfragmentary compression screws in oblique or comminuted patterns, and compression through the plate in transverse patterns. Implant removal is not routine, except for intolerance of the same for over 12 months after surgery [10].

9.8 Final Message

In summary, beyond the fact that the indications for surgical treatment are established in shortenings greater than 20 mm, angulations of the fracture greater than 30°, and skin tension over the displaced fragments, and the good results in the literature for conservative treatment, each case deserves a meticulous and detailed evaluation by the treating physician to balance the advantages and disadvantages of the decision in relation to functional demands, especially in pubertal pediatric patients and adolescents, a situation that is becoming more frequent today, with the aim that the patient and their caregivers make the best decision.

9.9 Authors' Advice

- The treatment of the vast majority of cases will be conservative, with excellent results, being only of surgical indication in exceptional cases.
- In case of requiring surgical treatment, the choice of intramedullary implant with elastic nail would have a good indication in comminuted fractures as it produces

the effect of internal splint by relative stability, the alignment, and length of the clavicle is recovered through fixation at the ends of the bone.

- In surgical treatment, the use of lateral traction on the axis of the bone and external rotation of the upper limb, or using percutaneous clamps or through minimal incisions, help to achieve reduction.
- The closure in a single plane that includes skin, cellular, fascia, and periosteum reduces the possibility of wound dehiscence in open fixation with plate.

References

1. Aliaga C, Henríquez E, Gómez A, Vásquez M, Schaufele P, Silva N. Functional and satisfaction evaluation in patients between 10 and 15 years old with overlapping diaphyseal fracture treated non-surgically. 54th Chilean Congress of Orthopedics and Traumatology. 2018. Santiago, Chile.
2. McGraw MA, Mehlman CT, Lindsell CJ, Kirby CL. Postnatal growth of the clavicle: birth to 18 years of age. J Pediatr Orthop. 2009;29(8):937–43. https://doi.org/10.1097/BPO.0b013e3181c11992.
3. McIntosh AL. Surgical treatment of adolescent clavicle fractures: results and complications. J Pediatr Orthop. 2016;36(Suppl 1):S41–3. https://doi.org/10.1097/BPO.0000000000000757.
4. Hughes JL, Newton PO, Bastrom T, Fabricant PD, Pennock AT. The clavicle continues to grow during adolescence and early adulthood. HSS J. 2020;16(Suppl 2):372–7. https://doi.org/10.1007/s11420-020-09754-8.
5. Hosseinzadeh P, Pokala N, Meyer Z, et al. Clavicles continue to grow beyond skeletal maturity: radiographic analysis of clavicle length in adolescents and young adults. J Pediatr Orthop B. 2020;29(2):195–9. https://doi.org/10.1097/BPB.0000000000000644.
6. Bae DS, Shah AS, Kalish LA, Kwon JY, Waters PM. Shoulder motion, strength, and functional outcomes in children with established malunion of the clavicle. J Pediatr Orthop. 2013;33(5):544–50. https://doi.org/10.1097/BPO.0b013e3182857d9e.
7. Gausden EB, Fabricant PD. Management of clavicle fractures in adolescents: a critical analysis review. JBJS Rev. 2018;6(9):e4. https://doi.org/10.2106/JBJS.RVW.17.00194.
8. Luo TD, Ashraf A, Larson AN, Stans AA, Shaughnessy WJ, McIntosh AL. Complications in the treatment of adolescent clavicle fractures. Orthopedics. 2015;38(4):e287–91. https://doi.org/10.3928/01477447-20150402-56.
9. Flynn JM, Skaggs DL, Waters PM. Rockwood and Wilkins' fractures in children. 8th ed. Philadelphia: Lippincott Williams & Wilkins; 2015.
10. Vander Have KL, Perdue AM, Caird MS, Farley FA. Operative versus nonoperative treatment of midshaft clavicle fractures in adolescents. J Pediatr Orthop. 2010;30(4):307–12. https://doi.org/10.1097/BPO.0b013e3181db3227.

Chapter 10
Proximal Humerus Fracture

Juan Fuenzalida and Humberto Galleano

10.1 Proximal Humerus Fractures

Proximal humerus fractures generally occur in adolescence, in relation to trauma during sports practices, by direct or indirect mechanisms. There is another group of fractures related to childbirth (obstetric trauma), or falls from the bed in preschoolers. Most of them correspond to Salter-Harris type I or II physeal fractures, and, due to the extraordinary growth and remodeling potential of the proximal humerus physis, they are mostly successfully treated with non-surgical methods, with excellent functional and anatomical results. We classify them according to their displacement by Neer and Horowitz. Surgical treatment is only indicated in fractures with severe displacements, and in children with advanced skeletal maturity.

10.2 Introduction

Proximal humerus fractures represent 2.2% of all pediatric fractures, and generally involve the proximal humeral physis, accounting for 3% of all physeal injuries in the pediatric patient. These fractures have their highest incidence between the ages of 11 and 15 years old, being four times more common in boys than in girls [1]. We see them related to moderate intensity mechanisms resulting from falls, direct

J. Fuenzalida (✉)
Hospital Luis Calvo Mackenna, Clínica Universidad de Los Andes, Clínica Indisa, Universidad De Santiago, Universidad de Los Andes, Santiago, Chile

H. Galleano
Universidad Católica de Asunción, Hospital de Especialidades Quirúrgicas Ingavi, Instituto de Previsión Social, Asunción, Paraguay

M. Sepúlveda O. (ed.), *Paediatrics Traumatology*,
https://doi.org/10.1007/978-3-031-89482-4_10

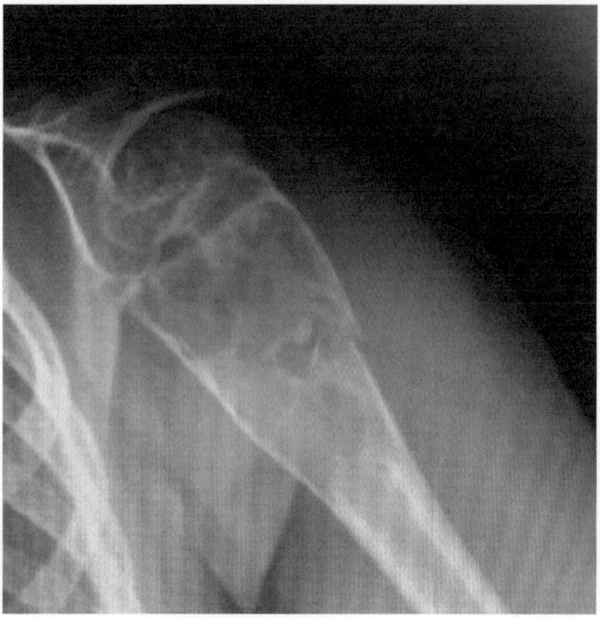

Fig. 10.1 Fracture in pathological bone. Fracture of the proximal humerus over an essential bone cyst

trauma during contact sports, gymnastics, bicycle falls, and high energy, such as traffic accidents.

This type of fracture in children under 2 years old continues to be important as an indicator of child abuse, being the second most frequently injured bone in these types of situations, so it should always be kept in mind when receiving a patient with this injury.

There is a group that is associated with fractures in pathological bone, due to the presence of tumors or bone cysts (Fig. 10.1), which should be considered in the diagnosis and for treatment.

The main method of treatment is immobilization with a sling or shoulder immobilizer, although, in fractures with severe displacement in older children, surgical treatment may be required [2].

10.3 Anatomy

The proximal epiphysis of the humerus is formed after the fusion at 7 years old of three independent ossification nuclei, the humeral head, which appears at 4–6 months old, the greater tubercle, which appears at 3 years old, and the lesser tubercle, which appears at 5 years old.

This physis maintains a high level of activity, so it is responsible for 80% of the longitudinal growth of the humerus, and reaches its definitive closure only at 16 years old, and sometimes up to 19 years old.

The glenohumeral capsule covers the entire articular surface and includes a large part of the medial portion of the proximal physis. In addition, the presence of a very thick periosteum, with ligamentous insertions in the area, provides great resistance and stability.

The muscles of the rotator cuff are inserted at the level of the epiphysis in the previously described ossification nuclei, and confer not only stability, but also the wide range of movement characteristic of this joint. The pectoralis major muscle inserts medially in the metaphysis near the physis, and the deltoid laterally, but more distally.

The fracture generally occurs proximal to the insertion of the pectoralis major and the deltoid, breaking the periosteum laterally to the proximal insertion of the biceps, which most of the time conditions the displacement of the diaphysis in adduction and towards proximal.

10.4 Injury Mechanism

The indirect mechanism that produces this fracture is a fall while trying to hold oneself up, supporting the hand on the ground, with the upper limb in extension, abduction, and external rotation of the shoulder. In the direct mechanism, the energy comes from a lateral or posterolateral direction at the shoulder or the upper part of the arm. Both situations require a moderate amount of energy to fracture the bone, as we see in typical sports and recreational activities of adolescence (gymnastics, contact sports, cycling, horse riding, etc.).

Due to the thickness of the periosteum in this age group, and the capsular and ligamentous insertions, most fractures of the proximal humerus are Salter-Harris (S-H) type I or II, the latter with a significant "Thurstan Holland" medial metaphyseal fragment, and generally are very stable. In addition, these particularities make shoulder dislocation associated with fractures an exception.

When the fracture occurs, the integrity of the medial and posterior part of the periosteum can make closed reduction difficult, due to interposition of this between the fragments.

According to Wolff's law, given the wide range of movement of the glenohumeral joint, and the great growth capacity of the proximal humeral physis, we can expect an extraordinary capacity for remodeling in proximal humerus fractures.

This stability, thanks to the components of soft parts, and the potential for bone remodeling, make it possible to treat these fractures conservatively, despite different degrees of displacement at this level, which are tolerable.

10.5 Diagnosis

In the newborn, the diagnosis is complicated by the absence of the ossification nucleus of the proximal humerus at this age, and it is given in the presence of a pseudoparalysis of the shoulder, after a dystocic birth, and after ruling out differential diagnoses such as shoulder septic arthritis, clavicle fracture, and obstetric brachial paralysis itself. On other pediatric ages, the diagnosis is based on clinical suspicion after a traumatic event, either direct or indirect, and after which functional impotence and pain around the shoulder are intense.

On physical examination, shoulder swelling is noted and bruising may be seen. When the fracture is very displaced, an anterior prominence around the axillary area becomes evident, which corresponds to the proximal metaphysis of the humerus. Both palpation of the area and mobilization of the joint are difficult to perform due to pain and local swelling.

With clinical suspicion, orthogonal radiographs should be requested in anteroposterior shoulder and axillary lateral projections, which are the most important for evaluating the fracture, in addition to a scapular "Y", not only to confirm the diagnosis and exclude other fractures around the shoulder, but also to classify it and decide the therapeutic approach (Fig. 10.2). Although most of the time all projections cannot be performed due to pain and functional impotence, we must insist on at least obtaining a good anteroposterior view that allows us to evaluate the glenohumeral joint, and an axial one to evaluate the axes.

The use of CT-scan or MRI are only indicated in the suspicion of more complex injuries, such as avulsions of the tuberosities, dislocations, suspicion of fractures in pathological bone, joint involvement, and very occasionally associated injuries (clavicle or elements of the scapula).

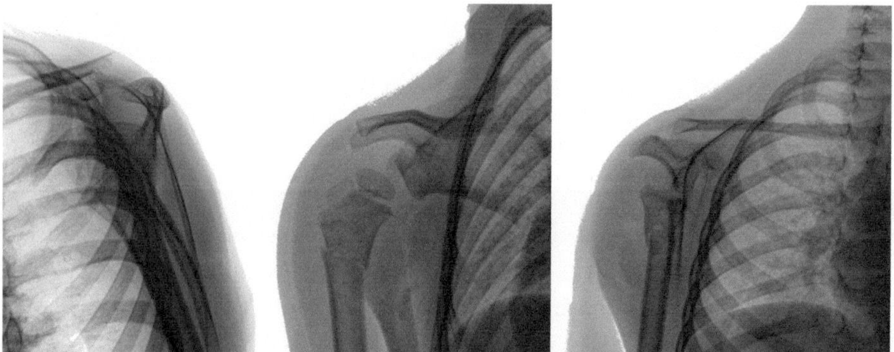

Fig. 10.2 Fracture of the proximal humerus in a 4-year-old child. Radiological projections scapular "Y", anteroposterior shoulder and anteroposterior shoulder in internal rotation

Ultrasound has been useful in cases of suspected fracture of the proximal humerus in the newborn due to the lack of ossification of the proximal humerus and for differential diagnosis of joint infections.

10.6 Classification

Proximal humerus fractures in children are classified according to the anatomical location in fractures of the physis, metaphyseal, of the trochin and trochiter.

Physeal injuries are classified according to Salter-Harris (Fig. 10.3). Type I are generally seen at early ages and in small patients. Most cases correspond to Type II, which are seen in teenagers, from the age of 11 years old. Type III or IV injuries occur rarely, in relation to severe and high energy accidents, as the great mobility of the proximal humeral epiphysis gives it some protection against this type of injury.

Neer and Horowitz classify these fractures based on the magnitude of displacement between the proximal portion and the diaphysis. Grade I have less than 5 mm of displacement; Grade II between 5 mm and 1/3 of the diameter of the diaphysis; Grade III between 1/3 and 2/3 of the diameter of the diaphysis; and Grade IV more than 2/3 of the diameter of the diaphysis.

The angulation at the time of classification does not modify it, although it can play an important role in decision-making, along with the bone age of the patient.

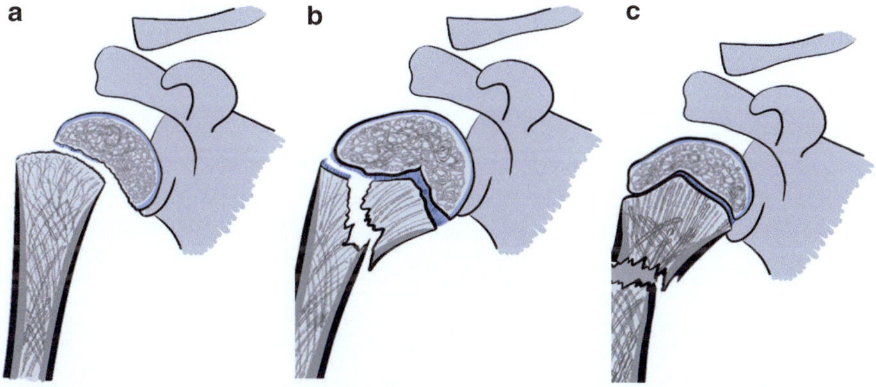

Fig. 10.3 Common traumatic injuries of the proximal humerus. (**a**) Salter and Harris type 1 fracture; (**b**) Salter and Harris type 2 fracture; (**c**) proximal metaphyseal fracture of the humerus

10.7 Treatment

The traditional initial treatment is non-surgical, due to the enormous potential for remodeling of the proximal humerus, and the thickness of the periosteum, which gives it stability. In addition, the characteristics of the great articular range that the joints in the upper limb allow to functionally compensate, making tolerable angulations and residual displacements in the proximal region of the humerus. The different non-surgical treatment options correspond to the use of a shoulder immobilizer or sling, bandage, or Velpeau cast, "U" splint associated with a sling, and hanging brachiopalmar cast. The fracture repair time is 3–6 weeks. By the third week there is stability of the fracture, and the immobilization can be removed, but not restart the sport yet. It is not a bad idea to use a sling in potential accident situations, such as school events and family recreational activities, removing the immobilization once you return to the controlled environment.

Simple immobilization, with the arm adhered to the body with a non-tension bandage, or the use of a safety pin that joins the sleeve of the clothes to the chest, to maintain in the position described, are sufficient for the treatment of a proximal humerus fracture in neonates. Do not forget to pad the armpit to avoid maceration. The repair produces an exuberant callus around the second week, from which no immobilization is necessary (Fig. 10.4).

According to the Neer-Horowitz classification, it can be suggested, for Grades I and II, conservative treatment, without attempt at closed reduction, at all ages, with the use of a shoulder immobilizer for 3–4 weeks. For Grades III and IV, an attempt at closed reduction is recommended to decrease pain and improve cosmetic deformity. In patients older than 10 years old, lesser remodeling potential is expected, with a correction of less than 30° in the axial axis. The reduction maneuver is performed after stabilizing the chest with a cinch that is held by an assistant,

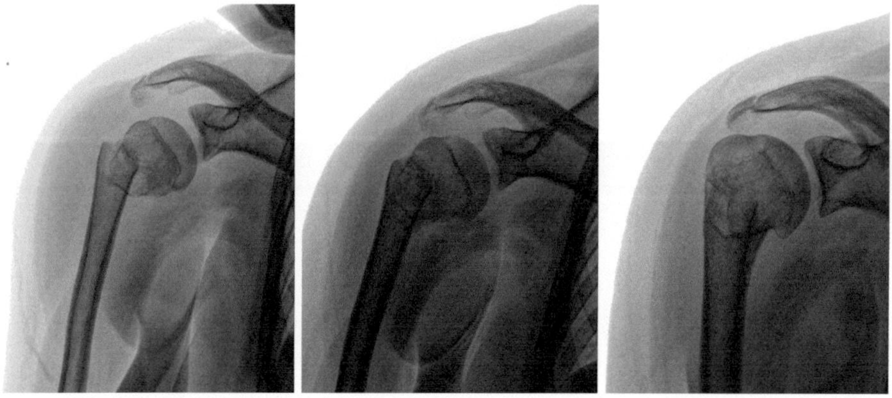

Fig. 10.4 Proximal humerus fracture in a 12-year-old girl. (**a**) Initial X-ray of the injury; (**b**) Radiographic control 1 month after the injury, where bone callus is observed; (**c**) Radiographic control 3 months after the injury

maintaining traction, abduction, anterior flexion and external rotation of the arm, under radioscopic vision. Many times the closed reduction can be difficult to obtain due to the interposition of tissues at the fracture, either from the periosteum of the humerus, the biceps tendon, the anterior portion of the deltoid muscle, and sometimes some comminuted fragment of the humerus.

There is currently no consensus in the literature about the absolute and relative indications for surgical treatment in fractures of the proximal humerus. Although in general, fractures with displacement in a skeleton that has little potential for remodeling (from 13 to 15 years) are considered surgical [3].

Dobbs suggests indications for surgical treatment in Grade III or IV fractures of Neer-Horowitz, according to age and degree of angulation: in patients under 7 years old and with angulation >75°, in patients between 7 and 11 years old with angulation >60° and in patients older of 11 years old with angulation >45°.

Other surgical indications are articular fractures (Salter-Harris III and IV), open fractures, neurovascular injuries, inability to achieve reduction and stability with closed maneuver, polytrauma (for better patient care), and neuromuscular diseases or paralysis, as they decrease the possibility of adequate remodeling [4].

Among the fracture fixation options we can find the use of Kirschner wires, elastic nails, cannulated screws, or plate and screws.

The reduction, either closed (Fig. 10.5), whenever possible, or open, when there is interposition of some anatomical structure, and subsequent percutaneous fixation with Kirschner wires, is a common treatment method. The wires are removed in the outpatient clinic, between the third and fourth week of the postoperative period.

The use of stable elastic intramedullary nailing technique, with flexible elastic nails, retrograde, requires more surgical time, greater blood loss, and often requires nail extraction in the future, but they allow less immobilization time and achieve greater stability.

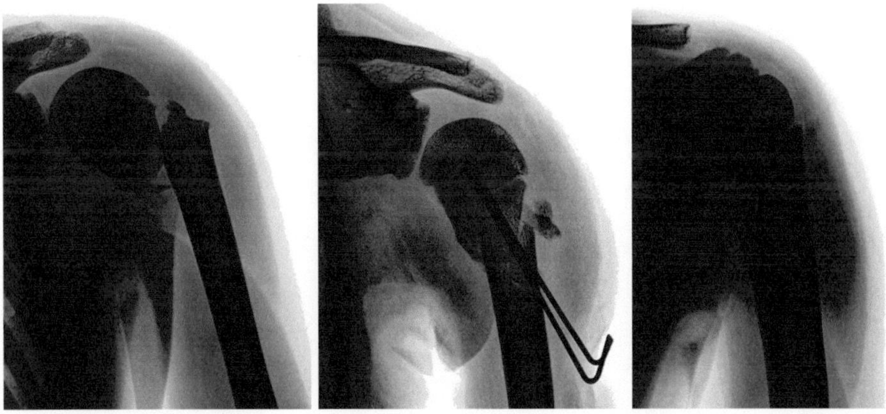

Fig. 10.5 (**a**) Radiographs of a 12-year-old boy with a displaced proximal humerus fracture. (**b**) Closed reduction and fixation with percutaneous Kirschner wires was performed. (**c**) Radiographic follow-up 1 year after the injury

Reduction and osteosynthesis with cannulated screws is used in fractures with a large metaphyseal fragment, which allows it. Finally, reduction and osteosynthesis with plates and screws is reserved for cases with mature skeletons very infrequently.

In case of requiring an open reduction, this is performed with the patient in dorsal decubitus, preferably in a "beach chair" position. A deltopectoral approach is performed, and an anterior arthrotomy, as needed, in the presence of intra-articular fragments. After the identification and removal of the anatomical structure that prevents reduction, usually the biceps tendon (Figs. 10.6, 10.7), the anatomical

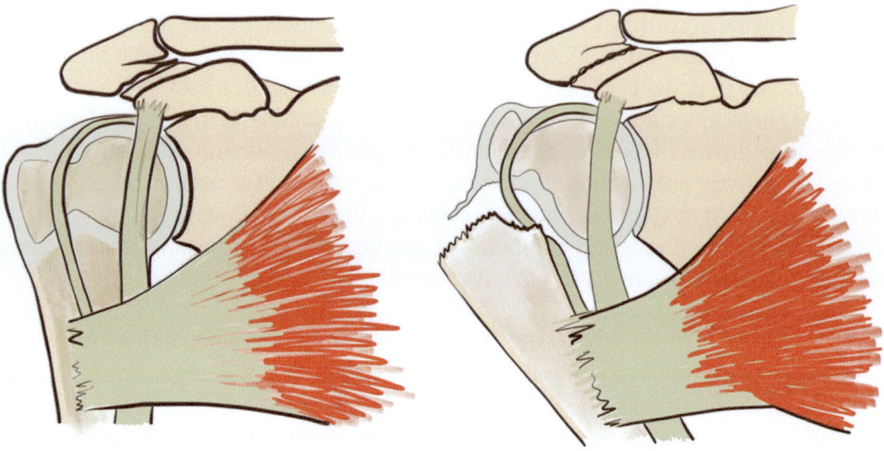

Fig. 10.6 Interposition of the biceps tendon at the level of the fracture site

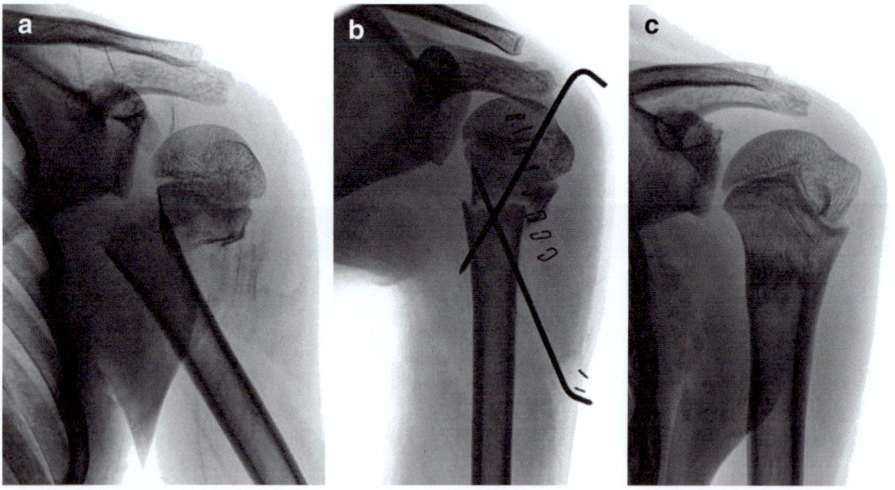

Fig. 10.7 Proximal humerus fracture (**a**), requiring open reduction because of soft tissue interposition, and posterior pin fixation (**b**). Follow-up at 6 months postoperatively (**c**)

reduction of the articular or metaphyseal fragments is achieved, and it is fixed with the chosen method. It is important to evaluate with orthogonal projection images to identify the possible intra-articular protrusion of the Kirschner wires and confirm the reduction [5].

10.8 Complications

Among the described complications, we find paralysis of the brachial plexus or peripheral nerve injury, which are usually related to the initial trauma. Do not forget the close relationship of the axillary nerve with the humeral neck on its posterior face.

We can also face a physeal injury, with shortening of the humerus, being up to 3 cm without functional repercussion, similar to a residual varus angulation, without major repercussion. Arterial injuries and humeral head necrosis are less frequent.

In the case of performing a surgical treatment, we can find infections in the path of the Kirschner wires, intra-articular migration of the same, fracture in its path, or acromial pinching caused by an anterograde wire positioning.

10.9 Special Situations

The fracture of the trochlea is generally an avulsion, either by overuse in repetitive throwing movements, or by a mechanism of external rotation force and adduction during a fall backwards, supporting the upper limb with the limb in extension, which produces a violent and sudden traction of the subscapular tendon. In the clinic, pain is evident with external rotation maneuvers of the shoulder. Axillary radiographs, along with the CT-scan, confirm both the injury and the displacement of the fragment. Conservative treatment with a sling is successful in non-displaced fractures, with surgical reduction, either open or arthroscopic, being the therapeutic option for those with greater displacement [6].

Shoulder dislocation associated with humerus fracture is very rare in pediatric age. It is mostly related to a high energy trauma. They are surgical injuries, looking for the dislocation reduction, either by closed or open means, then treating the fracture, according to the previously discussed criteria. Keep in mind that this injury significantly increases the risk of avascular necrosis of the humeral head, so we must follow these patients for a longer period.

The proximal humerus is an anatomical region where we can find fractures in pathological bone, due to simple bone cysts, aneurysmatic bone cysts, fibrous lesions, and sarcomas. Many times, simple bone cysts can heal spontaneously after a fracture, but not in aneurysmatic bone cysts. In the persistence of a simple cystic lesion after 3 months from the fracture, some treatment should be considered, whether curettage, graft, or tumor resection, with or without osteosynthesis. The risks or complications that this type of fracture presents include: refractures, physeal injuries, increase in lytic lesions, and recurrence of the cyst. In the suspicion of a malignant tumor, the patient should be referred to an oncological center, without intervening the fracture.

10.10 Final Message

The fracture of the proximal humerus in the pediatric patient is of low frequency. It should be suspected in direct or indirect traumas on the shoulder and upper limb. For its study, radiographs in two planes are usually requested. The most frequent treatment is conservative, with immobilization for a short period of time. Eventually, advanced images and surgical treatment with osteosynthesis are required.

References

1. Popkin CA, Levine WN, Ahmad CS. Evaluation and management of pediatric proximal humerus fractures. J Am Acad Orthop Surg. 2015;23(2):77–86. https://doi.org/10.5435/JAAOS-D-14-00033.
2. Shore BJ, Hedequist DJ, Miller PE, Waters PM, Bae DS. Surgical management for displaced pediatric proximal humeral fractures: a cost analysis. J Child Orthop. 2015;9(1):55–64. https://doi.org/10.1007/s11832-015-0643-2.
3. Pandya NK, Behrends D, Hosalkar HS. Open reduction of proximal humerus fractures in the adolescent population. J Child Orthop. 2012;6(2):111–8. https://doi.org/10.1007/s11832-012-0398-y.
4. Pahlavan S, Baldwin KD, Pandya NK, Namdari S, Hosalkar H. Proximal humerus fractures in the pediatric population: a systematic review. J Child Orthop. 2011;5(3):187–94. https://doi.org/10.1007/s11832-011-0328-4.
5. Herring J, Ho C. Upper extremity injuries. In: Herring J, editor. Tachdjian's pediatric orthopaedics. Philadelphia: Elsevier; 2014. p. 1253–8.
6. Samara E, Tschopp B, Kwiatkowski B, Vardar E, Lutz N, Zambelli PY. A single retrograde intramedullary nail technique for treatment of displaced proximal humeral fractures in children: case series and review of the literature. JB JS Open Access. 2021;6(1):e20.00119. Published 2021 Jan 25. https://doi.org/10.2106/JBJS.OA.20.00119.

Chapter 11
Humeral Shaft Fracture

Marco Morillo and Rodrigo Rivera

11.1 Humeral Shaft Fractures

Diaphyseal humeral fractures in pediatric patients are a low-frequency injury, representing 1 to 2% of all fractures in this age group. These injuries generally have a good prognosis, with good long-term functional outcomes and in the vast majority they are treated non-surgically [1]. However, in recent years, surgical management has been on the rise, especially in adolescent patients, where reduction and osteosynthesis have allowed excellent functional outcomes, with a quick return to daily and sports activities [2].

11.2 Epidemiology

Fractures of the humeral shaft in this age range are infrequent injuries, accounting for 1–2% of all fractures. They have an annual incidence of between 1.2 and 4.4 × 10,000, which corresponds to less than 5% of fractures in childhood. This injury has a bimodal presentation, with a higher frequency in patients under 3 years old and then in those over 12 years old. At an older age, it is predominantly related to accidents during sports practice [2, 3].

M. Morillo (✉)
Hospital Félix Bulnes, Santiago, Chile

R. Rivera
Hospital Dra. Eloísa Díaz de la Florida, Clínica Dávila Vespucio, Santiago, Chile

M. Sepúlveda O. (ed.), *Paediatrics Traumatology*,
https://doi.org/10.1007/978-3-031-89482-4_11

11.3 Mechanism of Injury

This fracture can be observed from newborn, with causes associated with the different ages of the child. In newborns, due to the adoption of different postures during childbirth, a fracture can occur due to hyperextension or rotation of the arm during passage through the birth canal, being associated with macrosomic newborns or in breech deliveries. In our experience, the evaluated cases are related to breech deliveries with shoulder retention, where the humerus fracture occurs when extracting the trapped limb [1].

In older children, it can be due to indirect impact, such as a fall with the upper limb extended, or direct, such as in traffic accidents or during play or sports activities. A mechanism that must be taken into consideration is non-accidental injuries, which implies a determined from the medical team to actively search for this cause. As the patient's age increases, sports accidents play a more frequent role. Finally, the fracture may be associated with structural bone alterations, such as pseudotumoral lesions, for example, a simple bone cyst (Fig. 11.1), malignant or benign bone tumors, osteogenesis imperfecta, and other metabolic disorders [1].

It is important to remember the characteristics of the immature skeleton, where it stands out as a growing system with the physis playing a fundamental role. Thus, the proximal humerus physis, the most active of this segment, contributes almost 80% of the longitudinal growth of this bone, so that fractures close to this growth cartilage have a great potential for remodeling.

Also, the presence of a thick periosteum provides greater stability, so that fractures typical of childhood, with incomplete fracture lines, can occur. It should be remembered that the radial nerve is close to the humeral shaft, as it runs through the

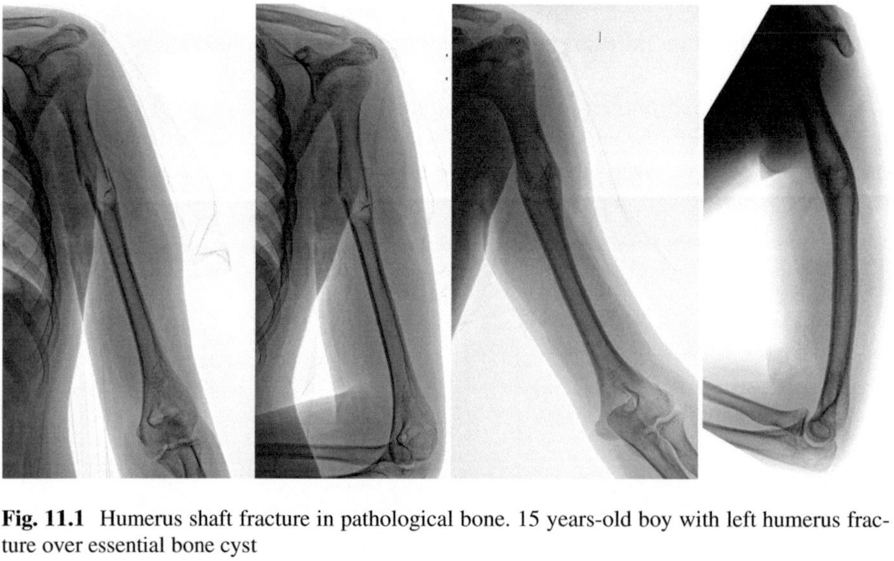

Fig. 11.1 Humerus shaft fracture in pathological bone. 15 years-old boy with left humerus fracture over essential bone cyst

torsion canal of the same, so it is not uncommon for damage to this neurological structure, both from the initial trauma and from reduction maneuvers and the surgery itself.

Finally, it is important to note that the arm has great mobility, especially given by the shoulder joint, so that minor deformities and residual shortening are easily compensated, with a low functional impact [2, 3].

11.4 Diagnosis

The clinical history plays a fundamental role, along with the physical examination and imaging studies, where the simple radiography is usually sufficient [1, 2].

In newborns, signs of a humerus fracture can be difficult to detect. The child may be irritable, or avoiding moving the affected arm, which is called "pseudoparalysis." It is necessary to know if there is a history of a difficult birth, fetal macrosomia, or difficulty in extracting the newborn. In these cases, a comparative imaging study with the healthy limb is very useful.

Older children can tell a story consistent with an injury to their upper limb and may present the classic signs of a fracture, such as localized pain, functional impotence, and even bruising and obvious deformity in this body segment. The doctor should perform a careful physical examination, from the clavicle to the wrist, comparing the affected limb with the contralateral one, avoiding overlooking concomitant injuries. It is important not to cause more pain to the patient, explaining the evaluation procedure to both the child and the parents.

For diagnostic confirmation, it is necessary to perform an imaging study. In most cases, a radiograph with projections in two different planes (Fig. 11.2) is sufficient. In the case of inconclusive radiological images, an ultrasound performed by an experienced radiologist can be useful to demonstrate a solution of continuity in the cortex or a subperiosteal hematoma. Computed tomography (CT) is useful in characterizing fractures in pathological bone, comminuted, or with articular extension. Finally, the study with magnetic resonance imaging (MRI) is reserved for cases with tumoral or infectious pathology. It should be considered that this study may require the use of general anesthesia, especially in younger patients.

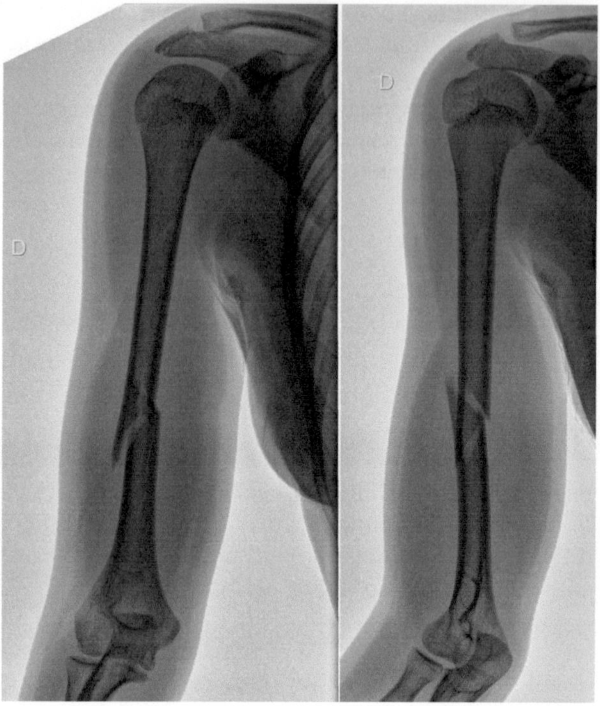

Fig. 11.2 Right humerus shaft fracture in a 13-year-old boy. Evaluated in anteroposterior and lateral radiological projections

11.5 Classification

Diaphyseal humerus fractures in children are descriptively classified according to their anatomical location: middle third, proximal third, or distal third. Since 2018, there is the AO classification of pediatric fractures, which is not widely used in the usual clinical setting, but rather descriptive for clinical studies.

It can also be described by the pattern type in radiographic images: transverse, short oblique, spiral, or comminuted (Fig. 11.3). It should be noted that spiral fractures have been identified in relation to accidents of small children with appliances, specifically vertical load centrifuges.

Another way to describe these fractures is in the category of open or closed, or it is present in a pathological bone. It is relevant to mention that if there is an ipsilateral forearm fracture, it is called "floating elbow," which will have implications for the treatment (Fig. 11.4).

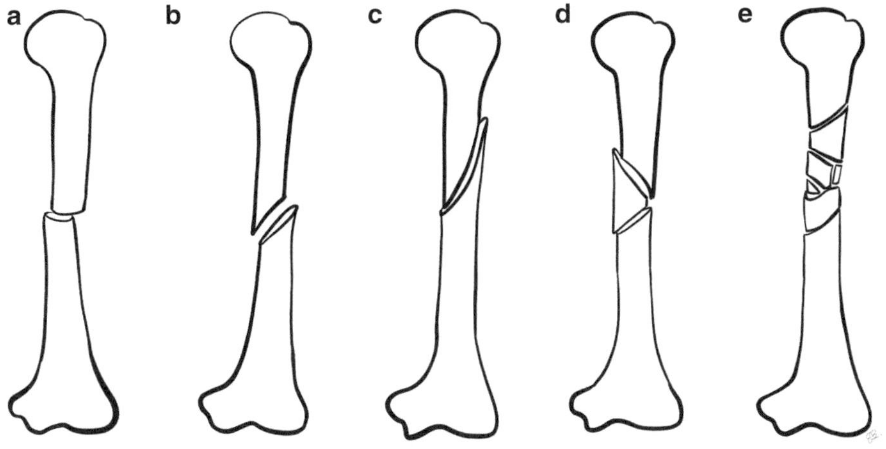

Fig. 11.3 Classification of humerus shaft fractures based on the description of the fracture pattern: (**a**) simple transverse; (**b**) short oblique; (**c**) long oblique or spiral; (**d**) butterfly fragment; (**e**) comminuted

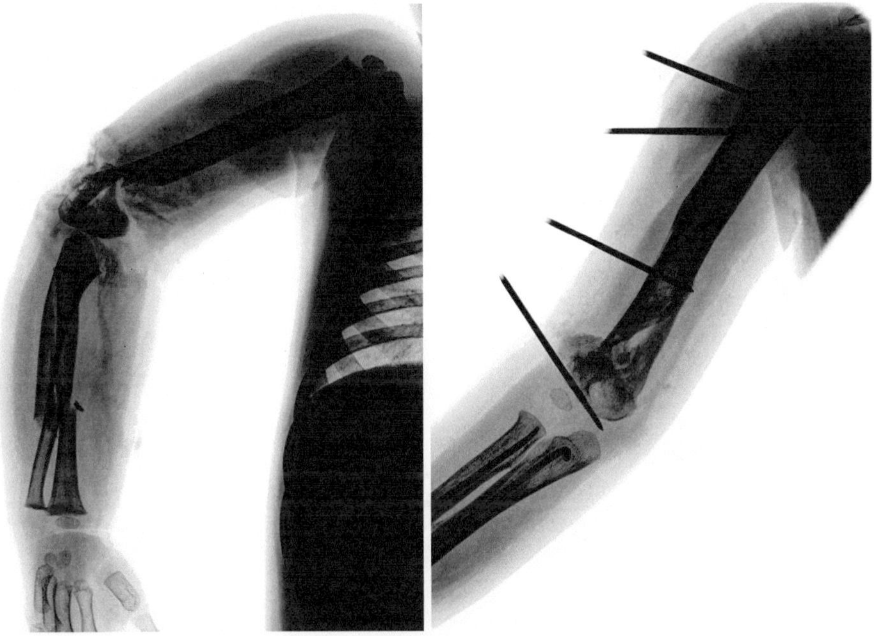

Fig. 11.4 X-rays of the upper extremity of a 4-year-old child, with a "floating elbow" injury: fracture of the humeral shaft and ipsilateral forearm, right. Treated with elastic stable intramedullary nailing to the forearm and an external fixator to humerus

11.6 Treatment Options

The treatment of these fractures is mainly non-surgical. It is essential to understand that the more proximal the fracture line is located in the diaphysis, closer to the proximal physis, the greater the potential for remodeling. Thus, displaced and shortened fractures up to 2 cm in this segment can be treated conservatively (Fig. 11.5).

There are multiple described immobilization options, which are used depending on factors such as the patient's age, their activity level, and associated conditions. In newborns, immobilization of the affected upper limb is sufficient, using regular clothing. In older children, shoulder immobilizers of size according to age are very useful, which allow their proper adjustment, and facilitate the patient's hygiene. In very active or restless patients, who have an unstable fracture, it is preferable to secure the immobilization with more rigid methods, such as plaster, either through a functional brace, or a hanging long-arm cast. Configurations such as the thoracobrachial plaster or the Velpeau type plaster are not commonly used today.

The surgical treatment of these injuries has an increase in its indication, especially in adolescent patients. It is indicated in open fractures, polytraumatized patient, bilateral fractures, floating elbow, fracture in pathological bone, vascular or neurological injury requiring repair.

Among the osteosynthesis alternatives to carry out the surgical treatment, we have the use of percutaneous Kirschner wires, endomedullary Kirschner wires, and elastic nails. Rigid nails require the physis to be closed to avoid complications in the growth zone, so they are reserved for special cases, mainly at the end of growth. Plates are indicated when it is necessary to approach the segment openly, for example, in the presence of an underlying condition in pathological bone, with the main

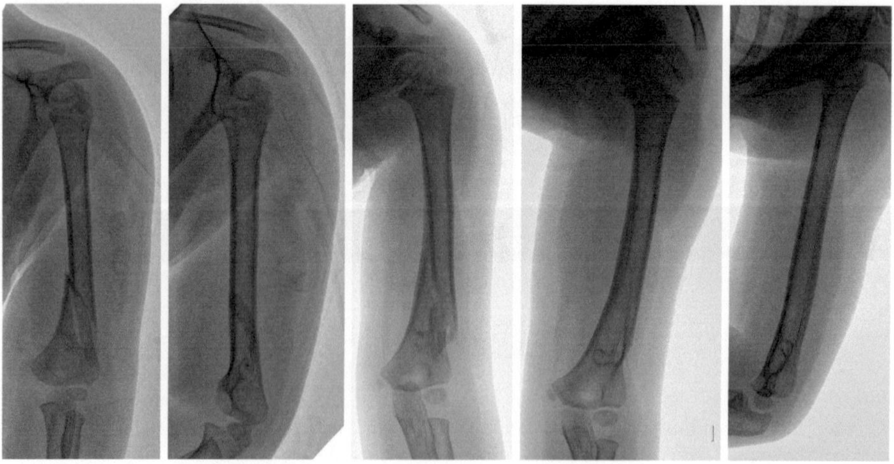

Fig. 11.5 Fracture of the left humerus in a 4-year-old girl, in which conservative treatment was performed. The evolution at 3 months and 1 year shows excellent result from conservative non-surgical treatment in these fractures

disadvantage of the loss of the fracture hematoma (Fig. 11.6). Another surgical possibility is the use of external fixation, especially in the case of open fractures, comminuted or with segmental loss [4–7].

Of all these osteosynthesis methods mentioned, elastic stable intramedullary nailing, either with titanium or steel nails, is the most used today for the surgical management of humeral shaft fractures in children. This technique has a low complication rate, is easy to learn, but requires the removal of the osteosynthesis elements in a second surgery, which must be explained to the parents and the patient. It can be carried out using an anterograde configuration, for managing distal third fractures, or retrograde, for stabilizing middle and proximal third fractures (Fig. 11.7). It is essential to respect the technical concepts of the method: nail entry at the same height, appropriate diameter (usually 30% of the medullary canal each), molding at the fracture line, and properly cut ends, under the skin.

Regarding rehabilitation in pediatric patients with surgically treated humeral shaft fracture, physiotherapy is recommended for early return to manual activities, through exercises of shoulder and elbow range of motion, fist strength, and pronosupination. Also, support with an occupational therapist for scar management can be of great help to avoid major aesthetic sequelae [8, 9].

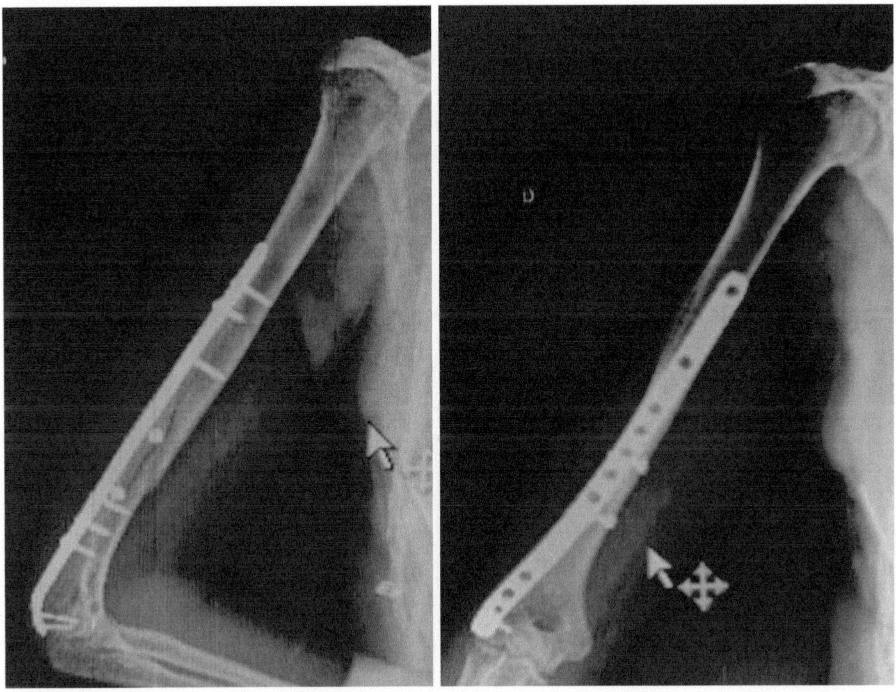

Fig. 11.6 Fracture of the right humerus of a 15-year-old boy, in whom surgical treatment was performed with open reduction and internal fixation with a plate

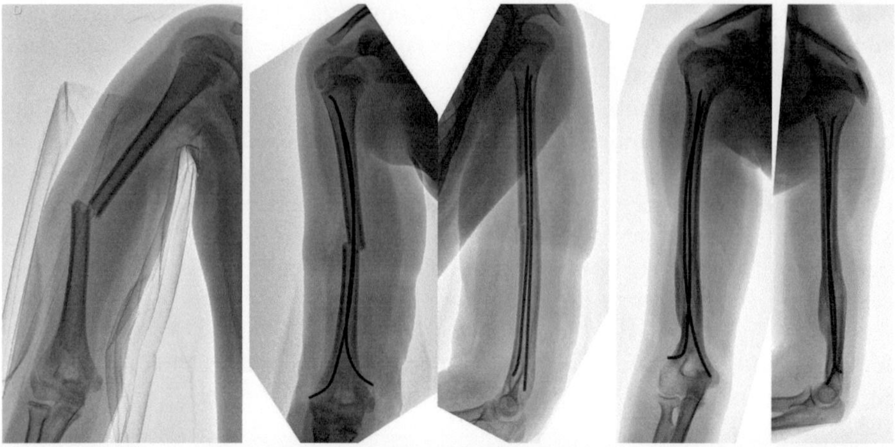

Fig. 11.7 Right humerus shaft fracture in a 12-year-old boy. Surgical treatment using elastic stable intramedullary nailing technique. It is observed the consolidation process after 4 months

11.7 Complications

Multiple complications are described in these fractures, but they are of low frequency in pediatric patients.

Among the most frequent we find radial nerve palsy. This is associated with a fracture of the distal third of the humerus that results in the entrapment of the radial nerve, called a Holstein-Lewis fracture. It has a good prognosis, as most of the time it corresponds to a radial nerve neuropraxia, due to primary contusion, at the time of the fracture, or secondary, during the reduction procedure. In the presence of a primary injury, observation is recommended for a period of 3 months. If no gradual recovery is observed, further study is recommended. In the presence of a secondary injury, the need for exploration will depend on what the surgeon did during the surgical procedure [10].

These fractures can consolidate with an axis alteration or shortening (Fig. 11.8). This is usually well tolerated in young children, due to the high degree of mobility of the limb.

Other less frequent complications are non-union, which is associated with open fractures that required surgical management, compartment syndrome, some associated vascular injuries, and infection, in relation to invasive management. Finally, cases of complex regional pain syndrome are reported, a complication that generally occurs in patients over 10 years old, without a clear cause, and that requires specific treatment with the rehabilitation team [11, 12].

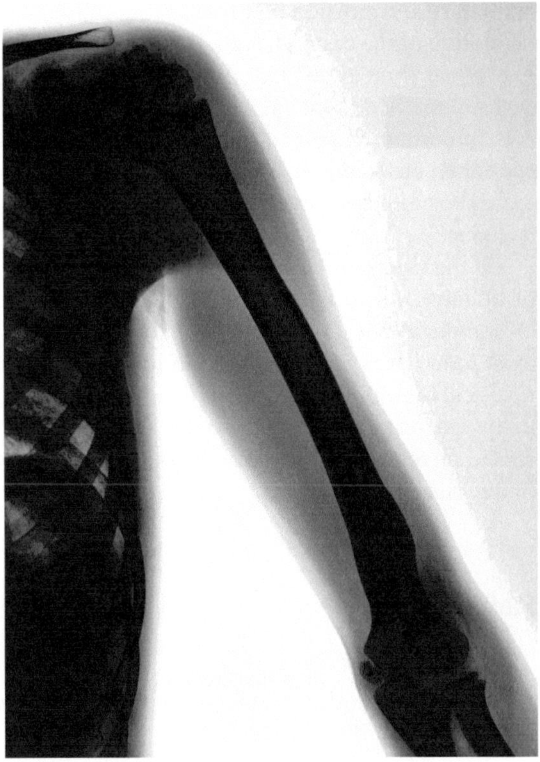

Fig. 11.8 Humerus diaphyseal fracture in a 10-year-old boy, consolidated in varus, in the process of remodeling

11.8 Final Message

Diaphyseal fractures of the humerus in children and adolescents are low-frequency injuries; however, it is important to recognize them promptly to start the appropriate treatment. Most cases require conservative treatment, with a variety of immobilization possibilities, which should be evaluated according to the patient's age, level of physical activity, parents' preference, as well as the possibilities for control and follow-up.

It is important to recognize the differential diagnoses in small children, where non-accidental injuries are of utmost importance. In these cases, there should be a specific protocol known by professionals to activate the social protection network as soon as possible.

11.9 Authors' Recommendations

It is essential to emphasize that the management of these injuries is preferably non-surgical, with functional immobilizations. This is because surgical treatment is constantly increasing, gaining more and more followers, especially due to the large amount of information and free access to it that parents have, who demand a quick resolution of the case. The aim is to avoid the use of rigid immobilizations with their functional limitations and associated discomforts, so it is understandable that the surgical method is the preferred by many specialists and also by parents. However, it is important to bear in mind that every surgical procedure has associated risks, economic costs, and usually the need for a second intervention for the removal of the osteosynthesis, situations that should be considered at the time of the treatment decision.

Of the osteosynthesis options available, the authors' recommendation is the use of titanium elastic nails, as it is a technique that is easy to perform, with a low rate of complications, and of lower cost compared to other osteosynthesis systems that exist today. It is recommended to remove these nails when the fracture consolidation is achieved, ideally before the year of operation, but not before 6 months, due to the risk of fracture. On the other hand, we believe that in adolescent patients with closed physis, solid locked nails are the best alternative, in centers with experience in their use.

References

1. Kraus R, Wessel L. The treatment of upper limb fractures in children and adolescents. Dtsch Arztebl Int. 2010;107(51–52):903–10. https://doi.org/10.3238/arztebl.2010.0903.
2. Ömeroglu H. Basic principles of fracture treatment in children. Eklem Hastalik Cerrahisi. 2018;29(1):52–7. https://doi.org/10.5606/ehc.2018.58165.
3. Hubbard EW, Riccio AI. Pediatric orthopedic trauma: an evidence-based approach. Orthop Clin North Am. 2018;49(2):195–210. https://doi.org/10.1016/j.ocl.2017.11.008.
4. Zhao CF, Gao QY, Zhang TJ, et al. Treatment of humeral shaft fractures in children with closed reduction and external fixation. Zhongguo Gu Shang. 2017;30(7):622–6. https://doi.org/10.3969/j.issn.1003-0034.2017.07.008.
5. Canavese F, Marengo L, Cravino M, et al. Outcome of conservative versus surgical treatment of humeral shaft fracture in children and adolescents: comparison between nonoperative treatment (Desault's bandage), external fixation and elastic stable intramedullary nailing. J Pediatr Orthop. 2017;37(3):e156–63. https://doi.org/10.1097/BPO.0000000000000843.
6. Marengo L, Rousset M, Paonessa M, et al. Displaced humeral shaft fractures in children and adolescents: results and adverse effects in patients treated by elastic stable intramedullary nailing. Eur J Orthop Surg Traumatol. 2016;26(5):453–9. https://doi.org/10.1007/s00590-016-1758-y.
7. Pogorelic Z, Kadic S, Milunovic KP, Pintaric I, Jukic M, Furlan D. Flexible intramedullary nailing for treatment of proximal humeral and humeral shaft fractures in children: a retrospective series of 118 cases. Orthop Traumatol Surg Res. 2017;103(5):765–70. https://doi.org/10.1016/j.otsr.2017.02.007.
8. Altintas B, Anderson NL, Boykin R, Millett PJ. Operative treatment of torsional humeral shaft fractures in throwers leads to an earlier return to sport: a survey of expert shoulder and elbow surgeons. Knee Surg Sports Traumatol Arthrosc. 2019;27(12):4049–54. https://doi.org/10.1007/s00167-019-05733-7.
9. Sahu RL. Percutaneous Kirschner wire (K-wire) fixation for humerus shaft fractures in children: a treatment concept. Niger Med J. 2013;54(5):356–60. https://doi.org/10.4103/0300-1652.122375.

10. Landry BW, Fischer PR, Driscoll SW, et al. Managing chronic pain in children and adolescents: a clinical review. PM R. 2015;7(11 Suppl):S295–315. https://doi.org/10.1016/j.pmrj.2015.09.006.
11. Weissmann R, Uziel Y. Pediatric complex regional pain syndrome: a review. Pediatr Rheumatol Online J. 2016;14(1):29. Published 2016 Apr 29. https://doi.org/10.1186/s12969-016-0090-8.
12. Abu-Arafeh H, Abu-Arafeh I. Complex regional pain syndrome in children: a systematic review of clinical features and movement disorders. Pain Manag. 2017;7(2):133–40. https://doi.org/10.2217/pmt-2016-0036.

Chapter 12
Humeral Condyle Fractures

Gino Martínez and Mauricio Silva

12.1 Humeral Condyle Fractures

Of all elbow fractures in pediatric patients, the lateral condyle fracture is the second most common, after supracondylar fractures, and represents between 12% and 20% of all upper limb fractures [1]. Generally, these fractures occur in children between the ages of 4 and 10 years old [1]. There are two mechanisms that can explain this fracture: a fall with the hand extended, the forearm supinated, and the elbow in extension (traction mechanism), or a fall in which the elbow suffers a valgus injury (impact mechanism) [1–3].

12.2 Classification

Multiple classification systems have been used to describe lateral humeral condyle fractures in pediatric patients, including the Milch [1], Jakob [3], Song [4], and Weiss [5] classifications.

The Milch classification [1] describes the anatomical location of the fracture; in type I, the fracture line is lateral to the trochlea and usually divides the capitellum; in type II (more common than type I), the fracture line extends medially and involves the trochlea, making the elbow unstable (Fig. 12.1a).

G. Martínez (✉)
Clínica Universidad de Los Andes, Santiago, Chile

M. Silva
Orthopaedic Institute for Children, David Gaffen School of Medicine at UCLA, Los Angeles, CA, USA
e-mail: msilva@mednet.ucla.edu

M. Sepúlveda O. (ed.), *Paediatrics Traumatology*,
https://doi.org/10.1007/978-3-031-89482-4_12

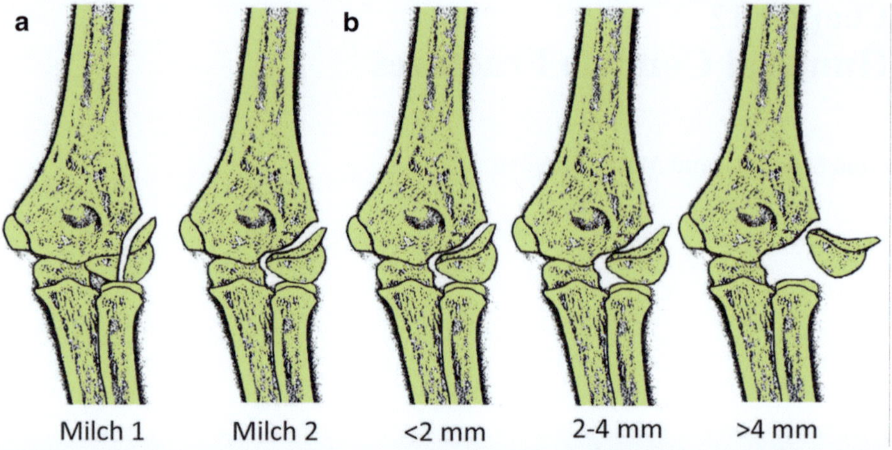

Fig. 12.1 (**a**) Milch's classification describes the anatomical location of the fracture; in type I, the fracture line is lateral to the trochlea; in the type II, the fracture line extends medially and envelops the trochlea, making the elbow unstable. (**b**) Weiss et al. describes a classification system based on displacement and congruity of articular cartilage: Type I, fractures have a displacement of <2 mm without alteration of the joint congruence; Type II fractures have a displacement >2 mm with a congruent articular surface; Type III fractures have a displacement >2 mm with an incongruent articular surface. (Orthopedic Institute for Children Image Bank)

Jakob [3] classifies fractures in relation to their displacement, with three specific types: non-displaced or type I, minimally displaced or type II, and completely displaced or type III.

Song [4] suggests a therapeutic algorithm for the management of lateral condyle fracture based on the radiological characteristics of the fracture, with a special emphasis on the internal oblique radiograph. Stage 1 fractures, those with a displacement <2 mm and a small metaphyseal fracture line, are generally stable. Stage 2 fractures, those with a displacement <2 mm and a solely lateral gap, may have compromised stability. Stage 3 fractures, those with a displacement <2 mm, but with medial and lateral gaps, are unstable. Stage 4 fractures have a displacement >2 mm, have no rotational component, and are unstable. Stage 5 fractures have a displacement >2 mm, have a rotational component, and are unstable. In general, he recommends surgical treatment for unstable fractures (Stage 3, 4, and 5). Recent studies have validated this classification, demonstrating high intra- and interobserver reliability [6].

Weiss [5] describes a classification system based on displacement and the congruence of the articular cartilage (demonstrated with arthrography) (Fig. 12.1b). Type I fractures have a displacement <2 mm without alteration of the articular congruence. Type II fractures have a displacement >2 mm with a congruent articular surface. Type III fractures have a displacement >2 mm with an incongruent articular surface. The authors recommend surgical treatment for fractures Type II and III, predicting fewer complications for fractures Type II. In general, patients with a fracture displacement between 2 and 4 mm benefit from an arthrography to determine the congruence of the joint surface and decide between a closed surgical treatment (no or minimal incongruity) or open (articular surface incongruity). Fractures with a displacement >4 mm are generally associated with joint incongruity and require a treatment that includes an open reduction. The Weiss classification system has been validated in the long term as a system that can predict the outcome of treatment [7].

12.3 Diagnosis

A patient with a fracture of the lateral condyle of the humerus usually presents with inflammation around the affected elbow. A bruise on the lateral aspect of the elbow suggests an unstable fracture, associated with a rupture of the brachioradialis muscle aponeurosis. The palpation on the lateral aspect of the affected elbow is painful, and it is possible to evidence a limitation of the elbow flexion-extension arc due to pain. It is important to examine the entire limb, including palpation of the shoulder and wrist, to be able to identify the presence of associated fractures. Similarly, it is important to perform a complete neurological and vascular examination of the affected limb, including the evaluation of motor and sensory functions of the hand, peripheral pulses, and capillary refill.

In general, the diagnosis of fractures of the lateral condyle of the humerus is made using simple radiographs. Three elbow projections should be obtained, including an antero-posterior, a lateral, and an internal oblique projection (Fig. 12.2). The

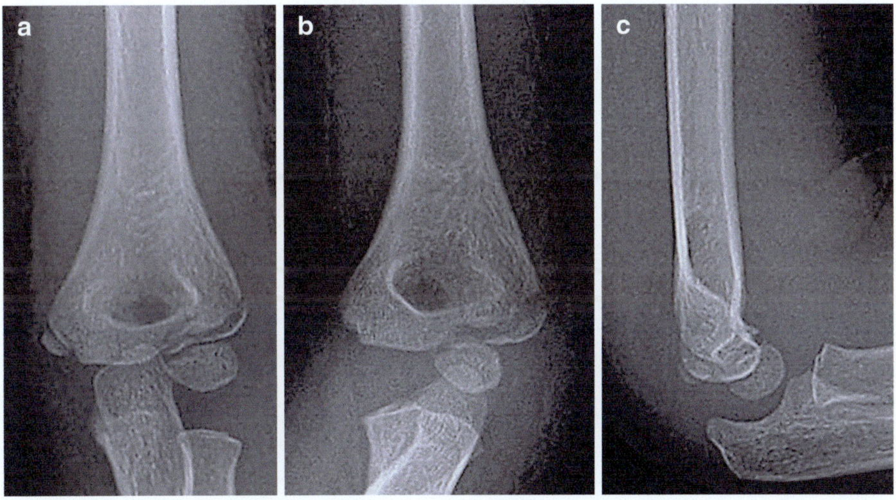

Fig. 12.2 The diagnosis of fractures of the lateral condyle of the humerus is performed using plain radiographs, including anteroposterior view (**a**), internal oblique view (**b**) and lateral view (**c**). The oblique internal view (**b**) provides a more precise assessment of the size of the fracture gap and the fracture pattern. (Orthopedic Institute for Children Image Bank)

internal oblique projection (Fig. 12.2b) provides a more accurate assessment of the size of the articular gap and the fracture pattern [8, 9].

The size of the fracture gap (or displacement) plays a determining role in the decision of the treatment to follow. This displacement is determined by the greatest distance (in millimeters) measured between the humerus and the fracture fragment in any of the three radiographic projections [10].

An additional factor in the decision of the treatment is determining if the lateral condyle fracture is associated with an elbow dislocation. This combination of injuries is rare (Fig. 12.3), but requires early identification to proceed to reduce the dislocation immediately and facilitate surgical treatment [11, 12].

In small patients, the distal humerus is cartilaginous and, therefore, cannot be visualized using simple radiographs. Arthrography can be used in these cases to help outline the articular surface involvement secondary to the fracture, and to determine the quality of the reduction, in cases where a closed reduction is chosen as treatment. Arthrography is obtained by injecting a contrast material into the elbow joint. This injection can be performed using a needle of a relatively large gauge (18 G) connected to a syringe through an extension. The anterolateral elbow portal or the posterior portal can be used. The contrast material should be diluted to 50% with saline solution. It is important to ensure (with a radiological image) that the needle is in an intra-articular position, before injecting a greater amount of the solution, to avoid extravasation of the contrast material. The extravasation of the contrast material makes it difficult to accurately assess the humeral joint surface. Once the intra-articular position of the needle is certain, a sufficient amount of the solution (2–3 cc) is injected. After the injection, the elbow is subjected to a full flexion-extension, which allows the contrast material to disperse uniformly within the elbow. The contrast material within the joint produces an outline of the distal humerus; in the presence of a displaced fracture, the material allows to determine the presence of gaps and/or articular steps.

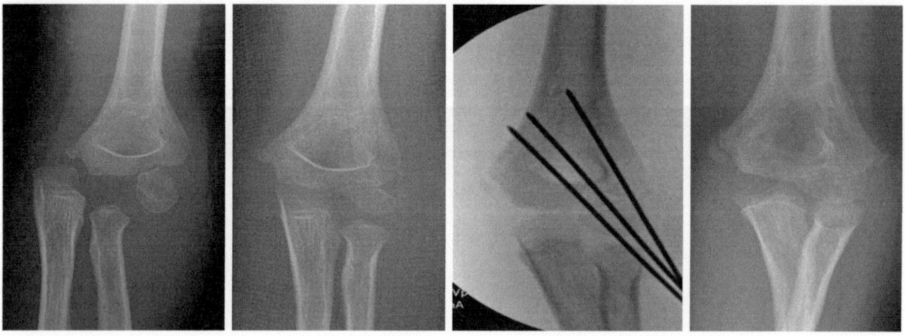

Fig. 12.3 Patient with a medial elbow dislocation associated with a displaced fracture of the lateral condyle. It is essential to make an immediate reduction of the elbow dislocation. Once the dislocation is reduced, the reduction and fixation of the fracture can be performed on a scheduled basis. (Orthopedic Institute for Children Image Bank)

In some cases, the use of advanced imaging may be useful to determine the degree of displacement of the lateral condyle fracture.

Computed tomography (CT-scan) allows a more accurate determination of fracture gap size, compared to simple radiographs. However, it is important to consider that it produces much higher radiation levels than simple radiography and may require the patient to undergo sedation. For these reasons, it is rarely used [13].

The potential advantage of magnetic resonance imaging is that allows for a precise evaluation of the integrity of the articular cartilage, especially in lateral condyle fractures with minimal displacement. Its use is not routine due to the need for sedation and associated secondary economic costs [14].

12.4 Conservative Treatment

In general, lateral condyle fractures with minimal displacement (<2 mm) can be treated without surgery, with a satisfactory clinical outcome [3–5, 14, 15]. Conservative treatment consists of immobilizing the elbow with a brachiopalmar cast, ideally with the wrist in extension and supination to relax the muscular insertions of the lateral condyle. It is important to evaluate the fracture with new radiographs obtained between 7 and 10 days after the application of the cast to ensure that there is no secondary displacement, which has been reported in up to 15% of lateral humeral condyle fractures treated non-surgically [16]. It is recommended to maintain the cast for a total of 4–6 weeks, after which it is removed, and progressive mobilization of the elbow is allowed, avoiding sports and contact activities for an additional period of 4 weeks.

12.5 Surgical Treatment

Surgical treatment is indicated in fractures with a displacement greater than 2 mm, with articular incongruity [4, 5, 10, 14]. Alternatives to anatomically reduce and fix the fracture include closed reduction with percutaneous fixation and open reduction with internal fixation. In general, closed reduction with percutaneous fixation, performed under general anesthesia, is indicated in fractures with a displacement between 2 and 4 mm. Open reduction with internal fixation is indicated for fractures with a displacement greater than 4 mm, or in those with an initial displacement between 2 and 4 mm in which closed reduction did not produce an anatomical reduction of the articular surface (Figs. 12.4, 12.5).

There is no general consensus on the type of fixation for these fractures. Traditional fixation includes the use of Kirschner wires introduced percutaneously, even though some authors recommend the use of compressive screws. Recent studies suggest that there are no major clinical differences between the two types of fixation (even though screws may provide greater compression on the fracture);

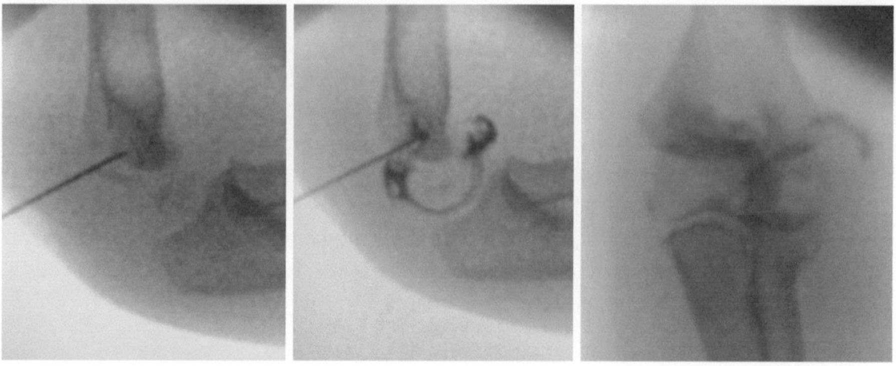

Fig. 12.4 Posterior elbow arthrography. Contrast is injected into olecranon fossa, intra-articular. In the anteroposterior X-ray projection, the integrity of the articular Surface can be evaluated

Fig. 12.5 Treatment algorithm based on Weiss classification

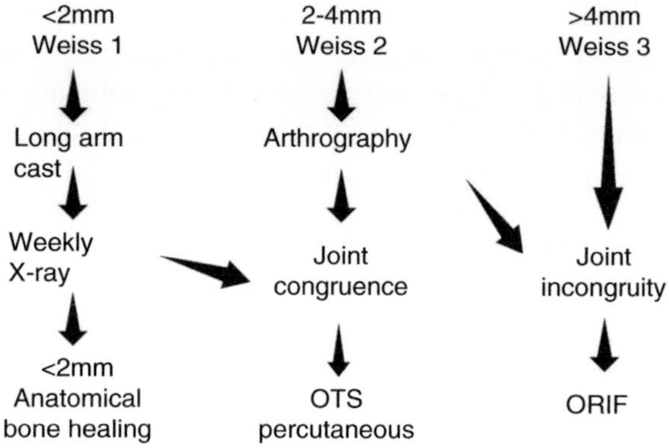

however, the use of screws requires a second surgical intervention to remove them [17–19].

Closed reduction and percutaneous fixation is indicated for fractures with a displacement between 2 and 4 mm. It consists of reducing the fracture by a mechanism of elbow flexion, forearm pronation, and direct compression on the lateral condyle, followed by percutaneous fixation using Kirschner wires (1.6 mm diameter). In some cases, the wires can be used to guide the reduction. In these cases, they are inserted only in the fracture fragment and are used as a lever to manipulate the fragment and facilitate the reduction. Ideally, 2–3 divergent wires should be used (ideally with a divergence greater than 60°), with their entry point in the lateral and distal portion of the fracture fragment, obtaining a bi-cortical fixation [20]. The goal is to obtain a stable fixation of the fracture with a residual displacement less than 2 mm. The quality of the fracture reduction can be evaluated using fluoroscopic images; however, accurate assessment of the integrity of the joint surface is essential and requires the use of arthrography. Generally, it is advisable to perform arthrography after the fracture has been percutaneously fixed. The contrast liquid within the joint allows confirmation that the articular surface is congruent, without the presence of residual steps (Fig. 12.6). Recent studies have questioned the utility of arthrography in the management of lateral condyle fractures that have undergone closed reduction and percutaneous fixation, indicating that the outcome of arthrography does not alter surgical management in fractures managed with this protocol [21, 22].

Open reduction and internal fixation is used in fractures with displacement greater than 4 mm. With the patient in a supine position on a regular surgical table, the affected elbow can be positioned over the C-arm of the fluoroscopy device (Fig. 12.7a), or over a lateral extension table (Fig. 12.7b).

A tourniquet should be applied to the affected arm, ensuring to use an appropriate size, which allows the most distal portion of the arm to be free. A lateral approach to the elbow is made with a 4–5 cm incision, centered over the lateral condyle, extending towards the radial head. Once the skin, subcutaneous tissue, and superficial fascia have been dissected, it is common to find that the interval of deep dissection that has been created by a defect in the musculature that connects directly with the fracture.

The insertion of the musculature into the fracture fragment should only be elevated in its anterior portion, avoiding any dissection in the posterior aspect of the fragment to avoid damage to its vascularization. The anterior capsule of the elbow is dissected to expose the joint surface of the fracture fragment. The periosteum of the proximal fragment can be carefully elevated from lateral to medial to facilitate visualization of the fracture and its reduction. Once the fracture is fully exposed, and the hematoma has been completely drained, the fracture is

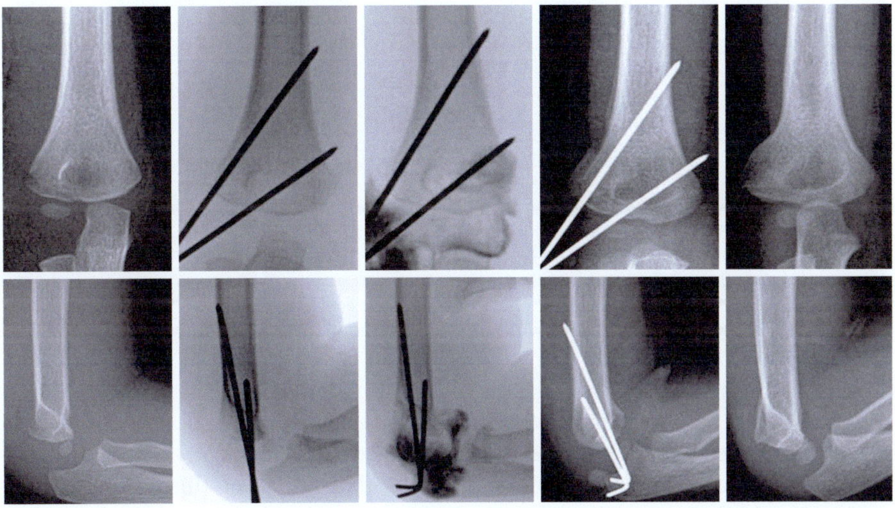

Fig. 12.6 X-rays of a patient with a fracture of the lateral condyle with a displacement of approximately 3 mm. The patient is subjected to closed reduction with percutaneous fixation using Kirschner wires. Once stable fixation is achieved, arthrography is performed to determine that the articular surface is congruent, without the presence from gaps to residual joint steps. (Orthopedic Institute for Children Image Bank)

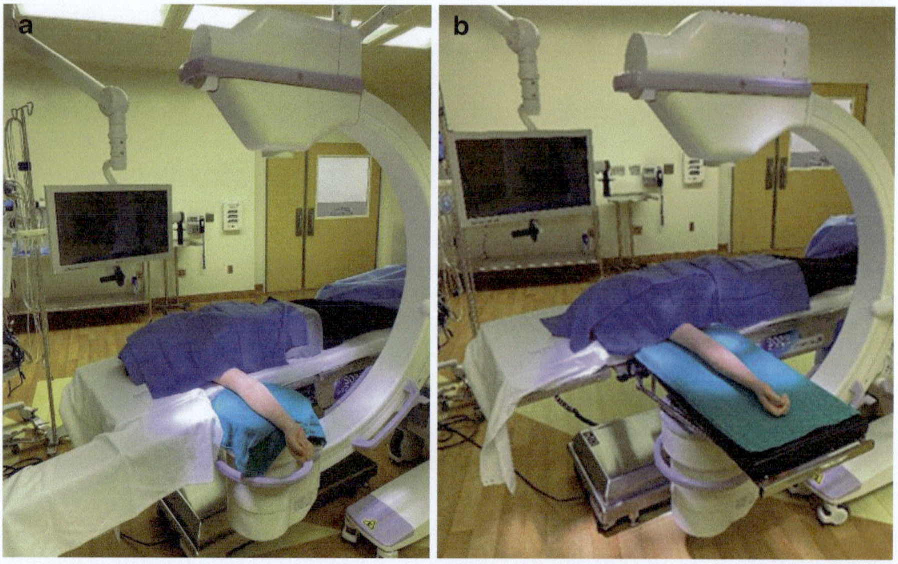

Fig. 12.7 With the patient in a supine position on a surgical table, the affected elbow can be positioned over the C-arm of the fluoroscopy (**a**), or on a lateral extensión table (**b**), depending on the surgeon preference. (Orthopedic Institute for Children Image Bank)

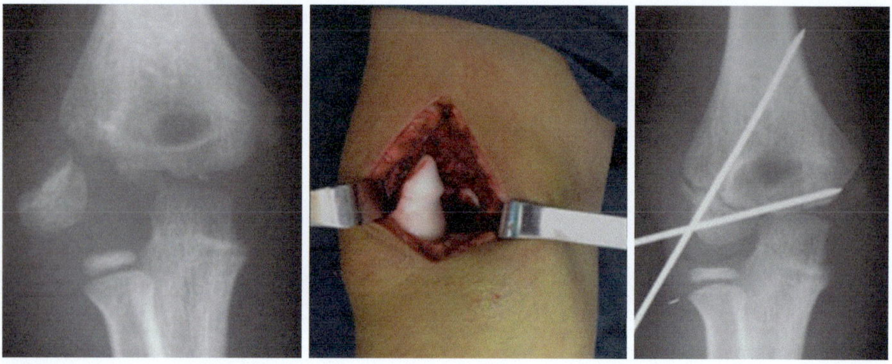

Fig. 12.8 Open reduction and osteosynthesis with divergent Kirschner wires on a fracture Type Weiss III, with a rotated fragment

reduced using a reduction forceps. To ensure an anatomical reduction, it is important to be able to observe the medial articular surface with the fracture fragment. An anatomical reduction requires that the joint line is completely restored and congruent. Once the anatomical reduction is achieved, and while it is maintained using the reduction forceps, the fracture is fixed with 2–3 Kirschner wires, as previously described (Fig. 12.8). It is important that the wires are introduced percutaneously, and not through the incision, to allow complete closure of it.

12.6 Postoperative Management

Postoperative management is similar for both patients who have received a closed reduction, and for those who have received an open reduction with internal fixation. An initial posterior splint or a short arm cast is used.

The patient should be evaluated 8–10 days after surgery with radiographs, to ensure that the anatomical reduction maintains, and the fixation is stable. If a posterior splint was initially used, it is replaced with a short arm cast during this visit. The Kirschner wires are kept in place until 4 weeks postoperative. It is advisable to leave them outside the skin for easy removal in the office, without the need for a new intervention [23, 24]. In this regard, it has been shown that leaving the wires under the skin not only requires a new intervention to remove them, but is also associated with a higher incidence of local complications and infection due to protrusion through the skin [23, 25].

The oral administration of analgesic medication prior to the removal of percutaneous wires does not result in a significant decrease in pain which, in general, is minimal [26, 27]. A new short arm cast is used for an additional period of 2 weeks until to complete a total of 6 postoperative weeks, after which it is removed and progressive mobilization of the elbow is allowed, avoiding sports and contact activities for an additional period of 4 weeks.

Clinical and radiological follow-up should continue until it is ensured that the range of motion has been recovered [28] and that the fracture has completely healed. In older patients, with greater ossification of the distal humerus, compressive screws can be used instead of Kirschner wires. These must be removed obligatorily in children with open physis, as they can cause epiphysiodesis and secondary deformities.

12.7 Treatment Outcomes

Compared to open reduction, closed reduction with percutaneous fixation of lateral condyle fractures of the humerus has proven to be a suitable alternative for fractures with a displacement less than 4 mm. In addition to offering the cosmetic advantage of not requiring a skin incision, closed reduction with percutaneous fixation offers clinical outcomes similar to those obtained with an open reduction and is associated with reduced surgical times [29, 30]. Compared to fractures treated with an open reduction, lateral condyle fractures treated with closed reduction and percutaneous fixation showed similar clinical outcomes, including recovery of the range of motion (99.2% vs. 99.7%), formation of a lateral spur (75% vs. 68%), complication rate (6.3% and 3.6%), and satisfactory outcomes (88.3% vs. 89.3%) [29].

Multiple case series have reported excellent results in the treatment of lateral condyle fractures using an open reduction [31]. Leonidou [31] reported excellent results in 105 patients treated with open reduction and internal fixation using Kirschner wires. In this series, excellent results were reported in 96% of the treated fractures. In general, a rapid recovery of the range of motion can be expected after 6 weeks from cast removal, followed by a slow and progressive recovery up to a year after the initial surgery [28].

There is some controversy regarding the need to perform the surgical treatment acutely or early, with studies suggesting that satisfactory results are observed when the surgical treatment is performed during the first 2 weeks after the initial injury, with surgical times, functional outcomes, and complication rates, comparable to those obtained in patients in which the fracture is managed acutely within the first 7 days after the injury. Open reductions performed later (>3 weeks after the initial injury) may result in a high rate of complications, including non-vascular necrosis of the lateral condyle, premature physeal arrest and functional limitations [3, 32].

12.8 Complications

A mal-union occurs when the fragment of the lateral condyle fracture consolidates in an abnormal or non-anatomical position, resulting in a varus or valgus deformity [33] (Fig. 12.9).

It is considered a late presentation when the lateral condyle fracture is evaluated for the first time more than 3 weeks after the original injury. A delay in consolidation is when the lateral condyle fracture shows no signs of consolidation between 6 and 12 weeks after the initial injury. Performing a late open reduction (>3 weeks after the original injury) for a displaced lateral condyle fracture is technically difficult. In these cases, the best results are obtained when the fracture fragment has a large metaphyseal portion, when a limited dissection is used to achieve the reduction (avoiding damage to the vascular supply of the fragment), and when the fracture gap is less than 1 cm (Fig. 12.10).

Even though it is ideal to obtain an anatomical reduction of the fracture fragment, a late reduction does not always manage to restore the anatomical joint surface. However, achieving healing of the metaphyseal portion of the fragment, with a partial realignment of the joint surface, provides the patient with the best

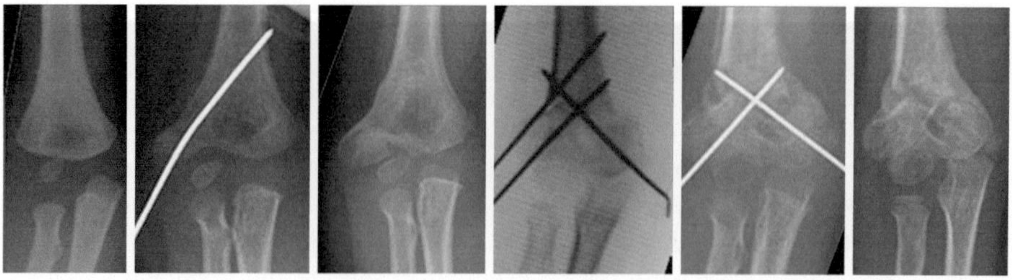

Fig. 12.9 A malunion occurs when the fracture fragment of the lateral condyle heals in an abnormal or non-anatomical position, resulting in a varus or valgus deformity. In this case, the patient was subjected to a corrective osteotomy, realigning the articular surface. (Orthopedic Institute for Children Image Bank)

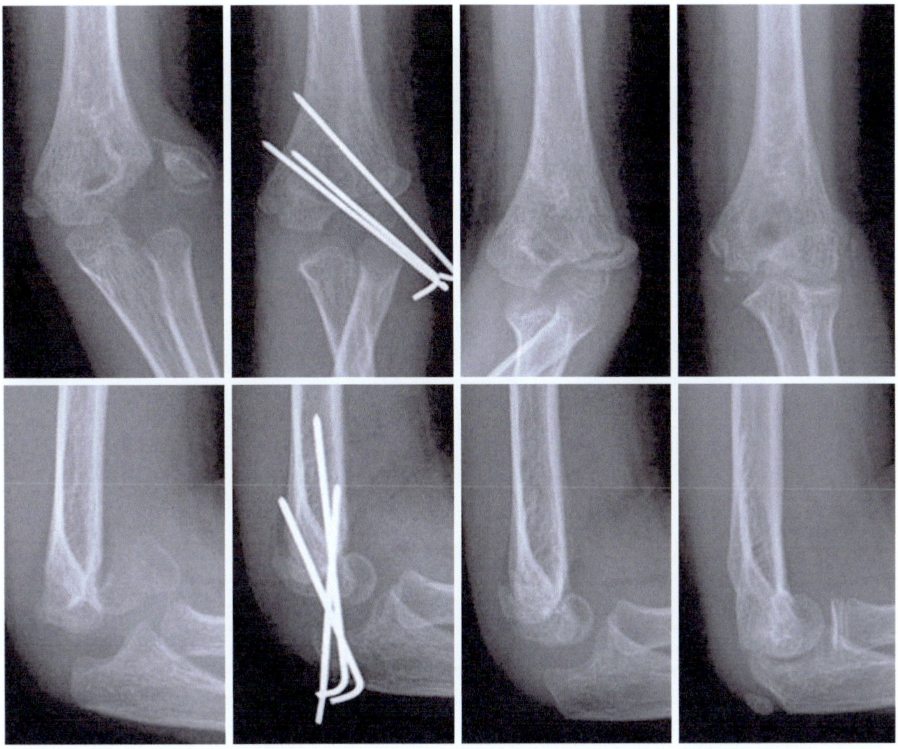

Fig. 12.10 Elbow radiographs of a girl who presented at 6 weeks after suffering a fall on his left elbow. Even if the reduction of the articular surface is not completely anatomical, it is obtained a partial realignment of the articular surface that allowed the patient to recover the range of motion and avoid a deformity in elbow valgus (Orthopedic Institute for Children Image Bank)

possibilities for recovery of the range of motion and prevents a progressive valgus deformity of the affected elbow [34, 35].

Non-union is defined as a lack of bone healing at 12 weeks after the original injury. Non-unions can be the result of an undiagnosed fracture (and therefore, untreated), of a fracture not surgically treated in which a late displacement occurred, or of a surgically treated fracture in which a re-displacement has occurred [36, 37] or a residual displacement greater than 1 mm has been noted after fixation [38]. Its incidence has been reported between 1% and 5% of lateral condyle fractures [10, 39, 40]. It is common for patients with a non-union of the lateral condyle to present pain upon palpation of the lateral region of the elbow, with deformity (usually in valgus), and some degree of limitation of the elbow's range of motion (Fig. 12.11).

There are multiple techniques described for the management of a non-union of the lateral condyle of the humerus, including open reduction with internal fixation with wires or screws (with or without bone grafts), and percutaneous fixation with a compressive screw [41–43].

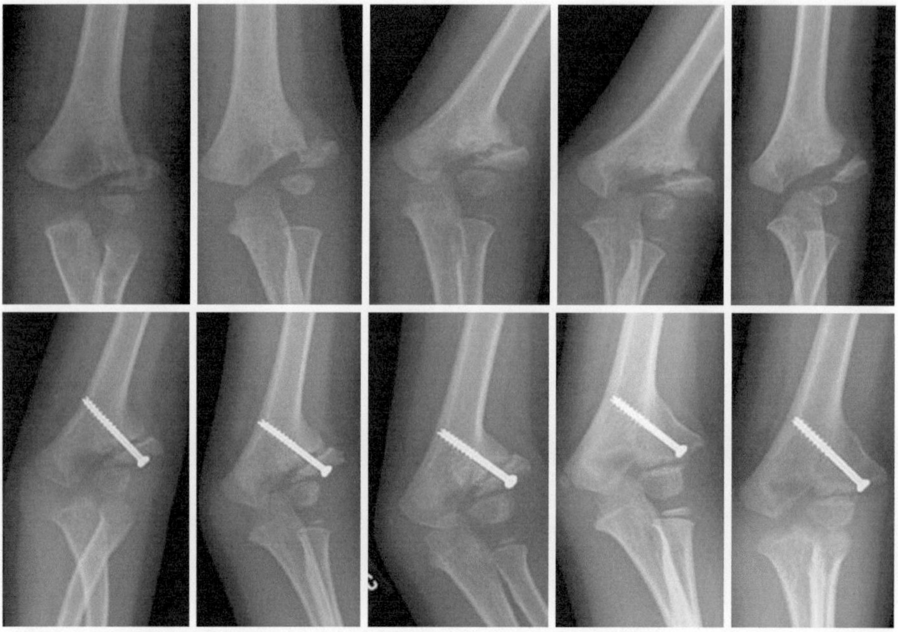

Fig. 12.11 It is common for patients with a non-union of the lateral condyle to present pain on palpation of the lateral region of the elbow, with deformity (usually valgus), and some degree of movement limitation. In this case a progressive valgus deformity was noticed. Non-union of the lateral condyle was managed with fixation percutaneously with a compression screw, achieving its consolidation. (Orthopedic Institute for Children Image Bank)

In general, if the fracture fragment has minimal displacement, percutaneous fixation with a compression screw is generally satisfactory, especially when surgery is performed within 16 weeks after the original fracture [42] (Fig. 12.12).

For fractures with greater displacement, open reduction of the non-union can be considered, with or without bone graft, and stable internal fixation [37]. In cases where the non-union is associated with a valgus deformity, in situ fixation of the non-union should be complemented with a corrective osteotomy [44]. Unaddressed valgus deformities of the elbow can result in elbow instability, with secondary chronic neuropathies of the ulnar nerve, due to elongation. In symptomatic patients, anterior transposition of the ulnar nerve should be considered to improve symptoms.

The "fish tail" deformity is a late complication associated with displaced fractures, caused by a central physeal closure that results in uneven growth of the humeral pallet, in which only its lateral ends grow [45]. Generally, it presents several years after the initial injury, and clinically it is characterized by a limitation of the elbow's range of motion, pain, presence of free bodies in the elbow, and a valgus deformity. Usually, the deformity is much more impressive on the radiograph than the actual clinical impact on the external anatomy of the elbow and its function. In cases where the presentation is asymptomatic, which are the majority, the patient

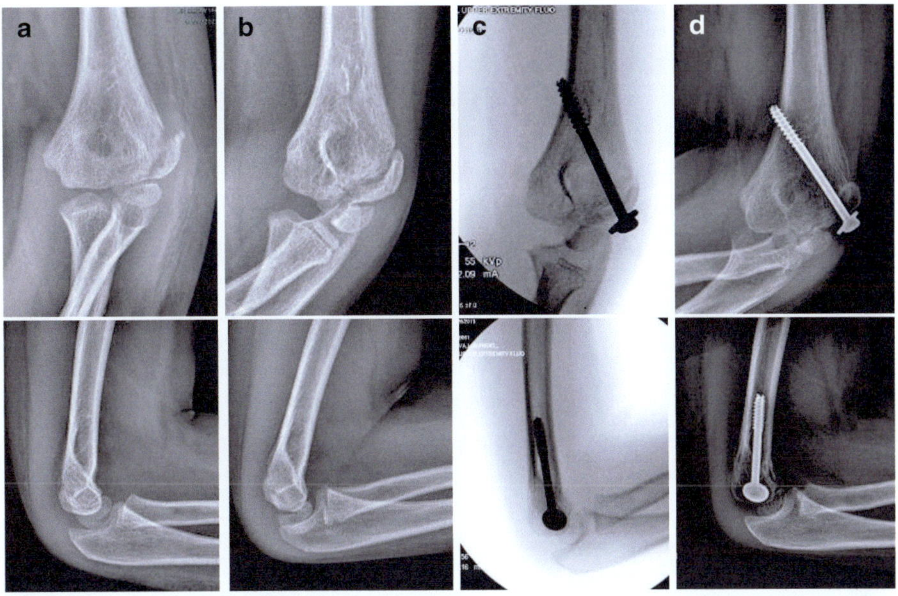

Fig. 12.12 Elbow radiographs of an 8-year-old girl who presented 3 weeks after a fall. (**a**) Initial radiograph. The patient received a brachiopalmar cast as treatment. (**b**) Radiographs obtained 2 months ses after the initial injury, demonstrating a delay in union. (**c**) Fluoroscopic images demonstrating treatment with percutaneous fixation with a compression screw. (**d**) Radiographs obtained 2 months after surgery, demonstrating complete healing of the fracture of the lateral condyle. (Orthopedic Institute for Children Image Bank)

can be observed. If associated with pain, surgical options can be considered that include the removal of free bodies, epiphysiodesis, or a distal humerus osteotomy.

Avascular necrosis of the distal humerus is a relatively rare complication, with an incidence reported at 1.4% [46]. In general, this complication is associated with displaced lateral condyle fractures (Weiss type III) that have been managed with open reduction and internal fixation. Fractures associated with a high-energy mechanism that produce a greater displacement of bone fragments have a higher risk of developing avascular necrosis of the distal humerus. Excessive dissection of the musculature that inserts into the lateral condyle, especially in its posterior portion, can affect the irrigation of the lateral condyle, and result in avascular necrosis. Most patients who develop avascular necrosis of the lateral condyle are asymptomatic, with almost complete recovery of the elbow's range of motion in the long term [46].

The natural history of avascular necrosis of the lateral condyle of the humerus is not fully described, even though there are reports of complete reconstitution of the capitellum-humeral surface [46] (Fig. 12.13).

The lateral spur is very common in patients with fractures of the lateral condyle of the humerus. There are reports indicating that 73% of patients with fractures of the lateral condyle present a lateral spur [47] (Fig. 12.14). It is more common in patients treated surgically (91%), but also occurs in patients

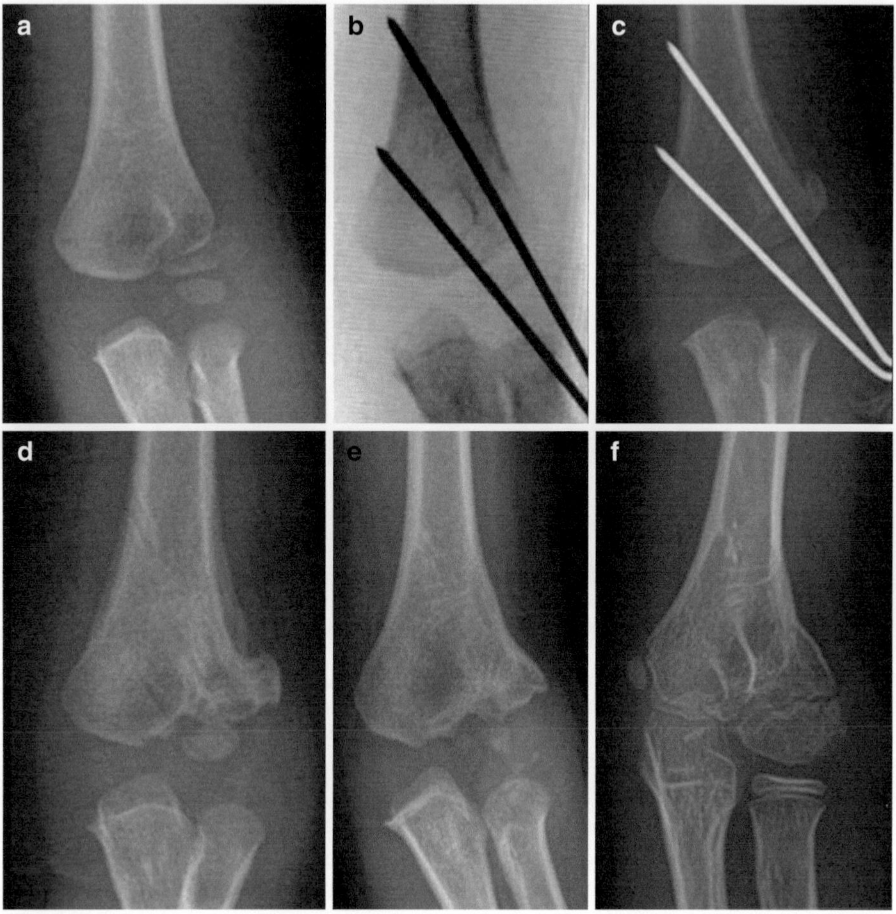

Fig. 12.13 X-rays of a 3-year-old girl who underwent open reduction and internal fixation of a fracture of the lateral condyle of the left elbow, 8 days after trauma (**a–b**). The Kirschner wires were removed 3 weeks after surgery (**c**). After 4 weeks, bone healing has improved, but an irregularity is noted in the medial portion of the lateral condyle (**d**). One year after initial surgery, X-ray shows fragments bone located between the humeral metaphysis and the head of the radius (**e**). X-rays at 5 years after initial surgery with complete reconstitution of the humeral condyle (**f**) (Orthopedic Institute for Children Image Bank)

undergoing non-surgical treatment (59%). In general, fractures associated with a high-energy mechanism, and therefore with greater displacement, tend to have a higher risk of developing a lateral spur. The lateral spur has cosmetic implications, as it can result in an apparent varus deformity, but it has no functional consequences for the patient.

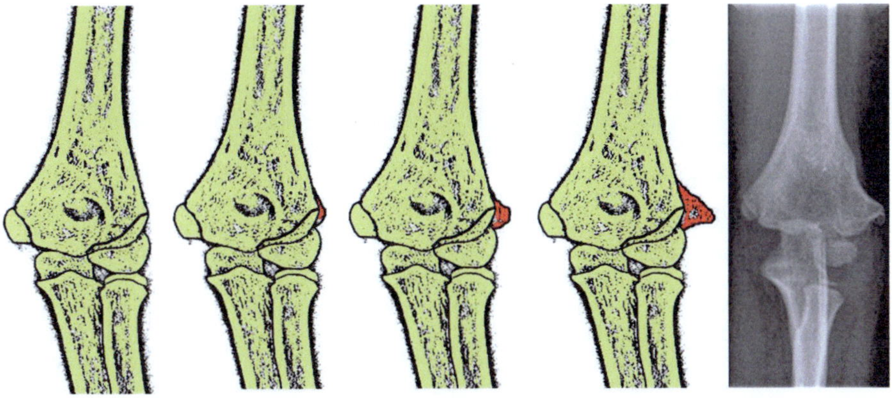

Fig. 12.14 The lateral spur occurs in 73% of patients with lateral condyle fractures. The severity of the spur depends on its size with relation to the size of the humerus. (Orthopedic Institute for Children Image Bank)

12.9 Final Message

The fracture of the lateral condyle of the humerus is the second most common elbow fracture in children. It is important to identify and treat them properly to preserve the integrity and joint surface congruence of the elbow. The treatment is conservative in non-displaced fractures (<2 mm) and surgical in displaced fractures (>2 mm) through open or percutaneous reduction and osteosynthesis, depending on the degree of displacement. Complications are common if not treated properly, with non-union being the main one.

References

1. Milch H. Fractures and fracture dislocations of the humeral condyles. J Trauma. 1964;4:592–607. https://doi.org/10.1097/00005373-196409000-00004.
2. Pirker ME, Weinberg AM, Höllwarth ME, Haberlik A. Subsequent displacement of initially nondisplaced and minimally displaced fractures of the lateral humeral condyle in children. J Trauma. 2005;58(6):1202–7. https://doi.org/10.1097/01.ta.0000169869.08723.c8.
3. Jakob R, Fowles JV, Rang M, Kassab MT. Observations concerning fractures of the lateral humeral condyle in children. J Bone Joint Surg Br. 1975;57(4):430–6.
4. Song KS, Kang CH, Min BW, Bae KC, Cho CH, Lee JH. Closed reduction and internal fixation of displaced unstable lateral condylar fractures of the humerus in children. J Bone Joint Surg Am. 2008;90(12):2673–81. https://doi.org/10.2106/JBJS.G.01227.
5. Weiss JM, Graves S, Yang S, Mendelsohn E, Kay RM, Skaggs DL. A new classification system predictive of complications in surgically treated pediatric humeral lateral condyle fractures. J Pediatr Orthop. 2009;29(6):602–5. https://doi.org/10.1097/BPO.0b013e3181b2842c.

6. Ramo BA, Funk SS, Elliott ME, Jo CH. The song classification is reliable and guides prognosis and treatment for pediatric lateral condyle fractures: an independent validation study with treatment algorithm. J Pediatr Orthop. 2020;40(3):e203–9. https://doi.org/10.1097/BPO.0000000000001439.
7. Nazareth A, VandenBerg CD, Sarkisova N, et al. Prospective evaluation of a treatment protocol based on fracture displacement for pediatric lateral condyle humerus fractures: a preliminary study. J Pediatr Orthop. 2020;40(7):e541–6. https://doi.org/10.1097/BPO.0000000000001491.
8. Song KS, Kang CH, Min BW, Bae KC, Cho CH. Internal oblique radiographs for diagnosis of nondisplaced or minimally displaced lateral condylar fractures of the humerus in children. J Bone Joint Surg Am. 2007;89(1):58–63. https://doi.org/10.2106/JBJS.E.01387.
9. Bland DC, Pennock AT, Upasani VV, Edmonds EW. Measurement reliability in pediatric lateral condyle fractures of the humerus. J Pediatr Orthop. 2018;38(8):e429–33. https://doi.org/10.1097/BPO.0000000000001200.
10. Silva M, Paredes A, Sadlik G. Outcomes of ORIF >7 days after injury in displaced pediatric lateral condyle fractures. J Pediatr Orthop. 2017;37(4):234–8. https://doi.org/10.1097/BPO.0000000000000640.
11. Silva M, Cooper SD, Cha A. Elbow dislocation with an associated lateral condyle fracture of the humerus: a rare occurrence in the pediatric population. J Pediatr Orthop. 2015;35(4):329–33. https://doi.org/10.1097/BPO.0000000000000270.
12. Lan X, Dai M, Zhang B, Huang G. Comparative study of lateral condyle fracture with or without posteromedial elbow dislocation in children. Int Orthop. 2018;42(3):619–24. https://doi.org/10.1007/s00264-018-3795-0.
13. Park DY, Cho JH, Lee DH, Choi WS, Bang JY, Yin XY. A 3-dimensional analysis of the fracture planes in pediatric lateral humeral condyle fractures for image-based pin positioning during fixation. J Orthop Trauma. 2017;31(10):e340–6. https://doi.org/10.1097/BOT.0000000000000914.
14. Horn BD, Herman MJ, Crisci K, Pizzutillo PD, MacEwen GD. Fractures of the lateral humeral condyle: role of the cartilage hinge in fracture stability. J Pediatr Orthop. 2002;22(1):8–11.
15. Bast SC, Hoffer MM, Aval S. Nonoperative treatment for minimally and nondisplaced lateral humeral condyle fractures in children. J Pediatr Orthop. 1998;18(4):448–50.
16. Knapik DM, Gilmore A, Liu RW. Conservative management of minimally displaced (≤2 mm) fractures of the lateral humeral condyle in pediatric patients: a systematic review. J Pediatr Orthop. 2017;37(2):e83–7. https://doi.org/10.1097/BPO.0000000000000722.
17. Ganeshalingam R, Donnan A, Evans O, Hoq M, Camp M, Donnan L. Lateral condylar fractures of the humerus in children: does the type of fixation matter? Bone Joint J. 2018;100-B(3):387–95. https://doi.org/10.1302/0301-620X.100B3.BJJ-2017-0814.R1.
18. Gilbert SR, MacLennan PA, Schlitz RS, Estes AR. Screw versus pin fixation with open reduction of pediatric lateral condyle fractures. J Pediatr Orthop B. 2016;25(2):148–52. https://doi.org/10.1097/BPB.0000000000000238.
19. Wendling-Keim DS, Teschemacher S, Dietz HG, Lehner M. Lateral condyle fracture of the humerus in children: Kirschner wire or screw fixation? Eur J Pediatr Surg. 2021;31(4):374–9. https://doi.org/10.1055/s-0040-1714656.
20. Bloom T, Chen LY, Sabharwal S. Biomechanical analysis of lateral humeral condyle fracture pinning. J Pediatr Orthop. 2011;31(2):130–7. https://doi.org/10.1097/BPO.0b013e3182074c5b.
21. Swarup I, Chan C, Mehta N, Lawrence JT. Does an elbow arthrogram change management after closed reduction of mildly displaced lateral condyle fractures in children? J Pediatr Orthop B. 2022;31(1):7–11. https://doi.org/10.1097/BPB.0000000000000811.
22. Vorhies JS, Funk S, Elliott M, Riccio A, Ramo B. The utility of intraoperative arthrogram in the management of pediatric lateral condyle fractures of the humerus. Orthopedics. 2020;43(1):30–5. https://doi.org/10.3928/01477447-20191031-01.
23. Das De S, Bae DS, Waters PM. Displaced humeral lateral condyle fractures in children: should we bury the pins? J Pediatr Orthop. 2012;32(6):573–8. https://doi.org/10.1097/BPO.0b013e318263a25f.

24. Raghavan R, Jones A, Dwyer AJ. Should Kirschner wires for fixation of lateral humeral condyle fractures in children be buried or left exposed? A systematic review. Orthop Traumatol Surg Res. 2019;105(4):739–45. https://doi.org/10.1016/j.otsr.2019.03.007.
25. Qin YF, Li ZJ, Li CK, Bai SC, Li H. Unburied versus buried wires for fixation of pediatric lateral condyle distal humeral fractures: a meta-analysis. Medicine (Baltimore). 2017;96(34):e7736. https://doi.org/10.1097/MD.0000000000007736.
26. Lim KB, Tan SS, Abdullah SN, Ong LL, Wong ML, Allen JC. Percutaneous pin removal in the outpatient clinic--do children require analgesia?: a randomized controlled trial. J Bone Joint Surg Am. 2014;96(7):597–602. https://doi.org/10.2106/JBJS.M.00806.
27. Sorenson SM, Hennrikus W. Pain during office removal of K-wires from the elbow in children. J Pediatr Orthop. 2015;35(4):341–4. https://doi.org/10.1097/BPO.0000000000000269.
28. Bernthal NM, Hoshino CM, Dichter D, Wong M, Silva M. Recovery of elbow motion following pediatric lateral condylar fractures of the humerus. J Bone Joint Surg Am. 2011;93(9):871–7. https://doi.org/10.2106/JBJS.J.00935.
29. Silva M, Cooper SD. Closed reduction and percutaneous pinning of displaced pediatric lateral condyle fractures of the Humerus: a Cohort Study. J Pediatr Orthop. 2015;35(7):661–5. https://doi.org/10.1097/BPO.0000000000000376.
30. Pennock AT, Salgueiro L, Upasani VV, Bastrom TP, Newton PO, Yaszay B. Closed reduction and percutaneous pinning versus open reduction and internal fixation for type II lateral condyle Humerus fractures in children displaced >2 mm. J Pediatr Orthop. 2016;36(8):780–6. https://doi.org/10.1097/BPO.0000000000000570.
31. Leonidou A, Chettiar K, Graham S, et al. Open reduction internal fixation of lateral humeral condyle fractures in children. A series of 105 fractures from a single institution. Strategies Trauma Limb Reconstr. 2014;9(2):73–8. https://doi.org/10.1007/s11751-014-0193-z.
32. Wattenbarger JM, Gerardi J, Johnston CE. Late open reduction internal fixation of lateral condyle fractures. J Pediatr Orthop. 2002;22(3):394–8.
33. Skak SV, Olsen SD, Smaabrekke A. Deformity after fracture of the lateral humeral condyle in children. J Pediatr Orthop B. 2001;10(2):142–52.
34. Abzug JM, Dua K, Kozin SH, Herman MJ. Current concepts in the treatment of lateral condyle fractures in children. J Am Acad Orthop Surg. 2020;28(1):e9–e19. https://doi.org/10.5435/JAAOS-D-17-00815.
35. Shrestha S, Hutchison RL. Outcomes for late presenting lateral condyle fractures of the humerus in children: a case series. J Clin Orthop Trauma. 2020;11(2):251–8. https://doi.org/10.1016/j.jcot.2019.09.012.
36. Liu TJ, Wang EB, Dai Q, Zhang LJ, Li QW, Zhao Q. Open reduction and internal fixation for the treatment of fractures of the lateral humeral condyle with an early delayed presentation in children: a radiological and clinical prospective study. Bone Joint J. 2016;98-B(2):244–8. https://doi.org/10.1302/0301-620X.98B2.34429.
37. Agarwal A, Qureshi NA, Gupta N, Verma I, Pandey DK. Management of neglected lateral condyle fractures of humerus in children: a retrospective study. Indian J Orthop. 2012;46(6):698–704. https://doi.org/10.4103/0019-5413.104221.
38. Salgueiro L, Roocroft JH, Bastrom TP, et al. Rate and risk factors for delayed healing following surgical treatment of lateral condyle humerus fractures in children. J Pediatr Orthop. 2017;37(1):1–6. https://doi.org/10.1097/BPO.0000000000000578.
39. Pace JL, Arkader A, Sousa T, Broom AM, Shabtai L. Incidence, risk factors, and definition for nonunion in pediatric lateral condyle fractures. J Pediatr Orthop. 2018;38(5):e257–61. https://doi.org/10.1097/BPO.0000000000001153.
40. Launay F, Leet AI, Jacopin S, Jouve JL, Bollini G, Sponseller PD. Lateral humeral condyle fractures in children: a comparison of two approaches to treatment. J Pediatr Orthop. 2004;24(4):385–91.
41. Park H, Hwang JH, Kwon YU, Kim HW. Osteosynthesis in situ for lateral condyle nonunion in children. J Pediatr Orthop. 2015;35(4):334–40. https://doi.org/10.1097/BPO.0000000000000353.

42. Knight DM, Alves C, Alman B, Howard A. Percutaneous screw fixation promotes healing of lateral condyle nonunion in children. J Pediatr Orthop. 2014;34(2):155–60. https://doi.org/10.1097/BPO.0000000000000077.
43. Prakash J, Mehtani A. Open reduction versus in-situ fixation of neglected lateral condyle fractures: a comparative study. J Pediatr Orthop B. 2018;27(2):134–41. https://doi.org/10.1097/BPB.0000000000000443.
44. Tien YC, Chen JC, Fu YC, Chih TT, Hunag PJ, Wang GJ. Supracondylar dome osteotomy for cubitus valgus deformity associated with a lateral condylar nonunion in children. J Bone Joint Surg Am. 2005;87(7):1456–63. https://doi.org/10.2106/JBJS.C.01545.
45. Narayanan S, Shailam R, Grottkau BE, Nimkin K. Fishtail deformity--a delayed complication of distal humeral fractures in children. Pediatr Radiol 2015;45(6):814–819. doi:https://doi.org/10.1007/s00247-014-3249-9.
46. Shabtai L, Lightdale-Miric N, Rounds A, Arkader A, Pace JL. Incidence, risk factors and outcomes of avascular necrosis occurring after humeral lateral condyle fractures. J Pediatr Orthop B. 2020;29(2):145–8. https://doi.org/10.1097/BPB.0000000000000698.
47. Pribaz JR, Bernthal NM, Wong TC, Silva M. Lateral spurring (overgrowth) after pediatric lateral condyle fractures. J Pediatr Orthop. 2012;32(5):456–60. https://doi.org/10.1097/BPO.0b013e318259ff63.

Chapter 13
Medial Epicondyle Fractures of the Humerus

María Jesús Figueroa and Julio Toledo

13.1 Medial Epicondyle Fractures of the Humerus

Medial epicondyle fractures represent 11–20% of all bone injuries in the elbow in the pediatric population [1]. These fractures occur most frequently between the ages of 9 and 14 years old and are four times more common in boys than in girls [1]. Approximately 50% of cases are associated with elbow dislocation, with the incarceration of the fragment being less frequent, between 5 and 18% of cases [2]. The association with ulnar nerve dysfunction has been reported in 10–16% of children with these fractures [3]. They are increasingly common injuries in the pediatric population, especially in children involved in high-performance sports activities from very early ages [4].

13.2 Anatomy

The ossification center of the epicondyle in the distal humerus is radiologically visible between the ages of 4 and 9 years old (Fig. 13.1) and is the last to merge with the rest of the distal humerus, between the ages of 15 and 20 years old [1].

The epicondyle is an apophysis of the posteromedial face of the distal humerus, being subject to traction forces, which can lead to avulsion. As an apophysis, it does not contribute to longitudinal growth [1, 5]. It corresponds to the point of origin of

M. J. Figueroa
Pontificia Universidad Católica de Chile, Instituto Teletón, Hospital Sotero del Río, Santiago, Chile
e-mail: Mufiguer@uc.cl

J. Toledo (✉)
Hospital Clínico Regional de Concepción, Concepción, Chile

M. Sepúlveda O. (ed.), *Paediatrics Traumatology*,
https://doi.org/10.1007/978-3-031-89482-4_13

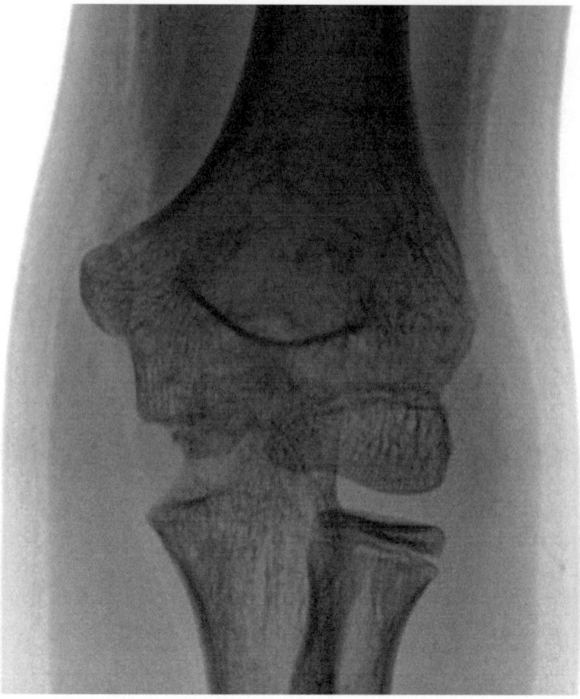

Fig. 13.1 Anteroposterior elbow X-ray of a 10-year-old child. The epitrochlea is seen as an ossification center on the medial border of the humeral palette

the flexor-pronator muscle mass of the forearm (Fig. 13.2), constituted by the Pronator teres, the Flexor carpi radialis, the Flexor digitorum superficialis, and the Flexor carpi ulnaris, playing a fundamental role in the biomechanics of wrist movements [6, 7]. Its lower and distal part is the point of origin of the ulnar collateral ligament, the main stabilizer of the elbow, and responsible for its stability in valgus. The anterior portion of the ligament is the most important for stability, especially in flexion and extension [2, 7].

In children under 8 years old, part of the insertion of the joint capsule may extend to the physeal line of the epicondyle. In older children, however, since the epicondyle migrates proximally, the fracture is typically extra-articular [1].

The ulnar nerve enters the ulnar tunnel posterior to the epicondyle. Its proximity puts it at risk of injury in fractures of this apophysis [1], so we must analyze its function during the physical examination.

The irrigation of the epicondyle comes from the ulnar collateral artery and a medial vascular arcade, which is an anastomosis between the superior and inferior ulnar collateral arteries and the posterior ulnar recurrent branch of the ulnar artery [1].

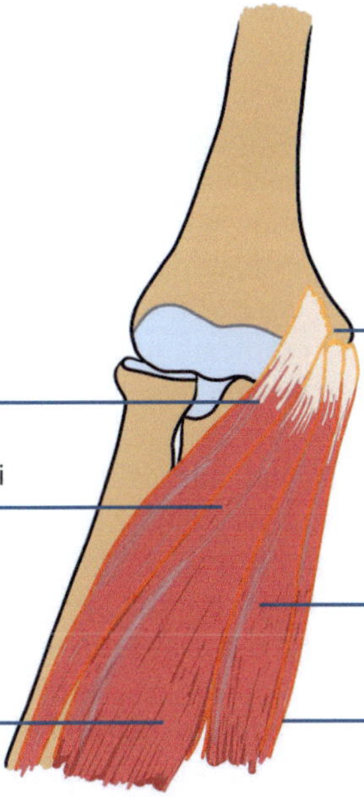

Fig. 13.2 Diagram of the muscle insertions at the level of the epitrochlea

13.3 Mechanism of Injury

Epicondyle fractures can result from two mechanisms of injury: direct trauma or avulsion.

Direct trauma corresponds to a blow in the posteromedial region of the elbow, where the fragment may end up comminuted [1].

Avulsion injury is the most frequent mechanism. It can occur in three situations [3, 8, 9]: avulsion and extension, with forced valgus stress on a locked elbow during a fall, possibly associated with wrist extension, which causes tension in the forearm flexor muscles; isolated avulsion, through the act of throwing a baseball (pitching) or in wrestling, where the sudden contraction of the forearm flexor muscles is capable of causing the collapse of the epicondyle; and associated with elbow dislocation, where the avulsive force of the ulnar collateral ligament, in posterior elbow dislocation produces traction.

13.4 Diagnosis

The patient with an epicondyle fracture usually presents increase in soft tissue volume and pain on palpation on the medial side of the elbow. Bone crepitus and deformity can be identified. The range of motion of the elbow may be compromised, with limitation secondary to pain, in the presence of an incarcerated fragment, or joint dislocation.

A careful examination of the rest of the extremity is mandatory, as this fracture may be associated with other injuries, including distal radius fractures, head and neck of the radius, coronoid process, and olecranon fractures [1].

A detailed neurovascular examination with special attention to the function of the ulnar nerve must be carried out, evaluating the abduction and adduction of the fingers, and sensation over the ulnar edge of the fifth finger [5] (Fig. 13.3).

Due to the complexity of elbow ossification, sometimes simple radiology does not quantify the real degree of fragment displacement, which makes decision regarding treatment difficult.

X-ray in anteroposterior, lateral and internal oblique projections are recommended for the diagnosis of an epicondyle fracture (Fig. 13.4). However, the predictive accuracy of displacement does not exceed 60% [5]. The disruption of the cortical contour in the anteroposterior projection, with loss of parallelism of both sclerotic margins of the apophysis and increase in the width of radiolucency in the apophyseal line should be evaluated. The oblique projection is particularly useful for evaluating displacement. The maximum displacement, typically anterior, is observed in an internal oblique projection (Fig. 13.5). The fat pad sign ("Fat pad") and capsular effusion are usually absent, as it is an extra-articular injury. If there is a large effusion, an elbow dislocation or other associated fractures should be suspected. The axial projection of the distal humerus has been shown to offer the best result between accuracy of displacement and the amount of radiation exposure [10]. It is performed with the humerus at 45° from the vertical, and the beam directed at 25° from the axis of the humerus, from superior to inferior.

All projections should be carefully evaluated for incarceration, especially in the case of an elbow dislocation. Whenever the medial epicondyle is seen at the level of the joint or is not observed, it should be considered at least partially incarcerated,

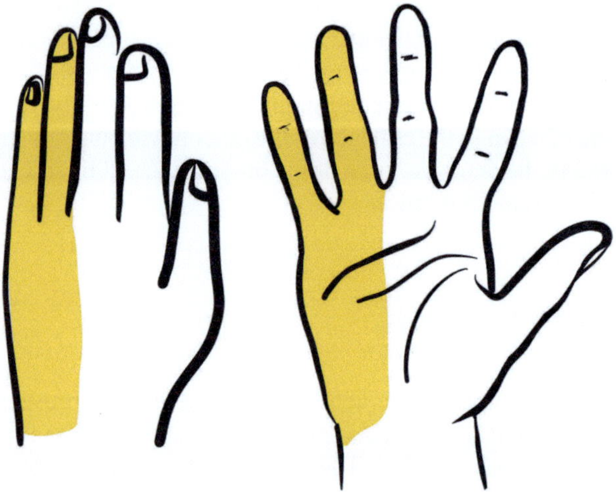

Fig. 13.3 Sensory innervation of the ulnar nerve, which must be evaluated in the presence of an epitrochlea fracture

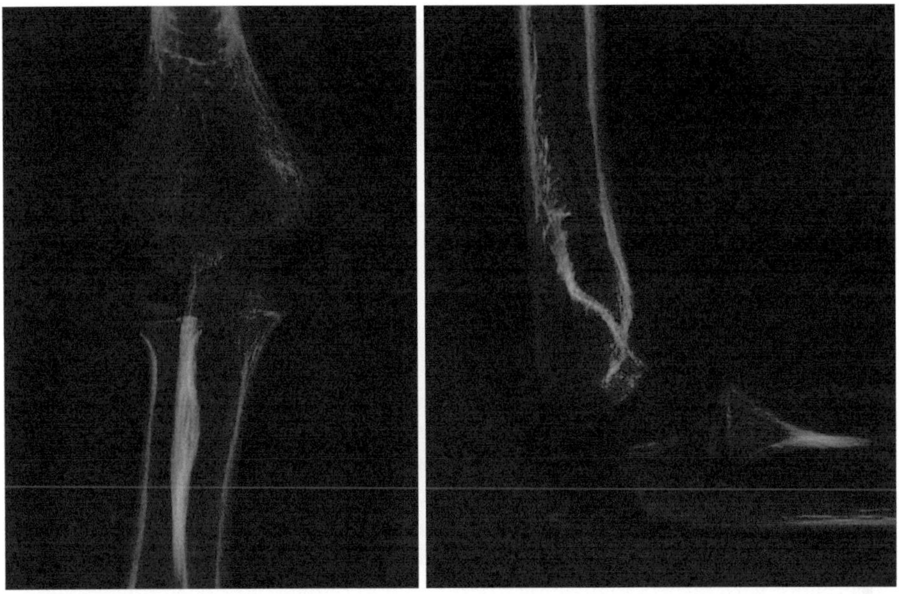

Fig. 13.4 Anteroposterior and lateral x-ray projections of an elbow of a 6-year-old child, with a displaced epitrochlea fracture

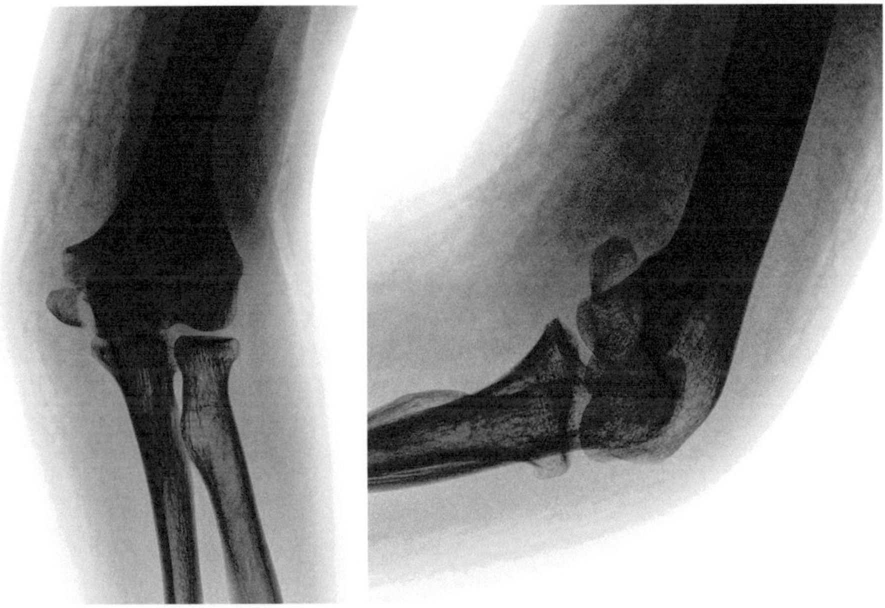

Fig. 13.5 Anteroposterior and internal oblique X-ray projections of an elbow a 12-year-old girl, with a displaced epitrochlea fracture. Can appreciate the significant anterior displacement

until proven otherwise. The incarcerated fragment is usually found between the trochlea and the notch of the semilunar facet of the olecranon [4].

It has been shown that even in radiographically non-displaced fractures, when studied with Computed Tomography (CT-scan), a displacement of up to 10 mm is evident. Other authors [8, 11] show that radiographs, in conventional anteroposterior projection, underestimate the displacement by an average of about 5.5 mm, and in the lateral projection it is difficult to observe displacement of <10 mm, thus questioning the value of these studies. In addition, some of these fractures may go unnoticed, due to superimposition of the fragment with the humeral trochlea. Even the use of oblique projections, recommended by some authors, which although improve the accuracy diagnostic, underestimate the degree of displacement, on average by 3.8 mm [6, 12].

The direction of displacement of the bone fragment is anterior, due to the force vector resulting from its muscular insertions. For this reason, the anteroposterior radiograph has low performance in describing the magnitude of the displacement. It has been recommended the study with CT-scan, and even with MRI, to quantify the magnitude and direction of the displacement, but the routine use of these studies does not occur in our practice, especially in the pediatric population [13]. In case of uncertainty with respect to diagnosis or optimal treatment, advanced images should be obtained. CT-scan is indicated in cases where the location of the epicondyle is not easily identifiable (Fig. 13.6), or the direction and magnitude of its displacement [4]. In athletes with suspicion of severe or chronic injuries, MRI can be considered because it provides information about the presence of pre-existing changes, as well as possible ligamentary injuries.

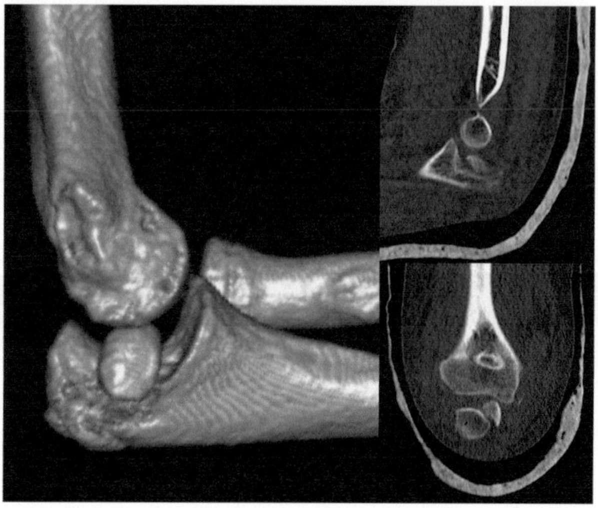

Fig. 13.6 CT-scan of an elbow with an epitrochlea fracture, with intra-articular fragment after reduction of an associated elbow dislocation. Incongruent secondary trochlear humerus with proximal ulna can be observed

13.5 Classification

Several authors have proposed classification systems for the medial epicondyle fracture, including Watson-Jones [9], Papavasiliou [14], Rang and Smith [14]. Because all are based on the anteroposterior radiograph, they have a descriptive value, but none of these is accepted. In general, most are based on the amount of displacement measured in millimeters, and the association with elbow dislocation, which has been shown to influence when deciding whether to opt for conservative management or surgery [5].

The Watson-Jones Classification [9] is the most used. However, despite its apparent simplicity, there is a high interobserver variability, up to 87% [15, 16].

It defines four types (Fig. 13.7): Type I, with less than 5 mm of displacement; Type II, with more than 5 mm of displacement; Type III, associated with the fractured epicondyle incarcerated within the joint (corresponding to a reduced elbow dislocation, associated to a fracture with great displacement); and Type IV, associated with elbow dislocation.

This injury in the AO pediatric classification corresponds to 13-M/7 m. It breaks down into: 1(humerus) 3(distal) M (metaphyseal)/7(epicondyle) m (medial). This classification has little clinical utility, and its function is mainly for data recording.

The Papavasiliou classification [14] has four types: Type 1, small avulsion; Type 2, complete fracture not incarcerated; Type 3, with incarcerated fragment; and Type 4, associated with elbow dislocation.

Finally, the Rang and Smith [14] classification also gives us four types: Grade I, apophyseal avulsion with minimal (<2 mm) or non-existent displacement; Grade II, apophyseal avulsion with displacement or rotation; Grade III, apophyseal avulsion

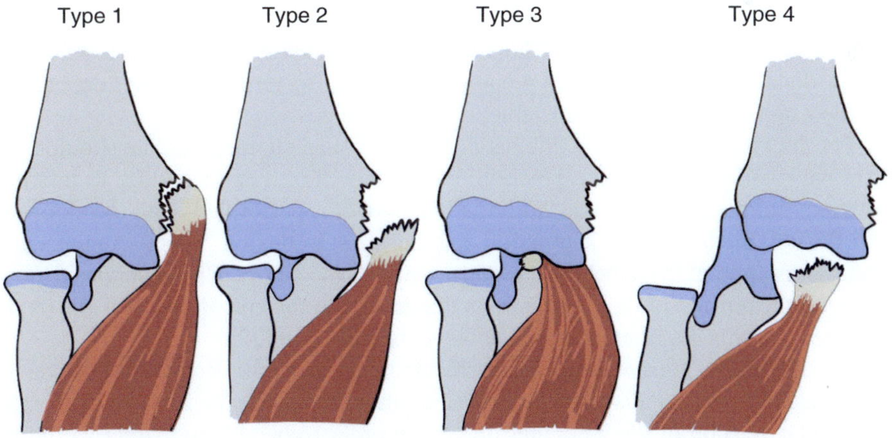

Fig. 13.7 Watson-Jones classification. Type I, less than 5 mm of displacement; Type II, with more than 5 mm of displacement; Type III, associated to the fractured epitrochlea incarcerated within the joint; and Type IV, associated with elbow dislocation

with intra-articular displacement of the fragment; and Grade IV, apophyseal avulsion in intra-articular location of the fragment and coexisting elbow dislocation.

13.6 Treatment

There is controversy in the management of displaced fractures and the degree of displacement from which surgical management is chosen. The majority of authors recommend surgical management when there is a displacement of the epicondyle by more than 5 mm [17]. There is no clinical or diagnostic parameter that justifies this cut-off point, but it has been shown in computer simulation studies that, with each 1 mm of displacement, the force of the wrist flexors decreases by 2% [17].

Orthopedic management can be successful, with low rates of complications, although there is a higher presence of instability, stiffness, and non-union in fractures associated with dislocation [18]. Currently, surgical treatment is increasingly chosen, due to the complications associated with conservative treatment, among which the instability in valgus of the elbow and non-union are important [6, 19, 20].

The indications for conservative management include minimally displaced fractures, low energy injuries, and stable elbow in valgus.

Conservative treatment consists of 3–4 weeks of elbow immobilization at 90° of flexion, trying to mold plaster with pressure exerted directly on the fracture [4]. Physiotherapy is considered as peremptory in cases associated with dislocation. In those patients in whom the injury mechanism suggests only isolated fracture, the decision to refer to rehabilitation is deferred until a first clinical and radiological control 2–3 weeks after the removal of the immobilization. In children with reckless behavior usually recovery does not require physiotherapy support.

The absolute indications for surgical management are open fractures, those associated with neurological injury, incarcerated fractures [20], or with a significant rotational component [6, 21]. The relative indications for surgery are recurrent elbow dislocation, displacement greater than 5 mm, fracture in "athletes dependent on their upper limb" [4] and unstable injuries in valgus.

For the surgical procedure, the patient is positioned supine, with the shoulder in external rotation, or in prone position, with elbow flexed and shoulder in internal rotation. For the reduction, the "milking" maneuver is performed, with the elbow at 90° flexion, the forearm in supination, and the wrist in flexion, a semi-compressive bandage is applied from the distal forearm towards the elbow. This generates a loosening of the tension of the muscle mass that inserts in the epicondyle and allows its advance towards the fracture site to achieve its reduction [22].

In case of the presence of an incarcerated fragment, the Roberts maneuver is described, where a valgus stress is applied on the elbow, with the forearm in supination and extension of the wrist and fingers, in order to be able to extract the intra-articular fragment. Considering that this situation is per se a surgical indication, the maneuver in general is not recommended, as it can cause iatrogenic injury and does not ensure an adequate reduction.

Fixation options include the use of cannulated screws, Kirschner wires, anchors, sutures, or the excision of the fragment and advancement of the soft tissues.

Fixation with a cannulated screw is a standard treatment in older children, close to skeletal maturity. Because the epicondyle is a posterior structure, the screw is placed obliquely, in direction from medial to lateral, and from posterior to anterior (Fig. 13.8). Partial thread screws (3.5–4.0 mm) are used, without the need for bicortical fixation, which is associated with a higher risk of iatrogenic injury to the radial nerve [23]. Until the age of 6 years old, the radial nerve crosses the distal lateral humerus at a distance (1 cm) proximal to the physis. Penetration of the olecranon fossa should be avoided, as the prominence of the implant may reduce elbow extension. Screw fixation could optimize its compression area with the help of a washer. However, Pace and Hennrikus [24] compared screw fixation with and without a washer in epicondyle fractures, showing that it does not decrease the risk of fragmentation, nor does it increase union rates in fixation reinforced with a washer, but its use is associated with a statistically significant increase in irritation, with the need to remove the implant.

Fixation with Kirschner wires (Fig. 13.9) is performed in young patients, with a fragment too small to perform osteosynthesis with another method. It has similar results to screw fixation, with no difference in range of motion, despite the longer immobilization time. The implant can be left under or over the skin, in which case the extraction of the implant can be performed as an outpatient procedure, avoiding the need for additional surgery. Care must be taken to avoid nerve injuries if the

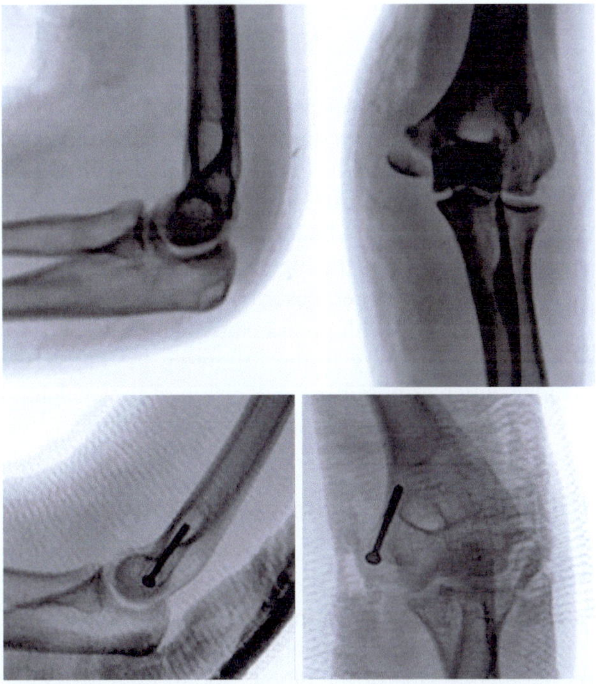

Fig. 13.8 Displaced epitrochlea fracture in a 14-year-old adolescent. Treated with open reduction and fixation with a cannulated screw with the interfragmentary compression

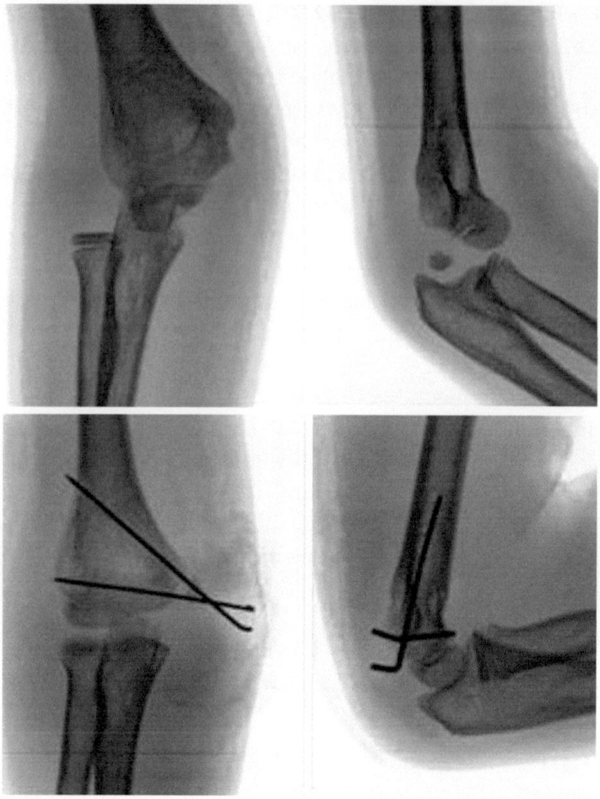

Fig. 13.9 Intra-articular incarcerated epitrochlea fracture in an 8-year-old girl. Open reduction and stabilization with Kirschner wires were performed

percutaneous wire enters at a distant entry point from the incision used to reduce the fracture. The ulnar nerve does not require routine exploration or mobilization [4].

The use of anchors has been compared with Kirschner wires, with statistically similar results in terms of bone healing and stability. The factor in favor of the use of anchors is being the fact that they do not require a new intervention to remove implants. Against it is the higher commercial cost [14].

A technique has been described with excision of the fragment and suture of the medial soft tissues with good results, but little used in practice, due to the presence of pain and instability in the follow-up [4, 17]. Therefore, it is recommended to avoid as much as possible the excision of the avulsion fragment.

13.7 Authors' Recommendations

A treatment scheme is recommended, based on displacement of the fragment, stability, and neurological compromise (Fig. 13.10).

In case of choosing for surgical treatment, we recommend making a skin incision on the medial side of the elbow, about 3 cm proximal to the epicondyle, with the

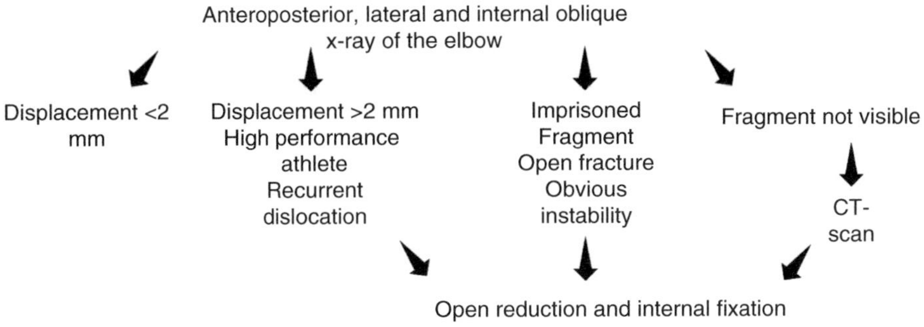

Fig. 13.10 Recommended flow chart for treatment of an epitrochlea fracture

elbow slightly flexed, a few millimeters anterior to the medial groove, up to 0.5–1.5 cm distal to the elbow joint. The fascia is opened parallel to the skin incision, and the connective tissue covering of the medial groove is divided for bone exposure and eventual visualization of the ulnar nerve. If necessary, the ulnar nerve is identified and tension-free rejected, protected with a rubber or elastic probe [25].

The fracture hematoma is drained and the fragments and bone surface are inspected. If the apophyseal fragment of the epicondyle is interposed in the humeral ulnar joint, it is carefully mobilized. After careful exposure and debridement of the fracture surfaces, the fragment is anatomically reduced. Manual reduction of the apophyseal fragment is achieved with a flexion of 45–60° of the elbow joint, with concomitant pronation of the forearm, and flexion at the wrist. The fragment is manually retained, and stabilized in place with a Kirschner wire in a transverse direction. The diameter of the Kirschner wire varies with age, from 1.4 to 2.0 mm. To secure the fragment against rotation, a second Kirschner wire is introduced, in an ascending oblique direction. Usually both wires are bent over the periosteum. However, the trend to externalize them by counter opening, and leave them extruded, avoiding a new surgical intervention, when removing them in outpatient care rooms, has been accepted. It is of great importance to ensure that no fragments or bone edges remain sharp in the groove of the ulnar nerve.

It is recommended to perform periosteal cartilaginous coping with resorbable material. The ulnar nerve is left in its groove and is not moved centrally. After the incision is closed, a long-arm cast is installed with 90° of elbow flexion and neutral rotational position [25].

To avoid stiffness after screw fixation, a short period of immobilization should be carried out, of 7–10 days, followed by early mobilization. This can then be accompanied by the use of an elbow stabilizer to reduce valgus stress on the fixation [4].

Because the epicondyle is an apophysis that does not contribute to the longitudinal growth of the distal humerus, leaving the screw in situ does not cause axis alterations. The screws should be removed if there is irritation of the ulnar nerve, or prominence related to pain. The percutaneous Kirschner wires should be removed between 3 and 4 weeks to reduce the risk of infection.

13.8 Complications

The non-union rate with conservative treatment is 50.8%, with most cases being asymptomatic. The non-union rate in surgical fixation depends on the type of fracture, from 0% to 7.5%, and significantly higher in incarcerated fracture (57%) [26].

The range of motion is reduced in both treatment modalities. There is an average reduction of extension reported of 15° in the non-surgical group, and 37° in the surgical group.

The elbow stiffness is probably due more to the damage to the periarticular soft tissues during the initial traumatic event, rather than to the surgery or the immobilization time. Even so, early mobilization after surgical management is essential [4].

Malunion, with cubitus valgus, post-epicondyle fracture has an incidence less than 10%. In the literature, it varies from 0% to 35.5%.

The prevention of elbow instability is a reason to suggest surgical management in athletes.

Ulnar nerve injury is rare. It is associated with the presence of elbow dislocation, and the highest rate is observed in incarcerated fragments. There is a debate about the appropriate treatment of preoperative ulnar nerve injuries. Transposition has been both recommended to increase the recovery rate, as well as discouraged due to the risk of ulnar nerve neuritis. Ulnar nerve paralysis after the reduction of the dislocation is a relative indication for surgical exploration and fixation [4].

An incarcerated fragment is not a surgical emergency and delays in surgery of up to 40 h have not shown any detrimental effect on the outcome, even in association with ulnar nerve paralysis. However, the reduction of the elbow joint remains an emergency and this should be prioritized [4]. It is assumed that the fragment would behave like a free body that would quickly induce mechanical blockage, necrosis, fibrosis, arthritis, and joint stiffness.

References

1. Rockwood and Wilkins' fractures in children 8th Edition. by John M. Flynn, David L. Skaggs, Peter M Waters; 2015. p.681.
2. Lotz B, Akilapa O, Karthik K. Delayed reconstruction following incarceration of the medial epicondyle in the elbow joint: A case report and review of the literature. JBJS Case Connect. 2018;8(3):e69. https://doi.org/10.2106/JBJS.CC.17.00239.
3. Patel NM, Ganley TJ. Medial epicondyle fractures of the humerus: how to evaluate and when to operate. J Pediatr Orthop. 2012;32(Suppl 1):S10–3. https://doi.org/10.1097/BPO.0b013e31824b2530.
4. Pathy R, Dodwell ER. Medial epicondyle fractures in children. Curr Opin Pediatr. 2015;27(1):58–66. https://doi.org/10.1097/MOP.0000000000000181.
5. Gottschalk HP, Eisner E, Hosalkar HS. Medial epicondyle fractures in the pediatric population. J Am Acad Orthop Surg. 2012;20(4):223–32. https://doi.org/10.5435/JAAOS-20-04-223.
6. Beck JJ, Bowen RE, Silva M. What's new in pediatric medial epicondyle fractures? J Pediatr Orthop. 2018;38(4):e202–6. https://doi.org/10.1097/BPO.0000000000000902.

7. Vergara-Amador E, Muñoz D, Vela RF. Anatomical description of the origin of the flexor and pronator muscles in the medial epicondyle of the humerus. Rev Cubana Ortop Traumatol. 2013;2725:199–208.
8. Haflah NH, Ibrahim S, Sapuan J, Abdullah S. An elbow dislocation in a child with missed medial epicondyle fracture and late ulnar nerve palsy. J Pediatr Orthop B. 2010;19(5):459–61. https://doi.org/10.1097/BPB.0b013e32833b6032.
9. Watson-Jones R. Fractures of the elbow. In: Wilson N, editor. Watson-jones fractures and joint injuries. 5th ed. Edinburgh, London and New York: Churchill Livingstone; 1976.
10. Souder CD, Farnsworth CL, McNeil NP, Bomar JD, Edmonds EW. The distal Humerus axial view: assessment of displacement in medial epicondyle fractures. J Pediatr Orthop. 2015;35(5):449–54. https://doi.org/10.1097/BPO.0000000000000306.
11. Blount WP. Injuries about the elbow: fractures of the medial epicondyle. Fractures in children. 1st ed. Baltimore: Williams & Wilkins; 1955. p. 55–61.
12. Watson-Jones R. Fractures and joint injuries. Baltimore: Williams & Wilkins; 1946.
13. Edmonds EW, Santago AC 2nd, Saul KR. Functional loss with displacement of medial epicondyle humerus fractures: a computer simulation study. J Pediatr Orthop. 2015;35(7):666–71. https://doi.org/10.1097/BPO.0000000000000371.
14. Rigal J, Thelen T, Angelliaume A, Pontailler JR, Lefevre Y. A new procedure for fractures of the medial epicondyle in children: Mitek(®) bone suture anchor. Orthop Traumatol Surg Res. 2016;102(1):117–20. https://doi.org/10.1016/j.otsr.2015.09.035.
15. Mehlman CT, Howard AW. Medial epicondyle fractures in children: clinical decision making in the face of uncertainty. J Pediatr Orthop. 2012;32(Suppl 2):S135–42. https://doi.org/10.1097/BPO.0b013e31824bdb78.
16. Pappas N, Lawrence JT, Donegan D, Ganley T, Flynn JM. Intraobserver and interobserver agreement in the measurement of displaced humeral medial epicondyle fractures in children. J Bone Joint Surg Am. 2010;92(2):322–7. https://doi.org/10.2106/JBJS.I.00493.
17. Stepanovich M, Bastrom TP, Munch J 3rd, Roocroft JH, Edmonds EW, Pennock AT. Does operative fixation affect outcomes of displaced medial epicondyle fractures? J Child Orthop. 2016;10(5):413–9. https://doi.org/10.1007/s11832-016-0757-1.
18. KKnapik DM, Fausett CL, Gilmore A, Liu RW. Outcomes of nonoperative pediatric medial humeral epicondyle fractures with and without associated elbow dislocation. J Pediatr Orthop. 2017;37(4):e224–8. https://doi.org/10.1097/BPO.0000000000000890.
19. Cruz AI Jr, Steere JT, Lawrence JT. Medial epicondyle fractures in the pediatric overhead athlete. J Pediatr Orthop. 2016;36(Suppl 1):S56–62. https://doi.org/10.1097/BPO.0000000000000759.
20. Josefsson PO, Danielsson LG. Epicondylar elbow fracture in children. 35-year follow-up of 56 unreduced cases. Acta Orthop Scand. 1986;57(4):313–5. https://doi.org/10.3109/17453678608994399.
21. Tarallo L, Mugnai R, Fiacchi F, Adani R, Zambianchi F, Catani F. Pediatric medial epicondyle fractures with intra-articular elbow incarceration. J Orthop Traumatol. 2015;16(2):117–23. https://doi.org/10.1007/s10195-014-0310-2.
22. Kamath AF, Cody SR, Hosalkar HS. Open reduction of medial epicondyle fractures: operative tips for technical ease. J Child Orthop. 2009;3(4):331–6. https://doi.org/10.1007/s11832-009-0185-6.
23. Nielsen E, Andras LM, Skaggs DL. Quantifying the location of the radial nerve in children for intraoperative use. J Pediatr Orthop. 2018;38(5):e292–5. https://doi.org/10.1097/BPO.0000000000001157.
24. Pace GI, Hennrikus WL. Fixation of displaced medial epicondyle fractures in adolescents. J Pediatr Orthop. 2017;37(2):e80–2. https://doi.org/10.1097/BPO.0000000000000743.
25. Haxhija EQ, et al. Treatment of avulsion injury of the epicondyle in children. Tec. Quir. Ortop. Traumatol. (ed. esp.) Vol. 16 núm. 3, 2007.
26. Stevenson RA, Perry DC. Paediatric medial epicondyle fractures of the distal humerus. Orthop Trauma. 2018;32:360. https://doi.org/10.1016/j.mporth.2018.07.014.

Chapter 14
Supracondylar Fracture of the Distal Humerus

Pía Franz, Unni Narayanan, and Matías Sepúlveda O.

14.1 Supracondylar Fracture of the Distal Humerus

Supracondylar fractures of the humerus are the most frequent fracture around the elbow in patients under 7 years old. The usual mechanism is a fall on the outstretched hand, with the elbow in hyperextension. It requires, in a high number of cases, surgical resolution, through closed reduction and percutaneous fixation with Kirschner wires, given the limited potential for remodeling of the residual deformities resulting without treatment. It is important to recognize the different fracture patterns, both by their mechanism and by the radiological study, as this allows for proper management, reducing associated complications.

14.2 Introduction

Supracondylar fractures of the distal humerus are the most common elbow fractures in pediatric age (75%), accounting for approximately 12–17% of all fractures in this period [1]. They account for 60% of humerus fractures in this population.

P. Franz
Valdivia, Chile

U. Narayanan
The Hospital for Sick Children (SickKids), Toronto, Canada
e-mail: unni.narayanan@sickkids.ca

M. Sepúlveda O. (✉)
Instituto de Especialidades, Universidad Austral de Chile, Clínica Alemana Valdivia, Valdivia, XIV Los Ríos, Chile
e-mail: contacto@matiassepulveda.com

M. Sepúlveda O. (ed.), *Paediatrics Traumatology*,
https://doi.org/10.1007/978-3-031-89482-4_14

They are observed more frequently in children under 10 years old, with a maximum incidence between 5 and 7 years old [2]. Most of the fractures occur on the left or non-dominant side, and recent studies report a similar incidence in men and women [3]. They are associated with neurovascular injuries in up to 5% of cases, and with ipsilateral distal radius fractures in up to 10%.

It should be noted that up to 80% of supracondylar fractures will require surgical treatment to achieve a good functional and aesthetic result, so it is essential to recognize the principles that guide these indications and the surgical techniques that achieve adequate stability of the most anatomical reduction possible.

14.3 Mechanism of Injury

The ossification of the distal humerus is a gradual process, which involves four ossification nuclei [4]: lateral humeral condyle, which is radiologically visible between 1–12 months old in girls and 1–26 months old in boys; epicondyle, which appears between 5–8 years old in girls and 7–9 years old in boys; trochlea, visible between 7–11 years old in girls and 8–13 years old in boys; and epicondyle, which is observed between 8–11 years old in girls and 9–13 years old in boys. The ossification nuclei of the epicondyle, condyle, and trochlea fuse together from the age of 10 years old in girls and 12 years old in boys, generating the distal humerus, which completes fusion with the distal metaphysis of the humerus at around 12–14 years old in girls and 13–16 years old in boys. This pattern of ossification allows for the existence of multiple injuries in the distal humerus of the pediatric patient, so it is fundamental to be aware of them (Fig. 14.1).

The supracondylar fracture of the humerus occurs because the bone anatomy of the elbow presents a point of weakness at this age, given by the olecranon fossa and the coronoid fossa, which present a thin bone wall, where the olecranon performs a hinge. Also, the distal humerus will present, in most cases, a structure mainly cartilaginous.

The mechanism of injury for a supracondylar fracture will depend on the position of the elbow at the time of the injury, and the direction towards where the body moves when falling. In this way, they are divided into fractures with the elbow in extension, which are the most frequent (98%), and fractures with the elbow in flexion (2%).

Supracondylar fractures in extension occur when the child falls with the hand extended, and the elbow performing a hyperextension, with the olecranon being forced into the olecranon fossa. This fulcrum results in a fracture over the olecranon fossa, with a distal fragment displaced posteriorly and proximally. In the event that the body weight shifts in external rotation over the elbow locked in extension, the proximal fragment damages the periosteum laterally, resulting in a posteromedial displacement of the distal fragment (Fig. 14.2). If the weight of the body falls in internal rotation posteriorly, the proximal fragment will cause damage to the periosteum medially, resulting in a posterolateral displacement of the distal fragment. This consideration is especially relevant when performing reduction maneuvers, trying to reverse the mechanism of displacement, and choosing the most suitable stabilization method, with fixation looking specially on the periosteum damaged.

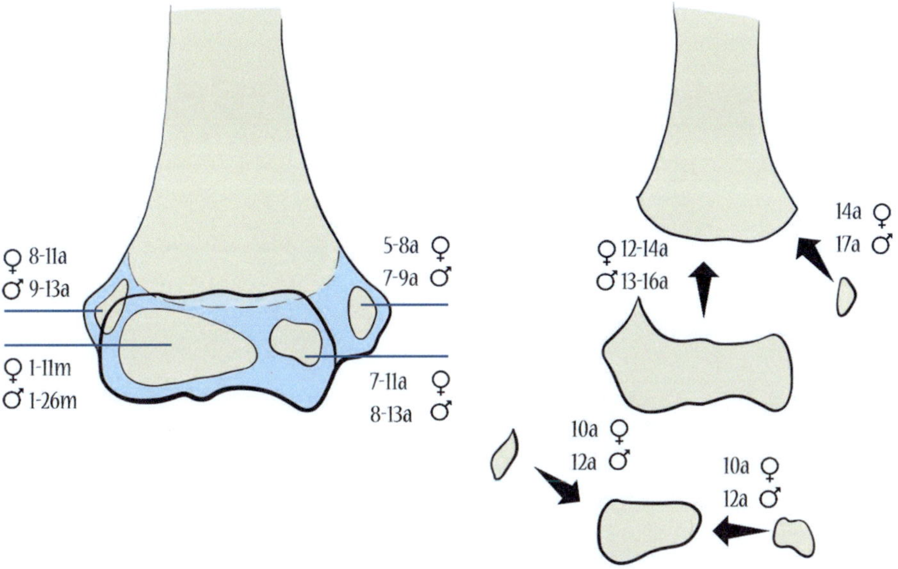

Fig. 14.1 Age of appearence of the ossification nuclei of the elbow and approximate ages of their union

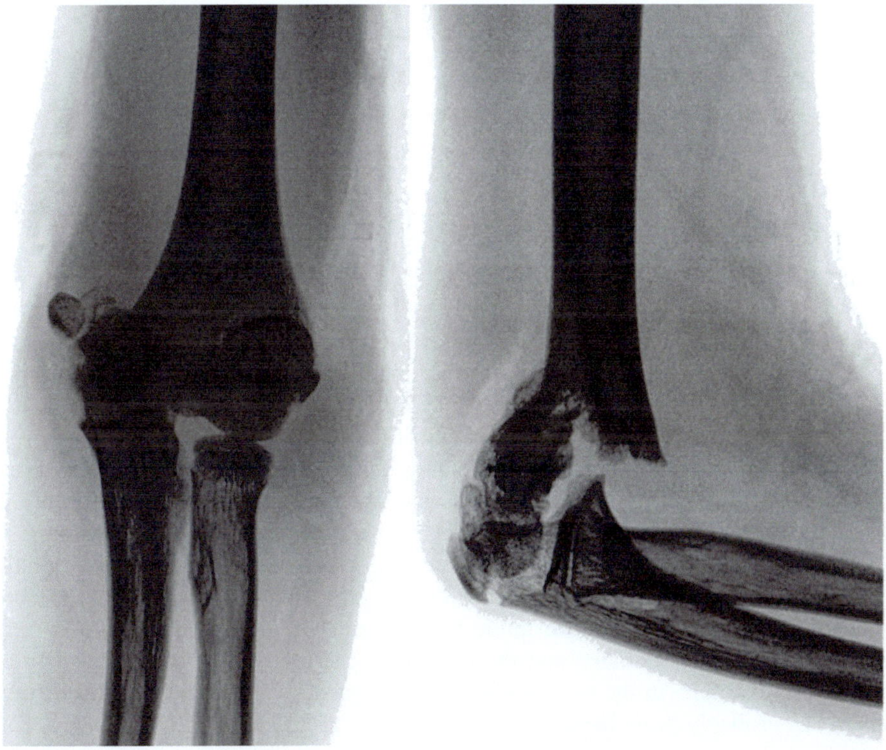

Fig. 14.2 X-ray of the left elbow with a supracondylar fracture in extension, with displacement of the distal fragment towards posteromedial

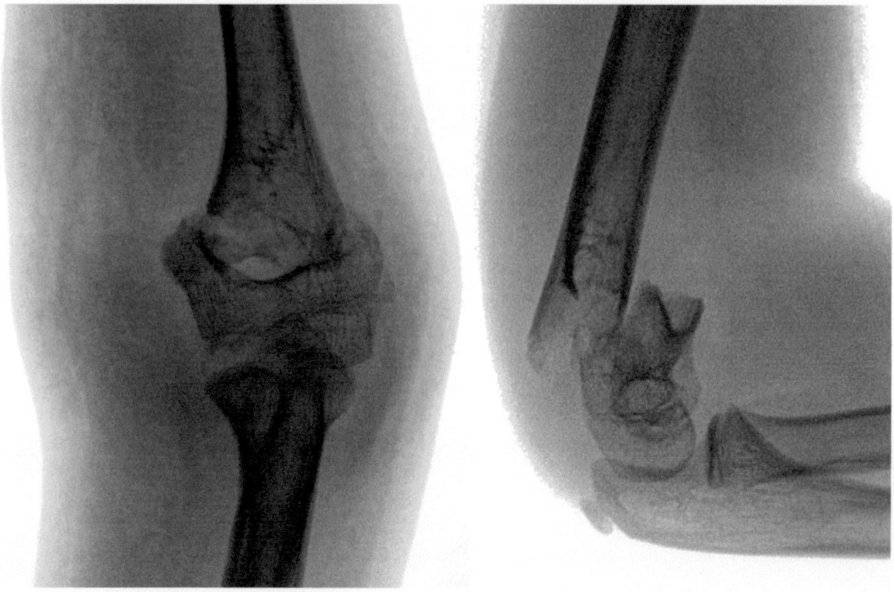

Fig. 14.3 Left elbow radiographs of a 10-year-old girl, with a supracondylar fracture of the humerus, due flexion mechanism

The supracondylar fracture with the elbow in flexion (2%) occurs when the patient falls directly on the elbow, hitting the olecranon against the floor, which pushes the distal fragment anteriorly [3] (Fig. 14.3).

14.4 Diagnosis

This injury should be considered in a patient who presents history of falling over the upper extremity with pain, swelling, and limited mobility of the elbow. As with all pediatric trauma, it is vital to be alert to characteristics in the history that may suggest a non-accidental injury, including a delay in seeking medical attention, inconsistent mechanism, and abnormal behavior of the child or caregivers.

A thorough physical examination, avoiding causing more pain, is essential to determine the mechanism and possible associated injuries. Usually, elbow deformity is observed due to swelling, increased volume, pain, and decreased range of motion.

It should be noted the presence of wounds or abrasions, umbilications of the skin that imply the passage of a bone fragment through the brachial muscle, and the location of hematomas, which will guide us to where the greatest damage occurred, including periosteal damage and the direction of displacement of the distal fragment. For example, in the presence of an anteromedial hematoma, the distal fragment has probably been displaced posterolaterally (Fig. 14.4).

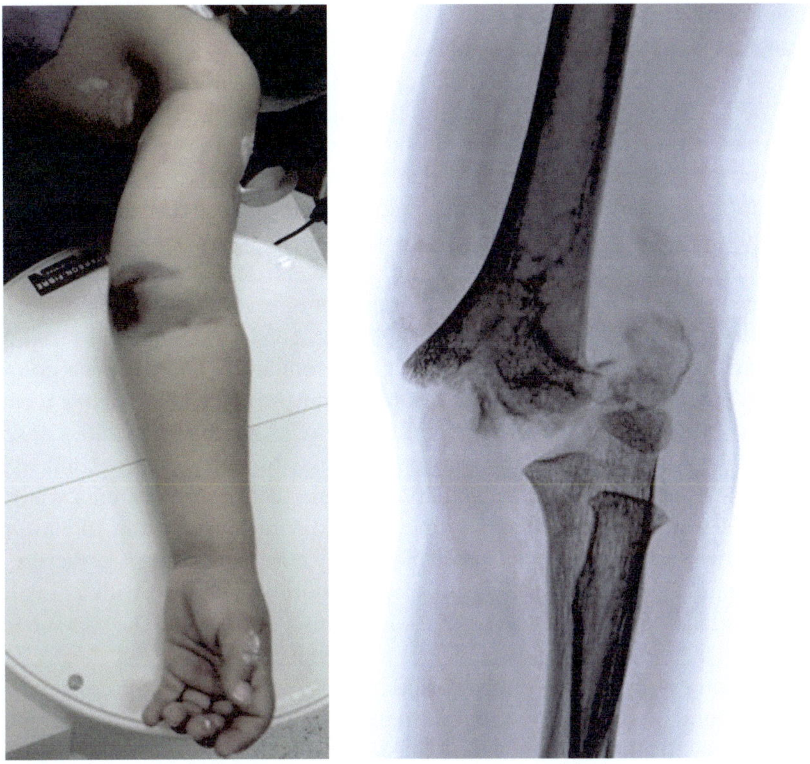

Fig. 14.4 Clinical image of an arm with medial hematoma in the left elbow, product of a supracondylar fracture in extension with posterolateral displacement

The presence of other fractures in the upper limb must be ruled out, the most frequently associated being distal radius and forearm fractures. The latter present a higher risk of developing compartment syndrome, so timely diagnosis and treatment are of vital importance.

Around 12–20% of displaced injuries are associated with a neurological deficit, with the anterior interosseous nerve, a motor branch of the median nerve, being the most frequently affected as it is stretched in a posteromedial displacement, followed by the radial nerve, mainly due to a posterolateral displacement, and the ulnar nerve in flexion mechanisms [5]. The sensory and motor function of each nerve should be examined individually.

For the evaluation of the radial nerve, we will look for sensitivity in the first interdigital space and mobility with wrist and finger extension. The median nerve is evaluated sensitively on the radial edge of the index finger and its motor function with the adduction of the thumb to the palm of the hand. The anterior interosseous nerve is evaluated by asking the patient to make the "OK" sign, with the remaining fingers in extension. Finally, the ulnar nerve is evaluated sensitively on the ulnar edge of the little finger, and motor function by performing ulnar and little finger extension and flexion, or flexion of the distal interphalangeal of the little finger (Fig. 14.5).

The physical examination should be repeated if necessary. In general, the neurological deficit identified at the time of the injury is temporary, and resolves in 6–12 weeks. However, a change in the postoperative neurological examination is more concerning, and may indicate that the affected nerve was injured during manipulation, or that it is trapped at the fracture site. In these cases, surgical exploration of the nerve may be necessary to avoid permanent damage [6].

It is important to evaluate the vascularity of the extremity by palpating the radial pulse. However, hand perfusion is a better indicator of severity in case of an injury. In most children, abundant collateral flow to the forearm and hand originates proximal to the fracture site, medially through the ulnar recurrent artery and the ulnar collateral artery, and laterally through the radial recurrent artery and the interosseous recurrent artery (Fig. 14.6). Despite the absence of radial pulse as a result of an injury or spasm of the brachial artery at the fracture site, the hand may be well perfused. Clinical indicators of distal perfusion include capillary refill less than 2 seconds, on a warm and pink hand. A child with an ischemic limb may experience significant forearm pain, loss of motor function, pain with passive finger extension, and/or paresthesias. The vascular status of the injured limb is classified as: normal, pulseless with a pink hand, and disvascular, which is described as pulseless with a white hand. The supracondylar fracture with a disvascular hand constitutes a surgical emergency [7].

The imaging study for this injury should include elbow radiographs in anteroposterior and lateral projections, the latter usually providing us with more information. These images will allow us to diagnose, classify, and guide subsequent management.

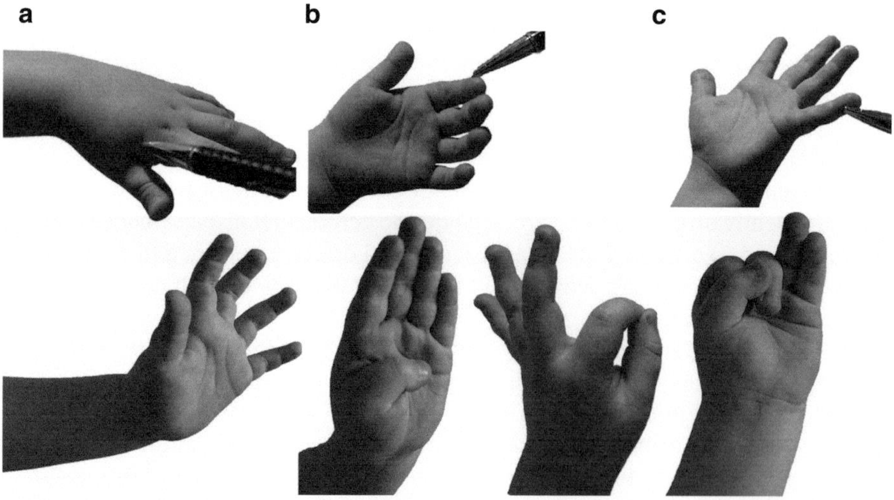

Fig. 14.5 Neurological examination at hand level. Assessment of sensory and motor function of radial nerve (**a**), median nerve (**b**), anterior interosseous nerve (**c**, motor only) and ulnar nerve (**d**)

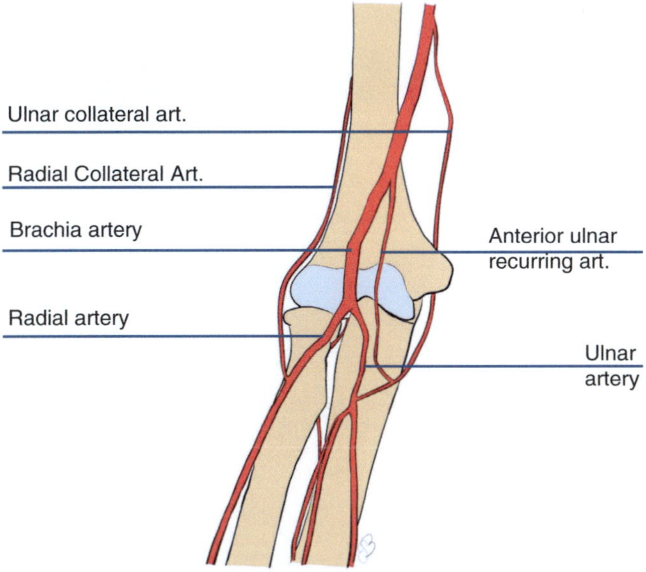

Fig. 14.6 Scheme of the vascular irrigation at the level of the right elbow, in an anterior view

In the anteroposterior (AP) radiograph, we will find a loss of anatomy, in the case of displaced fractures, while in non-displaced ones we usually see the fracture line. We can define displacement as medial, with periosteal damage laterally at the fracture focus, or lateral, with periosteal damage medially.

The Baumann angle, which is formed between the longitudinal axis of the humeral shaft and a line along the physis of the humeral condyle, should also be measured. Although it is a measure of alignment of the coronal plane of the distal humerus, it is not very reliable and should be used with caution. This angle is very sensitive to the position of the elbow when the radiograph is taken, and there is a wide variation in normal elbows, from 64° to 81° (Fig. 14.7).

In the lateral radiograph, we should look for the integrity of the humeral pallet, which is seen as an "hourglass," demonstrating continuity of the cortices (Fig. 14.8). We should observe that the anterior humeral line intercepts the capitellum in the center. If not, we will have a hinge displacement, anterior or posterior. The posterior displacement of the distal fragment, as occurs in extension injuries, causes the capitellum to be located posterior to the anterior humeral line (Fig. 14.8), the opposite occurring in fractures with a flexion mechanism. In the case of not finding great displacement, but if evidence of significant rotation of the distal fragment, we should consider the presence of a flexion fracture.

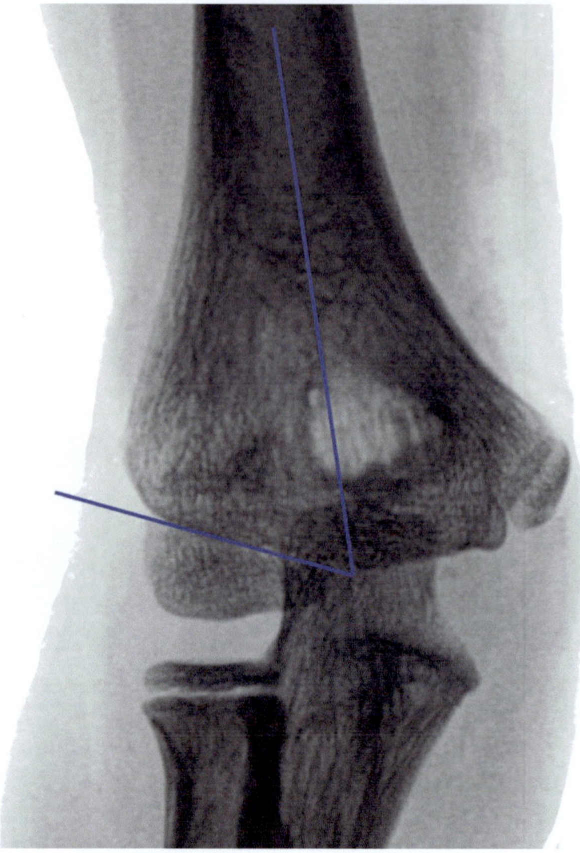

Fig. 14.7 Anteroposterior x-ray view of a right elbow. Baumann angle measurement, between the longitudinal axis of the humerus and the physeal line of the lateral condyle

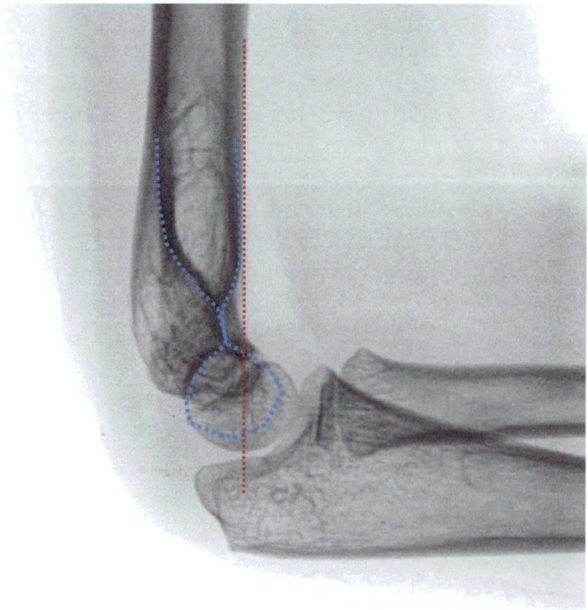

Fig. 14.8 Lateral elbow x-ray. It should be observed the continuity of the cortices of the humeral palett (blue line). The anterior humeral line must cross through the capitellum (red line)

In hidden fractures lines, we should look for the “fat pad” sign, which corresponds to the elevation of the fat at the level of the olecranon fossa, due to the presence of hematoma, which we can find in intracapsular fractures at the elbow level.

These projections will also help us rule out differential diagnoses such as humeral condyle fracture and radial neck fractures, among others.

14.5 Classification

Kocher (1896) classified supracondylar fractures according to their injury mechanism, into extension fractures (96%) and flexion fractures (4%).

The Gartland classification [8] is the most used system to describe extension type supracondylar fractures (Fig. 14.9). Type 1 corresponds to incomplete fractures without displacement, type 2 to incomplete fractures with an anterior hinge, and type 3 to complete fractures, with greater displacement.

Wilkins [9] modified the Gartland classification, dividing the fractures into subtypes A and B. Type 1A fractures are fractures without compression, while 1B fractures are those that present compression of the medial column, with varus deformity. Type 2A present posterior angulation, while 2B fractures present posterior angulation and frontal deviation. Type 3A corresponds to fractures with displacement of the distal fragment towards posteromedial (75–90%), and 3B fractures present posterolateral displacement.

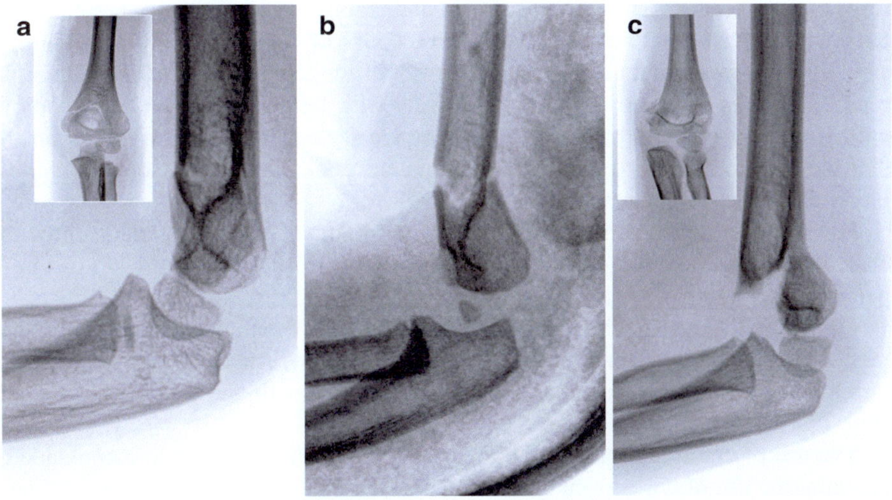

Fig. 14.9 Gartland classification for supracondylar fracture in extension. Type 1, incomplete without displacement (**a**), Type 2, incomplete with anterior hinge (**b**), Type 3, complete (**c**). According to AO Pediatric fracture classification, these are 13-M/3 (humerus, distal, metaphyseal), and divided in non-displaced, Type I (**a**) and Type II (**b**), and displaced Type III (**c**) and Type IV

Distinguishing between the subtypes allows the surgeon to predict which fractures can be successfully managed with reduction and cast, and which require reduction and fixation.

Leitch [10] proposed the addition of a type IV fracture to the Gartland classification. These are unstable both in flexion and in extension due to the complete periosteum damage, presenting great displacement and multidirectional instability. These fractures occur as a result of high energy trauma or by an excessive flexion force applied during the closed reduction maneuver.

Flexion fractures can be classified into type I or non-displaced fractures, type II with minimal displacement, with intact anterior cortex, and type III as displaced.

14.6 Treatment

The objectives are to restore the anatomy of the elbow, with normal function and appearance, using the safest and easiest method to reproduce.

Type 1 fractures, both in flexion and extension, can be treated with long-arm cast immobilization, at 90° of flexion and forearm in neutral, for 3 weeks. After removal, the patient usually presents elbow joint stiffness, which will recover progressively in 4–6 weeks, without the need of assistance for rehabilitation.

For type 2 extension fractures, it is recommended to evaluate the degree of angulation and displacement by the percentage of intersection of the capitellum by the anterior humeral line. If this line cuts more than 30% of the capitellum, we can perform conservative management, similar to type 1. If not, it is suggested to perform a closed reduction under anesthesia and stabilization with two percutaneous Kirschner wires (1.6–2 mm, depending on the size of the patient), from the lateral side, in order to avoid an extension deformity of the elbow (Fig. 14.10). Although type 2 fractures can be treated conservatively with long-arm cast without fixation with Kirschner wires, it should be radiographically evaluated in a week to verify that the position of the fragments is maintained. For this reason, some surgeons prefer to fix these fractures at the first moment.

For type 3, 4, or displaced in flexion, the treatment will be surgical, through closed reduction under anesthesia and stabilization with two (Fig. 14.11) or three percutaneous Kirschner wires (Fig. 14.12).

Occasionally, the Kirschner wires can be in a crossed configuration, one from the medial side and others from the lateral side of the elbow, especially in oblique fracture lines, high on the medial side, not possible to fix with wires only from lateral (Fig. 14.13).

The use of configurations with the wires from the lateral side is recommended, avoiding the use of wires from the medial side, as it is associated with a 6% of iatrogenic injury of the ulnar nerve [11].

It is essential to seek a closed reduction in order not to damage the irrigation of the distal humerus, in addition to avoiding the joint stiffness associated with an open reduction. In complex cases, such as highly unstable fractures, inverted oblique

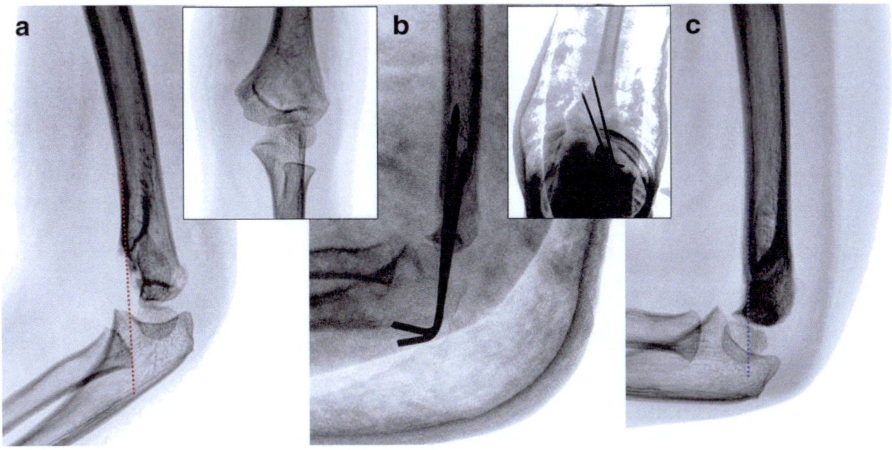

Fig. 14.10 Gartland type 2 fracture in extension. It can be seen that the anterior humeral line (red) does not cut capitellum (**a**). Closed reduction is performed and stabilization with 2 Kirschner wires from lateral entry (**b**). Radiological control at 2 months after surgery, with adequate axis correction (**c**)

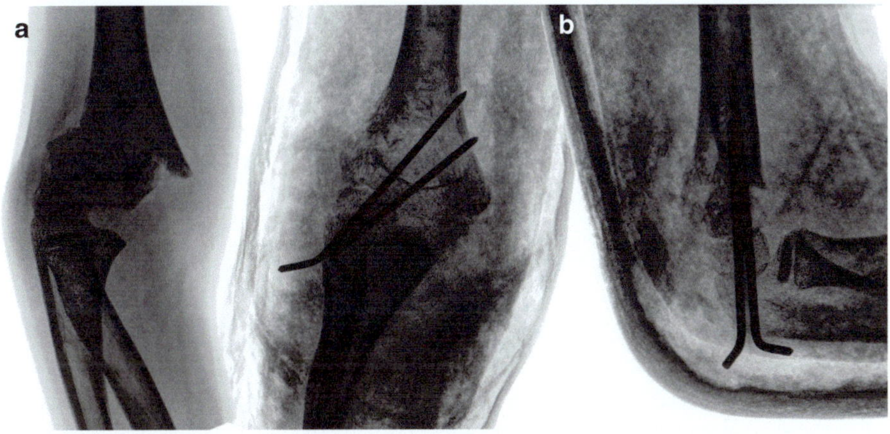

Fig. 14.11 Gartland type 3 fracture in extension (**a**). Closed reduction and fixation with 2 Kirschner wires from lateral, divergent (**b**)

fracture lines, comminuted or in flexion, we can use a lateral external fixator [12] to stabilize those fractures in which an anatomical reduction is not possible to achieve, and in this way, we avoid the open exploration of the elbow (Fig. 14.14).

In case associated with vascular injury, with the absence of radial pulse and good distal hand perfusion, reduction, and stabilization are recommended, and then the patient is kept under observation for at least 24 h, as over 95% recovery of distal perfusion is reported after fracture reduction. If, on the contrary, if there is no good distal perfusion, evidenced of a pale hand with decreased capillary refill, immediate surgical exploration is recommended once the fracture is stabilized [13].

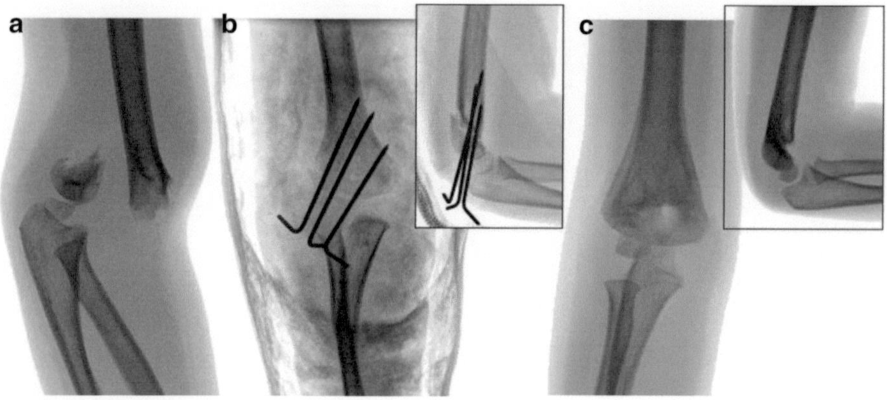

Fig. 14.12 Gartland type 3 fracture in extension (**a**). Closed reduction and fixation with 3 Kirschner wires from lateral side (**b**). X-ray analysis at 3 months shows a consolidated fracture, in anatomycal axis (**c**)

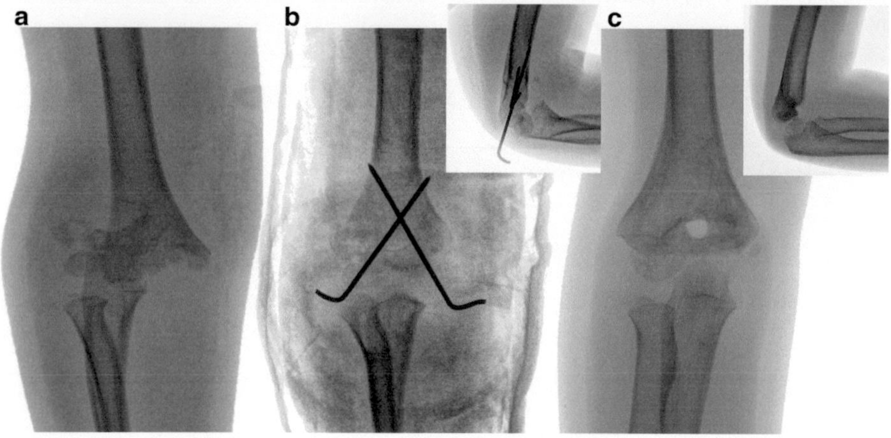

Fig. 14.13 Gartland type 3 supracondylar fracture in extension (**a**). It was decided to use Kirschner wires in a crossed configuration, for its stabilization (**b**). Control after 3 months with appropriate axis (**c**)

Surgical Technique for Reduction and Fixation with Percutaneous Pinning of an Extension Supracondylar Fracture.

The patient is positioned with the upper extremity on the fluoroscopy beam, or in highly unstable cases, on a lateral extension table, in order to rotate the X-ray machine around the elbow to evaluate the lateral projection, avoiding displacements of the reduction due manipulation on rotation.

The displacement of the fragments is verified under fluoroscopy. The mechanism of injury will help us understand where the main damage to the periosteum occurred, which in its undamaged segment will serve as a tension band when performing the closed reduction.

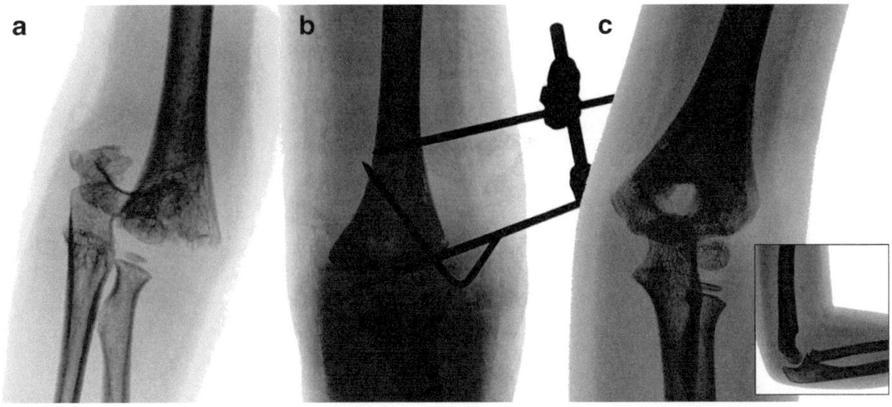

Fig. 14.14 Gartland type 3 supracondylar fracture in extension (**a**). Given high fracture instability, the use of an external fixator technique was required for its reduction and stabilization (**b**). Control after 3 months with appropriate axis (**c**)

If there is invagination of the proximal fragment into the brachial fascia, a "milking" maneuver is performed, seeking to reduce it. Then, maintain traction in longitudinal axis for a period of 3–5 min. In this way, we will recover the displacement towards proximal of the distal fragment, due to muscle contraction.

We continue seeking the alignment of the fragments in the frontal plane, through translation, under longitudinal traction. Finally, we align the lateral plane, pressing from the olecranon towards the front, pronating the forearm, as we flex the elbow. To evaluate the reduction in the lateral plane, we rotate the shoulder externally, with the elbow in maximum flexion.

It is important for stable closed reduction with Kirschner wires to achieve adequate bone contact, with a maximum of 10 degrees of rotation of the fragments, to avoid collapse into varus.

Once the fracture is reduced, we fix it in position with two or three divergent Kirschner wires, from the lateral side of the elbow. These wires must meet the following recommendations for greater stability: be of an adequate diameter (1.6–2 mm), fix the lateral and medial columns, enter the base of the capitellum, sufficiently separated at the fracture level, and that they pass through both cortices [10].

The stability of the reduction should be verified with fluoroscopy in four projections: anteroposterior, lateral, internal oblique, and external oblique, looking for continuity of the humeral cortices (Fig. 14.15). The criteria for appropriate reduction include continuity of the medial and lateral columns in the oblique projections, Baumann angle greater than 70°, and that the anterior humeral line intercepts the capitellum. The elbow should be extended to clinically confirm a carrying angle in slight valgus and similar to the uninjured side. Under continuous fluoroscopy, stability can be verified under flexion-extension maneuvers and internal rotation of the forearm. Once a stable reduction is confirmed, the elbow is protected with a long-arm plaster splint.

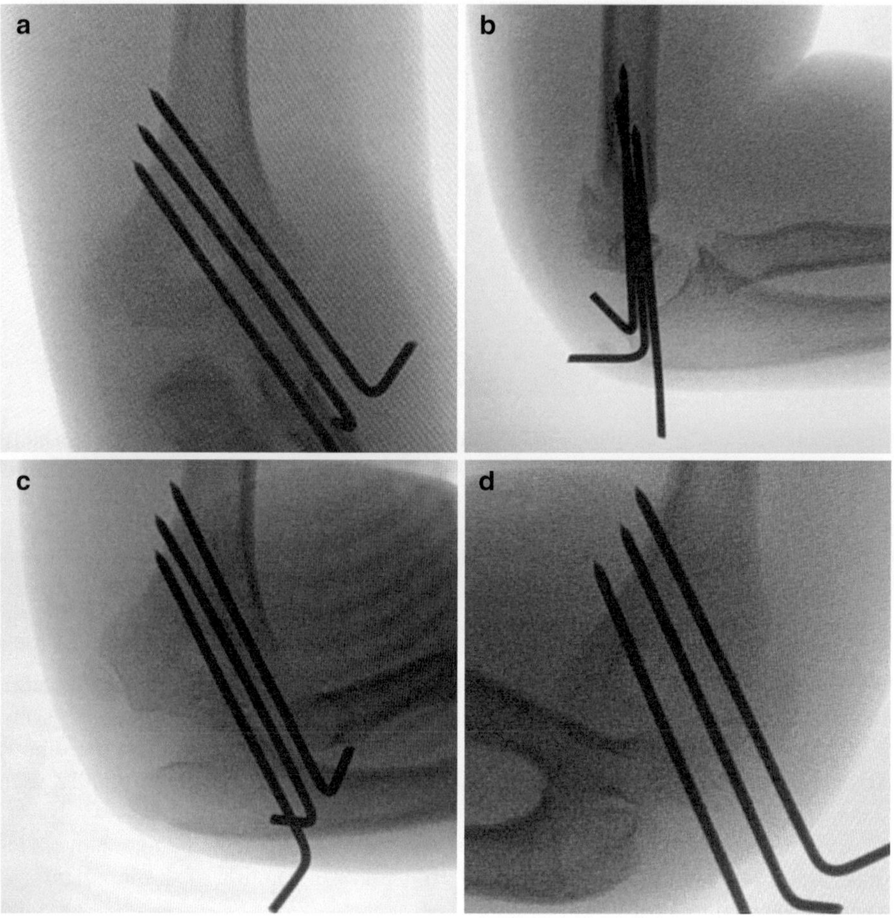

Fig. 14.15 Intraoperative verification of an anatomical reduction. X-ray views to evaluate antero-posterior plane (**a**), Lateral plane (**b**), External oblique, verifying medial cortex congruence (**c**) and internal oblique verifying lateral cortex congruence (**d**)

In this way, we will obtain a satisfactory result, with consolidation at 3 weeks, the adequate time for removal of the cast and the Kirschner wires, which is done in the ambulatory clinic. The normal range of motion of the elbow is recovered around 2 months after cast removal, usually without the need for rehabilitation.

14.7 Complications

Malunion in "Cubitus Varus" is one of the most frequent complications for supracondylar fractures of the humerus. An incidence of 2–3% is reported, and it can occur both after conservative as with surgical treatment. It is associated with an impaction of the medial column greater than 10°, with inadequate reduction, with a loss of reduction due poor stabilization, and in rarer cases, with physeal injuries.

This deformity is typically painless and does not affect the movement of the elbow. Over time it can be associated with posterolateral instability of the elbow, given by the medial displacement of the mechanical axis of the elbow, which results in asymmetric forces of the triceps that cause a chronic failure of the lateral collateral ligament [14].

Corrective osteotomy should be considered in patients with significant residual varus. The aesthetic deformity and the possibility of posterolateral rotational instability should be discussed with the parents. In general, surgery is performed after 1 year following the injury, when the range of motion of the elbow has stopped improving, and when the patient is old enough to cooperate with postoperative instructions. Multiple alternatives are described for this correction, such as performing a lateral closing wedge osteotomy and fixation with an external fixator (Fig. 14.16) [15]. Techniques such as dome osteotomy or step osteotomy may be necessary in patients with severe rotational or sagittal plane deformities.

Compartment syndrome is a rare complication of supracondylar fracture (0.3%), but with devastating consequences, such as Volkmann's ischemic contracture, which leads to a permanent functional deficit. It occurs most commonly due to hyperflexion of the elbow during cast immobilization, specially when this hyperflexion is necessary to maintain fracture reduction. This is one of the reasons why percutaneous fixation with Kirschner wires is recommended in those cases, as the elbow can be immobilized slightly extended, reducing this risk. Compartment syndrome is more common in patients with floating elbow and associated neurovascular injury.

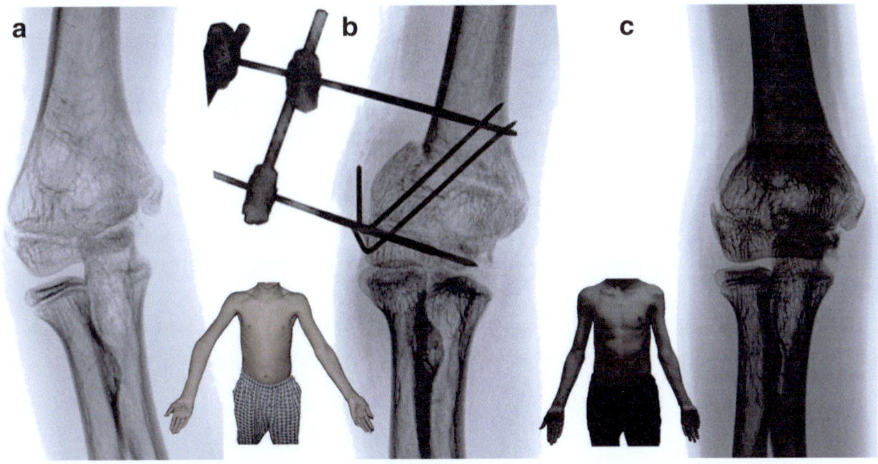

Fig. 14.16 11-year-old patient with cubitus varus secondary to a supracondylar humerus fracture (**a**). Closed wedge osteotomy and stabilization were performed with lateral external fixator (**b**), which is maintained for 5 weeks. Control at 3 months, with corrected transport axis and complete bone healing (**c**)

The traditional signs and symptoms associated with compartment syndrome in adults are not reliable indicators of the condition in pediatric patients. In them, suspicion should be raised in the face of the “3A’s”: Anxiety, Agitation, and increasing needs for Analgesics [6]. It is therefore important to observe the patient hospitalized for 12–24 hours after complex surgery to allow early detection. Neurovascular controls and monitoring signs and symptoms of increased pain should be frequent in scenarios where the risk of compartment syndrome is increased. The treatment will consist of a palmar fasciotomy of the forearm, from the elbow to the wrist.

Iatrogenic neurological injuries, particularly of the ulnar nerve, are associated with the insertion of Kirschner wires from medially. It is important to perform a mini open approach prior to their insertion to reduce the risks of this injury. The elbow should be extended when a Kirschner wire is required to be inserted from the medial side of the elbow, so that the ulnar nerve moves posteriorly, out of the path of the wire. Median nerve injuries are associated with the insertion of wires laterally. In general, the patient is observed until spontaneous recovery is achieved, which occurs in 80% of cases at 6–12 months. In the case of a positive Tinel’s sign, neuropathic pain or complete nerve paralysis, surgical exploration should be considered.

14.8 Final Message

Supracondylar fractures of the distal humerus are a complex situation, which generates great interest among pediatric trauma surgeons, both for their frequency, and for the importance of restoring the anatomy with the chosen treatment, given the limited remodeling potential of the area. Thus, an adequate diagnosis, based on imaging studies and the clinical signs described, will allow us to make a correct decision when proposing the treatment.

The closed reduction technique allows for achieving adequate anatomy in the vast majority of cases. This way, secondary aesthetic and functional problems can be avoided.

The stabilization of these injuries can be achieved with a lower risk, with percutaneous Kirschner wires from the lateral side of the elbow. This is supported by the rapid bone healing of the area, which allows wire removal on an outpatient basis after 3 weeks.

Without a doubt, a reduction as anatomical as possible, with good fixation, is fundamental to avoid a sequel of cubitus varus, often associated with this injury.

References

1. Khoshbin A, Leroux T, Wasserstein D, et al. The epidemiology of paediatric supracondylar fracture fixation: a population-based study. Injury. 2014;45(4):701–8. https://doi.org/10.1016/j.injury.2013.10.004.
2. Omid R, Choi PD, Skaggs DL. Supracondylar humeral fractures in children. J Bone Joint Surg Am. 2008;90(5):1121–32. https://doi.org/10.2106/JBJS.G.01354.
3. Cheng JC, Lam TP, Maffulli N. Epidemiological features of supracondylar fractures of the humerus in Chinese children. J Pediatr Orthop B. 2001;10(1):63–7.
4. Procell Villalobos CR, Cassis Zacarías N, Juárez Rojas CS, Cárdenas Turrent MB. Appearance of ossification centers in the elbow in Mexican children between 6 months and 12 years old. Acta Ortop Mex. 2008;22(6):347–9.
5. Campbell CC, Waters PM, Emans JB, Kasser JR, Millis MB. Neurovascular injury and displacement in type III supracondylar humerus fractures. J Pediatr Orthop. 1995;15(1):47–52. https://doi.org/10.1097/01241398-199501000-00011.
6. Badkoobehi H, Choi PD, Bae DS, Skaggs DL. Management of the pulseless pediatric supracondylar humeral fracture. J Bone Joint Surg Am. 2015;97(11):937–43. https://doi.org/10.2106/JBJS.N.00983.
7. Harris LR, Arkader A, Broom A, et al. Pulseless supracondylar humerus fracture with anterior interosseous nerve or median nerve injury-an absolute indication for open reduction? J Pediatr Orthop. 2019;39(1):e1–7. https://doi.org/10.1097/BPO.0000000000001238.
8. Gartland JJ. Management of supracondylar fractures of the humerus in children. Surg Gynecol Obstet. 1959;109(2):145–54.
9. Wilkins KE, Beaty JH, Chambers HG, Toniolo RM. Fractures and dislocations of the elbow region. In: Rockwood CA, Wilkins KE, Beaty J, editors. Fractures in children, vol. 4. Philadelphia, PA: Lippincott Williams and Wilkins; 1996. p. 653–904.
10. Leitch KK, Kay RM, Femino JD, Tolo VT, Storer SK, Skaggs DL. Treatment of multidirectionally unstable supracondylar humeral fractures in children. A modified Gartland type-IV fracture. J Bone Joint Surg Am. 2006;88(5):980–5. https://doi.org/10.2106/JBJS.D.02956.
11. Dekker AE, Krijnen P, Schipper IB. Results of crossed versus lateral entry K-wire fixation of displaced pediatric supracondylar humeral fractures: a systematic review and meta-analysis. Injury. 2016;47(11):2391–8. https://doi.org/10.1016/j.injury.2016.08.022.
12. Slongo T, Schmid T, Wilkins K, Joeris A. Lateral external fixation--a new surgical technique for displaced unreducible supracondylar humeral fractures in children. J Bone Joint Surg Am. 2008;90(8):1690–7. https://doi.org/10.2106/JBJS.G.00528.
13. Shah AS, Waters PM, Bae DS. Treatment of the "pink pulseless hand" in pediatric supracondylar humerus fractures. J Hand Surg Am. 2013;38(7):1399–404. https://doi.org/10.1016/j.jhsa.2013.03.047.
14. McKee MD, Kim J, Kebaish K, Stephen DJ, Kreder HJ, Schemitsch EH. Functional outcome after open supracondylar fractures of the humerus. The effect of the surgical approach. J Bone Joint Surg Br. 2000;82(5):646–51. https://doi.org/10.1302/0301-620x.82b5.10423.
15. Slongo T. Treatment of posttraumatic cubitus varus in children and adolescents. Supracondylar humeral osteotomy using radial external fixation. Oper Orthop Traumatol. 2015;27(3):194–209. https://doi.org/10.1007/s00064-015-0403-y.

Chapter 15
Radial Neck Fractures

Theddy Slongo

15.1 Introduction

In childhood, most fractures around the proximal radius are radial neck fractures, according to the AO Pediatric classification [1, 2] classified as types 21r-M and 21r–E. Real radial head fractures are rare and are not the primary focus of this chapter.

There is still a debate about the degree of angulation at which repositioning is necessary. We believe that this debate should no longer arise today, as we know that the proximal radius has a very low correction potential. On the other hand, we now have very simple, minimally invasive procedures at our disposal that, when used correctly, lead to excellent results. Therefore, over all the last years, the absolute gold standard for the treatment of all these fractures is the closed indirect reduction and internal fixation according to the elastic stable intramedullary nailing (ESIN) technique [3, 4]. Open reduction and internal fixation should be avoided as we see more problems such as AVN, unstable fixation, joint stiffness, and radioulnar synostosis with bad functional outcomes [5].

On the other hand, the ESIN method leads to a more frequent indication for an operative treatment, as the advantages of this technique are high. The functional postoperative treatment is one of the most important.

T. Slongo (✉)
Rüfenacht, Switzerland

M. Sepúlveda O. (ed.), *Paediatrics Traumatology*,
https://doi.org/10.1007/978-3-031-89482-4_15

15.2 Mechanism of Injury

To reproduce the injury mechanism of this fracture is difficult, even when there are some theories illustrated in some textbooks. In principle, the radial head is protected by the stable situation between the humerus and the ulna. Therefore, two main theoretical mechanisms are possible for most of the cases, (1) a "flexion type" fracture, where the radial head is in flexion in relation to the radial shaft due to high valgus stress on the extended elbow that leads to compression or fracture of the metaphyseal segment with angulation /dislocation of the radial head; (2) axial elbow dislocation, with or without valgus stress.

Since most injuries in this area are metaphyseal fractures, it can be assumed that the ligamentum annulare also plays a significant role. We often see that when the ligament is trapped in the fracture, pronation or supination is blocked and is only free again after "decompaction." This is extremely easy to demonstrate and perform with the ESIN method, since we push the radial head away from the metaphysis centrally in the bone (Fig. 15.1).

A special very rare situation, and therefore often overlooked, are radial neck fractures in which the radial head flips dorsally/backwards. It can be assumed that the fracture occurs during elbow dislocation but is not yet dislocated. If the elbow is spontaneously repositioned, the radial head remains stuck dorsally and flips backwards (Fig. 15.2).

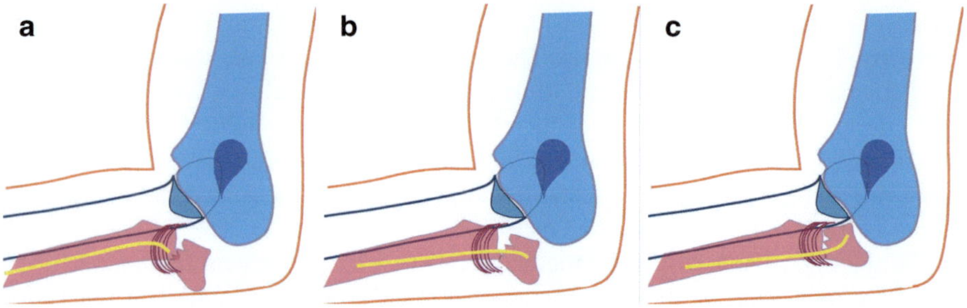

Fig. 15.1 Graphics that demonstrate how to imagine the ligamentum annulare as a hypomochlion. (**a**) The nail is in a waiting position; the ligament is trapped in the fracture. (**b**) By gently hammering on the nail after the tip has been turned toward the radial head, the fracture zone is freed from the ligament. (**c**) By rotating the nail, the fracture is reduced

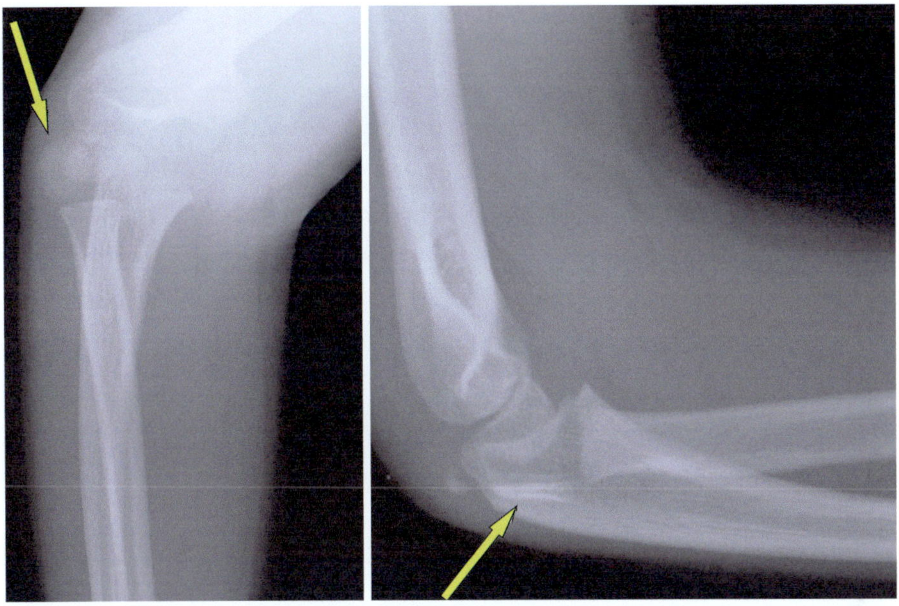

Fig. 15.2 AP and lateral X-ray of an injured elbow. The flipped radial head is clearly seen in the lateral view but also in the AP view (yellow arrow)

15.3 Clinical Evaluation and Radiology

One of the biggest problems of this fracture (respectively the fracture region) is to get an optimal X-ray, clear AP and lateral [6]. Most of the injury films we see are somewhat of oblique (Fig. 15.3) and does not allow a correct and adequate diagnosis or classification. Therefore, it is important to discuss with the radiologist how to perform correct X-rays and what we like to see. One of the options is using the image intensifier (Fig. 15.4).

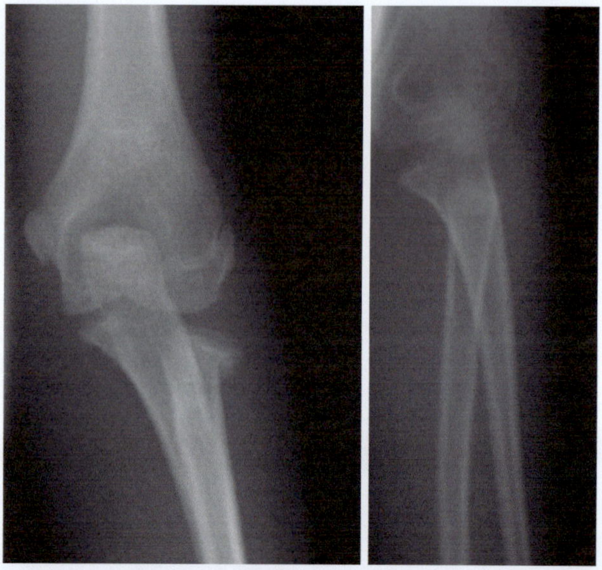

Fig. 15.3 For an optimal diagnosis, correct X-rays are mandatory. In this example, both planes are oblique, and the lateral image is not centered on the elbow

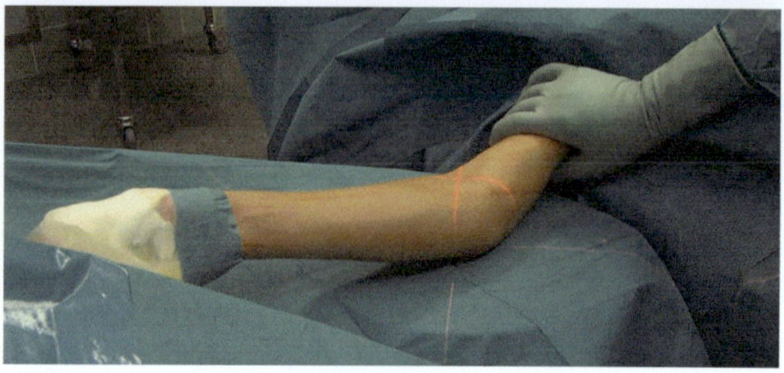

Fig. 15.4 An image intensifier with laser (red lines on the skin) facilitates the optimal positioning of the fractured segment and reduces irradiation (dosage and time)

15.4 Examples of Fractures for Non-operative and Operative Treatment According to the AO Pediatric Fracture Classification

According to the classification, all possible fractures are summarized in the following figures. In addition, it is an overview of the actual indication-philosophy and treatment modalities according to the fracture type.

1. Non-operative metaphyseal fractures, Fig. 15.5.
2. Operative metaphyseal fractures, Fig. 15.6.
3. Operative epiphyseal fractures, Fig. 15.7.

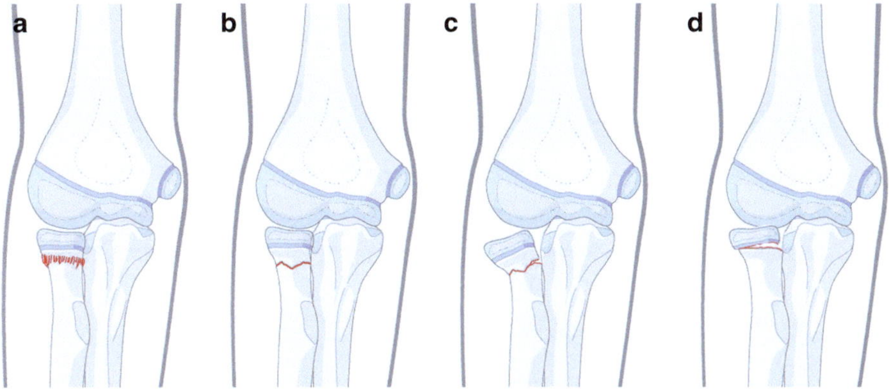

Fig. 15.5 These four graphics illustrate the different fracture morphologies we recommend for conservative treatment. (**a**) 21r – M/2.1, Buckle fracture; (**b**) 21r – M/3.1 I, complete fracture; (**c**) 21r – M/3.1 I, complete fracture, less than 25° angulation; (**d**) 21r – E/1.1 I

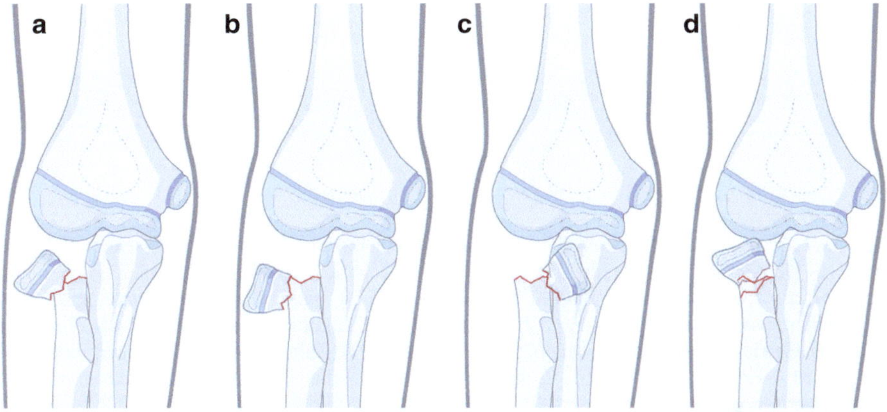

Fig. 15.6 These four graphics illustrate the different fracture morphologies of metaphyseal radial neck fractures we recommend for reduction and operative treatment (stabilization). (**a**) 21r – M/3.1 II, complete fracture, more than 25° angulation; (**b**) 21r – M/3.1 III, complete fracture, more than 25° angulation, fully displaced; (**c**) 21r – M3.1 III, complete fracture, more than 25° angulation, fully displaced to medial; (**d**) 21r – M/3.2 II, complete fracture multifragmentary, more than 25° angulation

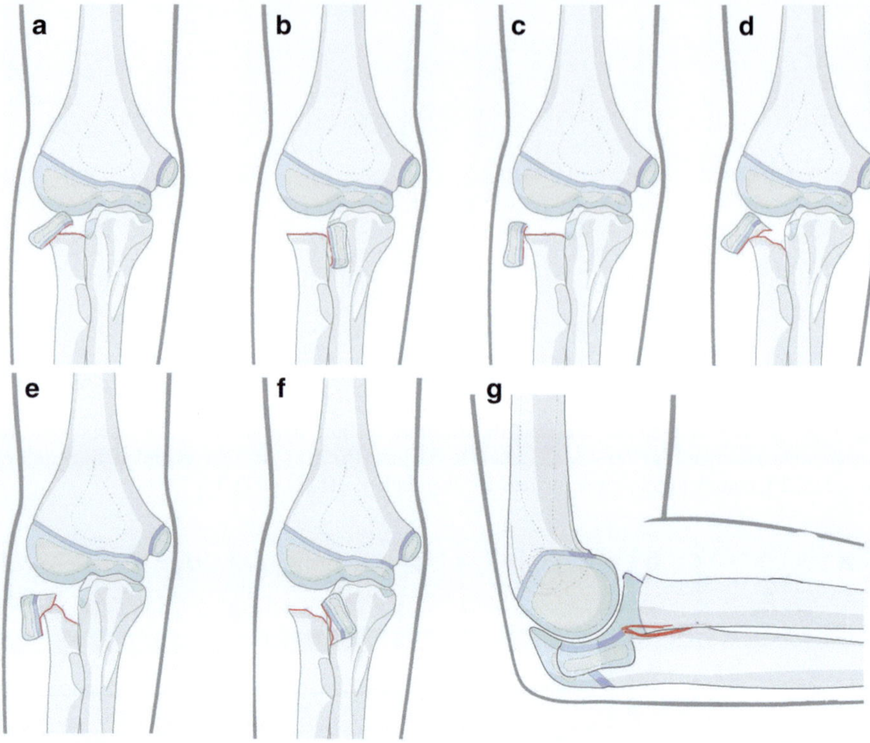

Fig. 15.7 The graphics illustrate the different fracture morphologies of epiphyseal radial neck fractures we recommend for reduction and operative treatment (stabilization). (**a**) 21r – E/1.1 II, Salter Harris 1, angulated more than 25°; (**b**) 21r – E/1.1 III, Salter Harris 1, angulated more than 25°, medial dislocation; (**c**) 21r – E/1.1 III, Salter Harris 1, angulated more than 25°; (**d**) 21 – E/2.1 II, Salter Harris 2, angulated less than 25°; (**e**) 21 – E/2.1 II, Salter Harris 2, angulated more than 30°; (**f**) 21 – E/2.1 II, Salter Harris 2, angulated more less than 25°, medial dislocation; (**g**) 21r, Salter Harris 1, extension type

15.5 Treatment Strategy

According to the fracture types, shown in the overview above, we have a base for the "decision making" process for the correct treatment. In our experience over the last 40 years, worldwide accepted and propagated by the pediatric trauma groups (as for example, the Pediatric AO Expert group), the operative preferable treatment technique for all fractures shown in overview should be the ESIN [7–9]. It is important to say that the ESIN technique is a method which can be applied not only with special nails. In this region for these fractures, this technique can be performed with 2.5 mm or 3.0 mm Kirschner wires [10].

For the non-operative treatment, a plaster cast immobilization is sufficient. We must know that the cast does only immobilize the elbow joint neither the fracture [11].

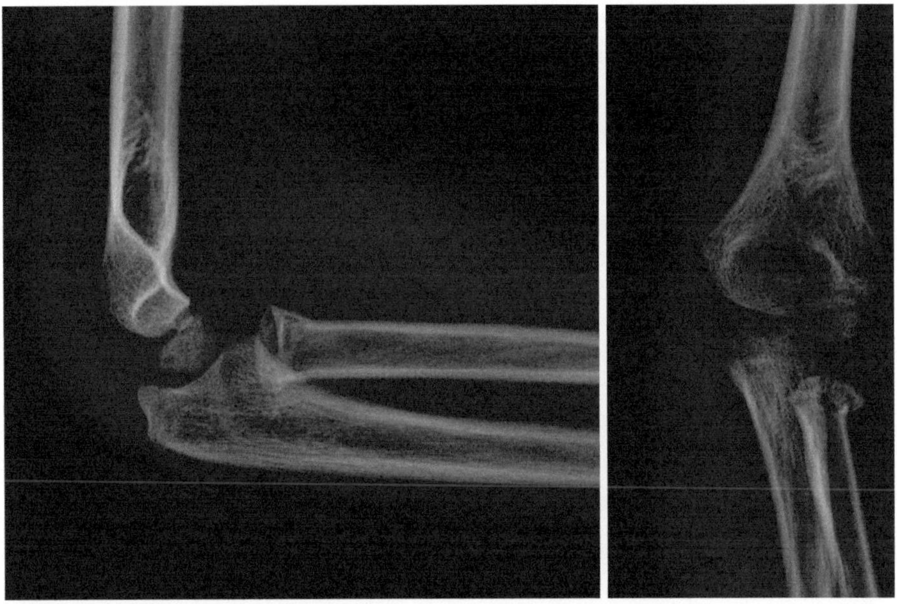

Fig. 15.8 AP and lateral X-ray of an 8-year-old girl. Images show a minimal angulated radial neck fracture, less than 30°. In the lateral view, we see only a minimal compressed zone without displacement

15.6 Conservative/Non-operative Decision Analysis

Conservative therapy will be illustrated using a typical case of an 8-year-old girl fallen on her extended arm of a climbing frame. She had immediately severe pain, and over the next minutes, a swollen elbow was seen. Due to the clinical examination and the case history, an AP and lateral X-ray of the elbow were performed. Figure 15.8 shows the AP and lateral X-rays of the elbow with a minimal angulated and displaced radial neck fracture, classified as AO 21 – M/3.1I Type.

15.6.1 Preoperative Considerations and Problem List

As we had no other injuries and the neuro-vascular situation was normal, according to our algorithm, this radial neck fractures type I is treated conservatively. We plan is to perform only immobilization of the elbow for 4 weeks in a long-arm cast.

15.6.2 *Basic Principles of Conservative/ Non-operative Treatment*

It's important to sow and to explain every step of your planned treatment as the child is not under anesthesia. The presence of the parent (at least mother or father) should be always possible and be a matter of course today.

Depending on the fixation you are using (plaster cast or fiber cast), it's important to have all material well prepared and ready. Depending on the clinic guidelines, the arm should be fixed in a circular cast or in a long-arm dorso-volar plaster splint. Since the arm can occasionally swell up very strongly, we prefer the fixation with dorso-volar plaster splints (Fig. 15.9). The easiest way to apply a neutral long-arm plaster splint (when no manipulation is required) is to hang up the arm on finger straps. This allows a stress-free working even you have no help and a 360° access to the arm [12].

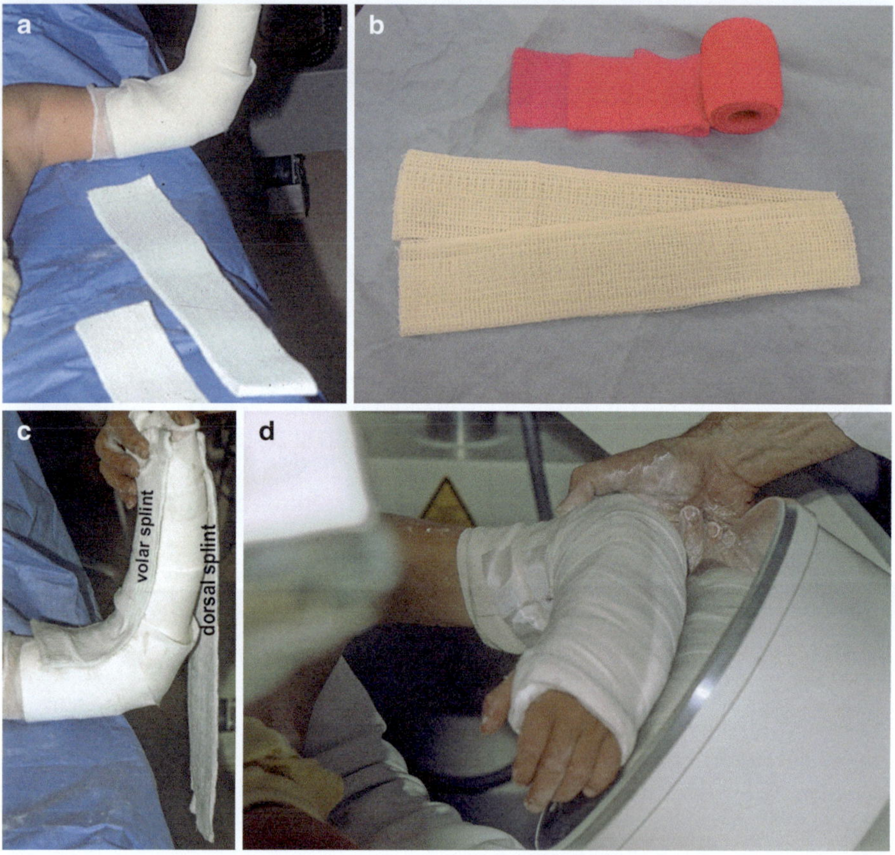

Fig. 15.9 Application of a long-arm dorso-volar long splint. (**a**) Preparation of a short (volar) and a long (dorsal) plaster of Paris Longette. (**b**) Same preparation if fiber cast is used. (**c**) The easiest way to apply the split is by starting with the volar splint and then the dorsal one, hanging the fore-arm on finger straps. (**d**) For optimal lateral X-ray with the arm in the cast, the C-arm must be rotated

15.6.3 Follow-Up and Avoiding Managing Problems/ Complications

Depending on the age of the child, an immobilization for 3–4 weeks is sufficient. In this case, the plaster splint was removed the first time after 2 weeks because of some pain at the olecranon region. The X-ray shows an additional fracture at the olecranon which was not recognized initially (Fig. 15.10). A new cast was applied again for 2 weeks, and after 4½ weeks, a good bone healing of both fractures is (Fig. 15.11).

In our hand, for such an unproblematic fracture, no follow-up was planned. The parents were requested for a visit if in 1 month the arm is not normal used.

15.6.4 Pitfall of Conservative/Non-operative Treatment

The injury film (Fig. 15.12) shows an elbow of an 11-year-old boy, injured his elbow at a fall with the bicycle. The child was sent to us for a second opinion after some months because of the limited elbow motion. The analysis of this X-ray shows the following problems: the elbow was little swollen, and the skin over the olecranon was scratched. Due to the clinical examination and the case history, an AP and lateral X-ray of the elbow were performed.

The AP and lateral X-rays of the elbow showed a minimal angulated and displaced radial neck fracture (AO 21 – M/3.1 I Type). In addition, we see a kind of "crash-zone," a sign of some instability. In this situation, conservative therapy was

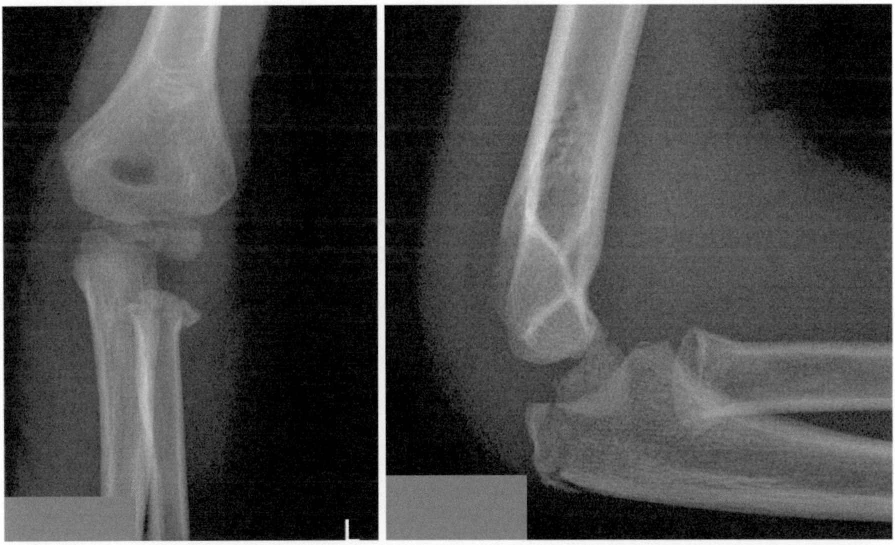

Fig. 15.10 (continue) A 8-year-old girl elbow X-ray made after 2 weeks of injury, without plaster cast because of unclear pain in the olecranon. We see now a not displaced olecranon fracture, which was not recognized initially

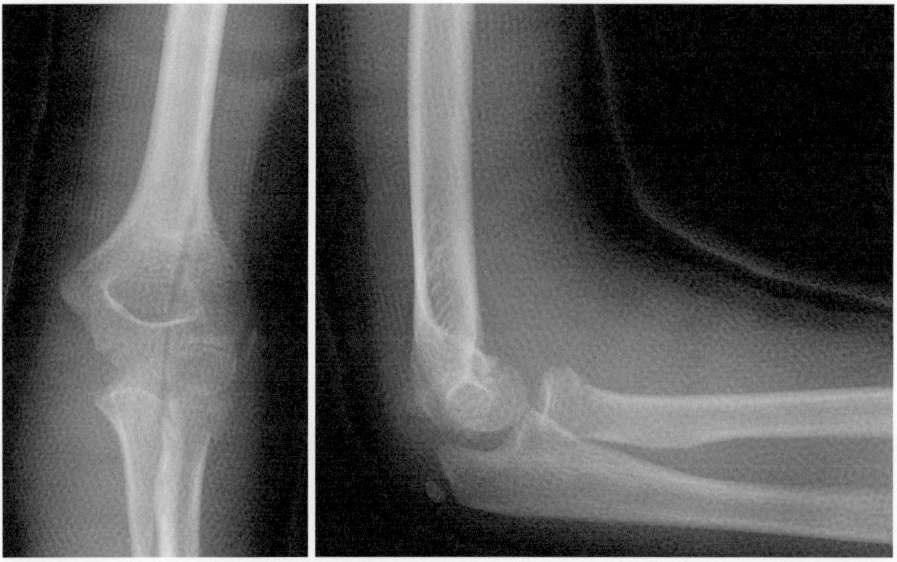

Fig. 15.11 (continue) A 8-year-old girl elbow X-ray made at 4½ weeks, where bone healing of both fractures is documented

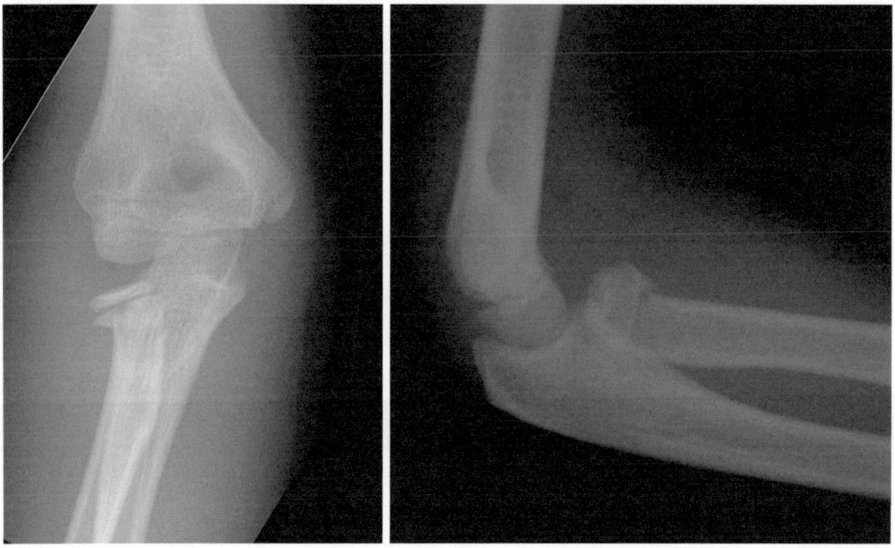

Fig. 15.12 AP and lateral X-rays of the elbow of an 11-year-old boy following a bicycle injury

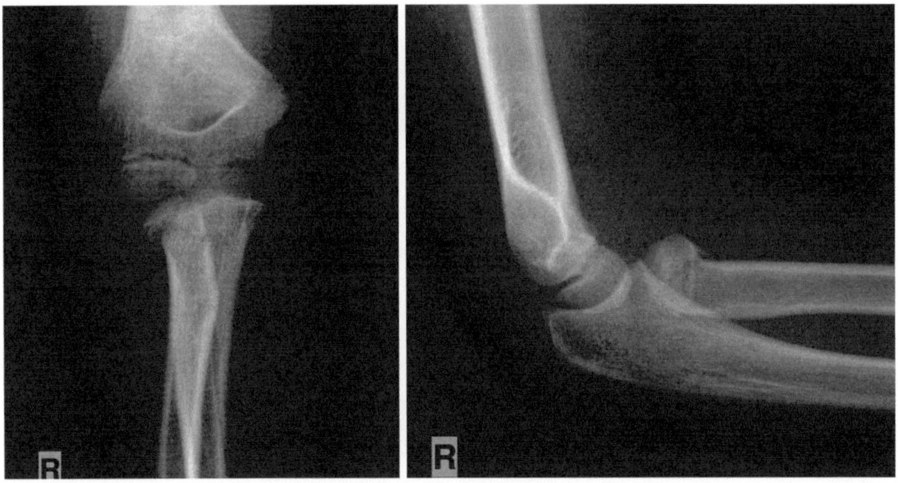

Fig. 15.13 (continue) First follow-up X-ray at day 3 in the cast (fiber cast) shows similar position of the head, but in addition we see some comminution, especially in the AP view

performed and the follow-up X-ray after 3 days (Fig. 15.13) shows a progressive subluxation of the radial head.

Was the decision for conservative therapy justified?

For unknown reasons, a first radiological control was scheduled after 3 days. The explanation to us was then that they would see if the fracture was stable or not at this moment.

At least at this time the treating surgeon should consider the stability of this fracture. We see now a small comminution zone in the metaphysis, which is a clear sign of potential instability. On the other hand, we recommend performing cast-free X-rays in this special situation, because the plaster or fiber cast does not fix the fracture, it's only an immobilization, mainly for pain control.

The 3-day follow-up X-ray was of a good quality, thanks to the immobilization with fiber cast. We already can see that the radial head has moved, providing that there must be a crashed zone.

Bone healing after 4 weeks is clearly visible (Fig. 15.14), with good callus formation. if we are critical, there is too extensive callus formation, which is not normal at this side. In addition, the radial head is no longer correctly centered. At least at this moment, a re-evaluation should be considered, as a revision and stable fixation.

The next X-ray evaluation was performed 5 months after the injury (Fig. 15.15). At this time, the child had limitation of pronation and supination. The flexion was 15° less to the non-injured side. During sports, the child had some pain in the elbow. X-ray shows the subluxation of the radial head and in addition, a bony fragment as a sign of a fracture of the border of the radial neck following forced impingement during sports activity.

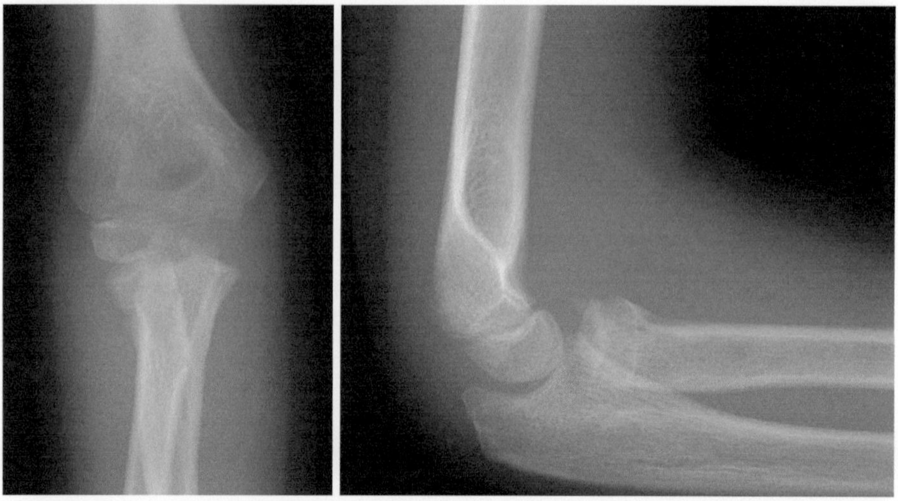

Fig. 15.14 (continue) After 4 weeks, the cast was removed. The X-ray shows a resent callus formation what can be interpreted that the trauma was more severe than initially recognized. In addition, we see a minimal dicentric radial head in both views

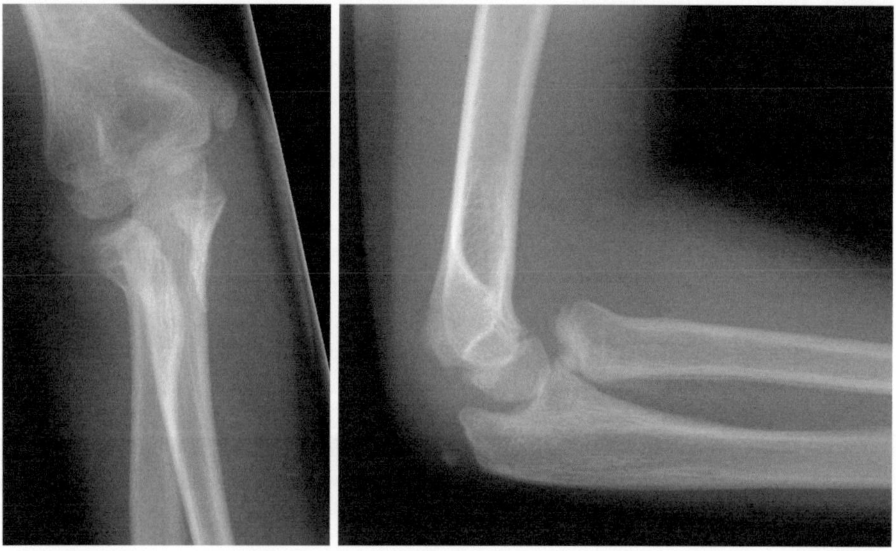

Fig. 15.15 (continue) X-ray control made after 5 months post-injury. Now the radial head is subluxated and we see in the lateral view a not consolidated bony fragment. We can still see the sclerotic zone of the proximal radioulnar joint. At this moment, it would be possible to correct the subluxation by angular ulnar osteotomy

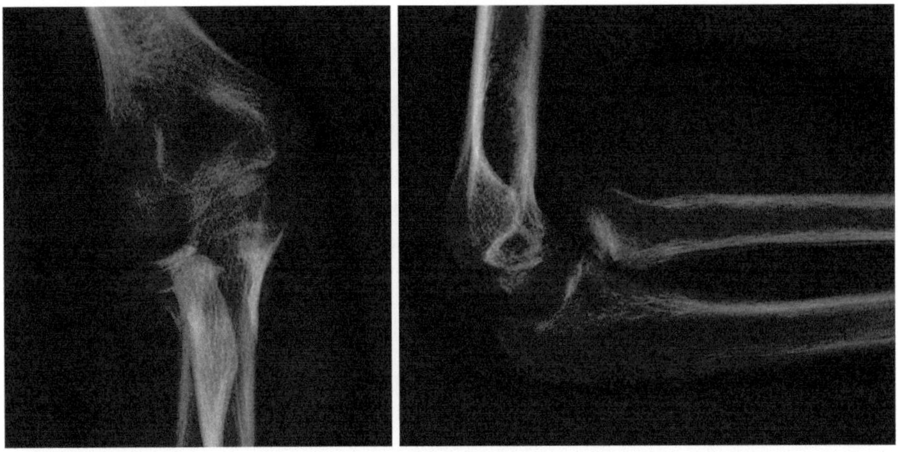

Fig. 15.16 (continue) X-ray control at 7 months post-injury. It shows the established subluxation of the radial head. The fragment is still visible. On the other hand, the concavity of the proximal radioulnar joint disappears a problematic sign for reduction

At this moment, an ulnar flexion osteotomy (like in missed Monteggia lesions) should be considered before the wrong joint situation is fixed and the radial condyle form gets flat. The last X-ray is at 7 months, when we have seen the child the first time in our clinic (Fig. 15.16).

This case shows very clear that even a stable fracture can dislocate or angulate in a plaster cast. In this specific situation, a plaster cast only immobilizes the elbow but it does not fix the fracture. The initial treatment was correct and the indication for immobilization as well. The problem was not to recognize that the fracture is not stable and not to react on this situation. Even an exact analysis of the initial injury film shows the comminution, what was seen in the first follow-up is a clear sign that it was a severe trauma.

15.7 Operative Treatment: ESIN Technique

Radial neck fractures with an angulation over 15–20°, and/or a displacement of more than 20–30% of the bone diameter, benefit from anatomical reduction and functional follow-up treatment.

The current opinion is that the indications are given practically regardless of age, but clearly according to the criteria of fracture morphology [13]. The graphics under heading in Figure 15.6 and 15.7 serves as a guide.

The treatment of these fractures with the ESIN technique, regardless of the implant choice (titanium original nails or corresponding Kirschner wires), is superior to all other treatment options and allows a closed procedure in most cases. The second significant advantage is the possibility of plaster-free follow-up treatment, which also leads to an improvement in the functional result. The only exception is the dorsally flipped radial head (Fig. 15.2).

The classical ESIN treatment (Elastic Stable Intramedullary Nailing) will again be presented using the case of an 11-year-old boy, fell from a tree (Fig. 15.17), clinically he had immediate severe pain in the elbow.

15.7.1 Preoperative Assessment and Treatment Strategy

As the child had no other skeletal injuries and the neurovascular situation was normal, we planned, according to our algorithm of Type II and II fractures, to operate this fracture, but not as an emergency intervention.

The degree of displacement of this fracture is a perfect indication to use the closed, indirect reduction with ESIN technique. On the other hand, as this fracture can be scheduled in the normal program, it allows to do this as a "teaching" operation, assisted by an ESIN-experienced surgeon.

For this operation, an image intensifier is mandatory. In addition, the adequate instruments and implants (nails 2.0 mm or 2.5 mm) must be available.

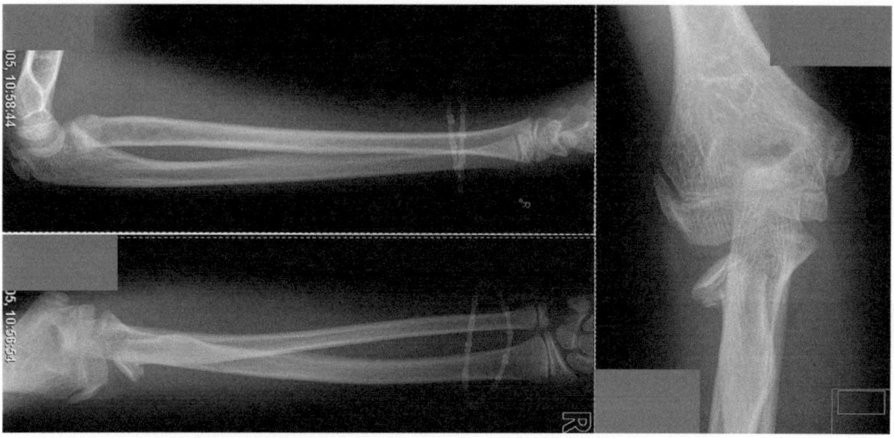

Fig. 15.17 AP and lateral X-rays of the elbow of an 11-year-old boy, with a more than 45° angulated radial head, which is additional translated more than 50% of the shaft diameter (21 – E/3.1 II), diagnosed as a Salter Harris II fracture

15.7.2 Basic Principles of the Treatment

1. Insertion of an elastic nail 2.0 mm or 2.5 mm, depending on the age/size of the child from the distal metaphysis of the radius
2. Advancement of the nail to the fracture line
3. Orientation of the nail tip toward the biggest angulation of the radial head and insertion of the nail tip in the head
4. A combination of external pressure to the radial head and internal reduction of the radial head by rotating the nail
5. Fixation of the reduced radial head
6. Free functional movement should be achieved
7. Plaster-free mobilization of the forearm postoperative

15.7.3 Surgical Steps

To position the sterile draped forearm with image intensifier (Fig. 15.18a) and identification of the distal entry point, today we recommend using the Lister's tubercle approach or the traditional dorso-radial approach. Figure 15.18b shows the level of the skin incision, today along the skin line transverse. This level should be checked under intensifier.

The skin incision is then performed and a blunt dissection up to Lister's tubercle: we must respect the retinaculum and the tendons as shown in Fig. 15.18c, d. Figure 15.18e shows the position of the awl, direct on the bone, a blind approach should be avoided. This entry point and the correct position of the awl must be checked under intensifier.

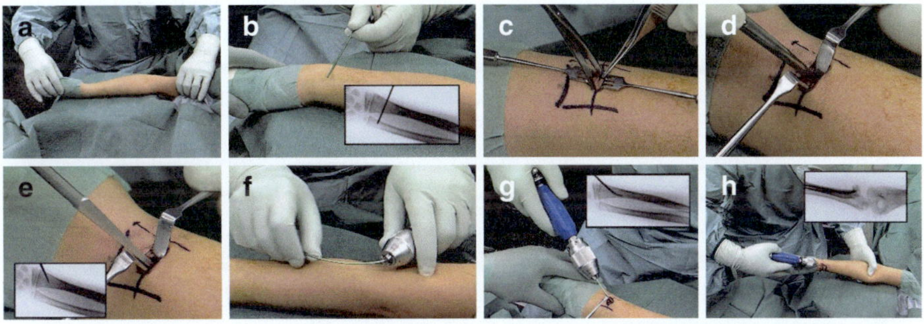

Fig. 15.18 Step-by-step of the correct ESIN insertion. (**a**) Correct positioning for the optimal view of the displacement. (**b**) Determine the entry point on the Lister's tubercle. (**c**) Transverse incision along the skin-folds (this is a cosmetically nicer scar). (**d**) Blunt preparation down to the bone, which must be visible. (**e**) Perforation of the bone with the awl under visual control. (**f**) Prebending of the first 5 cm of the nail. (**g**) Insertion of the nail and align the nail tip to the inner cortex. (**h**) After decompact of the annular ligament 180° rotation of the nail tip and direct reduction of the radial head

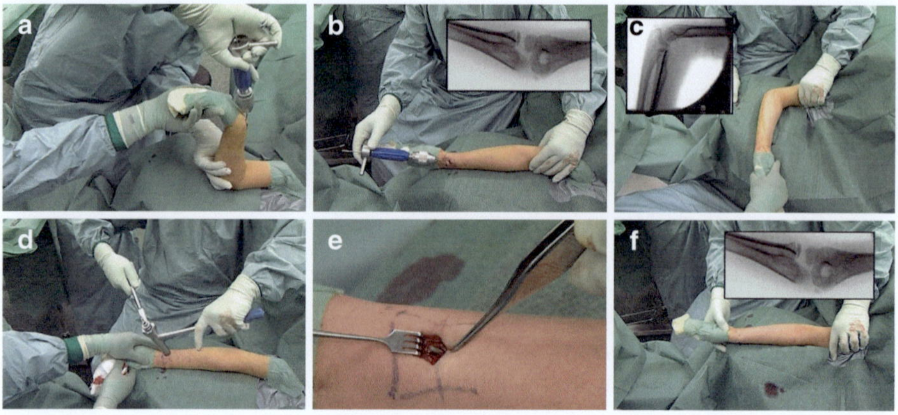

Fig. 15.19 Step-by-step documentation of the reduction maneuver. (**a**) The reduction maneuver is a combination of nail rotation and elbow flexion. (**b**) First X-ray control in extension and in (**c**) a lateral view. (**d**) Cutting of the nail with a bolt cutter. (**e**) The end of the nail should remain over the retinaculum, otherwise a rupture of a tendon can occur. (**f**) Last X-ray check after cutting in extension of the elbow

At the next step, the proximal third of the nail should be pre-bended (pre-contoured). This facilitated the nail insertion and the indirect head reduction once the nail has reached the radial head (Fig. 15.18f).

The pre-bended nail is now inserted under visual control. Check the alignment of the nail tip under one image intensifier shot (Fig. 15.18g).

In the next step, the nail is advanced under oscillating rotation up to the fracture; at this point, it's important to rotate under intensifier control in a way that we can see the most severe angulation/displacement of the fracture. The pre-bended nail tip must be orientated to the displaced/angulated fracture (Fig. 15.18h).

Once the nail is correctly orientated, it is inserted into the radial head by gentle hammer blows. A single perforation for a better grip of the nail doesn't cause any growth disturbances.

In the next step, the arm is flexed, the forearm is pronated, and at the same time the nail 180° rotated as shown in Fig. 15.19a.

Now we extend the elbow/forearm and check our reduction result under image intensifier; if the result is not perfect as shown in Fig. 15.19b, c, this maneuver can be repeated. In the most cases in the second maneuver, a perfect alignment can be achieved. Once the result is radiological perfect (and we should accept only perfect reduction with this technique), the nail is shortened (Fig. 15.19d).

It's important to shorten the nail in the correct length:

Tips

1. Use a bold cutter which avoids sharp ends (Fig. 15.19d)
2. Leave the nail end over the retinaculum; under the retinaculum, there is a high risk for tendon irritation/rupture

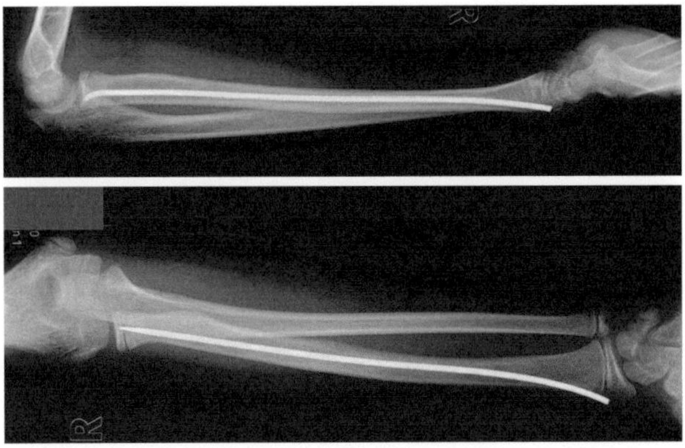

Fig. 15.20 (continue) An 11-year-old boy elbow X-ray control at 6 months from injury follow-up shows perfect bone healing, alignment, and function. The nails removal can be planned

3. Even a longer nail end does not irritate the extension of the hand (even you see a prominent buckle) and facilitates the nail removal (Fig. 15.19e)

After closure of the wound, a last X-ray check is made; in case of an incorrect reduction, the nail has been pulled back, and the reduction maneuver must be repeated (Fig. 15.19c, f). The series in Fig. 15.1 show the different steps of the reduction.

15.7.4 Postoperative Management and Outcome

An immobilization in an arm sling for 3–4 weeks is sufficient, depending on the age of the child. After 4 weeks, the first follow-up X-ray was made, showing a correct position and healing so that the child was allowed to return to sports (Fig. 15.20). We see the full bone healing and perfect alignment. Now the nail removal can be planned, depending on your local protocols, recommended after 6 months. No more controls were required in case the child has symmetrical range of motion and absolutely no restrictions.

15.8 Special Fractures and Situations

There are some special situations, where special considerations and tricks should be use. On these situations, it is important that a skilled surgeon who is performed this ESIN technique is present. On the other hand, as this fracture can be scheduled in the normal program, it allows to do this as a "teaching" operation, assisted by an ESIN-experienced surgeon.

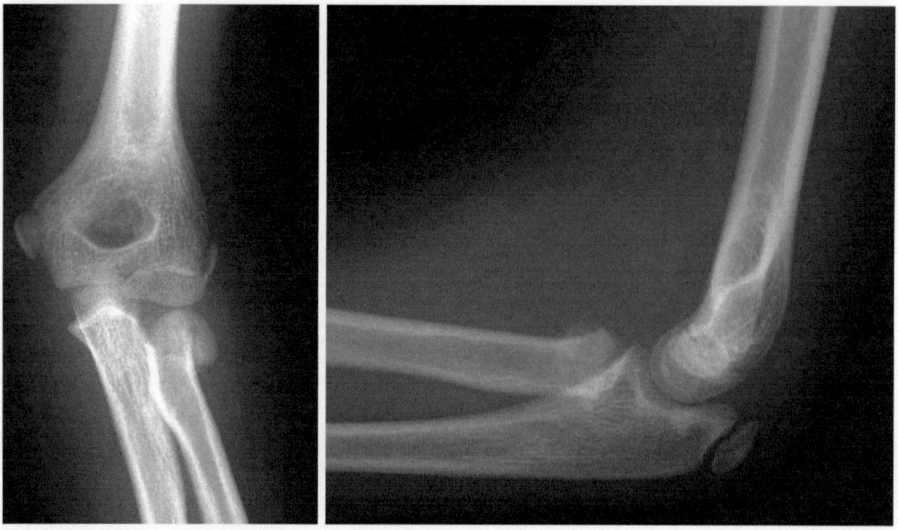

Fig. 15.21 AP and lateral X-ray of the elbow of a 10-year-old boy with nearly complete displaced radial neck fracture, recognize that the radial head is on the radial side of the radius

15.8.1 Completely Dislocated Radial Neck Fracture Without Contact of the Fracture Surfaces

The injury film shows the elbow of a 10-year old boy, sustained a traffic injury (Fig. 15.21). The arm was fixed between the car and his bicycle. Clinically, the elbow and forearm were very swollen. The fracture analysis shows a completely dislocated radius neck fracture, with the radial head resting laterally on the proximal radius. Despite the massive dislocation, it can be assumed that the vascularity to the radial head is preserved.

The treatment strategy was to reduce this type III fracture into a type II fracture in a closed manner, so that the complete reduction can be performed with the standard ESIN technique. Such a fully displaced radial neck fracture must not be an indication for an open reduction and internal fixation. Even such a complete displacement of this fracture is still a perfect indication to use the closed, indirect reduction and intramedullary stabilization ESIN technique.

The trick for reducing this fracture is using the tip of the well pre-bended nail tip to push the head fragment in a better position; once the neck fragment is pushed back to an acceptable position, then the nail tip can reach this fragment, and the reduction procedure is the same as in a type II fracture, all other steps are identically as described before (Fig. 15.22).

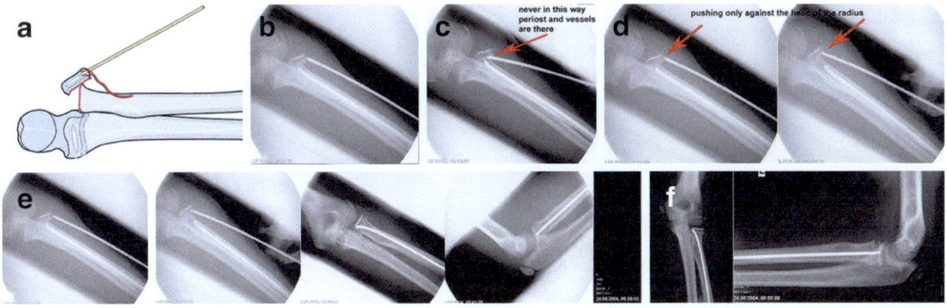

Fig. 15.22 In this situation, the elastic nail cannot reach the neck fragment; therefore, the "Joystick" technique is used. (**a**) Recognize the lateral intact periosteum where the remaining vessels for the head are located; by pushing with the tip of the Kirschner wire on the head, a damage of the vessels can be avoided. (**b**) Correct "pushing point" on the intensifier. (**c**) Wrong position of the Kirschner wire. The "Kapandji Technique" is not allowed at this point, as the remaining vascularity can be damaged. (**d**) Progress of pushing back the radial head in an optimal position for ESIN technique. (**e**) Reduction of the radial head by ESIN technique. (**f**) Final result with perfect alignment, the fracture is practically no longer visible

15.8.2 Dorsally Flipped, Completely Dislocated Radial Neck Fracture Without Contact of the Fracture Surfaces

Most of all radial neck fractures are so-called flexion fractures. That means, the radial head is displaced in flexion toward the radial metaphysis. In very rear cases, the radial head flips backwards, in extension. The theory of the pathomechanism can be that during an axial trauma to the elbow the radius makes a subluxation or a luxation. At this moment, a metaphyseal fracture happens but without displacement. In a second step, the radius shaft goes back to distal and the damaged metaphysis brakes, the redial head flips backwards.

Sometimes the dorsally flipped radial head fragment is difficult to see, especially in suboptimal X-rays (oblique or of bad quality). In such a fracture, the normal indirect reduction technique with the ESIN method is not possible. Therefore, an open reduction is required.

To avoid vascular damage of the radial head, we recommend a combined approach. Using a dorsal mini-open approach for visualization of the radial head, and a Joystick technique, to gentle pushed distally the radial head so that the fragment can get with the elastic nail and definitively reduced and fixed in the traditional ESIN technique. Figure 15.23 shows the X-ray of this very special condition and for better understanding of a graphic drawing.

The treatment strategy is to push back the flipped fragment in a better position and create a typical flexion fracture so that the radial head can be caught and reduced in a typical ESIN technique.

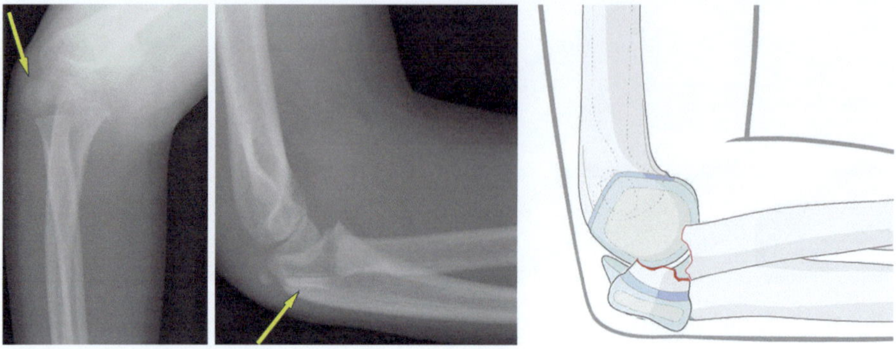

Fig. 15.23 X-ray of the elbow of an 8-year-old boy, injured on the playground, showing the flipped radial head (yellow arrows)

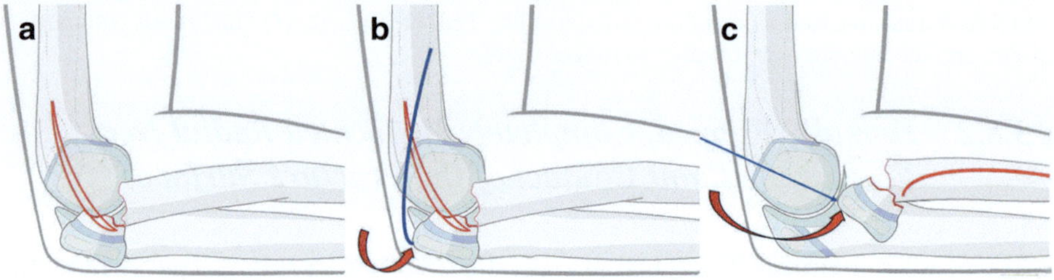

Fig. 15.24 This graphic demonstrates the technique for managing a flipped radial head. (**a**) Incision dorso-lateral over the lateral condyle. (**b**) With a bended Kirschner wire, or better with a dental hook, lifting up the radial head. (**c**) Pushing in a situation that the prepared nail can catch the head

To avoid additional damage of the periosteum and the remaining blood supply, we should avoid the classical approach to the proximal radius and radial head, respectively. The best way to get to the flipped radial head would be through a radial short incision on the most proximal side of the capsule insertion. Figure 15.24 shows our approach. This incision allows a good view to the dorsal joint over the radial capitulum, so that we can push back the radial head in front of the capitulum.

Before we can reduce the fracture with the tip of the well pre-bended nail tip, we must push the head fragment in a better position; once the neck fragment is pushed back to an acceptable position, then the nail tip can reach this fragment, the reduction procedure is the same as in a type II fracture (Fig. 15.25).

The basic principles for optimal treatment are the following steps:

1. Good visualization of the fracture under image intensifier
2. Apply of a sterile tourniquet (if available) is helpful
3. Now prepare the TEN for the typical insertion (we recommend using the Lister's tubercle approach) as shown in Fig. 15.18a–h
4. Advance the nail tip up to the fracture line (Fig. 15.18e–h)
5. Short dorso-lateral incision as shown in Fig. 15.24a

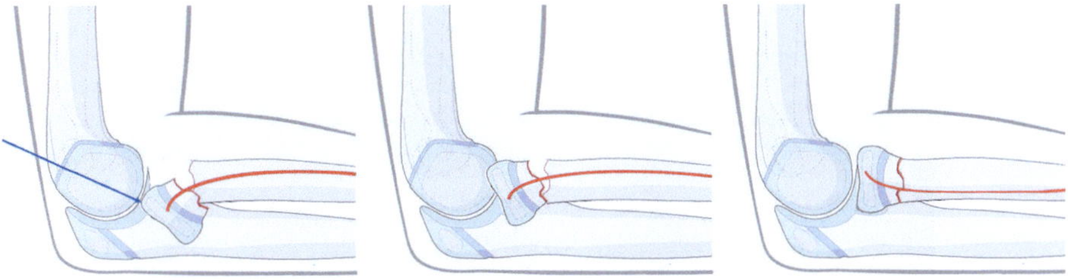

Fig. 15.25 Graphic visualization of the indirect radial head reduction

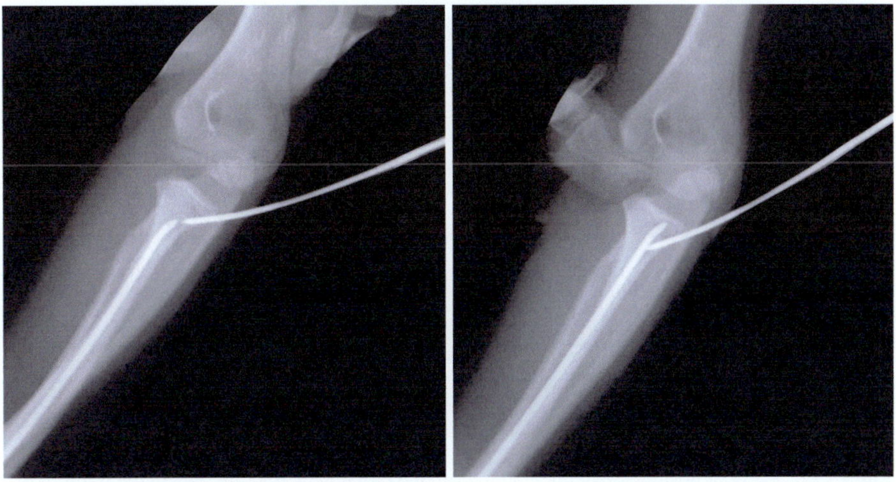

Fig. 15.26 Indirect radial head reduction seen in the intraoperative C-arm

6. Visualization of the flipped radial head fragment
7. With the help of a 1.6 mm K-wire which is bended at the tip as demonstrated in Fig. 15.24b, c (or better use a dental hook) lift up and push back the radial head toward the main radial fragment

   Trick: Try to dislocate the elbow again so that the radial shaft comes under the capitellum, in this position it's much easier and safer to push back the radial head. Then by pressing the radial head toward the main fragment, reduce the elbow again.
8. Figure 15.25 shows the situation after pushing back the radial head and reposition of the elbow
9. Now the positioned nail (which was in a "waiting position") is inserted in the head fragment by gentle hammer blows. The head must still be fixed/pushed by the K-wire, otherwise with the TEN the head flips back (Fig. 15.25)
10. By the typical rotation maneuver, the head is definitively reduced (Figs. 15.26 and 15.27)
11. Free functional movement should be achieved
12. Plaster-free mobilization of the forearm postoperative

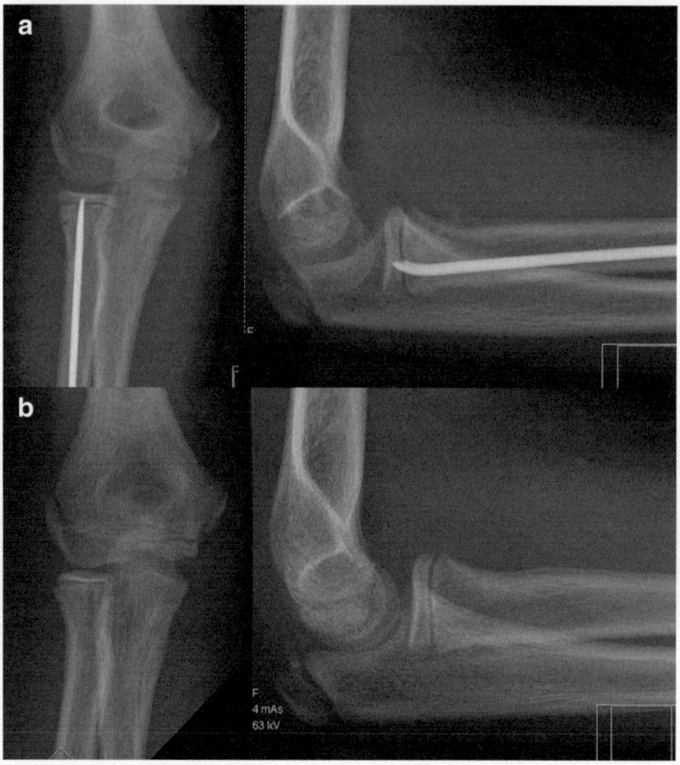

Fig. 15.27 X-ray of postoperative documentation of a radial neck fracture, where the fracture line is no longer visible (**a**). Follow-up after nail removal shows excellent outcome (**b**)

15.9 Summary

Radial neck fractures are not so frequent. Therefore, the closed management and safe fixation are demanding. Over the last 40 years, ESIN has been established as a method that allows us to reduce and securely fix virtually any radius neck fracture in a closed way, so that plaster-free, functional follow-up treatment is possible.

However, certain very simple points must be recognized and considered, including correct X-ray images, so that unnecessary further examinations such as CT can be avoided, precise analysis of the fracture to develop the right strategy, mastery of the correct technique; too often we see incorrect insertion points, implants that are not pre-formed accordingly, having the appropriate instruments and implants ready, precise information for parents/patients, and functional follow-up treatment.

References

1. Alongo T, Audigé L. AO pediatric comprehensive classification of long bone fractures (PCCF). J Orthop Trauma. 2018;32:S117–40. https://doi.org/10.1097/BOT.0000000000001065.
2. Joeris A, Lutz N, Blumenthal A, Slongo T, Audigé L. The AO pediatric comprehensive classification of long bone fractures (PCCF). Acta Orthop. 2017;88(2):129–32. https://doi.org/10.1080/17453674.2016.1258533. Epub 2016 Nov 24
3. González-Herranz P, Alvarez-Romera A, Burgos J, Rapariz JM, Hevia E. Displaced radial neck fractures in children treated by closed intramedullary pinning (Metaizeau technique). J Pediatr Orthop. 1997;17(3):325–31.
4. Dietz HG, Schmittenbecher PP, Slongo TF, Wilkins KE. AO manual of fracture management. Elastic stable intramedullary nailing (ESIN) in children. Stuttgart: Thieme; 2006.
5. Falciglia F, Giordano M, Aulisa AG, Di Lazzaro A, Guzzanti V. Radial neck fractures in children: results when open reduction is indicated. J Pediatr Orthop. 2014;34(8):756–62. https://doi.org/10.1097/BPO.0000000000000299.
6. Klitscher D, Richter S, Bodenschatz K, Hückstädt T, Weltzien A, Müller LP, et al. Evaluation of severely displaced radial neck fractures in children treated with elastic stable intramedullary nailing. J Pediatr Orthop. 2009;29(7):698–703. https://doi.org/10.1097/BPO.0b013e3181b76895.
7. Metaizeau JP, Lascombes P, Lemelle JL, Finlayson D, Prevot J. Reduction and fixation of displaced radial neck fractures by closed intramedullary pinning. J Pediatr Orthop. 1993;13(3):355–60. https://doi.org/10.1097/01241398-199305000-00015.
8. Schmittenbecher PP, Haevernick B, Herold A, Knorr P, Schmid E. Treatment decision, method of osteosynthesis, and outcome in radial neck fractures in children: a multicenter study. J Pediatr Orthop. 2005;25(1):45–50. https://doi.org/10.1097/00004694-200501000-00011.
9. Basmajian HG, Choi PD, Huh K, Sankar WN, Wells L, Arkader A. Radial neck fractures in children: experience from two level-1 trauma centers. J Pediatr Orthop B. 2014;23(4):369–74. https://doi.org/10.1097/BPB.0000000000000057.
10. Lascombes P. Embrochage centromédullaire élastique stable. Île-de-France: Elsevier Masson; 2006. https://doi.org/10.1016/S0246-0467(07)43343-8.
11. Vocke AK, Von Laer L. Displaced fractures of the radial neck in children: long-term results and prognosis of conservative treatment. J Pediatr Orthop B. 1998;7(3):217–22. https://doi.org/10.1097/01202412-199807000-00007.
12. Dresing K, Fernandez F, Schmittenbecher P, Dresing K, Strohm P, Spering C, et al. Bildgebung bei Kindern und Jugendlichen intraoperativ, bei ausgewählten Frakturen und im Verlauf nach konservativer und operativer Behandlung : Teil 2 der Ergebnisse einer bundesweiten Online-Umfrage der Sektion Kindertraumatologie der Deutschen Gesellschaft für Unfallchirurgie [Intraoperative imaging of children and adolescents, for selected fractures and in follow-up after conservative and operative treatment: part 2 of the results of a nationwide online survey of the Pediatric Traumatology Section of the German Trauma Society]. Unfallchirurgie (Heidelb). 2023;126(1):42–54. German. Epub 2021 Dec 16. https://doi.org/10.1007/s00113-021-01114-3.
13. Slongo T, Stranzinger E. Bildgebung in der Kindertraumatologie/Kinderorthopädie. Oper Orthop Traumatol. 2024;36:56–72. https://doi.org/10.1007/s00064-023-00839-1.

Chapter 16
Monteggia Fracture-Dislocation

Alejandro Baar and Jamil F. Soni

The Monteggia fracture-dislocation is a uncommon injury, but a high index of suspicion is needed in the presence of an isolated Ulna fracture. Delay in diagnosis and treatment lead to serious functional consequences. It corresponds to a fracture of the ulna associated with a radio-humeral dislocation. The Bado classification is the most commonly used, and it helps to explain the mechanism of injury and guide the treatment. In the acute stage, it is of paramount importance to make the diagnosis timely and then reduce the fracture of the ulna, which in turn, leads to, the reduction of the radio-humeral joint. Sometimes, internal fixation is necessary to stabilize the fracture. Those cases presented late are a challenge for the pediatric Orthopedic surgeon and require the use of complex reconstructive techniques, including ulnar osteotomies in most cases.

16.1 Introduction

The Monteggia fracture-dislocation was described in 1814 by Giovanni Batista Monteggia, as a fracture of the ulna, usually at the proximal end, associated with a dissociation of the proximal radio-ulnar joint, with a consequent dislocation of the radiocapitellar joint [1]. This injury corresponds to less than 1% of all pediatric forearm fractures and occurs mostly in the group age between 4 and 10 years old [2]. Despite its low frequency, these are complex injuries that can lead to serious functional sequelae if not identified and treated in time. The

A. Baar (✉)
Clínica Universidad de Los Andes, Santiago, Chile
e-mail: abaar@clinicauandes.cl

J. F. Soni
Pontifical Catholic University of Paraná, Curitiba, Brazil

M. Sepúlveda O. (ed.), *Paediatrics Traumatology*,
https://doi.org/10.1007/978-3-031-89482-4_16

diagnosis can be difficult, with an error rate reported in up to 50% of cases, especially when the dislocation is associated with a plastic deformity or greenstick fracture of the ulna [3, 4]. In addition, it has been reported that in up to 20% of cases, there reduction achieved at the acute setting is a lost [5].

16.2 Classification

Bado [6] has proposed a classification into four types, based on the direction of the radial head displacement and angulation of the ulna. This helps to understand the mechanism and allows to guide the management of the injury (Fig. 16.1).

Type I are the most common in children (70–75%), while type II are the most common in adults, but very rare in the pediatric population (6%). Type III follow in frequency to type I, and type IV are even less frequent.

In addition to these four classic types, new "Monteggia Equivalent" injuries have been described. Examples of this are the isolated dislocation of the radial head, and the associated fracture of the ulna and radial neck, among others.

Letts [7] proposed a specific classification for Monteggia pediatric injuries, dividing them into five types: A, B, and C present anterior dislocation of the radial head; D, presents posterior dislocation, and E, with lateral dislocation (Fig. 16.2).

Finally, Ring, Jupiter, and Waters [8] consider the Monteggia injuries as a proximal radio-ulnar dislocation associated with a forearm fracture. According to the authors, the most determinant for the treatment is the ulnar fracture, over the direction of the dislocation of the radial head.

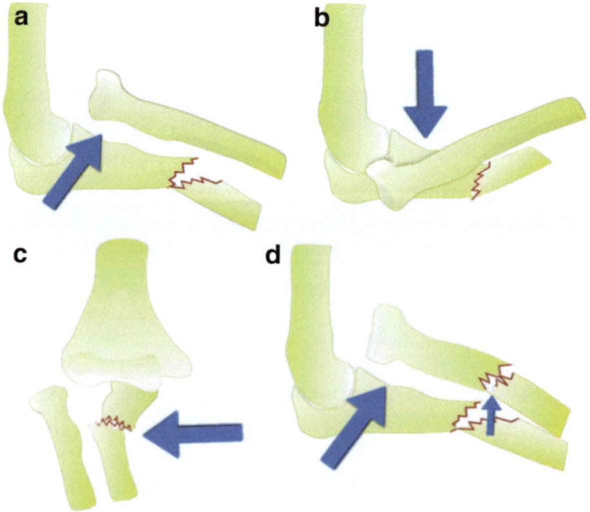

Fig. 16.1 Bado classification of Monteggia dislocation fractures. (**a**) Type I, with anterior dislocation of the radius and ulnar fracture with volar apex. (**b**) Type II, with posterior dislocation of the radius and ulnar fracture with ápex dorsal. (**c**) Type III, lateral dislocation of the radius, with ulnar fracture with apex lateral (Varus). (**d**) Type IV, anterior dislocation of the radius together with proximal radius and ulna fracture

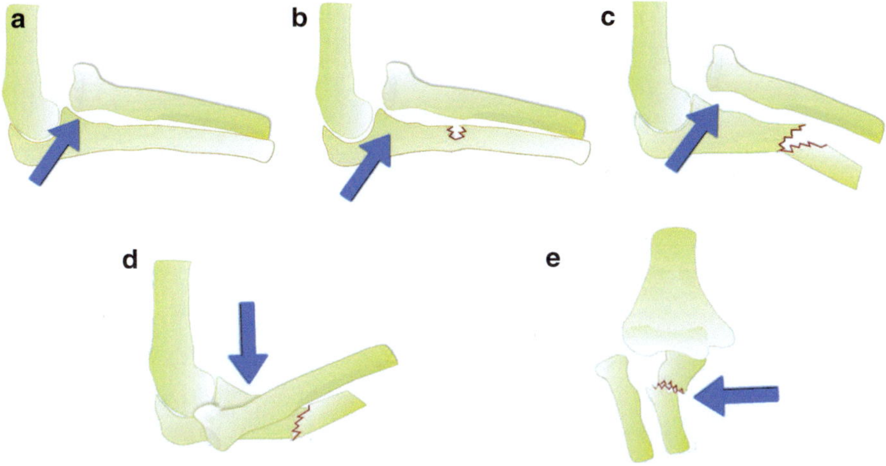

Fig. 16.2 Letts classification of Monteggia lesions. Types A, B, and C correspond to Bado type I. (**a**) Anterior dislocation of the radius with plastic deformation of the radius. (**b**) Anterior dislocation of the radius with a greenstick fracture of ulna. (**c**) Anterior dislocation of the radius with a complete fracture of the ulna. (**d**) Posterior dislocation of the radius with of dorsal apex fracture of the ulna (corresponds to type II of Bado). (**e**) Lateral dislocation of the radius and with lateral ápex fracture of ulna (corresponds to Bado III)

16.3 Mechanism of Injury

Depending on the mechanism, there will be different types of injury, according to what is described by Bado. For type I, three mechanisms are proposed: (1) direct trauma on the posterior edge of the ulna; (2) hyperpronation; and (3) hyperextension, this being the most accepted. Type II, according to experimental studies performed by Penrose [9], occur when the forearm receives a longitudinal load with the elbow at 60° of flexion. Type III are the result of varus forces, while type IV are a consequence of hyperpronation of the forearm.

Knowing the anatomy of the forearm, especially in its proximal portion, is very important when facing Monteggia injuries. The stability of the radio-capitellar joint is due to the reciprocity of the concave surface of the radial head with the convex surface of the capitellum. On the other hand, the bone geometry of the proximal radio-ulnar joint (PRUJ) provides minimal stability.

The radial head is elliptical in cross-section. In supination, the long axis of the ellipse is perpendicular to the proximal ulna, which causes the annular ligament and the anterior portion of the quadrate ligament to tense, stabilizing the PRUJ (Fig. 16.3). The arched shape of the radius allows for complete rotation of the forearm while maintaining stability in the PRUJ and distal radio-ulnar (DRUJ) joints. With the radius in supination, its arched shape tenses the oblique cord and the interosseous ligament, thus increasing the stability of the PRUJ.

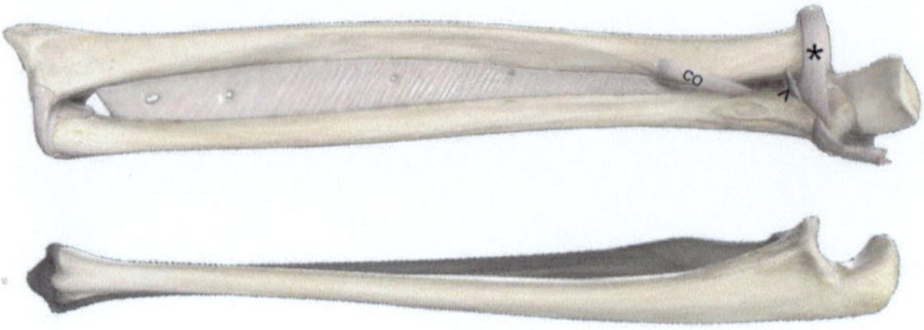

Fig. 16.3 Oseo-ligamentous anatomy of the proximal forearm. The asterisk (*) marks the annular ligament. The arrowhead indicates the quadrate ligament. "CO" corresponds to the oblique chord

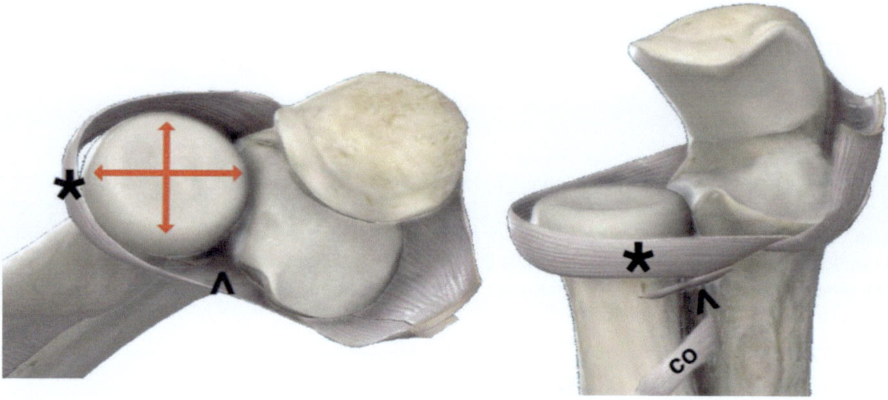

Fig. 16.4 Proximal radio-ulnar joint. The asterisk (*) denotes the annular ligament. The arrowhead indicates the quadrate ligament. "CO" corresponds to the oblique chord. The red arrows show that the transverse diameter of the head of the radius is greater than the antero-posterior

The main deforming muscular forces are the biceps brachialis and anconeus muscles. Finally, it is important to remember the ligaments that make up the PRUJ: the annular ligament, which is the main stabilizer of the PRUJ; the quadrate ligament, whose anterior and posterior edges tense in extreme supination and pronation, respectively; and the Weitbrecht ligament or proximal oblique cord, present only in 50% of forearms, and whose stabilizing function is under debate (Fig. 16.4).

16.4 Diagnosis

Depending on the amount of displacement, the clinical manifestations of a Monteggia injury can be more or less evident. The signs of a fracture (swelling, pain, deformity, pathological mobility, functional impotence, and/or bruising) are present. The neurovascular examination of the upper extremity is fundamental, especially the function of the posterior interosseous nerve, which can be assessed evaluating the extension of the thumb and the metacarpophalangeal extension of the fingers. This injury occurs preferably in type III injuries.

The radiological study of the forearm should always include the elbow and wrist joint. An isolated radio-capitellar dislocation is very rare and should alert the doctor to a possible fracture of the ulna, which could be a plastic deformation type. Likewise, an isolated fracture of the ulna should raise suspicion of a radio-capitellar dislocation.

Characteristically, a mid-diaphyseal line drawn on the radius should always project in the center of the capitellum, throughout the range of elbow movement. The loss of this relationship should alert the doctor to a Monteggia injury.

Unfortunately, up to 1/3 of missed Monteggia fracture-dislocations can end with pain, functional limitation, and restriction of movement (mainly flexion and supination), deformity, loss of strength, late-onset neuropathy, and arthritis [10].

A differential diagnosis to consider is congenital dislocation of the radial head. In these cases, the presence of a hypoplastic capitellum along with a convex and deformed radial head may suggest a congenital etiology. In addition, these are usually bilateral, and most of the cases have dislocated radial head. It can be associated with genetic syndromes, such as Ehlers-Danlos or Nail-Patella [11].

16.5 Treatment

The principles of treatment are the same, regardless of the type of fracture. The goal is to achieve alignment and recovery of the ulnar length, accompanied by the reduction of the radio-capitellar joint. Generally, by achieving the first, the second occurs spontaneously. The reduction should be performed with the patient anesthetized and under radioscopic control. If a satisfactory and stable reduction is achieved, a long-arm cast is used for 4–6 weeks. Usually, this treatment is suitable for incomplete fractures or plastic deformations of the ulna. The position for immobilization is with the forearm in neutral rotation and the elbow in 100–110° of flexion.

For the particular case of type II injuries, the position of the immobilization should be with the elbow at 60° of flexion.

For complete fractures of the ulna, it is usually necessary to perform internal fixation, either through a minimally invasive approach, with intramedullary nails (Fig. 16.5), or by open reduction and internal fixation with a plate and screws construct.

The surgeon must ensure a complete and stable reduction of the radio-capitellar joint. If not achieved after the reduction of the ulna, it is likely that the annular ligament has been interposed in the PRUJ, which necessitates a direct open approach, to clear the joint and possibly repair the damaged ligament.

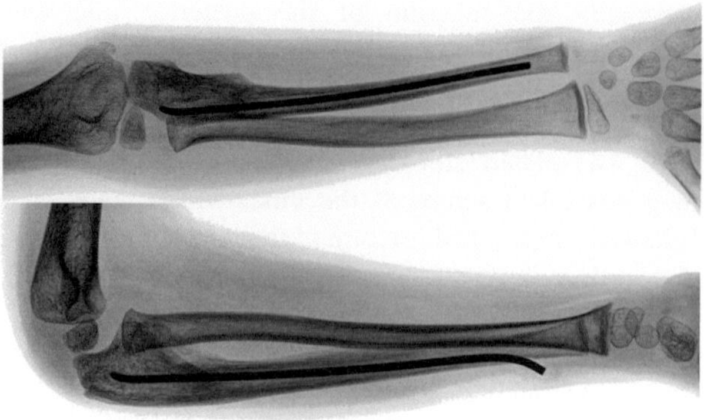

Fig. 16.5 Forearm X-ray of a 6-year-old boy, with a Monteggia luxofracture. The ulna was stabilized with an elastic intramedullary nail, distal entry, retrograde

16.6 Complications

In addition to the complications common to all fractures (neurovascular injury, compartment syndrome, and infections in case of open fractures), Monteggia's fracture-dislocation can present as a neglected injury, with a chronically radial head dislocation, either due to a failure of the initial diagnosis or after the loss of primary reduction. There is no consensus in the literature that defines the time to be considered chronic, although the period accepted by several authors is after 4 weeks from the trauma [5, 12].

As a result of the evolution of the neglected injury, the patient may present with pain, loss of pronation-supination arc, elbow stiffness, deformity, loss of strength, neuropathy, and secondary arthritis. Reconstructive surgery is indicated to prevent these complications, as long as the reduction of the radial head is possible.

Numerous surgical techniques have been described to address and correct chronic cases [12, 13], including open reduction, annular ligament reconstruction [14, 15], and resection of the radial head [12], among others.

The reconstruction of the annular ligament, as a single procedure, has shown to lead to poor results. Moreover, there is no evidence that it, as an adjuvant procedure, provides any futher benefit, Several studies have demonstrated that such reconstruction is associated with notching of the radial neck, which in turn, leads to limitation of pronation [14–17].

Although the series described consist of small samples and there is no standardization of the most appropriate treatment, there is consensus regarding the osteotomy of the ulna as the Gold Standard.

Inoue [18] and Hirayama [19] showed better results, with a lower index of re-dislocation and better morbidity when performing hypercorrections of the ulna compared to simple osteotomy. Regarding the type of osteotomy fixation, the use of plates have reported better results, due to the possibility to bend them, adapting to the new shape of the ulna [12, 19–23]. The use of stepped osteotomy, or "Z-shaped osteotomy," avoids the need of a bone graft [24]. Stabilization with an external fixator has the advantage of allowing a multiapical correction and simultaneously lengthening of the ulna [25, 26]. However, a common disadvantage is the inflammation and infection of the pin sites and patient discomfort, making it difficult to tolerate in some cases. Bor [27] reported, in a series of four cases, the correction and progressive lengthening of the ulna in chronic Monteggia injuries, without the need to open the joint or repair the annular ligament.

In general terms, the best results are obtained when the reconstructive procedure is performed within 1 year of the original injury [12, 13, 28]. According to various authors, it is possible to return the radial head to its position after a period of 6 months to 6 years from the original injury, in children under 12 years old and when there are no dysplastic changes [19, 20, 29–32].

16.7 Authors' Advice

The basic principle of Monteggia injury treatment is the reduction of the ulna. This maneuver leads to radio-capitellar reduction. If the reduction is unstable, fixation is required to ensure therapeutic success. In the acute setting, we recommend the fixation with intramedullary nails (Steinmann or elastic nails) and immobilization. In multifragmentary or very proximal fractures, we prefer to use plates and screws to maintain ulnar length. If a perfect radio-capitellar reduction is not possible, it is necessary to explore the joint and remove the interposed tissues.

In chronic cases, the ulna osteotomy is fundamental. We do not recommend the reconstruction of the annular ligament.

One of the authors (Soni [33]) has proposed a strategy of six steps for the treatment of chronic injuries (Fig. 16.6):

1. Lateral approach of the extended elbow toward the posterior edge of ulna.
2. Resection of joint fibrosis (radio-capitellar and ulno-humeral).
3. Transverse metaphyseal osteotomy of the proximal ulna.

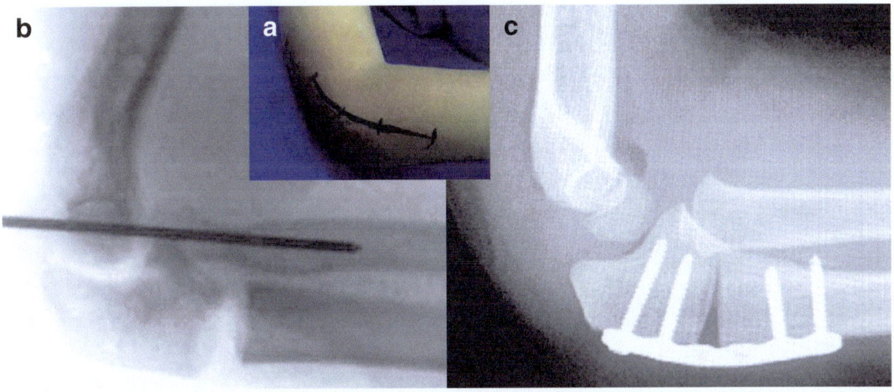

Fig. 16.6 A 6-step reconstruction technique. (**a**) Extended lateral approach to the posterior edge of the ulna. (**b**) Transitory fixation from posterior to anterior of the radio-capitellar joint. The osteotomy of the ulna is observed, with the necessary angulation and separation to keep the joint stable, reduced. (**c**) Fixation completed with plate and screws. The radio-capitellar transitory fixation has been removed

4. Reduction of the radial head, using temporary fixation with a 2 mm Kirschner wire, from posterior to anterior. This allows the necessary length and dorsal angulation of the ulna for stability after reduction.
5. Fixation with a 2.7 or a 3.5 mm plate and screws, bent according to the shape of the ulna after reducing the radial head.
6. Removal of the temporary fixation and examination of stability in flexion, extension, pronation, and supination.

Transcapitellar fixation should be avoided as a method of definitive stabilization, in the postoperative period, because it is commonly related to limitation of pronosupination, in addition to the risk of intra-articular breakage of the Kirschner wire.

As a standard postoperative treatment, a long-arm cast in a neutral position for 4 weeks is applied, avoiding supination, since pronation is the most commonly functional loss described.

On the other hand, the preferred method of treatment for neglected Monteggia injuries of the other author (Baar) consists of (Fig. 16.7):

1. Application of an external fixator, either monolateral (LRS Orthofix®) or circular hexapod type. The choice of one or the other depends on the size of the patient's forearm. When the ulna is very small, a circular external fixator is preferred, because it allows the use of transfixing wires without risking the Ulna from

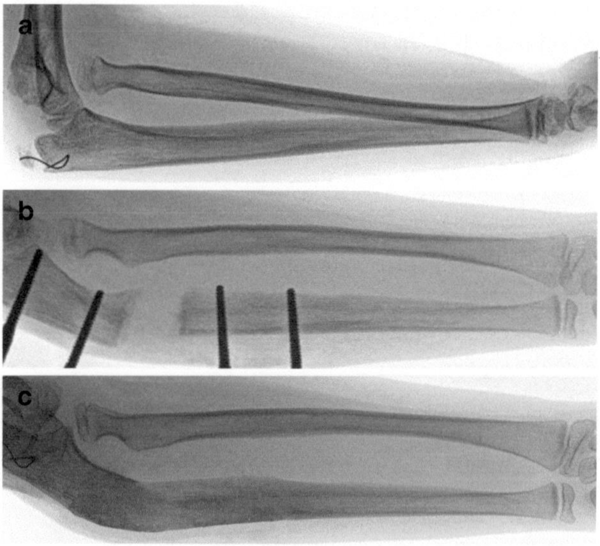

Fig. 16.7 Reconstruction technique with an external fixator and bone lengthening. (**a**) Forearm X-ray after 3 years from the initial injury. A wire cerclage is seen in olecranon, since the original diagnosis was fracture at this level, ignoring dislocation of the radial head. (**b**) Monolateral external fixator is observed in situ, with diastasis and angulation of the osteotomy focus. The radial head was progressively reduced. (**c**) Follow-up 1 year after the extrenal fixator was retired, with excellent bone healing at the osteotomy site. The radio-capitellar reduction is maintained

a fracture. The assembly is simple and consists of a 5/8 or 2/3 ring in the proximal region (leaving the cubital fossa free) and a complete distal ring, where, a radial-ulnar transfixing K-wire is placed, allowing dragging the radius distally along with the lengthening of the ulna. In patients whose ulna is thicker, the use a monolateral external fixator is recommended, with hydroxyapatite-coated screws of 3.5 mm,

2. Percutaneous osteotomy of the proximal region of the ulna.
3. With the fixation elements in each bone segment, the telescopic posts are disconnected in the circular external fixators, or the rail is removed when a monolateral is used.
4. The optimal position to maintain reduction is examined, and the necessary angulation and separation are recorded.
5. If a complete reduction of the radio-capitellar joint is not achieved, an arthrotomy is performed to remove the fibrotic tissue.

The patient does not require a longer hospital stay and is allowed to move the elbow at will. On the seventh postoperative day, bone distraction begins, progressing at a rate of 0.5–0.75 mm/day. Follow-up is with X-rays every 2 weeks. Once the reduction is achieved, the external fixator is maintained until consolidation.

16.8 Final Message

Monteggia injuries, although infrequent, can leave significant sequelae in forearm function. The greatest efforts should be made at the time of the initial consultation, requesting the appropriate X-rays and avoiding overlooking the radio-capitellar dislocation. The initial treatment aims to correct the deformity and shortening of the ulna. Although it is possible to do this in a closed manner, it tends to be unstable and may require internal fixation .

Chronic or inveterate cases are considered when more than 4 weeks have passed since the original injury. Treatment in these cases must be surgical, and ulnar osteotomy is the gold standard. Although there are various types of osteotomies and different fixation alternatives, the goal is to get a perfect and stable reduction of the radio-capitellar joint. The success rate largely depends on this. When dysplastic changes already exist, long time has passed since the original injury, or the patient is an older adolescent, the results with reconstructive techniques are discouraging.

References

1. Monteggia GB, editor. Instituzioni Chirurgiches, vol. 5. 2nd ed. Maspero: Milan; 1814.
2. Kay RM, Skaggs DL. The pediatric Monteggia fracture. Am J Orthop (Belle Mead NJ). 1998;27(9):606–9.

3. Gleeson AP, Beattie TF. Monteggia fracture-dislocation in children. J Accid Emerg Med. 1994;11(3):192–4. https://doi.org/10.1136/emj.11.3.192.
4. Goyal T, Arora SS, Banerjee S, Kandwal P. Neglected Monteggia fracture dislocations in children: a systematic review. J Pediatr Orthop B. 2015;24(3):191–9. https://doi.org/10.1097/BPB.0000000000000147.
5. Ramski DE, Hennrikus WP, Bae DS, Baldwin KD, Patel NM, Waters PM, et al. Pediatric Monteggia fractures: a multicenter examination of treatment strategy and early clinical and radiographic results. J Pediatr Orthop. 2015;35(2):115–20. https://doi.org/10.1097/BPO.0000000000000213.
6. Bado JL. The Monteggia lesion. Clin Orthop Relat Res. 1967;50:71–86.
7. Letts M, Locht R, Wiens J. Monteggia fracture-dislocations in children. J Bone Joint Surg Br. 1985;67(5):724–7. https://doi.org/10.1302/0301-620X.67B5.4055869.
8. Ring D, Jupiter JB, Waters PM. Monteggia fractures in children and adults. J Am Acad Orthop Surg. 1998;6(4):215–24. https://doi.org/10.5435/00124635-199807000-00003.
9. PENROSE JH. The Monteggia fracture with posterior dislocation of the radial head. J Bone Joint Surg Br. 1951;33-B(1):65–73. https://doi.org/10.1302/0301-620X.33B1.65.
10. Bae DS. Successful strategies for managing Monteggia injuries. J Pediatr Orthop. 2016;36(Suppl 1):S67–70. https://doi.org/10.1097/BPO.0000000000000765.
11. Almquist EE, Gordon LH, Blue AI. Congenital dislocation of the head of the radius. J Bone Joint Surg Am. 1969;51(6):1118–27.
12. Degreef I, De Smet L. Missed radial head dislocations in children associated with ulnar deformation: treatment by open reduction and ulnar osteotomy. J Orthop Trauma. 2004;18(6):375–8. https://doi.org/10.1097/00005131-200407000-00008.
13. Delpont M, Jouve JL, Sales de Gauzy J, Louahem D, Vialle R, Bollini G, et al. Proximal ulnar osteotomy in the treatment of neglected childhood Monteggia lesion. Orthop Traumatol Surg Res. 2014;100(7):803–7. https://doi.org/10.1016/j.otsr.2014.06.022.
14. Gyr BM, Stevens PM, Smith JT. Chronic Monteggia fractures in children: outcome after treatment with the bell-Tawse procedure. J Pediatr Orthop B. 2004;13(6):402–6. https://doi.org/10.1097/01202412-200411000-00011.
15. Bhaskar A. Missed Monteggia fracture in children: is annular ligament reconstruction always required? Indian J Orthop. 2009;43(4):389–95. https://doi.org/10.4103/0019-5413.55978.
16. Rahbek O, Deutch SR, Kold S, Søjbjerg JO, Møller-Madsen B. Long-term outcome after ulnar osteotomy for missed Monteggia fracture dislocation in children. J Child Orthop. 2011;5(6):449–57. https://doi.org/10.1007/s11832-011-0372-0.
17. Kim HT, Park BG, Suh JT, Yoo CI. Chronic radial head dislocation in children, part 2: results of open treatment and factors affecting final outcome. J Pediatr Orthop. 2002;22(5):591–7.
18. Inoue G, Shionoya K. Corrective ulnar osteotomy for malunited anterior Monteggia lesions in children. 12 patients followed for 1-12 years. Acta Orthop Scand. 1998;69(1):73–6. https://doi.org/10.3109/17453679809002361.
19. Hirayama T, Takemitsu Y, Yagihara K, Mikita A. Operation for chronic dislocation of the radial head in children. Reduction by osteotomy of the ulna. J Bone Joint Surg Br. 1987;69(4):639–42. https://doi.org/10.1302/0301-620X.69B4.3611173.
20. Belangero WD, Livani B, Zogaib RK. Treatment of chronic radial head dislocations in children. Int Orthop. 2007;31(2):151–4. https://doi.org/10.1007/s00264-006-0153-4.
21. Stoll TM, Willis RB, Paterson DC. Treatment of the missed Monteggia fracture in the child. J Bone Joint Surg Br. 1992;74(3):436–40. https://doi.org/10.1302/0301-620X.74B3.1587897.
22. Eygendaal D, Hillen RJ. Open reduction and corrective ulnar osteotomy for missed radial head dislocations in children. Strategies Trauma Limb Reconstr. 2007;2(1):31–4. https://doi.org/10.1007/s11751-007-0013-9.
23. Wang MN, Chang WN. Chronic posttraumatic anterior dislocation of the radial head in children: thirteen cases treated by open reduction, ulnar osteotomy, and annular ligament reconstruction through a Boyd incision. J Orthop Trauma. 2006;20(1):1–5. https://doi.org/10.1097/01.bot.0000189881.75421.92.

24. Peshin C, Ratra R, Juyal AK. Step-cut osteotomy in neglected Monteggia fracture dislocation in pediatric and adolescent patients: a retrospective study. J Orthop Surg (Hong Kong). 2020;28(3):2309499020964082. https://doi.org/10.1177/2309499020964082.
25. Hasler CC, Von Laer L, Hell AK. Open reduction, ulnar osteotomy and external fixation for chronic anterior dislocation of the head of the radius. J Bone Joint Surg Br. 2005;87(1):88–94.
26. Lu X, Kun Wang Y, Zhang J, Zhu Z, Guo Y, Lu M. Management of missed Monteggia fractures with ulnar osteotomy, open reduction, and dual-socket external fixation. J Pediatr Orthop. 2013;33(4):398–402. https://doi.org/10.1097/BPO.0b013e3182812762.
27. Bor N, Rubin G, Rozen N, Herzenberg JE. Chronic anterior Monteggia lesions in children: report of 4 cases treated with closed reduction by ulnar osteotomy and external fixation. J Pediatr Orthop. 2015;35(1):7–10. https://doi.org/10.1097/BPO.0000000000000203.
28. Nakamura K, Hirachi K, Uchiyama S, Takahara M, Minami A, Imaeda T, et al. Long-term clinical and radiographic outcomes after open reduction for missed Monteggia fracture-dislocations in children. J Bone Joint Surg Am. 2009;91(6):1394–404. https://doi.org/10.2106/JBJS.H.00644.
29. Horii E, Nakamura R, Koh S, Inagaki H, Yajima H, Nakao E. Surgical treatment for chronic radial head dislocation. J Bone Joint Surg Am. 2002;84(7):1183–8. https://doi.org/10.2106/00004623-200207000-00014.
30. Lädermann A, Ceroni D, Lefèvre Y, De Rosa V, De Coulon G, Kaelin A. Surgical treatment of missed Monteggia lesions in children. J Child Orthop. 2007;1(4):237–42. https://doi.org/10.1007/s11832-007-0039-z.
31. Oka K, Murase T, Moritomo H, Sugamoto K, Yoshikawa H. Morphologic evaluation of chronic radial head dislocation: three-dimensional and quantitative analyses. Clin Orthop Relat Res. 2010;468(9):2410–8. https://doi.org/10.1007/s11999-010-1283-y.
32. David-West KS, Wilson NI, Sherlock DA, Bennet GC. Missed Monteggia injuries. Injury. 2005;36(10):1206–9. https://doi.org/10.1016/j.injury.2004.12.033.
33. Soni JF, Valenza WR, Matsunaga CU, Costa ACP, Faria FF. Chronic MONTEGGIA fracture-dislocation in children surgical strategy and results. Acta Ortop Bras. 2019;27(5):244–7. https://doi.org/10.1590/1413-785220192705215273.

Chapter 17
Diaphyseal Fracture of the Radius and Ulna

Cristian Artigas and Dalia Sepúlveda

This chapter addresses forearm diaphyseal fractures, analyzing in detail the epidemiological data, pathophysiology, and mechanism of injury. It focuses on how to make a correct diagnosis and discusses treatments supported by the evidence currently available, complemented by the authors' experience. Finally, the most frequent complications will be reviewed, providing tips to avoid them.

17.1 Introduction

Forearm fractures are very common in pediatric age, representing 40% of all fractures at this stage of life [1, 2]. Of these, diaphyseal fractures represent between 13% and 20% [1], that is, 1 in every 5 patients evaluated for forearm fractures correspond to diaphyseal fractures. Thus, specifically, radius and ulna fractures account for 3–6% of total fractures in pediatric age [1–3].

From the 90s to the present, there has been a drastic change in the treatment of this injury, with a noticeable constant increase in treatment with internal osteosynthesis, specifically with the use of intramedullary elastic nailing, over the classic, conservative, or non-surgical management with casting. Cruz [4] analyzed a public database of pediatric trauma registry in the United States during the period 2000–2012, finding that the percentage of fractures treated with osteosynthesis increased from 59% to 70%. Sinikumpu [5], in Finland, also analyzed trauma in the

C. Artigas (✉)
Hospital Roberto del Río/Clínica Alemana, Santiago, Chile

D. Sepúlveda
COTI, Santiago, Chile
e-mail: dsa@cotichile.org

M. Sepúlveda O. (ed.), *Paediatrics Traumatology*,
https://doi.org/10.1007/978-3-031-89482-4_17

pediatric population from 1997 to 2009, finding that it increased from 10% to 30% the surgical management with internal osteosynthesis.

In our country we did not find epidemiological studies that record this change, however, what is demonstrated on scientific meetings of the Chilean Society of Orthopedics and Traumatology, and in high specialization courses in pediatric traumatology, indicate that this same trend exists at the national level.

17.2 Mechanisms of Injury

The most common mechanism associated with a diaphyseal fracture of radius and ulna is a fall with extension of the elbow and wrist, product of the child's protective reflex to cushion the fall [6]. If the fractures of the radius and ulna occur at a different level, it can be assumed that there was a rotational component, associated with the longitudinal force vector in extension of the upper limb [7]. Biomechanical studies have shown that the junction between the middle third and the distal third of the radius and ulna are the most vulnerable to fractures [6, 8].

It should be noted that the mechanism of a direct blow is less frequent, and usually fractures only one bone, usually the ulna, which the patient offers as a defense, for example, against an aggressor, without damaging the radiocubital joints at distal and proximal [9]. Non-accidental traumatic injury should be suspected in this type of injuries.

The fracture pattern is determined by the injury mechanism and by the properties of the bone. The diaphyseal bone is more resistant to the axial forces than to sagittal and torsional forces [10]. Therefore, the fracture pattern will behave differently, depending on the force vectors involved in the trauma.

It is necessary to remember that the bone of a pediatric patient behaves differently than the bone of an adult. The child bone tissue contains much more water and fewer minerals, being much more porous and elastic than adult bone. This makes it capable of absorbing a greater amount of energy prior to failure [11] and generates the existence of 2 types of special fractures, typical of the immature skeleton: plastic deformation and "greenstick" fracture.

The bowed fracture or plastic deformation occurs when subjecting the forearm to a trauma of low or moderate energy, with a deforming force that compromises a greater extension or surface of the bones (Fig. 17.1).

Multiple microfractures occur, generating a macro deformation, without an evident interruption of the cortices in the radiograph. It is important to have a high index of suspicion, both during the clinical examination and when analysing xray images. In the lateral radiographic projection of the forearm, the intact cortical of the ulna should follow a straight line (Fig. 17.2). If in doubt, radiographs of the opposite side can be requested.

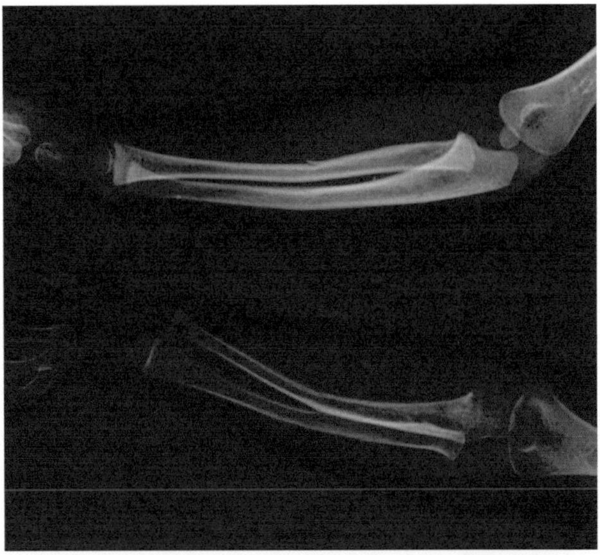

Fig. 17.1 Plastic deformity type of forearm fracture in a child of 3 years old, showing deforming curvature to a large extent in radius and diaphyseal ulna

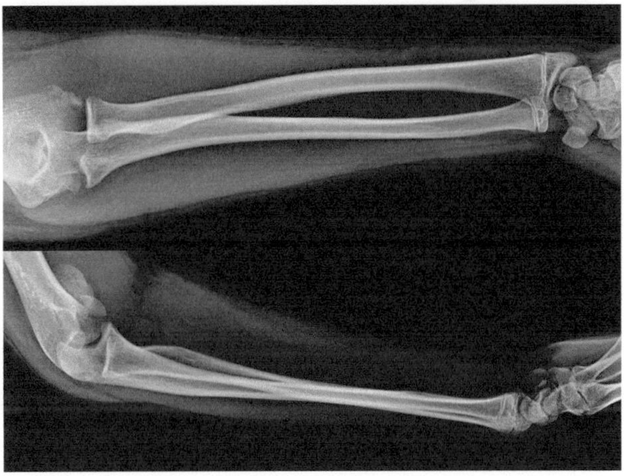

Fig. 17.2 Anteroposterior (AP) and lateral X-ray projections of the forearm. In the lateral view, the coronoid process points anteriorly, the radial styloid is not visualized, and the ulna follows a straight line. In the AP view, the radial styloid and the bicipital tuberosity should be visualized, but not the coronoid process and the ulnar styloid

The "greenstick" fracture occurs when the deforming force causes damage to both cortices of the affected bone, causing an incomplete fracture, which maintains the continuity of the cortex that receives the compressive force, with a complete loss of continuity of the cortex on the opposite side due to a distraction force (Fig. 17.3). It is the analogue, as its name says, to breaking a green stick from a tree with abundant water content, very flexible, and therefore does not lose its continuity (similar to breaking a celery stalk). It is considered an intermediate stage between plastic deformation and complete fracture.

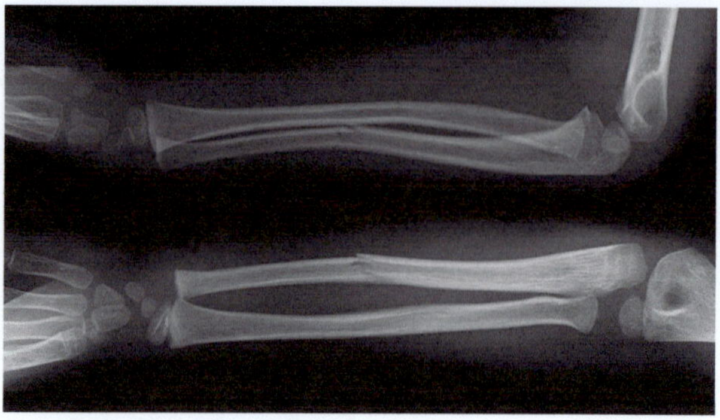

Fig. 17.3 "Greenstick" fracture of the forearm, evidencing complete failure of the cortex affected by a distraction force, and incomplete in the one affected by a compression force

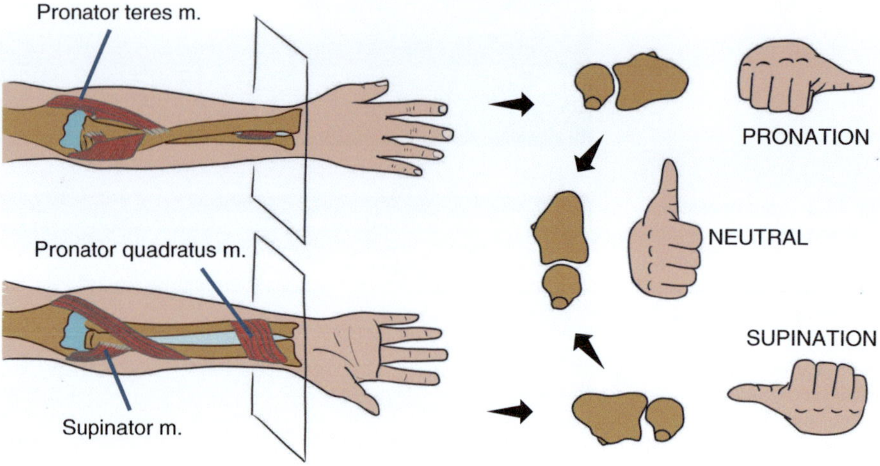

Fig. 17.4

17.3 Anatomy

Currently, the forearm is considered a joint, formed by the radius, the ulna, and the interosseous membrane, so its treatment should be understood in that way.

The normal biomechanics of the forearm is fundamental to develop several of the activities of daily life. While there is a capacity for compensation for residual deformities, at the expense of shoulder mobility, this is limited.

The average supination of the forearm is 85°, and its pronation is 75°. The radius, anatomically curved, rotates over the ulna, which remains fixed and straight in its position, acting as a pivot during this movement (Fig. 17.4). Most of the activities of daily life require at least a forearm movement arc that adds up to 100°, 50° of supination, and 50° of pronation [12].

17.4 Diagnosis

The diagnosis of a forearm fracture can be clinically evident in a mid-diaphyseal angulated fracture, or subtle clinical findings, for example, in an incomplete non-displaced fracture.

A detailed and thorough physical examination is necessary, which not only involves the forearm, but also includes the rest of the upper limb: clavicle, shoulder, arm, elbow, wrist, hand, and ipsilateral fingers, in search of concomitant injuries. Thus, the diaphyseal fracture of the forearm can be associated with a supracondylar fracture of the humerus, which is called "floating elbow" [13].

If the forearm fracture occurs in the context of a polytraumatized patient, this should be attended according to current recommendations (see Chap. 4). Skeletal injuries should be diagnosed during the primary and secondary survey, defining thus the best moment for its definitive treatment.

It is very important to evaluate the integrity of the skin. Small lesions, which appear as superficial abrasions, can be bone exposure wounds that communicate with the fracture site. An example of this are some ulna fractures, whose spicules pierce the skin from inside out, and then hide again under the soft tissues. Bone exposure should be suspected if bleeding persists after the exploration or if the blood presents fat droplets, indicators of bleeding from the bone tissue. The presence of air bubbles in the exit path of the bone can also be identified in the radiographs.

As for diagnostic support images, forearm radiographs in anteroposterior (AP) and lateral projections are more than enough to establish the diagnosis and treatment in practically all cases. It is important to obtain radiographs in optimal projections, which should include the complete wrist and base of the metacarpals at the distal end, and the complete elbow with the distal humerus at the proximal end. Sometimes, it may be necessary to request oblique projections or of the contralateral segment, to clarify doubts. Other exams, such as computed axial tomography (CT-scans), are not part of the usual study.

17.5 Classification

Traditionally, forearm diaphyseal fractures have been classified according to the region or anatomical zone of the diaphysis in which they occur, as well as based on the pattern of the fracture lines. By consensus, the diaphysis has been divided into three thirds, between the proximal and distal metaphyses of the radius and ulna. The metaphysis is defined and limited by a square, whose side corresponds to the sum of the length of the radius physis, plus the ulna physis. This square is projected onto the epiphyso-metaphyseal region, delimiting the beginning of the thirds toward the proximal in the diaphysis (Fig. 17.5).

In 2007, the "AO Trauma" group introduced a classification of pediatric long bone fractures [14], which followed the classic principles of fracture classification

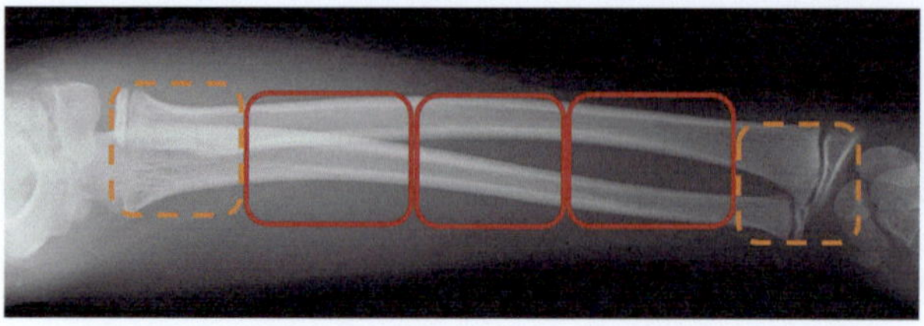

Fig. 17.5 Delimitation of the "thirds" of the forearm (red squares). The proximal and distal segments, metaphysio-epiphyseal, are delimited by a square with faces of length equivalent to the sum of the physes of the radius and ulna (Orange squares)

Table 17.1 Tolerable angular deformity in each segment of the diaphysis of the forearm, according to sex and age [16]

Angulation	Girl <8 years Boy <10 years	Girl >8 years Boy >10 years
Distal shaft	15°	15°
Mid shaft	15°	10°
Proximal shaft	15°	10°

in adults. The location No.2 corresponds to the radius and ulna, and the segment assigned to the diaphysis is No.2. Thus, all forearm diaphyseal fractures will always be "22." We will not delve further into this classification, which is openly available in "AO Surgery Reference" [15].

Along with the classification of the lesion, it is extremely important to be clear about the tolerable angular deformities according to location and age of the patient, defined, published and widely accepted in the classic study by Noonan and Price [16]. These values are shown in Table 17.1.

Regarding rotation, it is clinically very difficult to evaluate its magnitude in degrees. On the other hand, the ability of bone remodeling of a residual rotation is practically nil, even in pediatric bone tissue. This powerful reason leads to the suggestion of not tolerating any degree of rotational misalignment in forearm diaphyseal fractures.

17.6 Treatment

To indicate an appropriate treatment, it is necessary to consider various variables such as the patient's age, the energy involved in the trauma, the state of the soft tissues, the structural quality of the bone tissue (being different the treatment pathologic bone fracture), the existing angulations and/or displacements, the need or not to use implants for osteosynthesis and their availability, as well as the surgeon's experience in the surgical technique.

Treatment options range from immobilization with a cast molded in situ, the need to perform a closed reduction, with or without osteosynthesis, to the possibility of requiring an open reduction of the fracture.

The use of in situ casting, without the need for reduction maneuvers, is reserved for non-displaced, incomplete fractures, or those with minimal angulation and/or translation. The total treatment lasts between 6 and 8 weeks. It consists of the use of a long-arm cast for the first 3–4 weeks, then continuing with a short-arm cast for another 3–4 weeks. The follow-up of these patients must be strict, and at least one radiological check is advised within the first 10 days of treatment to assess the stability of the fracture and the integrity of the cast.

For it to be considered a well-performed treatment, the technique and principles of forearm casting must be respected, meeting the following requirements:

- Proper molding of the diaphysis, with 3-points support and counterforces
- A coronal section with an oval shape
- Proper marking of the interosseous membrane, separating the radius from the ulna
- Respect for the normal anatomical shape of the upper limb

This can be performed under sedation or with general anesthesia, depending on the local conditions of the health center. To perform a reduction under sedation, a procedure room and a professional team prepared to perform the procedure, including X-ray equipment to check the reduction, are required. In the case of using general anesthesia, the procedure is carried out in the operating room with the support of an anesthetic medical team and requires at least a transient hospitalization and a recovery room. The advantage of this situation is that the patient is asleep, with muscle relaxation and without pain. This is especially useful in smaller patients, or in those where the cast molding technique is demanding and requires very precise maneuvers.

Once the closed reduction of the fracture has been performed, outpatient follow-up must be strict, both to monitor the patient's tolerance to the plaster and to assess the maintenance of the achieved reduction. If there is a new displacement in the follow up visits or spaces are generated between skin and plaster, losing the containment capacity, it may be necessary to change the immobilizing cast. In unstable fractures or those at risk of instability (Table 17.2), closed reduction maneuvers are required (Fig. 17.6).

An alternative for when the reduction has been lost and angulations are generated above what is tolerated is to use the cast-wedging technique. This consists of making

Table 17.2 Characteristics that increase the risk of instability in forearm fractures

Instability
Complete fracture
Affects both bones (radius and ulna)
Convergence of bone segments at the fracture site
Oblique fracture line >30°

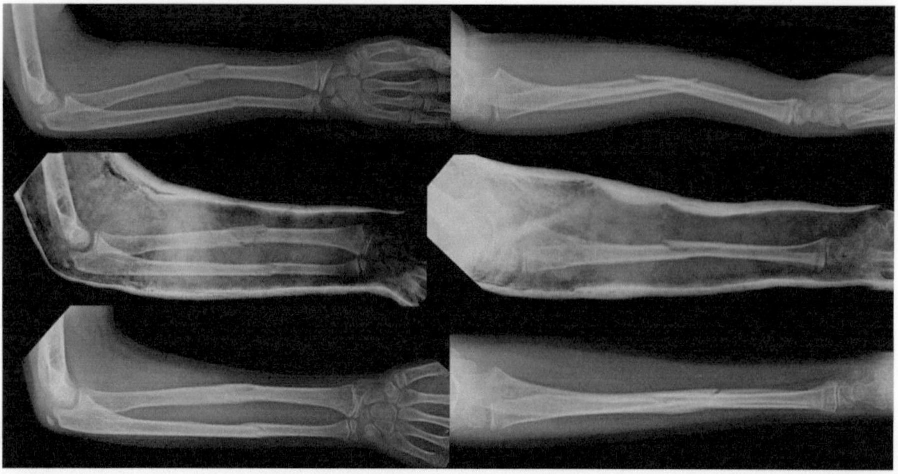

Fig. 17.6 A 12-year-old patient with an angulated diaphyseal fracture, in which a closed reduction and a molded long-arm cast were used

a linear cut in the semicircumference of the cast, on the opposite side of the apex of the deformity. Subsequently, an opening or space is generated at the level of the cut, which will be filled with a wedge or block of resistant material, seeking to align the cast and, therefore, the fracture. Another option is to make the cut at the apex of the deformity, then compress and close the generated space. This technique requires a lot of experience to define the cuts and magnitude of the wedges. In addition, it is important to know its correction limits to avoid damage to the skin and soft tissues.

In a fracture that cannot be stabilized by a well-molded cast, or in which the axes cannot be aligned, it will be necessary to perform a closed reduction or open reduction, with immediate osteosynthesis.

The closed reduction is achieved with the cooperation of an assistant, through traction-countertraction, rotation, and flexo-extension maneuvers, depending on the "personality" of the fracture. It is an act that requires technique and experience, and, even for experienced surgeons, it can be demanding. In most cases where closed reduction is not possible, soft tissues, such as the periosteum or part of the forearm muscle bellies, interfere.

If the surgeon chooses to perform an open reduction, a minimal incision should be used, to reach the fracture site, and in this way assist in the reduction that facilitates stabilization with internal fixation with intramedullary nails, or make a wide open approach when they consider the use of plates, especially in patients close to the end of bone growth. This will be determined according to the location of the fracture, if it is necessary to address one or both bones, and keeping in mind the neurovascular structures that run through the forearm.

Titanium elastic nails (TEN) for intramedullary nailing are nowadays the treatment of choice for diaphyseal fractures in which closed reduction failed or whose stability cannot be controlled only by immobilizing with a plaster cast. The technique was described by Metaizeau [17], and since then the principles remain the same. This technique consists of achieving a reduction, ideally closed, and stabilization by inserting a pre-tensioned nail into each bone of the forearm, of the same diameter, achieving an elastic stable intramedullary nailing system. In the forearm, the technique must achieve tensioning of the interosseous membrane, which generates greater stability to the construct. Stabilization with 2 nails must oppose the muscular deforming forces at the fracture site. Thus, the well-applied technique must control all instabilities, both in the axial, torsional, translational axes, as well as the forces in flexion. Nails of 2.0–2.5 mm are usually used, ideally equivalent to 2/3 of the isthmus of the canal of each bone. Nails of 1.5 mm may be necessary in smaller patients.

There are different configurations of stable elastic intramedullary nailing. The traditional one, initially described, is with a retrograde approach in the radius, from distal, to avoid damaging the deep branch of the radial nerve in the proximal third of the forearm, and anterograde to the ulna (Fig. 17.7). The molding of the nails must be taking into account that the apex of the pre-tensioning is ideally located at the level of the fracture site. This molding should be approximately 3 times the diameter of the canal of the affected bone.

The lateral distal approach is used for the radius. It allows an easy entry to the metaphysis in its widest distal portion. It has the risk of injuring the superficial sensory branch of the radial nerve, so it should be done with caution. AO trauma has proposed a new, dorsl approach to the distal radius over the Lister's tubercle. This approach would avoid the risk of injury to the radial nerve. However, there are cases described of extensor pollicis longus tendon injury due to the nail [18], so it is recommended to leave the curved end over the retinaculum. This approach is also the best option for fractures with palmar displacement.

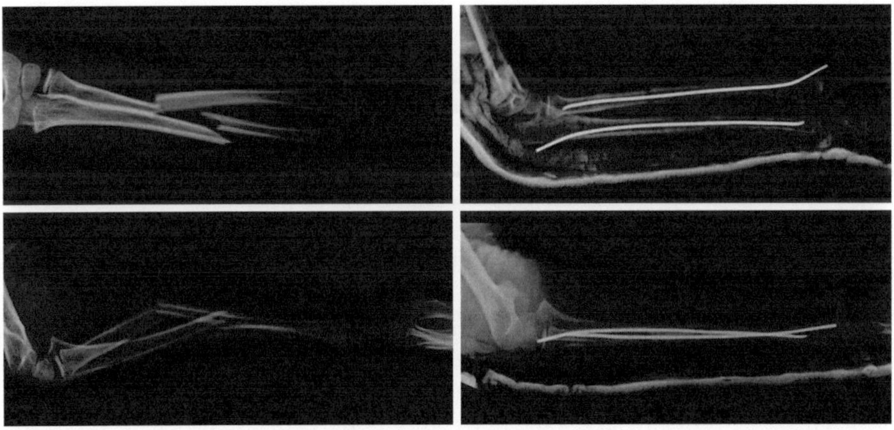

Fig. 17.7 An 8-year-old patient with a diaphyseal fracture of the radius and ulna, with transverse and short oblique fracture respectively. The Closed reduction failed. The pattern was not stable and internal fixation with elastic nails was performed

The nailing of the ulna can be with a traditional approach, anterograde, entering through the lateral cortice of the proximal ulnar metaphysis. AO trauma promotes a new approach for retrograde configuration, entering through the medial cortice of the distal ulnar metaphysis. The advantage of this entry point would be to facilitate the fracture reduction maneuvers, avoiding having to change the forearm position during the insertion both nails, which can be used as a reduction handle also allowing the surgeon a better visualization with the image intensifier throughout the procedure. The problem with this entry to the ulna is that the medullary canal at this level is narrower, so a very careful perforation of the cortical must be performed, which avoids the generation of a false path in the interosseous compartment of the forearm.

Once the reduction and insertion of both nails is achieved, the definitive cutting of these is proceeded. We recommend using a cutting tool specially designed for this, included in the surgical set of the nails. Doing it with other less precise implements can generate irregular and sharp edges, which could damage the adjacent soft tissues, causing chronic irritation that can even determine the appearance of a wound. Once the nail is cut, if it is considered that it is still too long, the nail is removed backward a few millimeters, cut again, and then pushed, to leave it protected under the skin.

Most surgeons prefer to leave a long-arm splint during the first month of the postoperative period. However, if the configuration of the nails is adequate and satisfactory stability is achieved, patients can be left with only a sling at this time. This should be evaluated by the treating physician for each specific case.

The removal of osteosynthesis material is not mandatory, but it is what is usually done. One of the main arguments for this is that it could be bothersome for future trauma surgery. Another common reason for removal is due to irritation of the soft tissues at the entry sites. In addition, cases are described where unfortunately, the inadequate pre-tensioning of the nails can generate a secondary deformity. Removal is not advised before 6 months post-surgery, for adequate formation and remodeling of the bone callus. If for various reasons, a significant amount of time has passed since the surgery and the nails are covered by bone tissue, or the entry points have significantly migrated from the initial insertion, it is very likely that extraction will be very difficult, even with the risk of significant complications, which is why we advise against removal in these cases.

The use of plates is restricted to patients with little or no remaining bone growth. They can be used when a closed reduction fails, and/or when there is great instability of the fracture. Plates and screws of 2.7 or 3.5 mm are usually used, with interfragmentary compression or bridging techniques, following the principles of regular trauma management. Although an anatomical reduction and adequate stability are achieved, it is necessary to perform larger approaches, compromise the biology of the bone tissue by stripping the periosteum, and lose the fracture hematoma. This leads to a significant alteration of the reparative process of children's bone tissue, which makes this treatment not the first choice in the pediatric patient.

Finally, another treatment option is the use of external fixation, which is always a very good alternative for the patient in whom the techniques of stabilization and conventional osteosynthesis are contraindicated, or because their condition does not allow them to be performed. Examples of these cases are those patients with significant soft tissue damage, fractures with great comminution, segmental bone loss, or with associated vascular injury that requires surgical repair. In fractures of a polytraumatized patient, stabilization with modular external fixators is the first choice, to allow the management of life-threatening associated injuries. It is important to emphasize that when we install an external fixator in pediatric patients, it should be considered that it can remain as definitive treatment until fracture healing. Thus you must be meticulous, respecting the basic principles of fracture reduction and stabilization using external fixation, seeking the best anatomical reduction.

17.7 Complications

The loss of reduction of a forearm fracture is probably the most common complication. It is described that its incidence is between 10% and 20% in the different series published [19]. The vast majority of fractures that will displace, do so within the first 15 days, which is why weekly radiological follow-up is recommended during the first 2 weeks from the start of treatment. The most common causes of this complication have to do with a deficient casting technique, so we must be demanding on this topic, striving to achieve good stabilization, using the containment through 3-points technique support, achieving to mold the forearm with an oval section, not round, padding adequately, not exaggeratedly, avoiding that the bandage becomes loose. It is also important to consider that with the passing of the days, the edema of the affected limb decreases, generating potential spaces between the skin and the cast, which could reduce its containment capacity despite good initial molding.

The delay in consolidation is defined as the absence of complete consolidation (4 visible cortices on radiographs) at 12 weeks after the fracture. Non-union is defined as the absence of complete radiological union at 6 months after the fracture [9]. Patients with an immature skeleton have a thick and richly innervated and irrigated periosteum, which, together with the biological potential of the fracture hematoma, make the delay in the bone healing and non-union very infrequent. However, in open fractures, or in those where the fracture site was reduced openly, with significant deperiostization, the risk of delayed consolidation or non-union is more frequent [9].

Loss of range of motion is the most feared complication, visible in the long term. In the pediatric patient, the ability to compensate for this loss with shoulder and scapular girdle mobility is important. Pronation is the most affected movement, being almost twice as limited as supination [20]. Loss of range of motion can occur even without an evident alteration of the bone axes, due to a fibrous scar of the interosseous membrane and/or interosseous ligament contracture [2].

A new fracture at the same level occurs on average within the first 6 months after the initial injury (Fig. 17.8). It is more common in men and in patients over 10 years [21]. Midshaft and proximal fractures are the ones with the highest risk of presenting a new fracture [22]. The treatment will depend on the initial one and the patient's age.

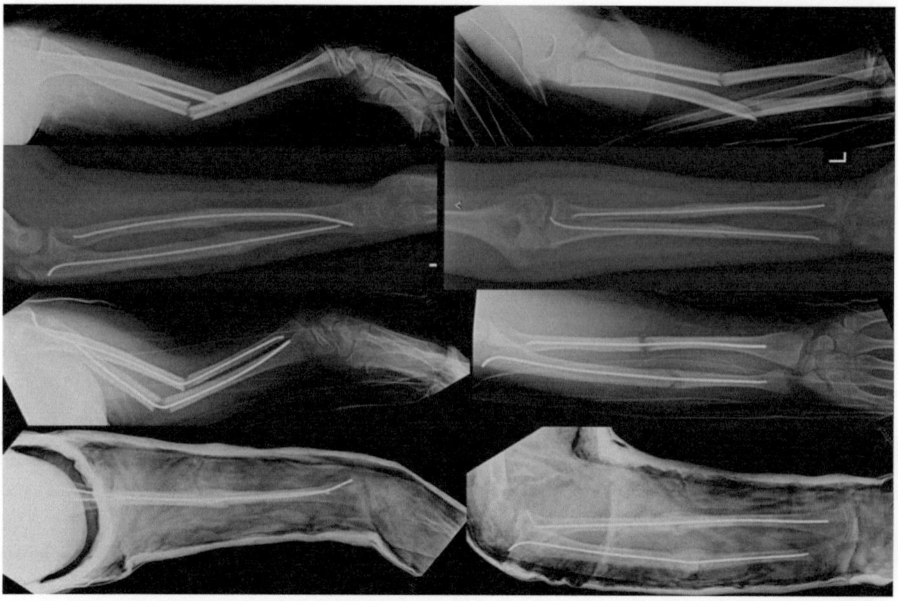

Fig. 17.8 A 12-year-old patient with forearm diaphyseal fracture. Treated with closed reduction and stable elastic nails. Four months after surgery, he suffered new fall, with a new fracture. Management by closed reduction is decided, leaving the nails in situ, with a molded cast

As previously mentioned, if the nails are not cut to the right length or with the appropriate instrument, they can protrude and cause functional alterations and pain, even at rest. In these cases, an erythematous area forms in relation to the tip of the nail. It can be very annoying and painful, especially when it occurs at the antegrade insertion at the elbow level in the ulna. If it is very symptomatic, the nail can be removed early.

A catastrophic complication is the forearm compartment syndrome, which has a frequency of between 1.5% and 7.5% in different series [23]. The forearm has 3 compartments, with the palmar one being the most affected. Risk factors for this complication include the presence of an open fracture [24], prolonged surgical times [24, 25], age under 10 years [26], surgery performed on the same day of the accident [3], and increased fluoroscopy times [25]. The latter is directly related to failed attempts at closed reduction during intramedullary nailing.

It is always necessary to have a high degree of suspicion in the face of this complication. A late diagnosis can have devastating consequences, even ending with a Volkmann's ischemic contracture. Today, there are devices capable of measuring compartmental pressure, but their availability is limited to some high-complexity trauma centers, so clinical diagnosis is fundamental. In our experience, the most relevant clinical sign is progressive pain, which does not change with position changes, dressing opening, and usual analgesia. In this scenario, we must be proactive, indicating the corresponding fasciotomy to the affected segment.

The most frequently compromised nerve in forearm diaphyseal fractures is the median nerve [27], although there may be involvement of other nerves crossing the forearm. Most injuries are neuropraxias that will resolve favorably spontaneously [19].

It is very important to objectify the neurological sensory and motor status of the affected limb, both at the time of the first evaluation and in the perioperative period, and clinical findings should be recorded in the medical record. Any change after surgery should alert the surgeon. If the neurological compromise persists after 3 months of injury in a fracture managed non-surgically, with absence of signs of clinical recovery, it is necessary to study the patient with nerve conduction tests and possible magnetic resonance imaging (MRI). If the fracture required stabilization with osteosynthesis and/or open reduction, the study of a possible neurological damage should be earlier.

17.8 Final Message

Diaphyseal fractures of the forearm in pediatric patients are very common. General trauma doctors and specialists in emergency services will find that at least 1 out of every 5 forearm fractures will be located in the diaphysis of the radius and/or ulna, so they will be frequent in their clinical practice.

It is extremely important to make a correct radiological diagnosis from the first moment, because both the optimal treatment and the best possible outcome of this depend on an accurate initial classification. This will help to decrease the problems and complications that will limit the pronosupination function of the forearm. For the correct treatment of the injury, whether conservative or surgical, it is necessary to consider all the variables described in this chapter.

17.9 Authors' Recommendations

Diagnosis

- Suspect a fracture in the presence of diaphyseal pain, even without evident deformity.
- Actively seek neurovascular integrity throughout the process.
- Demand well-taken radiographs, and visualize the straight ulna in the lateral projection.

Treatment

- Always consider bone maturity: the greater the potential for remodeling, the greater the flexibility to accept residual angular deformities.
- If you choose a conservative treatment with cast: follow the containment technique with support at three points, very well molded, achieving a coronal oval cut. Control with radiographs at 7 and 15 days.

- Pronosupination is significantly altered with greater residual angulations, so it is important to know the tolerated limits, especially in injuries located in the proximal third.
- Consider the possibility of a surgical reduction and immediate osteosynthesis, both in unstable fractures from the diagnosis, and in those where the treatment with casting has failed.

Follow-up

- Prioritize methods and treatment techniques that respect the biology of the fracture repair process.
- Stick to proven surgical principles and techniques with evidence. Do not innovate.
- Monitor the patient even until skeletal maturity, to ensure adequate functionality, maintaining a pronosupination of at least 50°/50°.

References

1. Rennie L, Court-Brown CM, Mok JY, Beattie TF. The epidemiology of fractures in children. Injury. 2007;38(8):913–22. https://doi.org/10.1016/j.injury.2007.01.036.
2. Patel A, Li L, Anand A. Systematic review: functional outcomes and complications of intramedullary nailing versus plate fixation for both-bone diaphyseal forearm fractures in children. Injury. 2014;45(8):1135–43. https://doi.org/10.1016/j.injury.2014.04.020.
3. Flynn JM, Jones KJ, Garner MR, Goebel J. Eleven years experience in the operative management of pediatric forearm fractures. J Pediatr Orthop. 2010;30(4):313–9. https://doi.org/10.1097/BPO.0b013e3181d98f2c.
4. Cruz AI Jr, Kleiner JE, DeFroda SF, Gil JA, Daniels AH, Eberson CP. Increasing rates of surgical treatment for paediatric diaphyseal forearm fractures: a National Database Study from 2000 to 2012. J Child Orthop. 2017;11(3):201–9. https://doi.org/10.1302/1863-2548.11.170017.
5. Sinikumpu JJ, Pokka T, Serlo W. The changing pattern of pediatric both-bone forearm shaft fractures among 86,000 children from 1997 to 2009. Eur J Pediatr Surg. 2013;23(4):289–96. https://doi.org/10.1055/s-0032-1333116.
6. McGinley JC, Hopgood BC, Gaughan JP, Sadeghipour K, Kozin SH. Forearm and elbow injury: the influence of rotational position. J Bone Joint Surg Am. 2003;85(12):2403–9.
7. Hsu ES, Patwardhan AG, Meade KP, Light TR, Martin WR. Cross-sectional geometrical properties and bone mineral contents of the human radius and ulna. J Biomech. 1993;26(11):1307–18. https://doi.org/10.1016/0021-9290(93)90354-h.
8. Blount WP, Schaefer AA, Johnson JH. Fractures of the forearm in children. JAMA. 1942;120(2):111–6. https://doi.org/10.1001/jama.1942.02830370023007.
9. Flynn JM, Skaggs DL, Waters PM. Rockwood and Wilkins' fractures in children. 8th ed. Philadelphia, PA: Lippincott Williams & Wilkins; 2015.
10. Carter DR, Spengler DM. Mechanical properties and composition of cortical bone. Clin Orthop Relat Res. 1978;135:192–217.
11. Currey JD, Butler G. The mechanical properties of bone tissue in children. J Bone Joint Surg Am. 1975;57(6):810–4.
12. Morrey BF, Askew LJ, Chao EY. A biomechanical study of normal functional elbow motion. J Bone Joint Surg Am. 1981;63(6):872–7.
13. Roposch A, Reis M, Molina M, Davids J, Stanley E, Wilkins K, et al. Supracondylar fractures of the humerus associated with ipsilateral forearm fractures in children: a report of forty-seven cases. J Pediatr Orthop. 2001;21(3):307–12.

14. Slongo T, Audigé L, Clavert JM, Lutz N, Frick S, Hunter J. The AO comprehensive classification of pediatric long-bone fractures: a web-based multicenter agreement study. J Pediatr Orthop. 2007;27(2):171–80. https://doi.org/10.1097/01.bpb.0000248569.43251.f9.
15. AO Foundation. AO surgery reference. https://surgeryreference.aofoundation.org/orthopedic-trauma/pediatric-trauma. Accessed 5 Jun 2022.
16. Noonan KJ, Price CT. Forearm and distal radius fractures in children. J Am Acad Orthop Surg. 1998;6(3):146–56. https://doi.org/10.5435/00124635-199805000-00002.
17. Ligier JN, Métaizeau JP, Lascombes P, Poncelet T, Prévot J. Treatment of diaphyseal fractures of both bones of the forearm in children using elastic stable pinning. Rev Chir Orthop Reparatrice Appar Mot. 1987;73 Suppl 2:149–51. French
18. Murphy HA, Jain VV, Parikh SN, Wall EJ, Cornwall R, Mehlman CT. Extensor tendon injury associated with dorsal entry flexible nailing of radial shaft fractures in children: a report of 5 new cases and review of the literature. J Pediatr Orthop. 2019;39(4):163–8. https://doi.org/10.1097/BPO.0000000000000897.
19. Neiman R, Maiocco B, Deeney VF. Ulnar nerve injury after closed forearm fractures in children. J Pediatr Orthop. 1998;18(5):683–5. https://doi.org/10.1097/00004694-199809000-00026.
20. Holdsworth BJ, Sloan JP. Proximal forearm fractures in children: residual disability. Injury. 1982;14:174–9.
21. Tredwell SJ, Van Peteghem K, Clough M. Pattern of forearm fractures in children. J Pediatr Orthop. 1984;4(5):604–8.
22. Baitner AC, Perry A, Lalonde FD, Bastrom TP, Pawelek J, Newton PO. The healing forearm fracture: a matched comparison of forearm refractures. J Pediatr Orthop. 2007;27(7):743–7. https://doi.org/10.1097/BPO.0b013e318142568c.
23. Pace JL. Pediatric and adolescent forearm fractures: current controversies and treatment recommendations. J Am Acad Orthop Surg. 2016;24(11):780–8. https://doi.org/10.5435/JAAOS-D-15-00151.
24. Blackman AJ, Wall LB, Keeler KA, Schoenecker PL, Luhmann SJ, O'Donnell JC, et al. Acute compartment syndrome after intramedullary nailing of isolated radius and ulna fractures in children. J Pediatr Orthop. 2014;34(1):50–4. https://doi.org/10.1097/BPO.0b013e31829527de.
25. Yuan PS, Pring ME, Gaynor TP, Mubarak SJ, Newton PO. Compartment syndrome following intramedullary fixation of pediatric forearm fractures. J Pediatr Orthop. 2004;24(4):370–5. https://doi.org/10.1097/00004694-200407000-00005.
26. Martus JE, Preston RK, Schoenecker JG, Lovejoy SA, Green NE, Mencio GA. Complications and outcomes of diaphyseal forearm fracture intramedullary nailing: a comparison of pediatric and adolescent age groups. J Pediatr Orthop. 2013;33(6):598–607. https://doi.org/10.1097/BPO.0b013e3182a11d3b.
27. Luhmann SJ, Schootman M, Schoenecker PL, Dobbs MB, Gordon JE. Complications and outcomes of open pediatric forearm fractures. J Pediatr Orthop. 2004;24(1):1–6. https://doi.org/10.1097/00004694-200401000-00001.

Chapter 18
Distal Radius Fracture

Juan Carlos Hernández and Verónica Vilches

Normal psychomotor development, the process of exploring new experiences, coupled with the increase in energy and violence of children's games have increased the frequency and complexity of fractures in pediatric patients. Distal forearm fractures are no exception to this reality. One in every four child will consult in an emergency service for a trauma event, a fifth of them will be diagnosed with a fracture, and of these, a third will correspond to a distal forearm fracture [1]. It is estimated that there are 210,000 forearm fractures per year in children in the United States [2], which shows the magnitude of this pathology and the need for standardized treatments that ensure an optimal result and without sequelae in patients, considering the quality scientific evidence when defining them.

18.1 Epidemiology

Forearm fractures represent 32% of childhood fractures [3], and 90% affect the distal third of the forearm [1]. The estimated incidence is 12–36/1000 children per year [4]. It occurs more frequently in males than in females, with a range of 42–64% in boys and 27–40% in girls, as described in the literature. The average age of occurrence is 9.9 years old, with the age of highest frequency between 10 and 11-years in females and 12 and 13 years in males [1].

J. C. Hernández (✉)
Hospital Roberto del Río, Clínica Indisa, Universidad del Desarrollo, Santiago, Chile

V. Vilches
Hospital Roberto del Río, Santiago, Chile

M. Sepúlveda O. (ed.), *Paediatrics Traumatology*,
https://doi.org/10.1007/978-3-031-89482-4_18

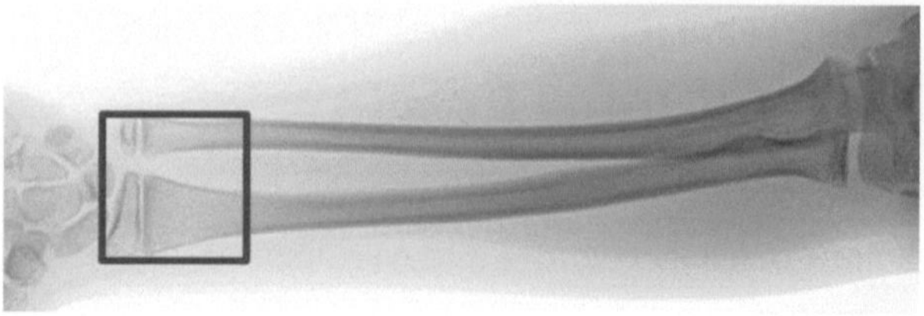

Fig. 18.1 The distal third of the forearm is defined as a square with faces of length equivalent to the width of the articular surface of the wrist in the anteroposterior plane

18.2 Mechanism of Injury

The mechanism of injury is still predominantly indirect, with a fall over the extended hand, with the wrist in hyperextension, which defines the displacement of the distal fragment toward dorsal [5]. However, we must not forget that a smaller percentage of fractures occur due to support of the wrist in flexion, which originates a displacement and angulation of the distal fragment to volar. The transmission of forces from the hand to the distal forearm occurs axially, 80% to the radius and 20% to the ulna.

Isolated fractures of the radius or ulna occur predominantly by direct mechanism [5]. In these cases, the dislocation of the radial head (Monteggia lesion) and the dislocation of the distal ulna (Galeazzi's injury) should be actively sought, through the appropriate radiological projections.

The forearm is made up of the radius, the ulna, and the interosseous membrane. It extends from the elbow to the wrist. Topographically, it is divided into proximal third, middle third, and distal third, the latter being the space between the distal radioulnar joint surface and the metaphyseal segment that reaches the width of the joint surface (Fig. 18.1).

As the ulna is straight and the radius is curved, the arc of pronation-supination movement is achieved. The normal range is 80–90° of supination and 75–80° of pronation, considering a functional pronosupination of 100° (50° of pronation and 50° of supination) [6]. This mobility decreases when there is a fracture, and this decrease is greater the more angulated and displaced it is.

18.3 Diagnosis

Usually, the patient can provide an account of a trauma event. Upon clinical examination, pain will be found when moving the forearm and/or upon direct palpation, with varying degrees of swelling and deformity, which will depend on the complexity of the fracture. Diagnostic confirmation is usually achieved with an X-ray study that should include at least two projections of the forearm, in the coronal (anteroposterior) and sagittal (lateral) planes, including the wrist and elbow joints (Fig. 18.2).

Occasionally, we may have the coexistence of fractures at different levels in the same segment, or in the adjacent one, especially a supracondylar fracture of the

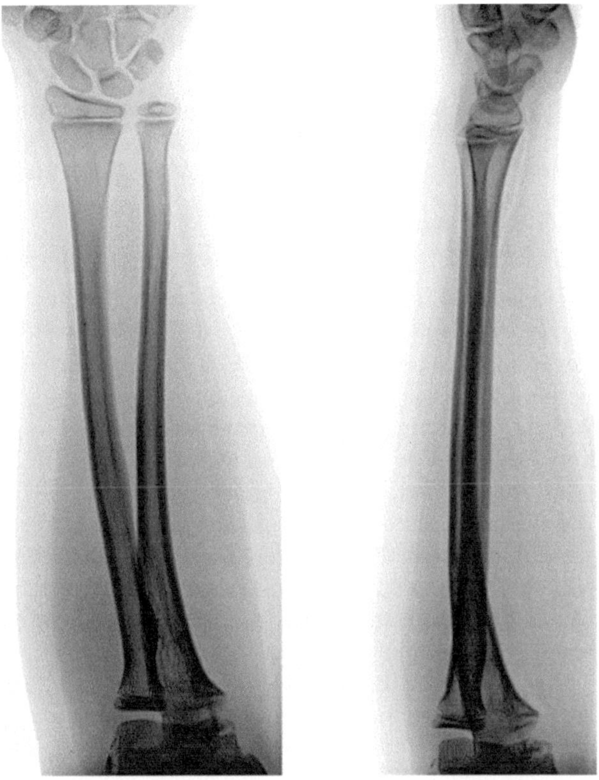

Fig. 18.2 Anteroposterior and lateral X-ray projections of the forearm, including elbow and wrist joints

distal humerus, so we must perform a thorough physical examination and require radiographs that include both adjacent joints in at least 2 planes.

Most of the time, this imaging study is sufficient for diagnosis and treatment planning, reserving the use of computed tomography (CT-scan) or magnetic resonance imaging (MRI) for cases where intra-articular involvement is suspected.

18.4 Classification

There are multiple ways to classify fractures at this level. According to the fracture line pattern, they can be transverse, comminuted, or oblique. According to the direction of angulation, they can be angled dorsally, palmarly, radially, or ulnarly. According to the resulting deformity, they can be incomplete (greenstick, torus, or bowed), angled, or displaced (the magnitude of displacement and/or angulation can be described). According to the involvement of soft tissues, they can be closed or open. If there is bone exposure, we classify it according to Gustilo-Anderson. If there is physeal involvement, the most commonly used classification is Salter and Harris.

In an attempt to unify these classifications, the AO has proposed a classification of distal forearm fractures specific for the pediatric population, which, although not widely used yet, allows unifying the different types of fractures, regardless of their topographic characteristics, displacement, and direction of angulation.

18.5 Treatment

Treatment has traditionally relied on the remodeling capacity of the child's skeleton, especially at the level of the distal radius, due to the high potential for correction with the longitudinal growth of the segment. For this reason, classic studies suggest initial conservative management even for angled and/or displaced fractures, without performing reduction maneuvers, according to some parameters of deformity magnitude at different ages (Table 18.1) [7].

However, today, and for different reasons attributable to the patient, their parents, and the medical team, this approach has been changing, not accepting treatments with initial deformities that rely solely on remodeling. This is reserved for those fractures that during the course of conservative treatment lose the axis within the values that are documented as tolerable by the remodeling capacity, considering the remaining growth of each patient.

In this context, the objectives of treating a fracture with altered distal radius axes are (1) to realign the proximal and distal segments of the fracture, with the least residual local deformity, in order to achieve consolidation in a correct axis in the different planes, which ensures the proper function of the segment in the future; (2) to maintain the reduction through an efficient method of stabilization, which may be conservative (through the use of casts) or surgical (through the use of osteosynthesis with Kirschner wires, screws, and very occasionally plates or external fixators).

The objective of fracture reduction is to restore normal anatomy, which will restore the function of the segment. However, sometimes this is not achieved, accepting residual local deformities whose magnitude will depend on several factors. The most important factor will be the patient's age, which is directly related to the remodeling capacity determined by the specific remaining growth. This allows us to tolerate angulations in the coronal and sagittal planes, regardless of the stabilization method used, but not so in the transverse plane, as rotational deformities do

Table 18.1 Parameters to determine deformity tolerance that can be considered for the choice of conservative treatment in distal radius fractures

	Proximal third	Middle third	Distal third
Angulation	<8 years, 10° >8 years, 0°	<8 years, 15° >8 years, 10°	<8 years, 20° >8 years, 10°
Rotation	<15°	<9 years, 45° >9 years, 15°	<30°
Translation	100%	100%	100%
Shortening	1 cm	1 cm	1 cm

not remodel correctly [7, 8]. For this, there are guidelines on the magnitude and direction of axis alterations and the ages at which they are tolerable, as described by the classic Price and Noonan tables, and recent consensus publications [7, 8].

In incomplete metaphyseal fractures, such as in a "torus" fracture, the treatment is to immobilize, by a short-arm cast, a short splint, or a removable wrist immobilizer splint. In this way, the repair of the injury is promoted, without pain, which usually in pediatric patients will be in 3–4 weeks.

In incomplete or complete metaphyseal fractures, with loss of their axis due to angulation, translation, or displacement, an adequate bone reduction must first be achieved, seeking to recover the anatomical axes, and then stabilize, maintaining the reduction until the fracture healing is achieved.

All reduction maneuvers are painful for the patient, so it is recommended to perform them without causing pain or anxiety to the child, or difficulties to the medical team, with patient sedation and radioscopic control of the reduction obtained. For the reduction maneuver, it is necessary to remember that the presence of a thick periosteum, characteristic of the pediatric patient, helps us in the stabilization of the fracture once reduced, so we must avoid damaging it with very energetic maneuvers. However, we must also know that the broken ends of this periosteum are capable of interposing in the fracture site and not allowing us to maintain the reduction of the fracture. For these situations, the maneuver chosen must consider the patient's age, the location of the fracture in the bone, and the orientation of the displacement.

A common mistake is to first try to reduce the shortening, by performing longitudinal traction, which reduces the overlap and can even restore the length. However, this maneuver compresses or crushes the fragments of the fracture between them, leaving the broken periosteum interposed between the corticals, or even in the fracture site, which destabilizes the reduction achieved (Fig. 18.3).

This leads to a not infrequent situation, in which after checking in the operating room a good stable reduction in a cast, in the postoperative control a displacement of the fracture is evidenced secondary to the instability produced by the soft tissues interposed in the fracture site.

To avoid this problem, it is recommended to perform the reduction maneuver by first increasing the deformity ("bayonet" maneuver), with axial traction, which allows restoring the length, preventing the periosteum from interposing in the fracture site. First, the deformity of the fracture is gently increased, usually by hyperextension for a fracture displaced dorsally, and then we move the fragment distally by traction, during which hyperextension is maintained, until the bone ends of the fracture contact. This manages to leave the damaged periosteum above the dorsal corticals of both fragments, and not in the fracture site. Once the length is achieved, the deformity is flexed, and the distal fragment is moved to palmar, achieving the reduction of the fracture, without interposition of soft tissues (Fig. 18.4).

Once a correct reduction is achieved, we must maintain it, stabilizing the fracture, which in most cases is done by a cast adapted to the anatomy of the forearm.

The shape of the cast should be oval, not cylindrical, following the axis of the first ray. A position with the wrist toward ulnar is recommended, seeking to reduce

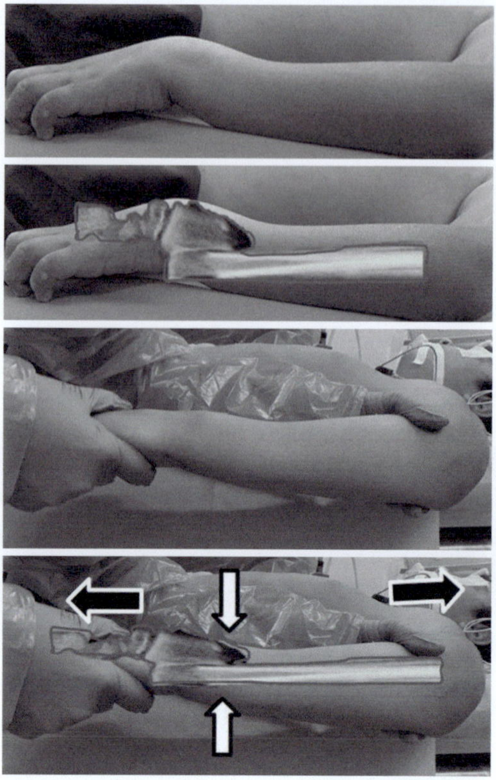

Fig. 18.3 Inadequate longitudinal traction maneuver, looking to correct shortening due to displacement

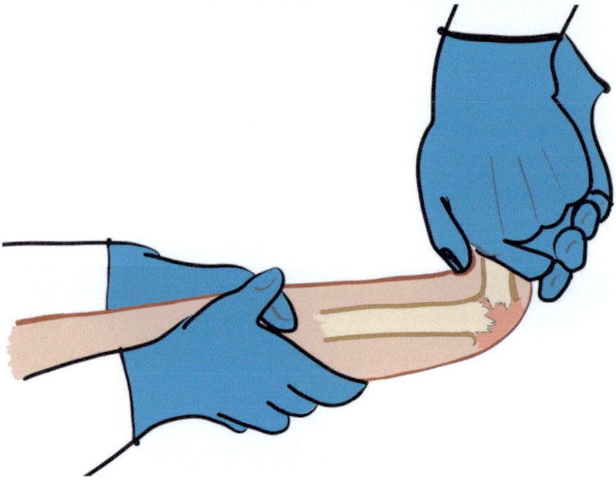

Fig. 18.4 Correct reduction maneuver, increasing the deformity in order to avoid interposition of periosteum at the fracture site while correcting the shortening

the possibility of translation of the distal fragment toward radial. There should be no remaining space or air between the cast and the skin, which is achieved by precise molding of the cast during installation and joining of the plaster bandages. The elbow should be straight at 90°, not curved, and with support from the cast at three points, which allows maintaining the reduction achieved (Fig. 18.5).

There are indicators that measure the quality of plastering technique by its molding, and that help predict the maintenance of the reduction within the cast during treatment (Table 18.2). The most commonly used is the "Cast index," which is a ratio between the diameter in the coronal plane and the sagittal plane, at the level of the fracture site. It should have an ideal value less than 0.7 (Fig. 18.6). The closer to one, the plaster has a rounder shape, less coincidence with the shape of the forearm, and therefore less containment of the fracture fragments, so the possibility of a loss of reduction increases.

It is important to emphasize that the molding and 3-point support of the cast allow maintaining the reduction of the fracture within it, which is fundamental as the post-trauma edema of the forearm is reduced because a space is generated between the skin and the cast that favors the displacement and/or angulation of the fracture. Thus, by a lever effect, the displacement of the fracture fragments is avoided, thanks to the adequate anti-deforming forces provided by the external stabilization.

The trick is not to "crush" the fracture, but to correctly mold the plaster. In the most common case, with dorsal displacement of the distal fragment, the plaster is molded with two dorsal support points with a palmar force vector, one proximal and one distal to the fracture, in addition to a support point at the fracture level by

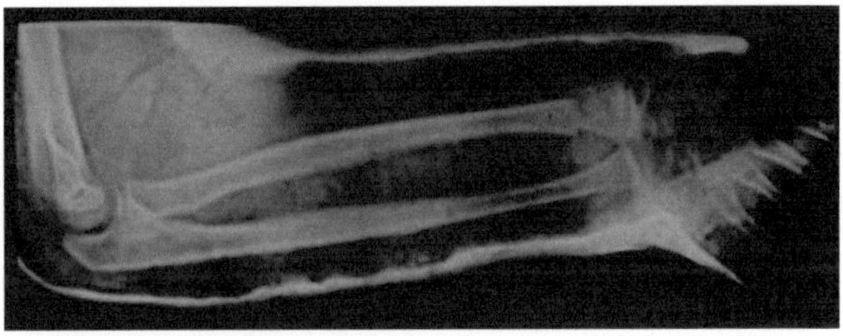

Fig. 18.5 Radiographic control of a well-positioned long-arm cast, with elbow at 90º, without air inside the cast

Table 18.2 Indicators to evaluate the quality of the casting technique

Index	Middle third	Ideal value
Cast index	Internal diameter of the cast in lateral view at the fracture level/internal diameter of the cast in AP view at the fracture level	<0.7
Space index	Radial space + ulnar space at fracture site + dorsal space + palmar space at the fracture site	<0.15
Padding index	Dorsal space at the fracture level on lateral view/maximal interosseous distance on AP view	<0.3
Canterbury	Cast index/Padding index	<1.1
3 points AP	Radial distal space + ulnar space at fracture site + proximal radial space/transverse contact area on AP view	<0.8
3 points lateral	Distal dorsal space + palmar space at fracture site + dorsal proximal space/transverse contact área on lateral view	<0.8

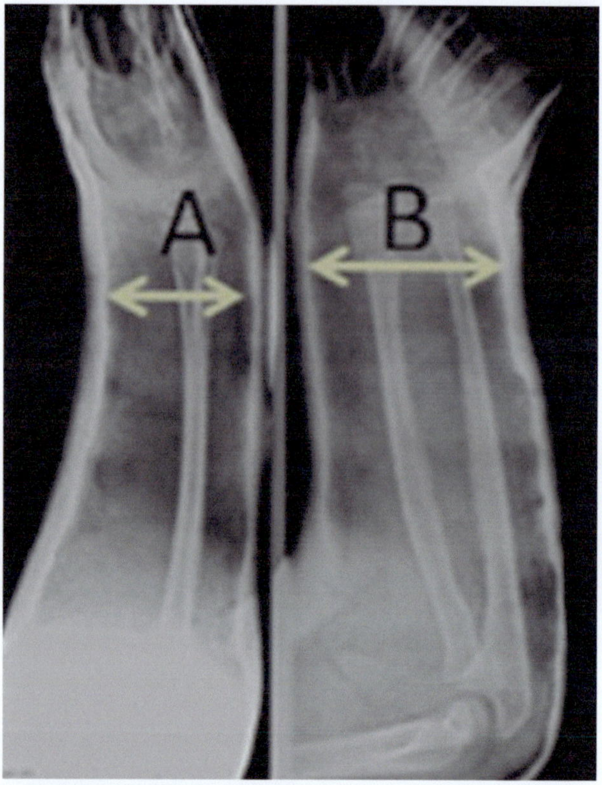

Fig. 18.6 Example of measuring the "Plaster Index." A/B should ideally be <0, 7

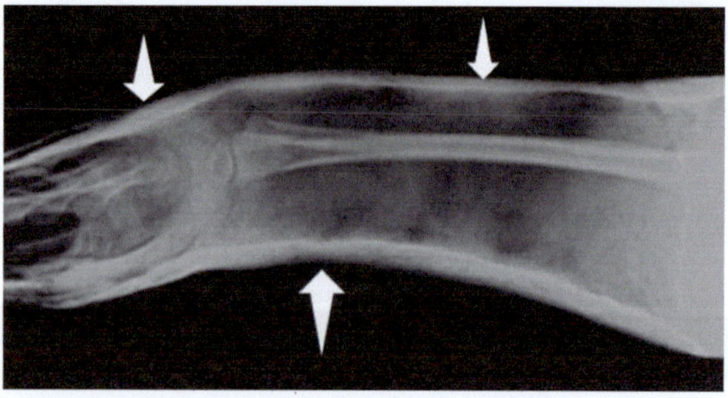

Fig. 18.7 Correctly molded plaster cast, with 3-points support, well positioned

palmar, with a dorsal force vector (Fig. 18.7). The position of the forearm within the plaster in the coronal plane has been discussed, with the reasoning to avoid the deforming forces of the pronator-supinator musculature, with publications for and against this idea. Our recommendation is to use casts in non-forced pronation of the forearm in distal third fractures.

Regarding the type of cast to use, there is a disparity of criteria in the literature [9] that support different positions, whether it is a short-arm cast or a long-arm cast. Our recommendation is to use initially a long-arm cast that blocks the deforming forces of pronosupination of the elbow musculature and reduces the risk of loss of reduction. This cast is maintained for 3–4 weeks, until sufficient callus has formed to maintain the reduction. After this period, a molded short-arm cast is installed, until the fracture healing is achieved, clinically and radiologically, which usually occurs in another 3–4 weeks. On the other hand, there are studies that show that non-conventional plasters, made of fiberglass or other synthetic materials, more resistant and durable, can be used from the beginning of the treatment, achieving sufficient immobilization to maintain the reductions within them [9].

Conservative treatment includes appropriate clinical and radiological control. Based on the time when the greatest amount of displacement of fractures previously subjected to a closed reduction and casting occurs, it is recommended that the first control be between 7 and 10 days [10]. If there has been a displacement of the reduction within the cast, and/or loss of its molding, we must correct this situation in this early control. The options are the installation of a new cast or performing a wedge on the cast. This consists of partially opening the cast at the fracture site (no more than 50% of the diameter), and placing a solid wedge of variable width, which when interposed between the ends of the open cast, separates it, modifying the axis of the bone in the desired direction [11]. This requires the presence of a soft bone callus and is performed with the patient awake, so it can generate pain. For this reason, some specialists do not recommend it, and it should be reserved for specific cases. In cases of anesthetizing the patient, a new plaster with the appropriate molding should be installed.

Undoubtedly, conservative treatment is the most common indication for treating fractures of the distal third of the forearm in the pediatric patients, and this is due to several factors: (1) the proximity of the fracture to the distal physis of the radius, which contributes the highest percentage of the longitudinal growth of this bone and leads to a great potential for remodeling of residual angular coronal and sagittal deformities; (2) the presence of a thick periosteum which favors remodeling, to a greater degree the more remaining growth the patient has and which also helps in the stabilization of the fracture; (3) residual deformities usually orient themselves in the plane of movement of the wrist joint, which favors remodeling and allows some non-anatomical reductions that at the end of growth will not have functional consequences of clinical significance; and (4) the biological characteristics of the immature skeleton that favor a rapid healing of fractures, reducing the possibility of joint stiffness due to prolonged immobilization.

The indication for surgical treatment for distal radius fractures is scarce, being more frequent in patients close to the end of growth. The recommended indications are as follows:

1. Fractures with articular involvement of the distal radius with greater than 2 mm articular steps or gap, which if consolidated in that position will lead to future joint degeneration, with the consequent arthritis. For this reason, we recommend the open anatomical reduction of the articular fracture line that allows us to ensure adequate congruence of the cartilage surface, and the stabilization of this with an osteosynthesis suitable for the size of the fragment: Kirschner wires,

interfragmentary screws (compression or situation), and occasionally plates. It is also possible to perform a closed reduction and percutaneous stabilization with arthroscopic assistance or the support of arthrography, which allows us to confirm the achievement of our objective.
2. The exposure in an open fracture requires performing an adequate surgical debridement and complementary antibiotic treatment. The method of stabilization will depend on the overall condition of the patient and of the fracture pattern, it can be with cast or with osteosynthesis.
3. Very unstable metaphyseal fractures or impossible to reduce due to interposition of soft tissues (periosteum or muscle). In these cases, reduction and percutaneous fixation can be performed with minimal osteosynthesis (Kirschner wires), or the opening of the fracture, release of the interposed tissues, reduction, and stabilization.
4. Failure in conservative treatment, understanding as such, the angulation and/or displacement during treatment with a cast of a magnitude not tolerable for adequate function in a skeleton close to the end of growth, with little capacity for remodeling [7].

18.6 Complications

The treatment of a fracture with casts has difficulties and complications, many of which will be generated by an inadequate position of the cast and lack of patient follow-up. The cast should be adjusted and molded to the shape of the forearm to not lose the achieved reduction, but it should not compress the limb, keeping in mind to install sufficient padding to protect the bony prominences and reduce the friction of the cast with the skin. However, excessive padding that prevents adequate molding increases the risk of displacement of fractures within the cast, which is variably described in the literature [12–15]. This may incline the surgeon to perform surgical treatment as a first choice to avoid this complication, generating unnecessary risks and costs.

The pressure of the cast on the limb should always be monitored, throughout the duration of the treatment, and especially during the first 24 h. If there is an increase in edema at the distal level, of the fingers, or an increase in pain or analgesic requirements by the patient, the cast must be fully opened, even when we run the risk of losing the fracture reduction. This is in order to avoid a compartment syndrome, a major complication, with catastrophic consequences.

The positioning of the plaster bandages when passing through the folds, especially in the first interdigital space, on the base of the thumb, must be careful, avoiding compression that will generate more edema. This can also cause friction wounds. For this reason, some authors propose including the thumb in all casts to avoid this problem. At the elbow fold, it is important to make a plaster bridge to avoid anterior compression by bandage passage, the risk of wounds, and/or compartment syndrome.

Another complication of conservative treatment are skin wounds from the insertion of various elements that patients use to scratch the itch they feel in the area under the cast like pencils, skewers, and toothpicks. To avoid this, it is essential to educate the adults responsible of the minor, explaining that this complication can lead to even more complex problems than the bone injury (Fig. 18.8).

When it has been necessary to use some osteosynthesis, this can also generate complications such as granulomas and infection at the entry point of percutaneous Kirschner wires. This is common, with the consequent loosening of the bone tissue, and the risk of losing the fracture reduction.

There can be complications resulting from the energy that caused the fracture, regardless of the treatment used, and that damages the physis of the radius or ulna. This causes early physeal closures and/or physeal bars, which will generate alterations of the axis and/or length of the segment. This will be more evident as the patient grows, with the associated functional alterations, so it is recommended to follow up for at least 2 years in the high-risk fractures. This physeal damage can also occur iatrogenically, by the fixation method used or by the multiple drilling through the physis during the installation of Kirschner wires. There can also be growth plate damage due to forced manipulation of fractures with physeal

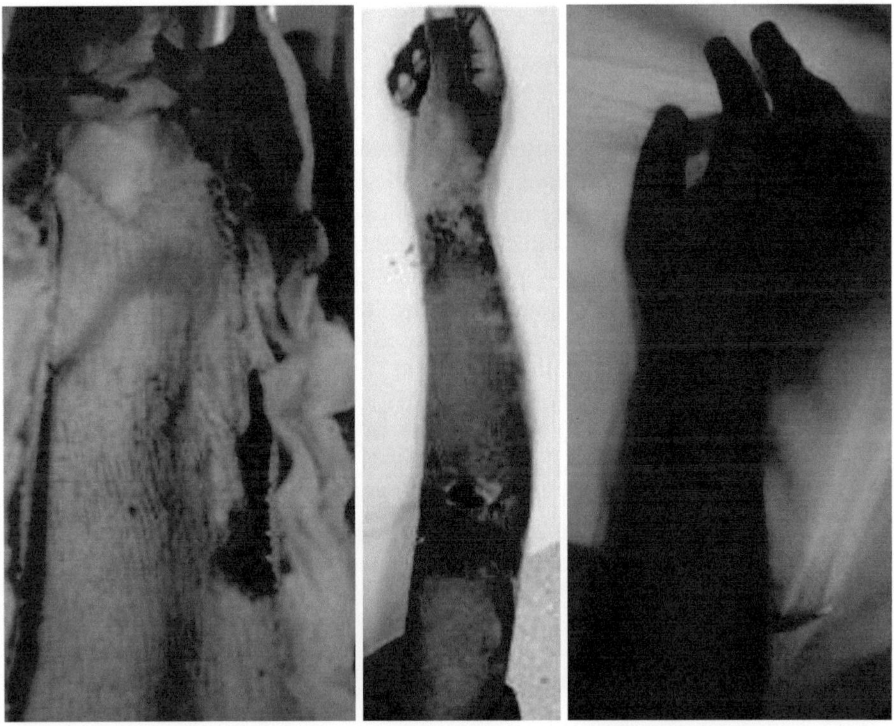

Fig. 18.8 Cases of complications due to foreign bodies (for example, lid of a pencil) inside the cast, causing significant injuries

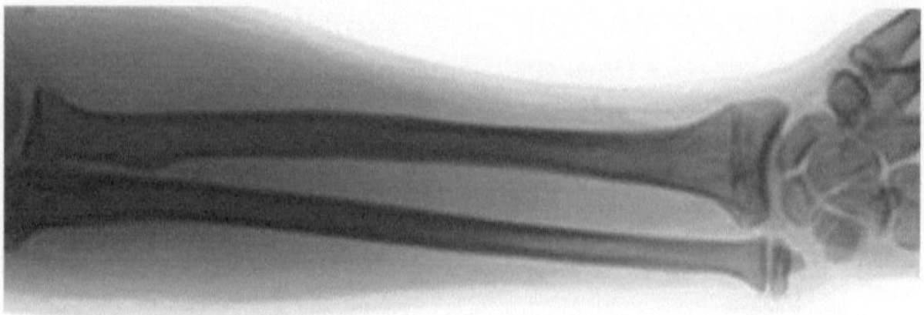

Fig. 18.9 Patient with distal radius fracture presenting physeal closure, after a closed reduction performed 10 days after the injury

involvement of late diagnosis, so it is recommended to avoid manipulation in fractures of physeal involvement after 7–10 days of the injury (Fig. 18.9).

Finally, there can be problems with bone healing such as mal-union, secondary to displacement of the reduced fracture or incomplete remodeling at the end of growth. Depending on the magnitude of the angulation or displacement, it will lead to a functional alteration, which may be unacceptable and will require reconstructive surgery. Much less common, but of greater complexity in its treatment, is the non-union, which is usually associated with bone tissue pathologies, such as neurofibromatosis.

18.7 Final Message

Forearm fractures are very common in pediatric patients, with distal third fractures being the majority. The usual mechanism of injury is indirect, with wrist support in hyperextension. There can be incomplete fractures for conservative treatment, with forearm immobilizations for 1 month, or complete fractures with or without physeal injury. If there is displacement or initial axis alteration not tolerable, painless reduction maneuvers and proper stabilization should be performed. This is achieved in most cases with a long-arm cast, molded with 3-points support, and with strict follow-up. Occasionally, surgical stabilization methods will be required, usually minimal osteosynthesis is associated with a closed reduction. The open reduction is reserved for those fractures with articular injury of the distal radius or in the impossibility of an adequate reduction and/or conservative stabilization. Whatever the treatment to be used, we must be alert to avoid complications, or to detect them early for their proper management.

Do not forget that the treatment of choice for distal third forearm fractures is conservative, and that the cast is a very good stabilizer for most of these injuries, but it requires time and patience for proper posture and control.

18.8 Authors' Recommendations

1. Relate the injury mechanism to the fracture pattern.
2. Always consider the possibility of conservative treatment as the first option.

3. The appropriate reduction maneuver will be according to the fracture mechanism.
4. Cast technique: patience and time. Practice it.
5. Always provide information to parents about complications and cast care.
6. Perform strict control before 10 days in the case of conservative treatment.

References

1. Lempesis V, Jerrhag D, Rosengren BE, Landin L, Tiderius CJ, Karlsson MK. Pediatric distal forearm fracture epidemiology in Malmö, Sweden-time trends during six decades. J Wrist Surg. 2019;8(6):463–9. https://doi.org/10.1055/s-0039-1692471.
2. Acree JS, Schlechter J, Buzin S. Cost analysis and performance in distal pediatric forearm fractures: is a short-arm cast superior to a sugar-tong splint? J Pediatr Orthop B. 2017;26(5):424–8. https://doi.org/10.1097/BPB.0000000000000382.
3. Ravier D, Morelli I, Buscarino V, Mattiuz C, Sconfienza LM, Spreafico AA, et al. Plaster cast treatment for distal forearm fractures in children: which index best predicts the loss of reduction? J Pediatr Orthop B. 2020;29(2):179–86. https://doi.org/10.1097/BPB.0000000000000678.
4. Naranje SM, Erali RA, Warner WC Jr, Sawyer JR, Kelly DM. Epidemiology of pediatric fractures presenting to emergency departments in the United States. J Pediatr Orthop. 2016;36(4):e45–8. https://doi.org/10.1097/BPO.0000000000000595.
5. van Delft EAK, Vermeulen J, Schep NWL, van Stralen KJ, van der Bij GJ. Prevention of secondary displacement and reoperation of distal metaphyseal forearm fractures in children. J Clin Orthop Trauma. 2020;11(Suppl 5):S817–22. https://doi.org/10.1016/j.jcot.2020.07.016.
6. LaStayo PC, Lee MJ. The forearm complex: anatomy, biomechanics and clinical considerations. J Hand Ther. 2006;19(2):137–44. https://doi.org/10.1197/j.jht.2006.02.002.
7. Noonan KJ, Price CT. Forearm and distal radius fractures in children. J Am Acad Orthop Surg. 1998;6(3):146–56. https://doi.org/10.5435/00124635-199805000-00002.
8. Chia B, Kozin SH, Herman MJ, Safier S, Abzug JM. Complications of pediatric distal radius and forearm fractures. Instr Course Lect. 2015;64:499–507.
9. Seiler M, Heinz P, Callegari A, Dreher T, Staubli G, Aufdenblatten C. Short and long-arm fiberglass cast immobilization for displaced distal forearm fractures in children: a randomized controlled trial. Int Orthop. 2021;45(3):759–68. https://doi.org/10.1007/s00264-020-04800-w.
10. Bowman EN, Mehlman CT, Lindsell CJ, Tamai J. Nonoperative treatment of both-bone forearm shaft fractures in children: predictors of early radiographic failure. J Pediatr Orthop. 2011;31(1):23–32. https://doi.org/10.1097/BPO.0b013e318203205b.
11. Samora JB, Klingele KE, Beebe AC, Kean JR, Klamar J, Beran MC, et al. Is there still a place for cast wedging in pediatric forearm fractures? J Pediatr Orthop. 2014;34(3):246–52. https://doi.org/10.1097/BPO.0000000000000091.
12. Laaksonen T, Puhakka J, Stenroos A, Kosola J, Ahonen M, Nietosvaara Y. Cast immobilization in bayonet position versus reduction and pin fixation of overriding distal metaphyseal radius fractures in children under ten years of age: a case control study. J Child Orthop. 2021;15(1):63–9. https://doi.org/10.1302/1863-2548.15.200171.
13. Syurahbil AH, Munajat I, Mohd EF, Hadizie D, Salim AA. Displaced physeal and metaphyseal fractures of distal radius in children. Can wire fixation achieve better outcome at skeletal maturity than cast alone? Malays Orthop J. 2020;14(2):28–38. https://doi.org/10.5704/MOJ.2007.008.
14. Khandekar S, Tolessa E, Jones S. Displaced distal end radius fractures in children treated with Kirschner wires—a systematic review. Acta Orthop Belg. 2016;82(4):681–9.
15. Truong W, Howard A, Georgiadis A. Displaced distal radius fractures in children: to reduce or not to reduce? To pin or not to pin?. JPOSNA. 2020 [cited 2022 Jun 4];2(2). https://www.jposna.org/ojs/index.php/jposna/article/view/77

Chapter 19
Fractures of the Phalanges of the Hands

Jorge Gamboa

Fractures of the phalanges of the pediatric hand are very common in the trauma emergency consultation. Their proper diagnosis is fundamental to avoid future sequelae. The phalanges have a significant capacity for remodeling, especially in the sagittal plane. Most of these injuries are of conservative treatment, although it is important to recognize some that, if poorly treated, can leave sequelae. It is very important to make the surgical decision at the right time to avoid complications. The method of surgical fixation should be as closed as possible, with Kirschner wires being the preferred method of osteosynthesis.

19.1 Introduction

The hand, due to its characteristics as a tool for exploration and exposure to the environment, is the main area of the body injured in the child population [1]. Children use their hands to explore the environment, with little awareness of the risks of their surroundings.

Hand fractures in the pediatric age are common, reaching an incidence of over 624/100,000 patients per year. Characteristically, a bimodal curve is observed, with a higher frequency in small patients, and another increase in incidence in the adolescent [2]. The most frequently injured hand will be the dominant one, and they are more common in men than in women, at a percentage of 66%. The most frequently injured finger is the little finger, with 52%, and the most injured phalanx is the proximal, with 67%.

The emergency trauma surgeon must be trained to evaluate the injuries, their complications and choose the least invasive treatment for each one. Due to the

J. Gamboa (✉)
Hospital San Borja Arriaran, Clínica Alemana de Santiago, Santiago, Chile

M. Sepúlveda O. (ed.), *Paediatrics Traumatology*,
https://doi.org/10.1007/978-3-031-89482-4_19

patient's pain and the parents' nervousness, it is especially difficult to perform a thorough physical examination. For this reason, it is necessary to calm the patient, in order to be able to perform the physical examination and evaluate both bone and associated soft tissue injuries.

The smaller the patient, the greater their remodeling potential will be, which plays in favor of the prognosis of the injuries. The physis will be our ally, because the greater the remaining growth, the greater the expected remodeling. On the contrary, in the injuries where there is damage to this structure, the sequelae and progression of deformities will be greater.

Deformities in the plane of movement will remodel more easily, while in rotational ones, remodeling will be very scarce (or null), so they should generally not be tolerated. Clinodactyly deformity will be the main sequel and must be avoided at all costs. It will be evident when making a fist, being able to observe the overlap of the deformed finger over the others (Fig. 19.1).

The treatments will basically be conservative, while surgical indications will be the exception.

In the adolescent, the situation changes due to the expected remodeling will be less, and fractures that are more unstable. Because of this, surgical indications increase. In these patients, we will be able to perform a more complete physical examination and evaluate the movement of the fingers actively. The injuries will be related more to the practice of sports performed with the hand such as basketball, volleyball, handball, among others. Also with falls at speed, either running or using skate, bicycle, and similar.

It is very important to note that, in both groups described, the injuries we find, their diagnosis, and their treatment will differ greatly, so it is very important to have these concepts clear when evaluating injuries and proposing a treatment.

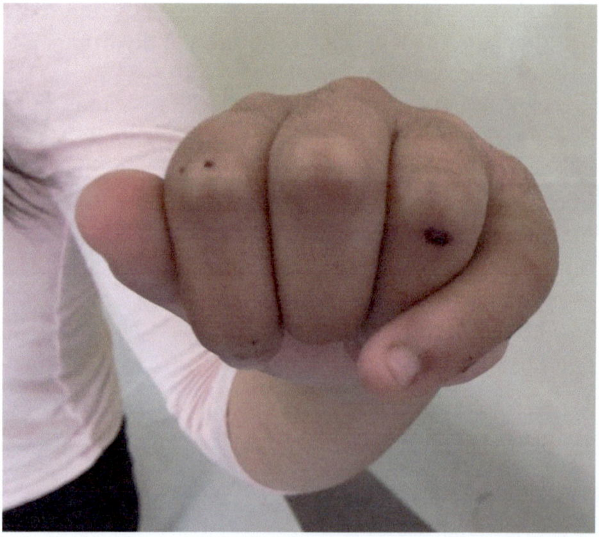

Fig. 19.1 Photograph of the hand of an 8-year-old girl, with rotation of the little finger due to a fracture of the proximal phalanx

19.2 Anatomy

The proximal and middle phalanges present a similar anatomy, and therefore fractures manifest with a similar pattern in them.

There are associated structures that act on the bone fragments, causing specific deforming forces, which must be considered for the proper management of the fracture.

The volar plate, a thin fibrous tissue that is inserted from the subcondylar area of the neck to the epiphysis of the respective phalanx, can hinder the reduction of the fracture by entrapment between the bone fragments or the joint, by rotation of the condyle (Fig. 19.2), or hyperextension of the proximal interphalangeal, as in the "swan neck" deformity.

The superficial flexor and deep flexor tendons cause deformities with flexion forces. They must be taken into account for the proper immobilization of the fingers, if conservative management is decided.

The extensor tendons, which are inserted at the level of the epiphysis of the middle and distal phalanx, produce deforming forces in extension.

The periosteum helps to maintain the stability of fractures, especially diaphyseal, preventing further displacement. It can hinder the reduction in very displaced fractures, especially of the base of the proximal phalanx or diaphyseal.

The physis in the fingers, excluding the thumb, is located at the base of the phalanges [3]. This is a weak point of the phalanx; therefore, a large percentage of

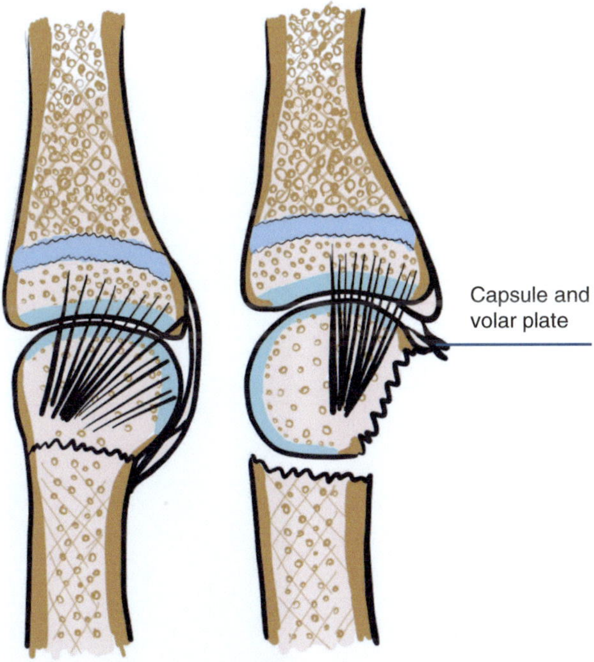

Fig. 19.2 Rotation of the distal fragment in a subcapital fracture of a phalanx, trapping the capsule and volar plate in the joint

fractures will involve this structure. They present in various ways, according to the Salter-Harris classification. Its injury can leave different types of deformities or shortening as a sequel, depending on whether its involvement is partial or total.

19.3 Mechanism of Injury

There are different forces that act on the phalanges to generate the varied patterns of fractures. In practice, these forces do not act individually but combined.

Torsional forces will cause fractures mainly at the level of the diaphyses, resulting in oblique features. They are observed when the patient's finger is trapped in a position and the hand rotates on it, or when the finger is rotated on the hand. They can also act at the level of the neck of the phalanges, causing its fracture.

The axial compression force causes a classical fracture pattern at the level of the condyles (Fig. 19.3), usually with articular cartilage involvement. It is seen in the practice of sports such as volleyball or basketball, where the ball impacts the finger in extension. When it receives this force associated with a lateral vector, an intra-articular epicondylar feature tends to occur. In older patients, fractures with articular crushing can occur.

Lateral forces, a situation where one of the fingers moves to one side as the hand advances in speed, cause its hyperabduction. This force mainly creates a fracture at the base of the phalanx, especially the proximal one (Fig. 19.4). One of the most frequent fractures is that of the base of the little finger, although it can also be seen in the other fingers that are less exposed.

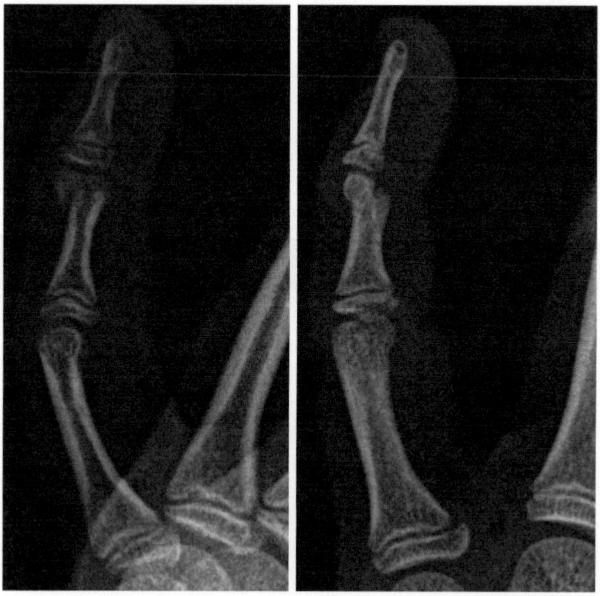

Fig. 19.3 Fracture of condyles of the middle phalanx of the little finger, of a 7-year-old girl

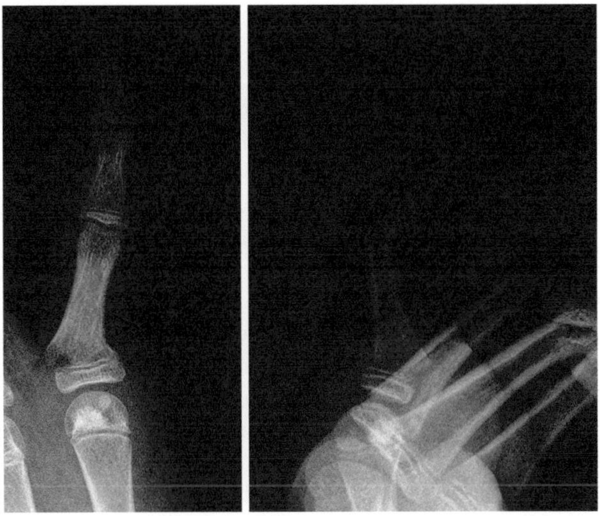

Fig. 19.4 Salter-Harris type 2 fracture of the proximal phalanx of the little finger in the hand of a 9-year-old child

Finally, injuries can be the result of a direct blow. In this case, the force will be exerted, either by an object (hockey stick, hammer, etc.), or by the fall of a heavy structure on the finger. The injuries will be of various kinds, according to the level of trauma, being able to cause comminution at the level of the fracture and/or significant injury to the soft tissues. Also in case of great trauma, it can permanently injure the physis, as in the case of a Salter-Harris type 5 fracture.

19.4 Diagnosis

To make an adequate diagnosis, various considerations must be done. One of the most important is the caracteristic of the accident, which will give us an idea of the degree of injury we can find.

The mechanism of the injury will inform us if it was produced with an object, sports practice, or direct blow.

The time from injury is very important, as if it takes a few days, it will present less pain and local swelling than in the case of being acute. Upon physical examination, we will find local swelling, pain, and bruising, which are the most common signs. In the case of deformity and significant functional impotence, it should make us think that there is a displaced fracture.

Among the imaging tests, an X-ray will be the most requested, often the only one necessary to make an accurate diagnosis. Other complementary diagnostic methods, such as computed tomography (CT-scan), ultrasound, or magnetic resonance imaging (MRI), will help us evaluate associated injuries.

The X-ray of the hand is the main diagnostic tool in hand fractures in the pediatric patient [4]. Many times its interpretation is a challenge. It is important to emphasize that when evaluating a suspected fracture of a finger, the radiograph should be of that segment, and not of the entire hand. In the case that the anteroposterior and lateral projections do not adequately show the feature or displacement, they can be complemented with oblique projections (Fig. 19.5). It is very important that the lateral radiograph should be strict, as this projection is fundamental to evaluate the rotation of the fragments.

The use of computed tomography (CT-scan) is limited in the child population, given its significant level of radiation. Its use is reserved, basically, to evaluate fractures with articular compromise in which it is necessary to visualize the displacement or degree of comminution.

Hand ultrasound is a highly operator-dependent examination and is requested to evaluate associated injuries. In the case of avulsive fractures, it provides us with information about the ligamentous or tendinous insertion. It also gives us information about the rupture of the volar plate, in hyperextension interphalangeal injuries.

Finally, magnetic resonance imaging (MRI) is only required when we want to rule out associated injuries or complications, such as post-traumatic avascular necrosis, its use being exceptional.

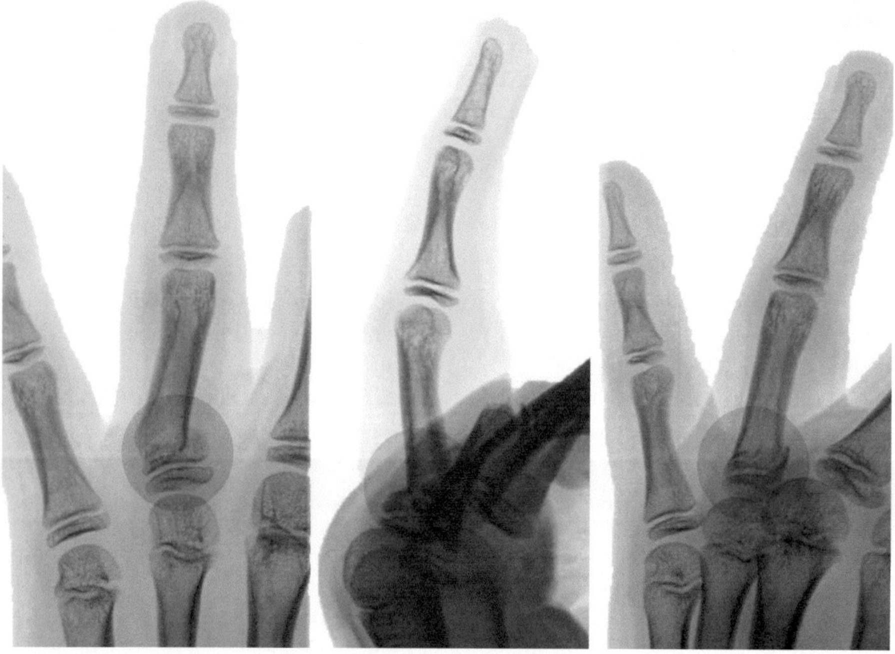

Fig. 19.5 Anteroposterior, lateral and oblique X-ray projections of the finger ring of an 8-year-old boy, with a fracture of the proximal phalanx

19.5 Treatment

19.5.1 Unicondylar Phalangeal Fractures

These fractures occur by a mechanism of axial and angular force on the head of the phalanx. A shearing feature will produce the proximal and volar displacement of the condyle [5]. In the lateral X-ray, a double shadow image will be observed, due to the described displacement (Fig. 19.6).

An articular step will occur, which is very poorly tolerated, should not exceed >0.5 mm. One of the most feared complications of this type of fracture is clinodactyly. This deformity is produced by the lateral inclination of the joint, when a single condyle is displaced. The patient should be examined by flexing the fingers and observing the angular inclination of the affected one, which will mount on the adjacent one. It is very important to compare the contralateral side, because some patients present a functional deformity of their fingers, especially in the ring finger.

If the patient presents >0.5 mm, or if rotation is observed, it should be reduced. The maneuver is performed with local anesthesia, moving the condyle to its original position, and it is immobilized with a digital splint. It is very important not to solidify with the adjacent one, since in this position it is very difficult to observe the obtained alignment. The reduction is evaluated with a control X-ray. If it is satisfactory, it should be checked weekly, for 2 weeks. If there is displacement in the weekly

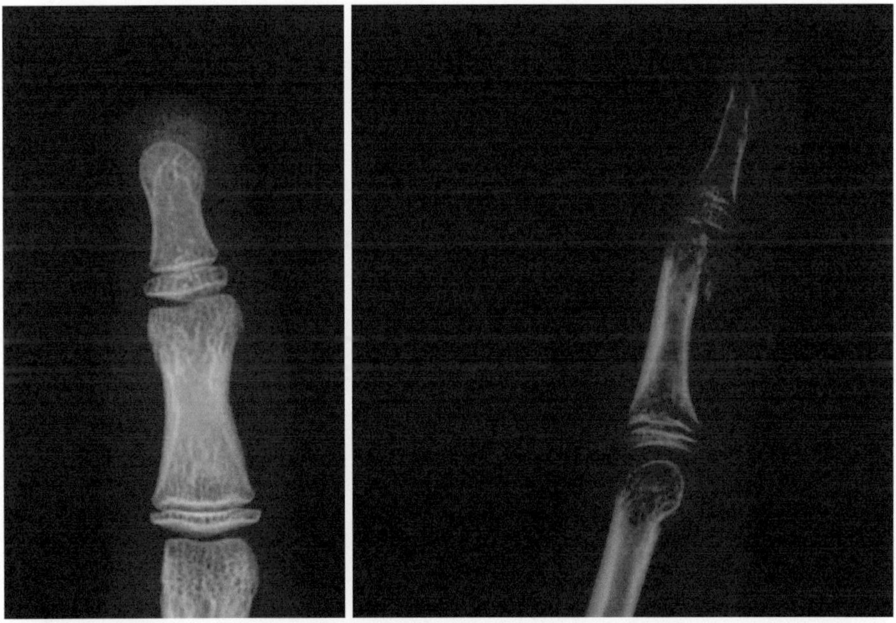

Fig. 19.6 Unicondylar fracture of the middle phalanx of the index finger. The lateral X-ray view shows a double contour image that demonstrates the displacement of the distal fragment

control, it is cataloged as unstable and must be stabilized with osteosynthesis in the operating room.

The recommended fixation method in pediatric patients is through 1 or 2 percutaneous Kirschner wires of 0.8–1 mm, depending on the size of the phalanx. The configuration of the wires prior to their insertion should be evaluated, avoiding repeated passage at the articular level [3]. These are inserted parallel or divergent, depending on the fracture line. Once the stable fixation of the fracture is verified, it is immobilized for 3–4 weeks, depending on the age of the patient. It should be checked for 2 weeks, to observe complications such as infection and/or loss of reduction. The use of mini fragment screws, in an open or ideally percutaneous manner, is an alternative in adolescents (Fig. 19.7). It allows for early mobility of the fracture in higher demand patients.

19.5.2 Subcapital Fractures of Phalanges

In this area of the phalanx, an anatomical weakness is presented, so they are common in the child population [6]. Their classification can be seen in Fig. 19.8. The mechanisms of production are entrapment in doors, that is usually observed in small

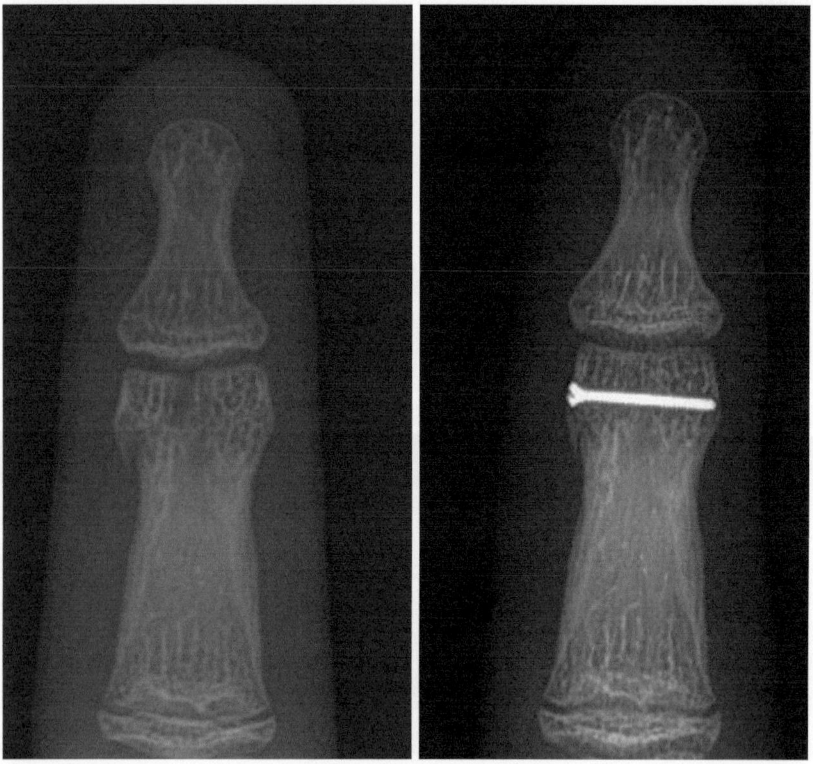

Fig. 19.7 Unicondylar fracture of the middle phalanx, with open reduction and stabilized with a compression screw

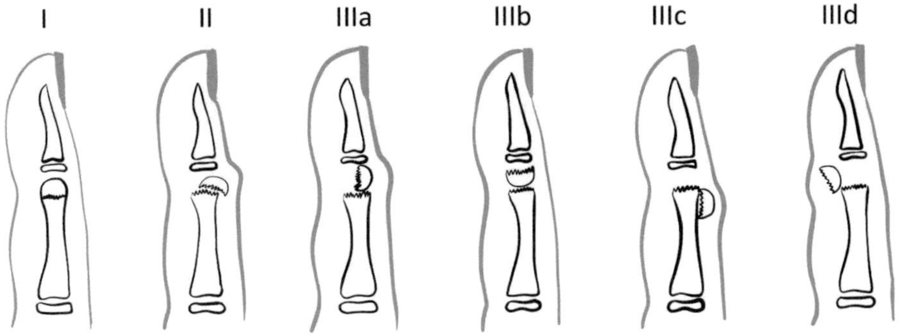

Fig. 19.8 Classification of subcapital phalanx fractures. Type I, no displaced; Type II, displaced with cortical contact; and Type III, displacement without cortical contact

children. Another common mechanism is the forced rotation of the finger when turning the hand with it fixed. Due to the small size of the distal fragment and the insertion of the collateral ligaments, they are always considered unstable.

In the radiological evaluation, the displacement of the fracture will be seen, especially in the lateral radiograph, where the rotation of the fragment can be observed. Characteristically, a double shadow image is seen when one condyle is projected over the other. Evaluating this displacement is very important because a rotation at this level will cause a clinical mal rotation with functional compromise when making a fist (Fig. 19.1).

Displaced fractures, especially rotated ones, should be reduced with local anesthesia. Once reduced, an X-ray should be taken of the affected finger, avoiding fixing it to the adjacent finger, to evaluate the rotation in the lateral radiograph. The finger is immobilized and radiographically controlled for 2 weeks. Complete immobilization for 4 weeks before starting progressive movement. If it cannot be reduced or loses the reduction in the controls, it must be reduced in the operating room and fixed with crossed percutaneous wires (Fig. 19.9). An important point is that the surgical decision should be made before 2 weeks, due to the rapid fracture healing, which will make it difficult to reduce it in a closed manner and avoid open reduction which can cause avascular necrosis or injury to the collateral ligaments.

19.5.3 Bicondylar Fractures of Phalanges

This fracture involves both condyles and is mainly produced by an axial force on the distal end of the phalanx. In small children, they are very infrequent. They usually occur in adolescents, and due to their joint involvement, they can leave sequelae. The displaced ones are very difficult to immobilize due to their high instability. They must be anatomically reduced, which in most cases will need to be done in the operating room. They can be reduced in a closed manner and fixed with percutaneous Kirschner wires. In case of needing an open reduction, they can also be fixed

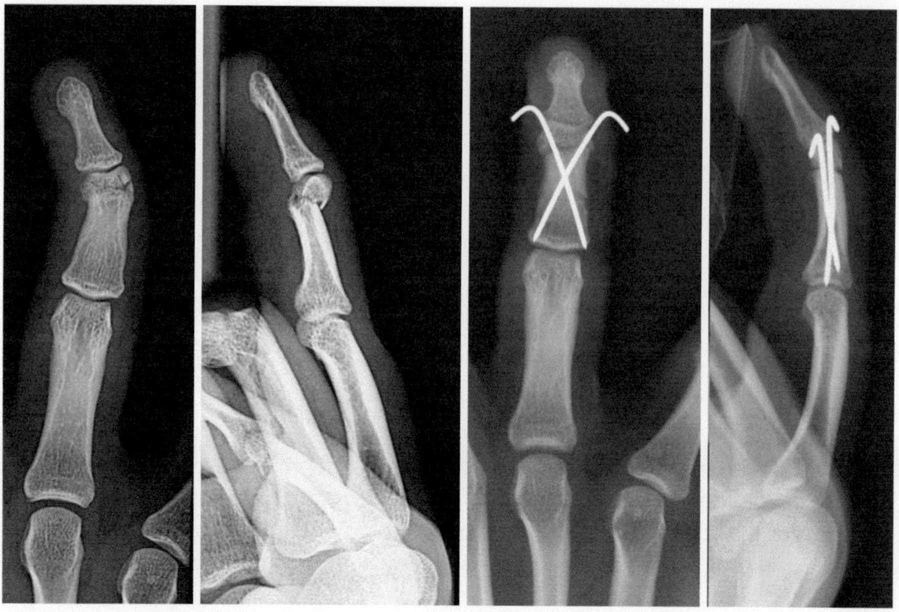

Fig. 19.9 Subcapital fracture of the middle phalanx of the index finger of a14-year-old girl, resolved with closed reduction and fixation with Kirschner wires

with wires or screws. In fractures that present comminution, with a difficult fixation, a dynamic traction device can be used.

19.5.4 Comminuted Fractures of Phalanges

Comminuted fractures are rare in the child population, due to the characteristics of immature bone tissue. The treatment alternatives should be very well considered, since a surgical procedure can add more damage. Many times it is better to wait for bone consolidation and perform an alignment osteotomy later. The potential for remodeling, either angular or of the joint surface, is often sufficient to leave no functional sequelae.

19.5.5 Diaphyseal Fractures of Phalanges

In younger children, they are associated with mechanisms of direct contusion, such as entrapment in doors or a blow with a blunt object. In this situation, transverse or short oblique fractures younger will occur, with significant local swelling and pain.

Due to the existence of the periosteum, in most cases they are stable and can be managed in a conservative manner, either with immobilization alone, or with reduction and subsequent control.

Fractures located in the diaphysis of the middle and proximal phalanx primarily occur in adolescents. The mechanism is the forced twisting of the finger, which is observed in adolescents associated with sports or accidents. Due to its mechanism, it will lead to oblique and spiral fractures [7]. These fractures are characteristically unstable, and while they can be reduced in a closed manner in the emergency room, great care must be taken when evaluating the result and stability of immobilization. If an adequate reduction is not achieved, the instability of the fracture or the presence of some interposed tissue must be considered. In these cases, or if we observe a loss of reduction in the control, it should be reduced and fixed in the operating room. The first choice for its fixation will be percutaneous, with Kirschner wires perpendicular to the fracture line. If it cannot be reduced in a closed manner, it should be opened and fixed with Kirschner wires or screws (Fig. 19.10).

Another common fracture is that of the base of the diaphysis. Its production mechanism is the hyperabduction of the finger in the coronal plane. The fracture will be observed on the frontal X-ray, and if it is displaced, reduction can be performed with local anesthesia and splinting. This easy-to-perform procedure will usually be sufficient, with rare occasions where it will need to be reduced in the operating room, usually due to the interposition of soft tissues.

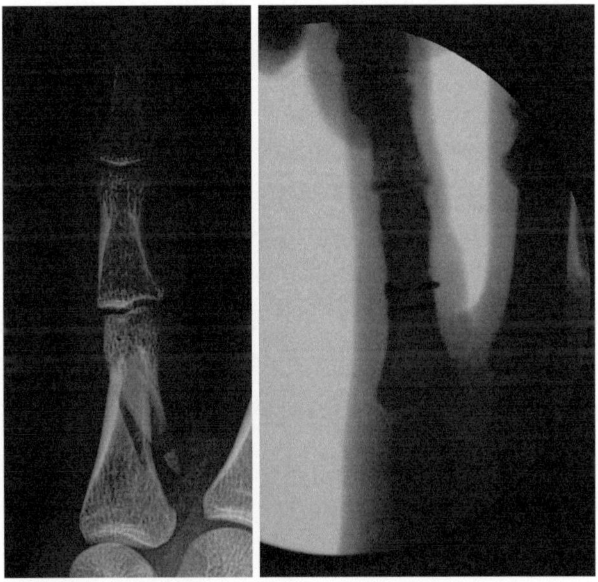

Fig. 19.10 Spiroid fracture of the proximal phalanx of the index finger, stabilized with 2 screws with interfragmentary compression

19.5.6 Fractures of the Base of the Middle and Proximal Phalanges

The production mechanism of a fracture at the base of the proximal phalanx is by an axial and lateral compressive force, on the head of the metacarpal [8]. This fracture is mainly observed in the adolescent population, and in the case of fragments with >25% displacement, surgical treatment is recommended. It is possible to attempt a percutaneous reduction with Kirschner wires, but if it is done openly, it is preferable to use mini fragment screws.

The base fractures in the middle phalanx occur by different mechanisms. The fracture on the palmar face is produced by hyperextension, pulling the insertion of the volar plate on the epiphysis of the base of the phalanx. Its treatment is conservative, using a digital splint for a week, followed by a solidarity bandage for 2 weeks. This allows early movement, reducing the residual stiffness of these injuries.

The fracture on the dorsal face is produced by avulsion of the central band of the extensor (Fig. 19.11). This injury can be evaluated with the Elson test. The finger to be examined is flexed at the level of the proximal interphalangeal joint at the right angle of the edge of a table, and this position is firmly held. The patient is asked to try to extend the proximal interphalangeal joint. The extensor pressure perceived by the examiner is exerted by the central band, while the distal interphalangeal joint remains without hyperextension. If it is injured, it requires repair.

Another mechanism observed at this level are fractures associated with dislocations, which can produce palmar or dorsal fragments, depending on the direction of the dislocation (Fig. 19.12). In the case that they are displaced, the percentage of the

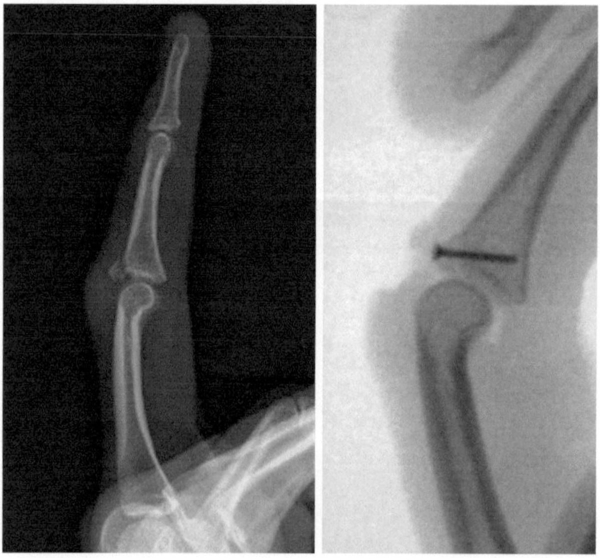

Fig. 19.11 Dorsal avulsive fracture of the base of the middle phalanx. Requires open reduction and screw fixation

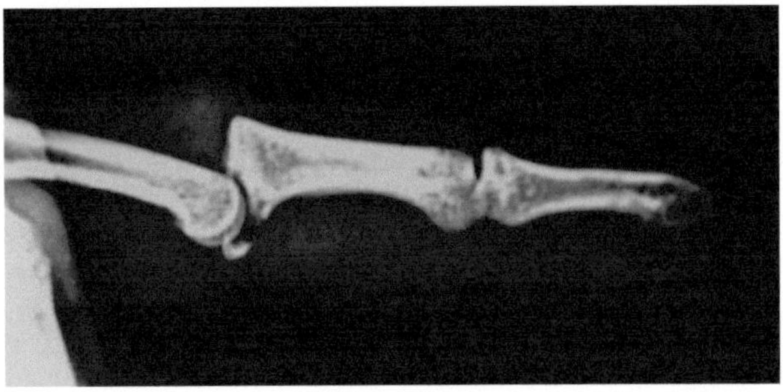

Fig. 19.12 Fracture of the base of the middle phalanx, avulsive due to extension

articular cartilage surface compromise must be evaluated. If this percentage is >25–30%, if it is associated with an articular step, or if subluxation is observed, a reduction maneuver will be required. This should be performed in the operating room and preferably in a closed manner. If this is not possible, it will be done openly, taking care not to injure the soft parts around the joint.

19.6 Complications

Phalange fractures in the pediatric population have a good prognosis, and the vast majority are conservatively treated. It is very important to know how to diagnose those injuries that will leave sequelae if we do not treat them properly [4].

Among the complications that we can find is the mal union, which occurs due to late consultation or lack of adequate weekly control of the patient in treatment, which must be monitored during the first 2 weeks after surgery or closed reduction of the fracture.

Another complication that we can see is avascular necrosis of the distal fragment, which is caused by an inadequate approach to the fracture, excessive periosteal stripping, or late intervention (after 2 weeks) in an open manner [9].

References

1. Vadivelu R, Dias JJ, Burke FD, Stanton J. Hand injuries in children: a prospective study. J Pediatr Orthop. 2006;26(1):29–35. https://doi.org/10.1097/01.bpo.0000189970.37037.59.
2. Nellans KW, Chung KC. Pediatric hand fractures. Hand Clin. 2013;29(4):569–78. https://doi.org/10.1016/j.hcl.2013.08.009.
3. Sivit AP, Dupont EP, Sivit CJ. Pediatric hand injuries: essentials you need to know. Emerg Radiol. 2014;21(2):197–206. https://doi.org/10.1007/s10140-013-1158-0.
4. Goodell PB, Bauer A. Problematic pediatric hand and wrist fractures. JBJS Rev. 2016;4(5):e1. https://doi.org/10.2106/JBJS.RVW.O.00028.
5. Karl JW, White NJ, Strauch RJ. Percutaneous reduction and fixation of displaced phalangeal neck fractures in children. J Pediatr Orthop. 2012;32(2):156–61. https://doi.org/10.1097/BPO.0b013e3182423124.

6. Market M, Bhatt M, Agarwal A, Cheung K. Pediatric hand injuries requiring closed reduction at a tertiary pediatric care center. Hand (N Y). 2021;16(2):235–40. https://doi.org/10.1177/1558944719850635.
7. Yeh PC, Dodds SD. Pediatric hand fractures. Tech Orthop. 2009;24(3):150–62.
8. Boyer JS, London DA, Stepan JG, Goldfarb CA. Pediatric proximal phalanx fractures: outcomes and complications after the surgical treatment of displaced fractures. J Pediatr Orthop. 2015;35(3):219–23. https://doi.org/10.1097/BPO.0000000000000253.
9. Liao JCY, Chong AKS. Pediatric hand and wrist fractures. Clin Plast Surg. 2019;46(3):425–36. https://doi.org/10.1016/j.cps.2019.02.012.

Chapter 20
Fingertip Injuries

Macarena Morovic and Paulina de la Fuente

Injuries to the fingertips are among the most common found in the pediatric population and can present in various ways, from a simple laceration to a complete amputation of the segment. Without proper treatment, these injuries can leave significant sequelae, both functional and aesthetic. The treatments available today cover a wide range of techniques that help reduce these complications, so a proper recognition of the type of injury and early management are fundamental to achieving good results.

20.1 Introduction

The fingertip is a highly specialized structure that provides tactile and sensory function, which allows interaction with the environment during exploration and manipulation [1–3]. However, this capability makes it particularly prone to injuries [1], therefore being a significant cause of emergency services consultation, and if not managed properly, can leave significant functional and aesthetic sequelae.

The goals of treatment will be to preserve length, maintain sensitivity, allow early mobilization, and restore function in a timely manner with adequate aesthetic results.

M. Morovic (✉)
Hospital Base Valdivia, Clínica Alemana Valdivia, Universidad Austral de Chile, Valdivia, Chile

P. de la Fuente
Clínica Alemana, Santiago, Chile

M. Sepúlveda O. (ed.), *Paediatrics Traumatology*,
https://doi.org/10.1007/978-3-031-89482-4_20

20.2 Epidemiology

These injuries are the most common of the hand, accounting for approximately 2/3 of all hand injuries in pediatric patients [3, 4].

In countries like the United States, approximately 700,000 pediatric patients are treated each year just for fingertip injuries related to door traumas, and children under 5 years old, especially boys, have the highest annual rate of finger amputations (18.8/100,000 inhabitants) [3].

20.3 Pathophysiology

The mechanisms of injury are diverse; however, most of these occur within the home. The most common are [2] as follows:

- Crushing injuries due to compression forces. Correspond to the most common type of injury in children, generally caused by the abrupt closing of doors and/or windows on the finger [2, 5]. These can present as a closed or open injury, associated or not with distal phalanx fractures.
- Laceration injuries, generally secondary to a household instrument (knife, scissors, cans) or work tools (saw).
- Avulsion injuries that occur when the nail plate separates from the surrounding structures, leaving the nail bed exposed.
- Amputations, which involve both the loss of soft tissues and the partial or complete loss of the distal phalanx.
- Flexion/extension forces lead to avulsion injuries of the distal tendon.

It is important to mention that most of these injuries are preventable, so it is essential to raise awareness among the population and take measures to reduce them.

Since the main injury mechanism is crushing by abrupt closing of doors and/or windows, various devices currently available on the market can be used, which prevent the closing abrupt from these, such as a side stop on the hinge or at the top/bottom of the door (even a towel over the door is sufficient).

20.4 Anatomy

Anatomically, the fingertip is defined as the portion distal to the insertion of the deep flexor tendon and the extensor on the distal phalanx, or on the interphalangeal when we refer to the thumb [2]. It is composed of the nail complex, the pulp, and the distal phalanx.

20.4.1 The Nail Complex

The nail complex is composed of the nail plate, the nail bed, the eponychium, peronychium, and hyponychium [1] (Fig. 20.1).

The nail plate corresponds to a layer of keratin that protects the back of the fingertip. It stabilizes the distal portion of it, providing resistance to the pulp, thus contributing to the manipulation of small objects and fine touch [1, 6].

The nail bed consists of two parts: the germinal matrix and the sterile matrix. The former is responsible for the growth of 90% of the nail, while the latter contributes to its thickening and adherence. The junction between these two structures is the lunula, the visible portion of the germinal matrix [1]. The matrix has multiple longitudinal fibers that anchor the dermis to the periosteum of the distal phalanx.

The eponychium and peronychium form the proximal and lateral soft tissue edges of the nail, respectively. The hyponychium marks the transition between the adhered nail and the free one, acting as a mechanical barrier that prevents the accumulation of foreign bodies between the nail and the bed [1].

20.4.2 The Pulp

The pulp is divided into a distal portion and a proximal one (Fig. 20.2). The distal portion is related to the nail plate and is characterized by having radial osteocutaneous partitions that give it stability and resistance to deformation, thus allowing adherence (in the same way as the grooves of a tire) [6]. Together with the counter support provided by the nail plate, it achieves a fine grip when picking up small

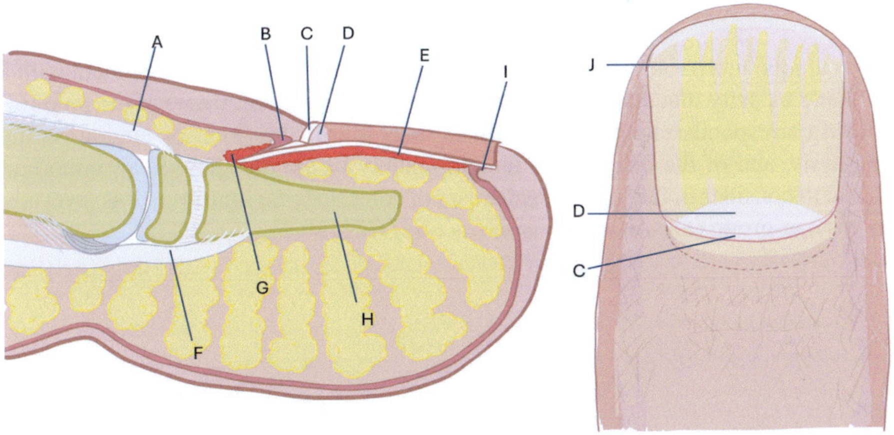

Fig. 20.1 Nail complex. (**a**) Extensor tendon; (**b**) nail fold; (**c**) eponychium; (**d**) lunula; (**e**) sterile matrix; (**f**) deep flexor tendon; (**g**) germinal matrix; (**h**) distal phalanx; (**i**) hyponychium; (**j**) nail body

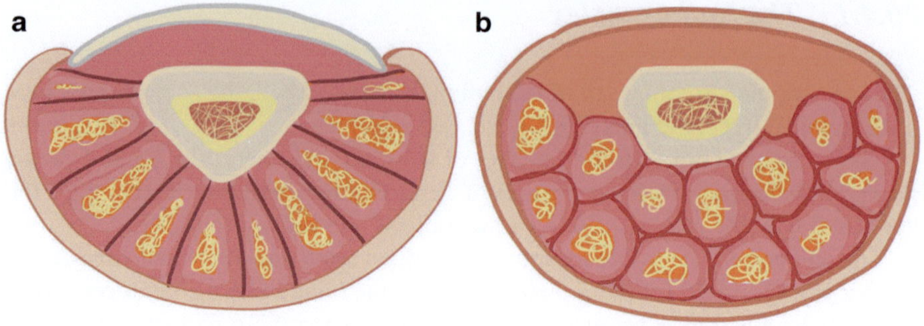

Fig. 20.2 Anatomy of the pad of a finger. (**a**) Distal pulp, with the radial osteocutaneous septums; (**b**) proximal pulp, with lobed septums

objects [1, 6]. The proximal portion, unlike the previous one, presents lobulated partitions, which gives malleability and the ability to adapt the contour when picking up larger objects [6].

The irrigation of the pulp occurs through an anastomotic arch given by the digital palmar arteries, distal to the insertion of the flexor tendon, and from where the longitudinal arteries of the pulp originate, which then anastomose with the dorsal vessels. Generally, the central artery is the largest. Venous drainage of the fingers is generally dorsal; however, distal to the distal interphalangeal joint, the venous vessels are predominantly palmar [6].

The innervation is given by the divisions of the digital palmar nerves at the level of the palmar fold of the distal interphalangeal.

20.4.3 The Distal Phalanx

It has unique morphological characteristics, presenting a diaphyseal segment with a palmar concavity that corresponds to the convexity of the soft tissue of the pulp [6]. It also corresponds to the point of distal insertion of the extensor tendon on the epiphysis, and of the deep flexor tendon, mainly in the metaphysis, an important aspect to consider in the injury mechanism of some specific injuries at this level and in this age-group (e.g., Seymour type fracture) (Fig. 20.3).

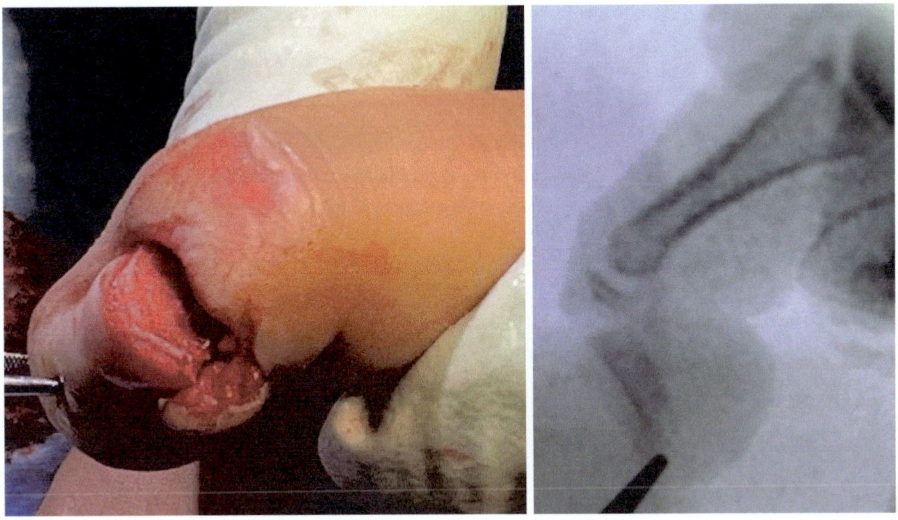

Fig. 20.3 Seymour fracture, with juxta-epiphyseal displacement of distal phalanx, bone exposure and laceration of the nail bed, product of the insertion of the extensor tendon in the epiphysis, and the flexor tendon in the metaphysis

20.5 Diagnosis

Generally, it is performed without anesthesia to accurately assess the motor and sensory function. The range of motion of the distal phalanx should be objectified, looking for a probable tendon injury, and a two-point discrimination test should be performed on both sides of the fingertip to assess sensitivity [4].

Capillary refill and finger color allow for the assessment of the vascular state, while an evident deformity may indicate a fracture or dislocation.

The size, location, and geometry of any skin coverage defect of the fingertip, the degree of nail bed involvement, and the presence or absence of exposed bone should be determined [1, 4].

The radiological study is performed with X-rays of the affected finger in three projections: anteroposterior, lateral, and oblique.

20.6 Classification

The classification of Evans and Bernardis [7], known as PBN classification (pulp, nail, bone), describes the involvement of the fingertip, nail, and bone, being the most used. It assigns an ascending numbering according to the greater involvement of each of the structures. The value 0 indicates no injury, while 7 or 8 implies total loss, for each segment (Table 20.1).

Table 20.1 Evans and Bernardis classification, describing the degree of involvement of the pulp, nail, and bone

	Pulp	Nail	Bone
0	No injury	No injury	No injury
1	Laceration	Laceration of sterile matrix	Plume
2	Flattening	Laceration of sterile matrix and germinal	Comminuted not Articular
3	Transverse distal loss	Flattening	Articular
4	Partial los dorsal oblique	Nail proximal dislocation	Displaced from the Base
5	Loss dorsal	Loss distal 1/3	Tip open fracture
6	Oblique	Loss of two- thirds	Loss distal half
7	Lateral loss	Lateral loss	Subtotal los
8		Complete loss	Complete loss

20.7 Treatment

The objectives of the treatment of fingertip injuries are to preserve and repair. For this, an attempt should be made to maintain the length, preserve the nail for an acceptable aesthetic result, and achieve a stable and painless skin coverage.

20.7.1 Subungual Hematoma, Remove and Repair or Trephine and Drain?

Subungual hematomas result from compression, crushing, or attrition injuries. Type III evidence recommends removing the nail, to explore and repair the nail bed if there is a displaced tuft fracture [8]. However, if the edges of the nail fold are intact and (if present) the fracture is not displaced, then the optimal management is controversial. Traditionally, the treatment was based on the size of the hematoma [9], being drained if it compromised more than 50% of the nail, and more than 25% if it was associated with fracture. Simple trephination of the nail plate, to drain the hematoma, with intact folds and nail margins, has produced equal or superior results, compared to the extraction of the nail and formal reconstruction of the nail bed [10, 11]. In addition, trephination or conservative management has shown similar cosmetic results and similar complication rates, regardless of the size or a non-displaced fracture.

Trephination consists of making a hole in the surface of the nail with a hypodermic needle to release the trapped blood, achieving good results in relation to pain relief, function, and cosmetics [11, 12]. Drainage ideally should be performed on the same day of the trauma.

It is not recommended to lift the nail if it is well adhered, for the exploration of the nail bed, since the longitudinal growth of it requires between 70 and 140 days.

Baden [11] postulates that after an injury, it takes approximately 3 weeks until the growth begins again, which explains the hypertrophy present within the nail in the elongation process. Then, the regeneration progresses at a faster pace during the next 2 months, with a total healing time of 4 months.

20.7.2 Traumatic Onychectomy, Should the Nail be Replaced or Discarded?

After repairing the nail bed, 96% of surgeons replace the nail plate, while 4% prefer to discard it [13]. It has been argued that nail replacement confers some advantages. Firstly, it acts as a mold to allow the growth of the new nail over normal anatomy. It also stabilizes some associated distal phalanx fractures. In addition, replacing the proximal portion of the nail plate prevents the formation of scars between the proximal nail fold and the germinal matrix, which can produce a permanently split nail. Consequently, it is recommended to stabilize the proximal nail fold with a nail plate, for 2–3 weeks.

This surgical dogma has been questioned by evidence of increased morbidity accompanying nail plate replacement. Replacing the nail plate has a higher complication rate (17.6%) than discarding the nail plate and applying a non-adherent dressing (Mepitel) (5%). These complications included postoperative infection, persistent pain, delayed wound healing, and excessive granulation. Prophylactic antibiotics would not significantly influence infection rates. The method of fixing the nail plate would cause inflammation and edema, which can be associated with laceration of the nail fold at the sites of tight sutures. However, studies suggest that nail plate replacement may not be solely responsible for complications and increased morbidity, highlighting the need for high-quality studies to establish definitive indications and management strategies.

An ongoing multicenter randomized controlled trial (Nail bed INJury Analysis [NINJA] trial) aims to determine whether the nail plate should be replaced after nail bed repair in children. A preliminary study agreed with an earlier study, which showed that nail plate replacement was associated optimizing with a higher incidence of infection, complications, and postoperative pain, but did not reach statistically significant differences, probably due to a small sample size. The definitive trial is expected to report results of greater statistical weight. Ultimately, the goal is to minimize morbidity, exposure to multiple operations, and the amount of necessary follow-ups, while optimizing outcomes.

There are two possible situations, having a recovered nail or it being lost.

If the native nail is recovered, it is suggested to wash it profusely with antiseptic solution, and reinsert it into the nail sac, fixing it with separate nylon points to the eponychium and paronychium, without sutures on the free edge of the nail.

In the case of not having the native nail, it is recommended to replace it with synthetic material, ideally the same size and thickness as the original nail. An acetate sheet or a silicone plastic sheet can be used (for example, a portion of a urine collection bag, a portion of a syringe, and a serum drop). The new substitute nail is carved, fixed with separate nylon points to the nail sac and to the eponychium and peronychium to maintain the anatomy of the lateral channels. The free edge of the substitute nail should not be fixed to the skin.

20.7.3 Nail Bed Injury, Suture or Adhesives?

Nail bed lacerations can be simple, star-shaped, or crush injuries (Fig. 20.4). The latter two often involve fragmentation of the nail plate. The success of nail bed repair decreases with the delay of the repair procedure, with intervention recommended within 2–3 days from the injury, ideally as soon as possible. The repair of star-shaped lacerations can have good results, while crush injuries have a worse prognosis due to the additional contusion of the nail bed [14]. Although examples of management protocols for these injuries have been described, the surgical technique is widely debated. Absorbable sutures are practical, as they do not they need to be removed. In a survey, hand surgeons preferred an interrupted suture technique (85.1%) using polyglactin 910 as material (Vicryl-Rapide) (83.3%) [13]. Medical adhesives are an alternative to primary repair with sutures, for nail bed injuries. 2-octyl cyanoacrylate (Dermabond) can bind broken nail plate fragments and wound margins,. Preliminary research suggested that adhesives achieved an acceptable cosmetic appearance, but were limited in their comparisons with standard suturing, the objectivity of their outcome measures, and their small sample sizes. Subsequent studies highlighted the effectiveness of Dermabond in relation to suture, such as similar breakage resistance, and a shorter average tourniquet time required. Its disadvantages are the risk of chronic infection, granuloma formation and foreign body reaction, and tissue tattooing. Therefore, the widespread adoption of its use requires a more solid evidence base. Thus, despite its advantages, surgeons prefer an eight-shaped suture (45.1%) to secure the nail plate under the nail fold, over the use of adhesives (20.7%) [13].

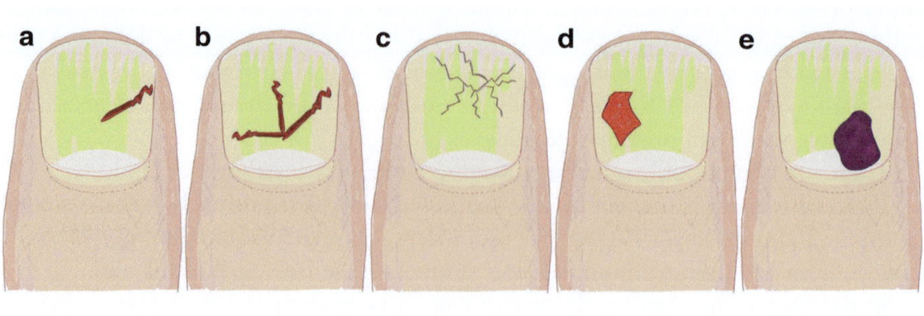

Fig. 20.4 Types of nail bed lacerations. (**a**) Simple; (**b**) starry; (**c**) crush; (**d**) avulsion; (**e**) subungual hematoma

20.7.4 Avulsion or Nail Bed Defect, Suture or Graft?

Nail bed avulsions that present with the avulsed tissue attached to the nail plate can be sutured in place. Small defects, <2 mm, heal by second intention, with the nail bed acting as a cover and a splint. A substitute introduced into the space (if it is >2 mm) can prevent scar formation, particularly for full-thickness germinal matrix injuries. Options include a dermal replacement template (Integra or Matriderm), partial thickness skin graft, partial thickness nail bed graft, and full-thickness nail bed graft. The last two are preferred, but can cause a deformity at the donor site. The graft can be taken from non-injured areas of the affected finger or from other intact fingers for larger defects. For pediatric nail bed defects of more than 3 × 3 mm, partial thickness nail bed grafts taken from the injured finger or the hallux are recommended, although objective evaluations of this are lacking.

20.7.5 Distal Phalanx Fracture, Repair and Fixation or Suture?

More than 50% of all nail bed injuries are associated with a distal phalanx fracture. Non-displaced distal tuft and distal phalanx fractures are treated with nail bed repair and nail plate replacement. Displaced fractures and fractures proximal to the nail fold are surgically stabilized using one or two 0.8 mm Kirschner wires (Fig. 20.5).

For exposed Seymour fractures, the principles of managing exposed fractures are recommended, along with antibiotics due to frequent infectious

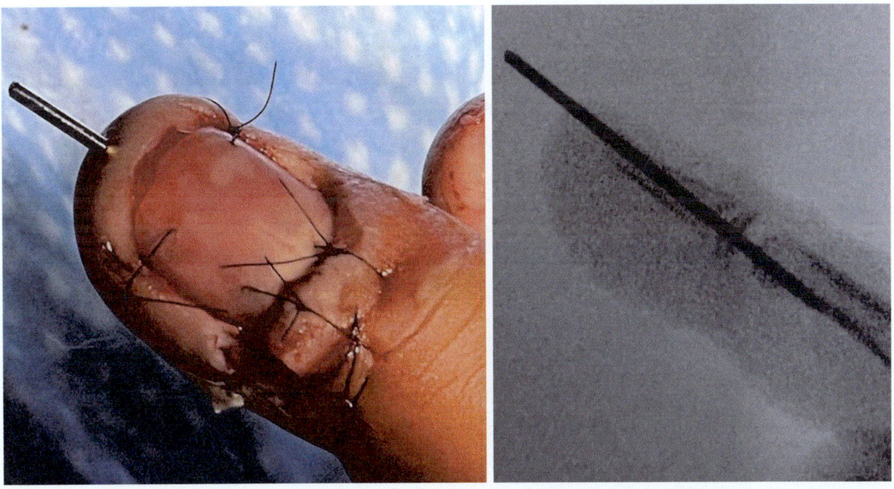

Fig. 20.5 Seymour fracture treated with surgical cleansing, reinsertion of the nail, nail fold repair, and stabilization with Kirschner wire

complications. However, for nail bed tears associated with distal phalanx fractures, the use of vertical eight-shaped sutures, with tension bands, without formal nail bed repair or fracture stabilization, is described as a simple, minimally traumatic and equally effective option. Comminuted fractures often have small bone fragments attached to the nail bed. The repair of the nail bed injury allows the approximation of these bone fragments. The replacement of the nail plate has often been used as a splint for fracture healing, although there are synthetic alternatives if the nail is not available.

20.7.6 Amputation, Conservative Treatment, Revision Amputation, Flaps, or Reimplantation?

The management of fingertip amputations depends on the level of the injury and the integrity of the remaining structures.

Conservative treatment consists of using a semi-occlusive dressing and second intention closure of the distal phalanx lesion. It can cause nail deformity (hook nail), in cases of lack of palmar tissue. It has been documented that sensitivity recovery after second intention healing is superior to other surgical methods, and two-point discrimination approximates normal after healing [13]. In pediatric patients, it is indicated in PNB P3, N0 or 5, B1 or 57 lesions.

In a significant loss of soft tissue on the palmar side, complete amputation (i.e., shortening and closure) is the simplest procedure, with the fastest recovery, in selected patients. The important thing in this procedure is the complete ablation of the nail bed, to avoid hook nail deformity, and the identification and transverse section of the digital nerves as proximal as possible to the level of amputation, to avoid the formation of a neuroma.

The reconstruction of a tissue loss may require shortening of the exposed bone, replacement of skin or nail bed, local flaps, or reimplantation. If the lesion exposes the distal phalanx, bone shortening and suturing of the remaining skin using local flaps over the distal phalanx is a standard reconstructive technique. Mobilization and advancement of the local flap is a useful option, and the selection of the flap modality is guided by the orientation and configuration of the wound.

20.7.7 Local Flaps

Atasoy flap/V-Y flap: It is a triangular palmar advancement flap, V-Y design indicated in amputations distal to the nail groove, with transverse or oblique dorsal features. One advantage is that it provides sensitivity. The use of this flap is contraindicated in patients with palmar oblique amputations and greater palmar tissue loss. The distal edge of the wound is the base of the flap; the apex of the flap should extend to the distal interphalangeal fold (Fig. 20.6). Then, an incision is made in the skin and subcutaneous tissue, including the fibrous septa that anchor the pulp tissue to the bone, and thus maintain the distal anastomotic arch of the digital arteries. The flap can be advanced up to 6 or 10 mm over the defect and is fixed with non-absorbable suture, creating a Y-shaped repair.

Kutler flap/Lateral V-Y. It is a triangular lateral advancement flap indicated in amputations distal to the nail groove, with transverse or oblique dorsal features, with greater palmar than dorsal tissue loss. It also provides sensitivity. The distal edge of the wound is the base of the flap. The apex of the flap should extend to the distal interphalangeal fold. The flap is similar to the Atasoy, except that two flaps are used with bases on the radial and ulnar sides of the wound, safeguarding the lateral digital artery (Fig. 20.7). Unlike the Atasoy flap, this can provide up to 12 mm of advancement.

Venkataswami flap: Oblique triangular flap indicated in amputations with lateral palmar bevel in triphalangeal fingers and thumb. The flap achieves an advancement of up to 2.5 times the defect, but requires careful technique (Fig. 20.8).

Fig. 20.6 Atasoy or V-Y flap scheme

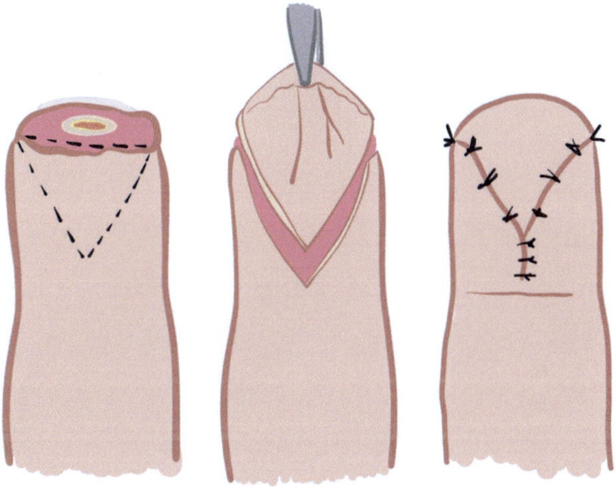

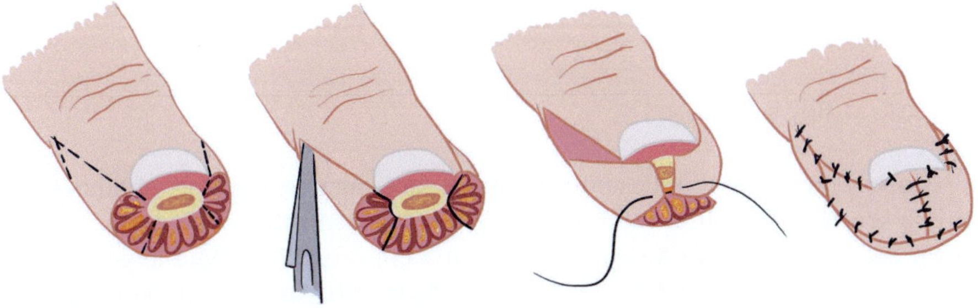

Fig. 20.7 Kutler or lateral V-Y flap scheme

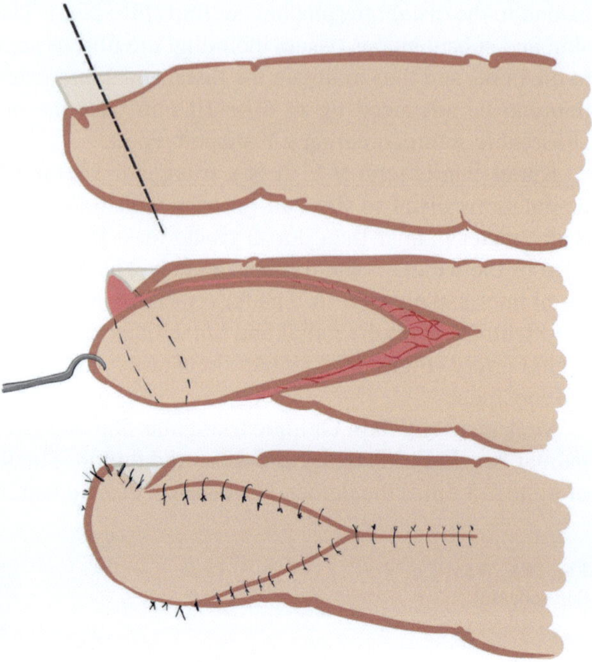

Fig. 20.8 Venkataswami flap scheme

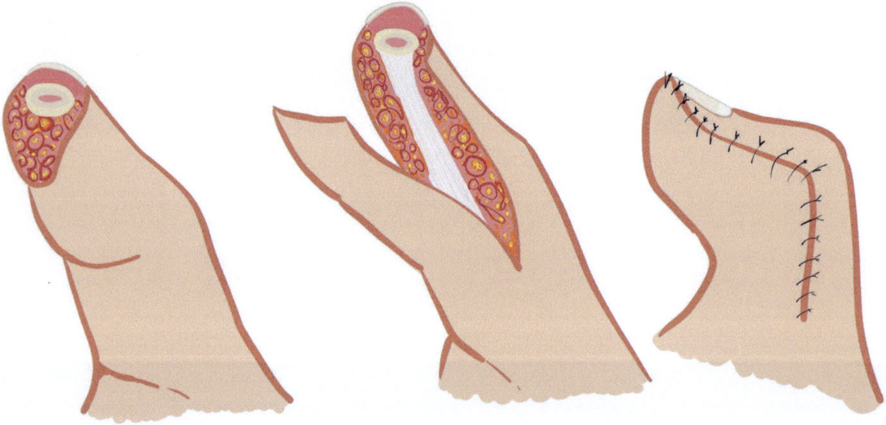

Fig. 20.9 Moberg flap scheme

Moberg flap: This is indicated in thumb amputations with palmar oblique bevel. It is a sensitive flap. It is used when a V-Y advancement flap cannot adequately cover the defect and this measures less than 2 cm (Fig. 20.9). Mid-axial incisions are made on both the radial and ulnar side of the thumb, extending proximally to the metacarpophalangeal fold. The flap is dissected with palmar skin, including the neurovascular bands. It is separated from the flexor tendon and advanced over the defect. It may be necessary to flex the interphalangeal joint to facilitate wound coverage.

Regional flaps: Regional flaps use tissue that is not adjacent to the defect. These flaps are useful when the wound is too large to allow coverage with a local flap. The commonly used regional flaps include the cross-finger flap, the thenar flap, and the thenar-H flap. In these techniques, a pocket flap is made for the fingertip and depends on the blood flow from the donor site, to allow the flap to incorporate into the native site. This type of technique requires a second intervention to separate the fingertip from the donor site, 3–4 weeks after the initial procedure. The disadvantage of these regional flaps is that they require a prolonged period of immobilization while incorporating, which can cause stiffness or contractures in the interphalangeal joints of the injured finger.

Cross-finger flap: It can be used to cover palmar tissue loss in any finger. The flap is designed as a rectangle over the middle phalanx of the donor finger, with the hinge side located next to the injured finger. The incision extends through the subcutaneous tissue, preserving the extensor tendon's paratenon. The flap is reflected on the hinge and sutured to the injured finger. A full-thickness skin graft is applied at the donor site. Similarly, a reverse cross-finger flap can be used to cover dorsal soft tissue defects.

Thenar and thenar-H flap: It is used for palmar defects of the index and ring fingers, only because the ulnar fingers often fail to comfortably reach the thenar eminence. The thenar flap is designed with the radial edge parallel and adjacent to the metacarpophalangeal joint fold of the thumb. The base of the flap is proximal and can be up to 2 cm wide. The flap is raised with its underlying subcutaneous tissue, taking care to protect the radial digital nerve. The flap is then sutured to the fingertip defect and covered with a total skin graft at the donor site. For a thenar-H flap, the flap is designed as an "H" on the thenar eminence, creating two flaps, one with a distal base and another with a proximal base. These flaps are sutured to the fingertip. Once the flap is separated, a full-thickness skin graft is applied to the defect.

Island flaps: Island flaps with a neurovascular pedicle can also be used to cover the fingertips. These flaps have two advantages: they provide sensitivity to the fingertip and can avoid the prolonged period of immobilization required for a cross or thenar flap. However, island flaps are technically more demanding than other regional flaps, and studies have not yet shown that these flaps produce better results despite the apparent advantages.

Small distal finger amputations survive as reinserted composite grafts in pediatric patients, with more successful results than in adults. The amputated tip is sutured to the stump without the need for formal microvascular repair. It is important to perform a careful repair of the nail bed and reduce and stabilize any fracture, for example, with Kirschner wires. The most likely outcome of composite grafts is partial survival; graft success is unlikely in those over 4-year-old and in crush injuries. In older patients, tip amputations can be degreased and replaced as a "cap" graft, with greater success. To perform this technique there must be at least 2 mm of healthy germinal matrix, and 6 mm of exposed and healthy bone, to leave the periosteum and the nail bed to be reimplanted in close contact.

20.8 Final Message

Pediatric fingertip injuries pose a significant challenge to health care, particularly if not properly managed. Currently, there is a lack of high-quality level I evidence. Randomized studies (for example, the NINJA trial [14]) are crucial to guide best practices.

Optimal care provision requires the combination of different treatment indications with appropriate management strategies, with the adoption of outcome measures informed by the patient specific for pediatrics. These should be promoted along with specific prevention mechanisms, to reduce the burden of these common injuries.

References

1. Peterson SL, Peterson EL, Wheatley MJ. Management of fingertip amputations. J Hand Surg Am. 2014;39(10):2093–101. https://doi.org/10.1016/j.jhsa.2014.04.025.
2. Pencle FJ, Doehrmann R, Waseem M. Fingertip injuries. [Updated 2022 Aug 7]. In: StatPearls [Internet]. Treasure Island (FL): StatPearls Publishing; 2022. https://www.ncbi.nlm.nih.gov/books/NBK436006
3. Venkatesh A, Khajuria A, Greig A. Management of pediatric distal fingertip injuries: a systematic literature review. Plast Reconstr Surg Glob Open. 2020;8(1):e2595. https://doi.org/10.1097/GOX.0000000000002595.
4. Kawaiah A, Thakur M, Garg S, Kawasmi SH, Hassan A. Fingertip injuries and amputations: a review of the literature. Cureus. 2020;12(5):e8291. https://doi.org/10.7759/cureus.8291.
5. Weir Y. Fingertip injuries in children: a review of the literature. Emerg Nurse. 2018;26(3):17–20. https://doi.org/10.7748/en.2018.e1795.
6. Merle M, Dautel G. Emergency surgery of the hand; 2016.
7. Evans DM, Bernardis C. A new classification for fingertip injuries [published correction appears in J Hand Surg [Br] 2000 Aug;25(4):414. Bernadis, C [corrected to Bernardis, C]. J Hand Surg Br. 2000;25(1):58–60. https://doi.org/10.1054/jhsb.1999.0305.
8. Patel L. Management of simple nail bed lacerations and subungual hematomas in the emergency department. Pediatr Emerg Care. 2014;30(10):742–8. https://doi.org/10.1097/PEC.0000000000000241.
9. Simon RR, Wolgin M. Subungual hematoma: association with occult laceration requiring repair. Am J Emerg Med. 1987;5(4):302–4. https://doi.org/10.1016/0735-6757(87)90356-1.
10. Gellman H. Fingertip-nail bed injuries in children: current concepts and controversies of treatment. J Craniofac Surg. 2009;20(4):1033–5. https://doi.org/10.1097/SCS.0b013e3181abb1b5.
11. Roser SE, Gellman H. Comparison of nail bed repair versus nail trephination for subungual hematomas in children. J Hand Surg Am. 1999;24(6):1166–70. https://doi.org/10.1053/jhsu.1999.1166.
12. Seaberg DC, Angelos WJ, Paris PM. Treatment of subungual hematomas with nail trephination: a prospective study. Am J Emerg Med. 1991;9(3):209–10. https://doi.org/10.1016/0735-6757(91)90077-w.
13. Mennen U, Wiese A. Fingertip injuries management with semi-occlusive dressing. J Hand Surg Br. 1993;18(4):416–22. https://doi.org/10.1016/0266-7681(93)90139-7.
14. Sierakowski A, Gardiner MD, Jain A, Greig AV, Nail bed INJury Analysis (NINJA) Collaborative Group. Surgical treatment of paediatric nail bed injuries in the United Kingdom: surgeon and patient priorities for future research. J Plast Reconstr Aesthet Surg. 2016;69(2):286–8. https://doi.org/10.1016/j.bjps.2015.10.025.

Part III
Lower Extremity Trauma

Chapter 21
Pelvic Injuries in the Pediatric Patient

Fernando Inostroza and Lenin Colmenares

Pelvic fractures in pediatric patients are uncommon, accounting for no more than 0.2% of all fractures in this age-group. The pelvis in pediatric patients presents different anatomical characteristics from adults; they have growth cartilages and a thick periosteum, and the skeleton has greater elasticity. These particular conditions mean that there can be avulsion injuries, fracture patterns that compromise the pelvic ring differently from adults, and intrapelvic injuries without an evident compromise of the pelvic ring.

The cause of pelvic fractures in pediatric patients is primarily related to traffic accidents, in which the child is a pedestrian, and secondly as a passenger in a vehicle involved in an accident [1].

Therapeutic measures range from rest and protected walking with crutches in the case of avulsions, to the use of external fixation in unstable fractures of the pelvic ring. The medical team that receives these patients must have a clear understanding of what a pelvic fracture in a child means and be able to recognize those types of fractures that increase the suspicion of associated injuries, which can compromise the patient's life more than the fracture itself.

F. Inostroza (✉)
Hospital Hernán Henríquez Aravena, Universidad de La Frontera, Temuco, Chile
e-mail: fernando.inostroza@ufrontera.cl

L. Colmenares
Hospital Regional de Talca, Dr. Cesar Garavagno Burotto, Talca, Chile

M. Sepúlveda O. (ed.), *Paediatrics Traumatology*,
https://doi.org/10.1007/978-3-031-89482-4_21

21.1 Anatomical Factors

The pelvis in children is more elastic than in adults, because its structure contains cartilaginous components, and the bone structures have a higher water content, which gives it a great capacity for deformation, so that they can present injuries that constitute a plastic deformation, as happens in other areas of immature skeleton [2].

Associated with these bone characteristics, we find that the sacroiliac joints in infants are more elastic and the pubic symphysis is thicker. The infant pelvis is capable of absorbing and dissipating the energy of trauma, before a fracture occurs. This explains that fractures in various areas of the pelvis associated with ligamentous injuries are rare in pediatric patients, so unstable fractures are uncommon.

This greater elasticity means that intrapelvic organs can be injured in the absence of an evident fracture, and a higher level of energy is required to produce a displaced injury of the pelvic bones. Therefore, a high level of energy from the trauma should always be considered, despite finding a simple pelvic fracture or with little displacement.

Another fundamental anatomical consideration is that the blood vessels of infants have a smaller caliber and their vascular reactivity is high, greater vasoconstriction that prevents significant bleeding. The thick and well-adhered periosteum to the bone prevents significant displacements and buffers the surfaces of spongy bone, avoiding major bleeding.

The pelvis in children presents multiple physes and cartilaginous areas with endochondral ossification, which should be considered when evaluating the images obtained so as not to confuse them with fracture sites. The triradiate cartilage is open, and its injury can cause a serious alteration in the development of the acetabulum.

21.2 Epidemiology

Pelvic fractures in pediatric patients are rare. The incidence ranges from 0.3% to 3.5% in different publications [3].

The average age at which a pelvic fracture occurs in children under 14-years-old is 8-years-old, and in children under 16-years-old, it is 9-years-old. The age distribution of pelvic fractures [4] is 1–5 years-old, 6.6%, 6–10 years-old, 10.5%, 11–14 years-old, 15.3%, and 15–17 years-old, 18.4%. The sex ratio is 1.4:1 male/female.

21.3 Etiology

The cause of pelvic fractures in pediatric patients corresponds to high-energy trauma. In 60% of cases, the child is a pedestrian who is hit by a motor vehicle, and in 20% of cases, the infant is a passenger in a vehicle involved in a traffic accident. Falls from height are the mechanism in 10% of cases [4]. Sports activities cause avulsion injuries of secondary ossification centers in the pelvis, due to muscle pulls.

21.4 Associated Injuries

Pediatric patients with pelvic fractures present associated injuries in 78% of cases [5]. There are on average 5.2 associated injuries at the time of hospital admission [6]. The most frequent are traumatic brain injury (TBI, 44%), fractures in the extremities (42%), thoracic injuries (27%), and abdominal and urogenital injuries (17%) [5]. An important consideration is that TBI causes 75–77% of deaths in children with pelvic fractures [7]. The most frequent abdominal injuries are those of the liver and spleen, with significant bleeding that can compromise the patient's life, which makes it important to perform an eco-FAST in those patients with hemodynamic instability, to decide on an urgent laparotomy.

We must remember that associated injuries are common in pelvic fractures, and often these injuries determine emergency surgical treatments because they put the patient's life at risk, more than the pelvic fracture itself.

21.5 Classification

The most commonly used classification in pediatric patients is the modified Torode-Zeig [8] (Fig. 21.1):

Type 1: Avulsion fractures.
Type 2: Iliac wing fracture without pelvic ring involvement.
Type 3A: Fracture of the anterior area of the pelvic ring.
Type 3B: Fracture of the anterior and posterior area of the pelvic ring.
Type 4: Multiple fractures of the pelvis causing instability of the pelvic ring.

In this classification, type 3B is related to associated injuries, a greater need for blood transfusions, admission to the intensive care unit, and a longer hospital stay. Type 3A is an anterior injury that can be associated with genitourinary injuries. The difference between both is difficult to establish in an anteroposterior radiograph of the pelvis, so it will be necessary to perform inlet and outlet X-ray projections of the pelvis, or a computed tomography (CT scan). Type 4 injuries are the most severe, with the highest morbidity and mortality.

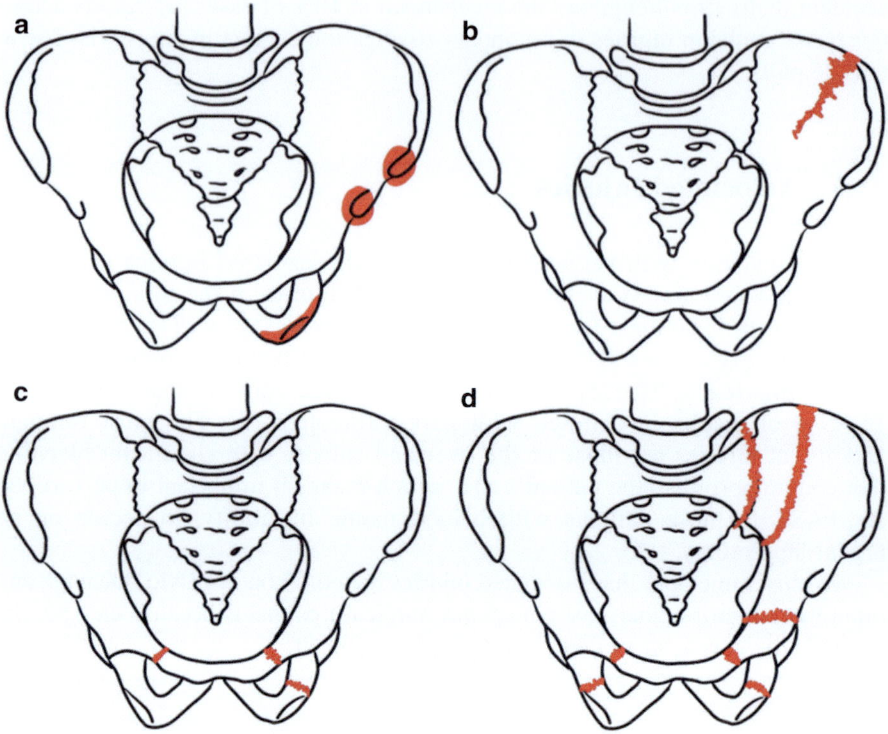

Fig. 21.1 Torode-Zieg classification scheme for pelvic fractures in pediatric patients. (1) Avulsion fractures; (2) fracture of the iliac wing without pelvic ring involvement; (3) anterior arch fracture; (4) unstable pelvic ring fracture

21.6 Diagnosis

The evaluation of a patient in whom a pelvic fracture is suspected should be carried out in the context of each case. In those patients who have suffered a high-energy trauma, the ABC of trauma according to ATLS should be started.

Once the patient is stabilized, the inspection should be done without their clothes, paying attention to asymmetries of the pelvis, difference in length of the lower limbs and look for different coloration of them. The soft tissues around the pelvis should be evaluated for erosions, hematomas, or volume increases. It is important to examine the urinary meatus and the vagina for bleeding and to evaluate the distal pulses in both limbs, noting differences, if any. It is important to perform an orderly neurological examination and to protect the patient against hypothermia, using some type of body heating system. On palpation, painful bone points should be sought, without performing maneuvers in search of instability of the pelvic ring, as they could cause more bleeding.

The anteroposterior X-ray projection of the pelvis is easy to obtain and quickly available for interpretation, with low levels of radiation (Fig. 21.2). However, the interpretation of the exam is difficult due to the presence of cartilaginous areas in the pediatric pelvis.

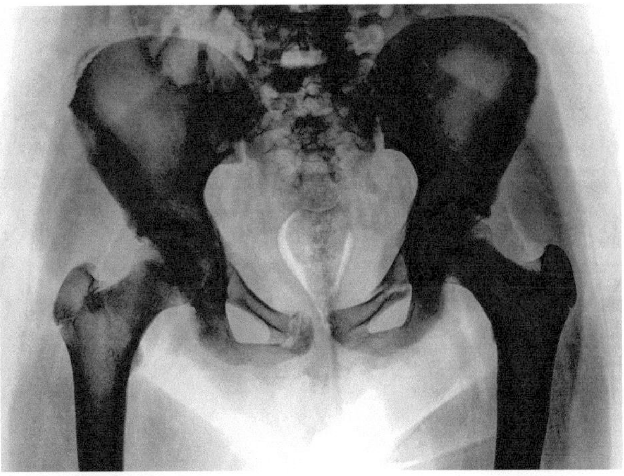

Fig. 21.2 AP pelvic X-ray of a 10-year-old girl with a Torode-Zieg 3B type pelvic ring injury

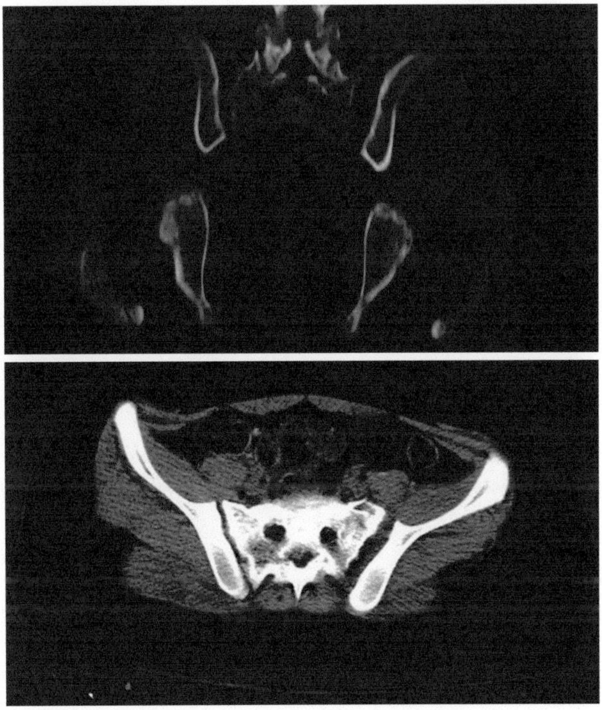

Fig. 21.3 Computed tomography of the pelvis of an 11-year-old girl with a posterior ring injury, left sacroiliac dislocation

It is important to consider the patient's hemodynamic status at the time of obtaining the radiograph. In pediatric patients with suspicion of pelvic fracture and hemodynamic instability, a routine thoraco-abdomino-pelvic CT scan should be performed. The CT scan has a high sensitivity for detecting pelvic fractures and is the method of choice for evaluating the sacrum, the sacroiliac joints, and the acetabulum in infants (Fig. 21.3).

In pediatric patients, the CT scan should be limited only to those cases in which the severity of the trauma warrants it, and not as a screening exam.

Other pelvic X-ray projections, such as Inlet, Outlet, Judet, and Iliac wing (Fig. 21.4), and an MRI may be useful later, in the planning of definitive surgical treatment, but not in the initial emergency evaluation.

It should be noted that MRI is very useful in the diagnosis of lesions at the level of sacroiliac joints in children who present cartilaginous components, and in the fractures of the acetabulum that have the open triradiate cartilage.

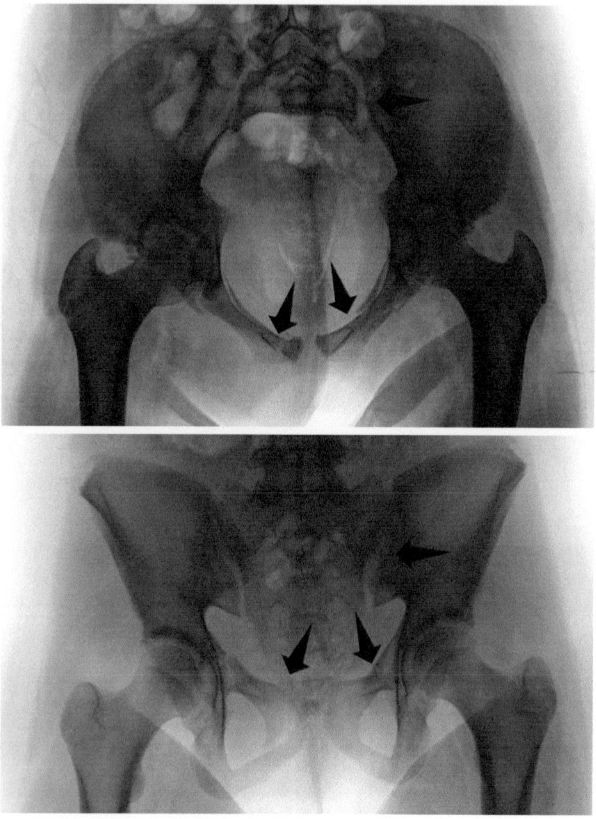

Fig. 21.4 Inlet and outlet X-ray views of the pelvis of a 10-year-old girl, with a Torode-Zieg 3B type pelvic ring injury

21.7 Treatment

Once the clinical evaluation and the imaging study have been completed and the pelvic fracture is diagnosed, the treatment will depend on the type of fracture and the associated injuries. Most of other fractures that occur in combination with the pelvic fractures can be treated in a deferred emergency.

It is essential to recognize instability in the pelvis in presence of multiple fractures that will require the intervention of a specialist, who will determine the need for surgical stabilization. Unstable pelvic fractures or with significant displacements will be eligible for surgical reduction and internal fixation; however, most pelvic fractures do not require surgical treatment. Between 70% and 95% of pelvic fractures in pediatric patients can be treated without the need for surgical intervention [5, 9–11].

21.7.1 *Stable Injuries*

Stable injuries are Type 1, 2, 3A, and 3B according to Torode-Zeig.

- Type 1 fractures usually occur from sports activities, which generate an avulsion of secondary ossification centers that are attached to muscles. These can be treated with rest for 4–6 weeks, analgesia, and protected walking with crutches (Fig. 21.5).
- Type 2 fractures, which occur from a lateral impact, are treated with rest for 6–8 weeks, analgesia, and exceptionally through surgical reduction and osteosynthesis in those very displaced (Fig. 21.6).

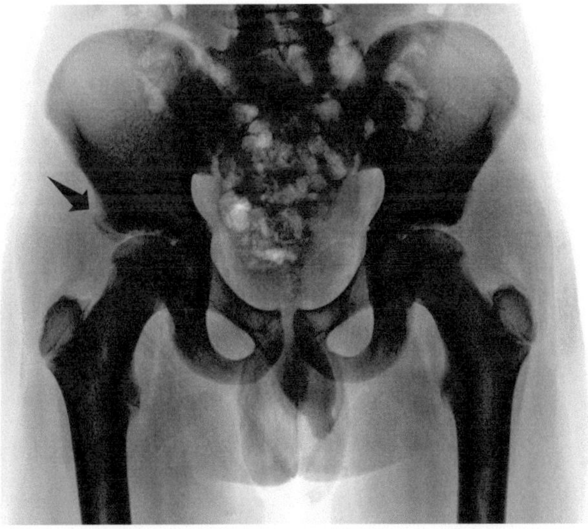

Fig. 21.5 Anteroposterior X-ray view of the pelvis of a 13-year-old boy, with a Torode-Zieg 1 type pelvic ring injury, iliac spine avulsion anteroinferior, with conservative treatment

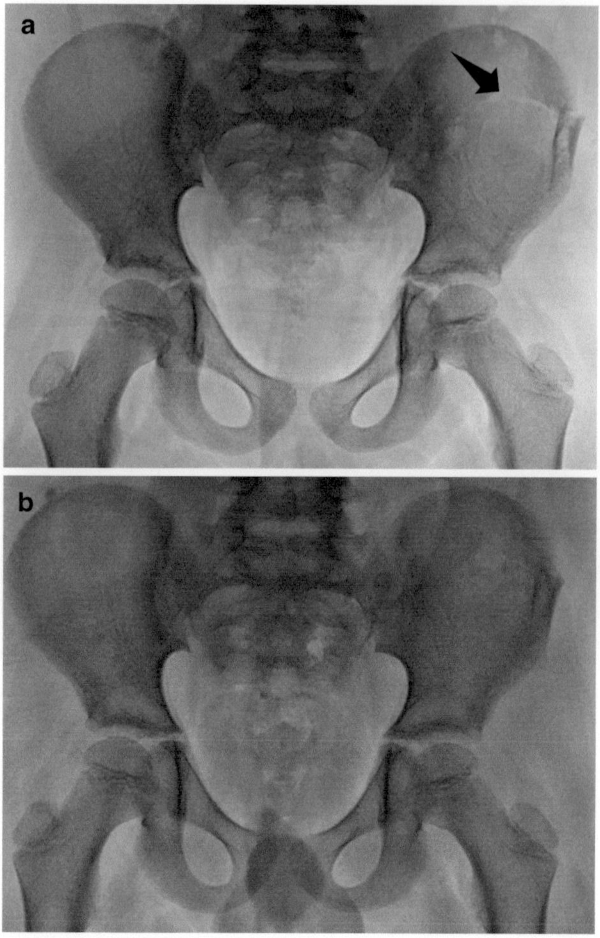

Fig. 21.6 (**a**) Anteroposterior X-ray view of the pelvis of an 11-year-old boy, with a Torode-Zieg 2 type pelvic ring injury. (**b**) Complete consolidation of 8 weeks of evolution

- For type 3A fractures, in which there is only unilateral anterior involvement, the treatment will be bed rest for 6–8 weeks, analgesia, and protected walking with crutches as tolerated.
- Type 3B fractures are more difficult to diagnose in the anteroposterior X-ray view of the pelvis, so it is necessary an Inlet and Outlet X-rays projections or a CT scan, and that despite being stable in relation to the pelvis, there are patients who may present hemodynamic instability due to vascular injuries from the posterior disruption of the sacroiliac joint. These patients may need vascular repairs or embolization of the compromised vessels. In hemodynamically stable patients, they will be treated with bed rest for 6–8 weeks, analgesia, and protected walking according to tolerance.

21.7.2 Unstable Injuries

Unstable fractures in a patient who is in a general stable condition can be treated in a deferred manner, while those who present hemodynamic instability must be treated urgently, based on the principles of ATLS.

In patients with pelvic fractures and hemodynamic instability, it is essential to identify associated injuries that may participate actively in its cause, that is, thoraco-abdominal injuries.

Type 4 fractures can be found in three modalities:

- Double anterior fractures, where a fracture of both pubic branches on both sides of the pubic symphysis, or fracture of both pubic branches plus disruption of the pubic symphysis. The recommended treatment is bed rest for 4 weeks, analgesia, and start of protected walking from 5 to 8 weeks, according to tolerance. Osteosynthesis is exceptional, for those very displaced or clinically unstable fractures (Fig. 21.7).

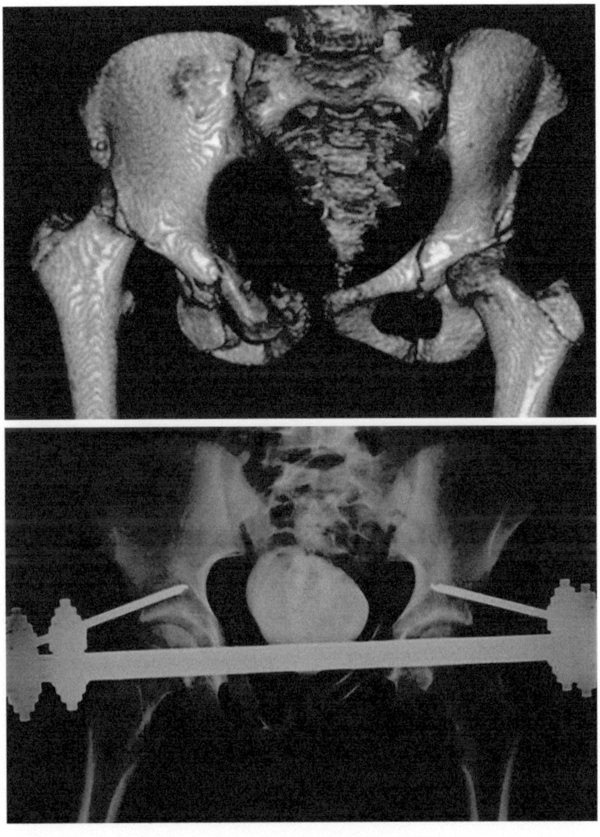

Fig. 21.7 (**a**) CT scan reconstruction images of the pelvis of a 5-year-old girl, demonstrating an injury Torode-Zieg type pelvic ring 4. (**b**) Stabilization with external fixator supraacetabular

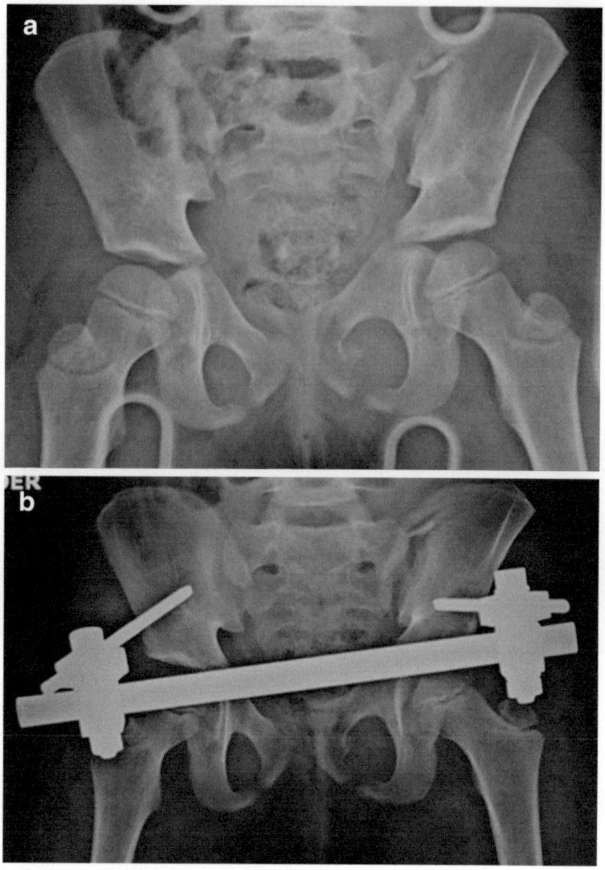

Fig. 21.8 (**a**) Anteroposterior X-ray view of the pelvis of an 11-year-old girl, demonstrating a Torode-Zieg type 4 pelvic ring injury. (**b**) Stabilization with supraacetabular external fixator

- Anterior and posterior fractures, which affect the anterior ring and the sacroiliac joint or the cartilaginous elements adjacent to the joint. This combination of anterior and posterior injury is seen on the anteroposterior X-ray of the pelvis. They are unstable injuries, associated with hemodynamic compromise, and should be managed by pelvic belt or external fixator, ideally supraacetabular (Fig. 21.8). Hemodynamically stable patients with little displacement can be treated with bed rest for 6–8 weeks, analgesia, and resumption of walking in a protected manner.
- The anterior and posterior fractures that compromise both sides of the pelvis are the most serious and constitute a major problem for their treatment, because most of these patients present associated injuries, and often exposure of one of the fractures. The treatment should be aimed at solving the general instability of the patient and specifically of the pelvis, to stabilize the fractures by combination of external and internal fixation.

21.8 Final Message

The immature skeleton of the pediatric patient generates significant differences in relation to injury patterns and the intrinsic stability of the pelvis, which should always be considered when evaluating and planning the treatment of these injuries.

Although the vast majority of these injuries are non-surgical treatment, one must alert to the need to stabilize the pelvic ring in cases of hemodynamic instability, significant deformity, and requirements for mobilization of a polytraumatized patient.

References

1. Reichard SA, Helikson MA, Shorter N, White RI Jr, Shemeta DW, Haller JA Jr. Pelvic fractures in children - review of 120 patients with a new look at general management. J Pediatr Surg. 1980;15(6):727–34. https://doi.org/10.1016/s0022-3468(80)80272-7.
2. Forestier-Zhang L, Bishop N. Bone strength in children: understanding basic bone biomechanics. Arch Dis Child Educ Pract Ed. 2016;101(1):2–7. https://doi.org/10.1136/archdischild-2015-308597.
3. Gänsslen A, Heidari N, Weinberg AM. Fractures of the pelvis in children: a review of the literature. Eur J Orthop Surg Traumatol. 2013;23(8):847–61. https://doi.org/10.1007/s00590-012-1102-0.
4. Zwingmann J, Lefering R, Maier D, Eberbach H, Neumann M, Strohm PC, et al. Pelvic fractures in severely injured children: results from the TraumaRegister DGU. Medicine (Baltimore). 2018;97(35):e11955. https://doi.org/10.1097/MD.0000000000011955.
5. Chia JP, Holland AJ, Little D, Cass DT. Pelvic fractures and associated injuries in children. J Trauma. 2004;56(1):83–8. https://doi.org/10.1097/01.TA.0000084518.09928.CA.
6. Galano GJ, Vitale MA, Kessler MW, Hyman JE, Vitale MG. The most common traumatic orthopedic injuries from a national pediatric inpatient population. J Pediatr Orthop. 2005;25(1):39–44. https://doi.org/10.1097/00004694-200501000-00010.
7. Amorosa LF, Kloen P, Helfet DL. High-energy pediatric pelvic and acetabular fractures. Orthop Clin North Am. 2014;45(4):483–500. https://doi.org/10.1016/j.ocl.2014.06.009.
8. Shore BJ, Palmer CS, Bevin C, Johnson MB, Torode IP. Pediatric pelvic fracture: a modification of a preexisting classification. J Pediatr Orthop. 2012;32(2):162–8. https://doi.org/10.1097/BPO.0b013e3182408be6.
9. Tosounidis TH, Sheikh H, Giannoudis PV. Pelvic fractures in pediatric polytrauma patients: classification, associated injuries and early mortality. Open Orthop J. 2015;9:303–12. Published 2015 Jul 31. https://doi.org/10.2174/1874325001509010303.
10. Spiguel L, Glynn L, Liu D, Statter M. Pediatric pelvic fractures: a marker for injury severity. Am Surg. 2006;72(6):481–4.
11. DeFrancesco CJ, Sankar WN. Traumatic pelvic fractures in children and adolescents. Semin Pediatr Surg. 2017;26(1):27–35. https://doi.org/10.1053/j.sempedsurg.2017.01.006.

Chapter 22
Hip Fractures in Children and Adolescents

Laura Montes and Catalina Larraín

Hip fractures are extremely rare among childhood lesions incidence, accounting for less than 1% of the total fractures at this age range. Unlike most fractures presenting in pediatric age, which usually have a favorable prognosis, this injury is associated with high rates of complications and a reserved prognosis evolution. This is due both to the severity of the associated injuries by the injury mechanism and to the direct result of the hip fracture. Proper management is essential to avoid its potential complications, among which avascular necrosis, coxa vara, non-union, premature physeal closure, and lower limb length discrepancy can be mentioned.

22.1 Introduction

Hip fractures in pediatric age are rare injuries and account for less than 1% of all fractures in childhood and adolescence [1]. Their incidence increases in those over 11 years old. An incidence of more than 100 hip fractures in adults is reported for each similar fracture in pediatric age. In contrast to adult patients, in skeletally immature patients, the most common cause is high-energy trauma, such as a fall from height or traffic accident. For this reason, about 30–85% is associated with a traumatic brain injury (TBI), facial trauma, splenic laceration, retroperitoneal hemorrhage, and/or perineal injuries. Other associated musculoskeletal injuries are also common, such as pelvic and acetabular fractures, hip dislocation, and ipsilateral

L. Montes
Hospital Universitario Donostia, San Sebastián, Spain

C. Larraín (✉)
Clínica Alemana de Santiago, Santiago, Chile
e-mail: clarrainb@alemana.cl

M. Sepúlveda O. (ed.), *Paediatrics Traumatology*,
https://doi.org/10.1007/978-3-031-89482-4_22

femur fracture [2]. Hip fractures are associated with high rates of complications and can have an unfavorable evolution. This is due both to the severity of the associated injuries and to the complexity of the injury itself [3]. It should be noted that fractures associated with low-energy mechanisms should make us suspect pathological bone fractures, as well as non-accidental trauma in children prior to walking age.

22.2 Pathophysiology

Most of the complications associated with hip fractures in pediatric age occur due to the anatomical peculiarities of the hip in the skeletally immature patient. The longitudinal growth of the proximal femur takes place mainly through a continuous growth plate, which spans from the major trochanter apophysis to the femoral head, passing through the upper portion of the femoral neck. This physeal bridge is susceptible to injury by a fracture at that level, producing growth alterations secondary to a physeal closure, with the consequent angular deformities of the proximal femur or growth disturbance.

The secondary ossification center located in the femoral epiphysis begins to ossify around 6 months old in males and 4 months old in females. The fusion of the proximal femoral epiphysis with the femur neck occurs in both sexes around 18 years old. The ossification center of the major trochanter is evident at 4 years old and joins the femoral metaphysis approximately at 14 years old in females and 16 years old in males. This ossification center is responsible for the appositional growth of the major trochanter and also contributes to the growth of the intertrochanteric metaphyseal area of the femur and femoral neck.

The vascular anatomy of the hip, specifically at the level of the proximal femur, has been studied in depth due to its importance in multiple pathologies. In the case of hip fractures, its understanding is fundamental to comprehend the high rate of avascular necrosis that occurs in them.

When the physis of the femoral head is present, it constitutes a barrier to the passage of blood vessels from the femoral neck, so there is practically no intraosseous circulation through it to the ossified epiphysis of the femur head. The artery of the round ligament contributes scarcely to the total irrigation of the femoral head, and in adults, it provides only 20% of the total. Therefore, the main vascular contribution to the femoral epiphysis comes from small vessels that enter over the physis, directly into the proximal femoral epiphysis; the main ones being the ascending lateral cervical artery (branch of the lateral circumflex femoral artery) and the posteroinferior branch of the medial circumflex artery (Fig. 22.1). These blood vessels penetrate the articular capsule, so they are also called subsynovial intracapsular arteries. They are located outside the bone, which makes them susceptible to collapse when there is a significant increase in intra-articular pressure, as in the case of an intracapsular fracture. In addition, their close relationship with the femoral neck puts this vascular system at risk of direct injury when a displaced fracture occurs.

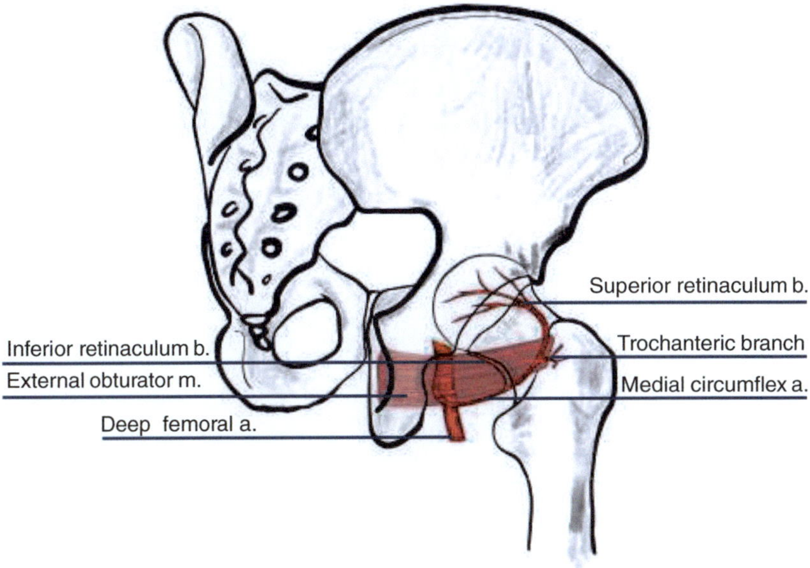

Fig. 22.1 Scheme of the irrigation of the femoral neck and femoral head, from a posterior view, in presence of a physis still open

22.3 Diagnosis

It is important to obtain information about the mechanism of injury, medical history, and look for concomitant injuries. Since most cases are the result of high-energy mechanism accidents, the primary evaluation will include airway management, cardiovascular stabilization, and detection of life-threatening injuries (head, neck, chest, abdomen, and pelvis injuries) [1].

Clinically, the patient presents with groin or thigh pain, functional impotence, with the inability to weight-bearing. The affected limb is in external rotation and abduction. If the fracture is displaced, there may be shortening of the limb. If there is a posterior dislocation of the femoral head, the hip will be in a position of extension, adduction, and internal rotation. Non-displaced fractures may go unnoticed, presenting only painful limping and limitation to passive mobilization of the joint, especially to internal rotation. The clinical history and physical examination of the patient can help differentiate a hip fracture from other pathologies with similar clinical findings. The differential diagnosis should include Legg–Calvé–Perthes disease, a slipped capital femoral epiphysis, stress fractures, osteoarticular infections, juvenile autoimmune pathology, and transient synovitis of the hip in small patients. It is always important to consider in a hip fracture without a history of high-energy trauma, the suspicion of a non-accidental injury. With the anteroposterior pelvic (Fig. 22.2) and axial X-ray projections of the affected hip, it is usually sufficient to detect, and even classify the fracture. It is advisable to avoid the use of the Lauenstein projection to not increase the displacement of the fracture.

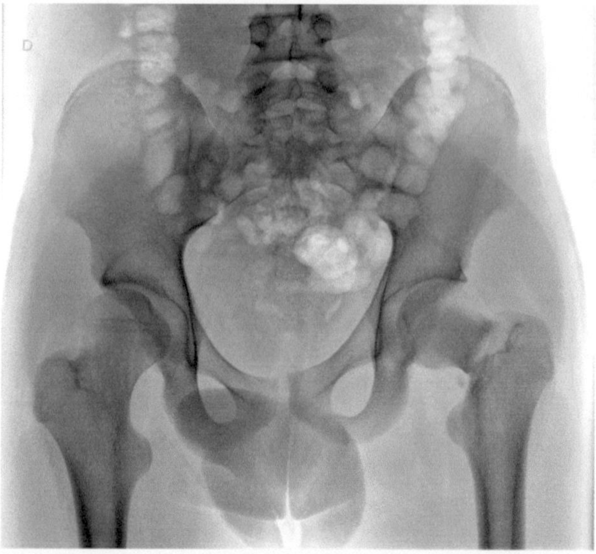

Fig. 22.2 Anteroposterior pelvis X-ray of a 14-year-old boy, with a left hip fracture

The use of computed tomography (CT scan) is useful in the suspicion of a non-displaced fracture or fractures in pathological bone. In cases of complex fractures, with great fragmentation, the study and three-dimensional reconstruction allowus a better characterization of the fracture and preoperative planning.

Magnetic resonance imaging (MRI) is useful in the suspicion of fractures not diagnosed by other methods, as in stress injuries or in pathological bone, where it also provides information about its tissue characteristics. In addition, in some cases, it can provide us with information about the vascular status of the femoral head, especially with the use of perfusion studies [4].

Another study is the Technetium (Tc99) three-phase scintigraphy, which currently has limited use, being reserved for the study in younger patients, high clinical suspicion of injury and without radiological evidence, in whom the use of MRI is desired to be avoided, because usually requires sedation in small children. Therefore, it is useful for the detection of hidden femoral neck fractures and some associated musculoskeletal alterations.

22.4 Classification

The fracture classification system in pediatric age described originally by Delbet and popularized by Colonna [5] is the most used one. It is based on the anatomical location of the fracture, dividing them into four types (Fig. 22.3). It was modified by Parker and Pryor [6] adding a fifth type of fractures. These authors highlight the need to describe each type of fracture as non-displaced or displaced, as complications occur particularly, although not exclusively, in the group with displacement.

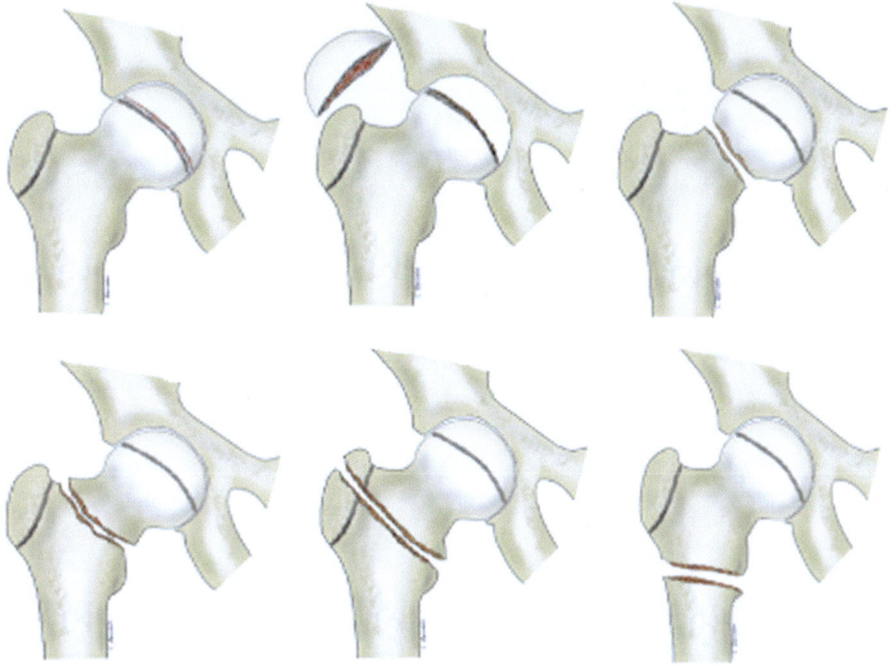

Fig. 22.3 Modified Delbet classification. (**a**) Type IA, transphyseal without dislocation of the epiphysis; (**b**) Type IB, transphyseal with dislocation of the epiphysis; (**c**) Type II, transcervical; (**d**) Type III, basicervical; (**e**) Type IV, intertrochanteric; (**f**) Type V, subtrochanteric

The five types of hip fracture in pediatric age described by Delbet and modified by Parker and Pryor are as follows:

Type I: Transphyseal fracture equivalent to an epiphysiolysis of the femoral epiphysis. It can occur without dislocation (IA) or with dislocation of the epiphysis (IB). It is the least common of the four types (10%), but the one with the highest risk of avascular necrosis (AVN) and worse outcomes.

Type II: Transcervical fracture. They constitute 50% of all hip fractures and are the most common type of hip fracture in the pediatric patient.

Type III: Cervicotrochanteric or basicervical fracture. They are the second most common type of hip fracture in the pediatric patient (25–30%).

Type IV: Intertrochanteric fracture. Less common, constituting 6–15% of hip fractures in the pediatric patient.

Type V: Subtrochanteric fracture. These are those located between 0 and 5 cm from the lesser trochanter. It is a frequent location of fracture in pathological bone.

A special group of injuries in pediatric age are the overuse fractures of the femoral neck. These are rare to find in infants, and often the only symptom is pain at the inguinal or thigh level. They can be related to intense sports practice and repetitive movements. In these injuries, X-rays show sclerosis of the lower portion of the

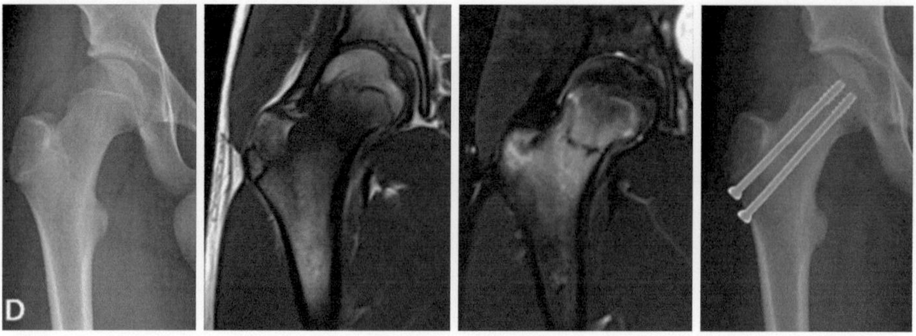

Fig. 22.4 A 14-year-old adolescent, with a stress fracture of the femoral neck, confirmed by magnetic resonance imaging (MRI). Treatment was performed before stabilization with osteosynthesis

Table 22.1 Frequent causes of pathological bone fracture in childhood

Pathological bone
Unicameral bone cyst
Aneurysmal bone cyst
Fibrous dysplasia
Osteomyelitis
Langerhans cell histiocytosis
Osteogenesis imperfecta
Osteopenia
Metabolic diseases
Malignant tumors

neck, due to the constant attempt to bone tissue repair. The diagnosis can be confirmed by bone scintigraphy or MRI. The treatment will be aimed at reducing physical activity, which can be associated with immobilization, with a monopodal pelvipedal cast. Depending on the age and activity of the patient, it may be necessary to perform osteosynthesis (Fig. 22.4).

Finally, we can find fractures in pathological bone, which are usually the result of a low-energy mechanism. They present with little displacement of their fragments and may have areas of bone fragmentation due to low quality tissue (Table 22.1). These lesions are usually located in the cervicotrochanteric and subtrochanteric region of the femur. The treatment focuses on recovering the acute injury. Biopsy, curettage, and tissue graft are usually performed simultaneously with the reduction and definitive stabilization of the fracture (Fig. 22.5).

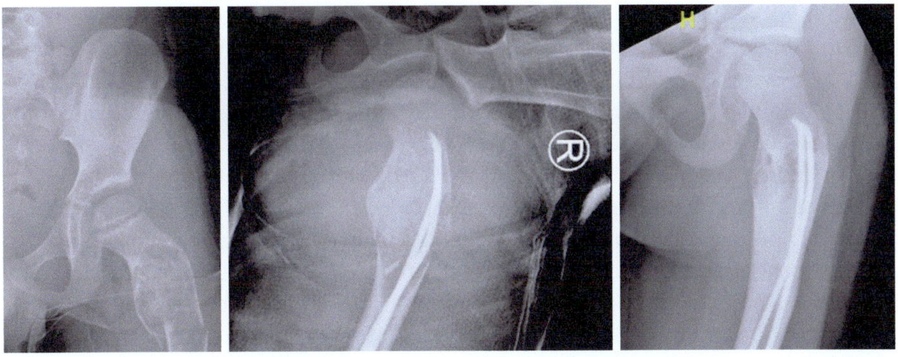

Fig. 22.5 Subtrochanteric fracture of the femur in a 5-year-old child, product of bone fragility due to the presence of an essential bone cyst. He was fixated with elastic stable intramedullary nails, with complete consolidation at 2 years follow-up

22.5 Treatment

The treatment and its prognosis for hip fractures in pediatric age depend on the age, the general conditions of the patient, the location of the fracture, the displacement, and the stability of the lesion.

The treatment of these injuries should be considered an emergency in most cases, especially in Types I-II-III of Delbet, as in them the restitution of the anatomy could normalize the reversible vascular damage of the intracapsular fractures. For this reason, their treatment should be carried out within the first 24 h, with the aim of reducing the risk of AVN.

The indication of capsular decompression, in order to decrease the pressure on the vessels at the capsular level, continues to be a controversial topic, with no consensus in the literature. It has not yet been it has been sufficiently demonstrated that this procedure reduces the incidence of AVN [1, 2]. However, we recommend the decompression of the intra-articular hematoma in Type I, II, and III fractures, as a routine procedure, once the fracture has been reduced and stabilized [7]. The methods for performing this decompression can be aspiration with a thick gauge needle, through a sub-adductor or anterior approach to the hip, or an open capsulotomy, through a small anterior incision. Regarding the decompression technique, there is no evidence of a significant difference between puncture and open decompression [8].

The treatment for Type IA fractures, that is, transphyseal without dislocation, non-displaced in children under 2 years old, is by a pelvic spica cast, without internal fixation. These fractures usually displace in varus and external rotation, so the cast should be placed in abduction and 10° of internal rotation. In children under 3 years old who require reduction, the use of internal fixation with 2 or 3 smooth Kirschner wires, 2 mm in diameter, crossing the physis, is recommended. We suggest cutting and bending them flush with the bone, leaving them covered under the skin. The cast is maintained for a period of 6 weeks.

In children older than 3 years old, the use of internal fixation with cannulated screws of 4–7 mm, crossing the physis, is recommended. These are installed through a lateral approach, centered on the femoral neck. We recommend installing two guide wires before the insertion of the first screw, to avoid displacement, or rotation, when it is advanced through the fracture lines. Drilling is performed up to the physis, without crossing it. The screws should be left no less than 5 mm from the subchondral bone. It is suggested to avoid positioning the screws in the anterolateral quadrant of the epiphysis and the posterior drilling of the femoral neck, in order to reduce the risk of vascular injury.

Type IA fractures that are displaced require reduction maneuvers. Under general anesthesia, a gentle traction maneuver should be applied, then abduction and finally internal rotation, with the hip at 45° flexion. After anatomical closed reduction, the need for osteosynthesis should be assessed according to age. If after gentle maneuvers reduction is not achieved, an open reduction is performed, usually through a Smith-Petersen anterior approach or Watson-Jones anterolateral approach, with subsequent use of internal fixation.

In the case of a Type IB injury, open reduction and internal fixation are recommended. The approach will be dictated by the position of the femoral epiphysis. If it is anterior or inferior, a Watson-Jones approach is recommended. If it is posterior, a posterior approach is recommended. This type of injury is extremely rare, presenting a high rate of complications. Currently, there are some case reports approached through a surgical hip dislocation, achieving a complete direct visualization of the hip, the retinacular vessels, and the irrigation of the femoral epiphysis [9].

For non-displaced Type II fractures, it should be considered that, although good results are described with immobilization with a pelvic spica cast with strict radiological control, these are intrinsically unstable fractures, with a high incidence of AVN, coxa vara, and secondary displacement [10]. For this reason, we recommend internal fixation with Kirschner wires or cannulated screws, depending on the age and size of the patient.

For displaced Type II fractures, we must perform a reduction under general anesthesia, through traction, abduction, and pressure toward the posterior of the greater trochanter, with internal rotation of 20°. If an open reduction is necessary, an anterolateral Watson-Jones approach is recommended. These fractures should be stabilized with internal fixation, Kirschner wires, or cannulated screws, depending on the

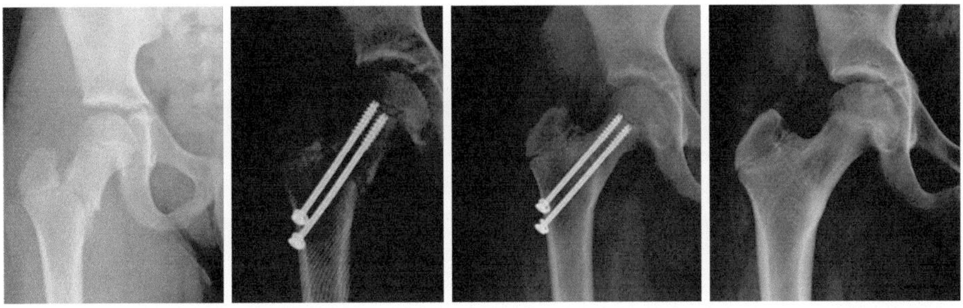

Fig. 22.6 Delbet Type III fracture, in a 7-year-old girl, was treated surgically with reduction and stabilization with cannulated screws, showing adequate consolidation at one year after surgery

age and weight of the patient. In younger children, less than 8 years old, 2–3 screws of 4–4.5 mm are recommended. Above 8 years old, 6.5 mm screws are recommended. If possible, crossing the physis should be avoided, but always considering that the primary goal is to achieve stable fracture fixation, over the integrity of the physis, given the minimal impact on the total length of the limb.

Non-displaced Type III fractures, depending on the size and tolerance of the patient, can be treated with a spica cast and close radiological control. If necessary, it can be protected with internal fixation, with cannulated screws, without crossing the physis. Displaced Type III fractures require a closed reduction or, if necessary, open, through a Watson-Jones anterolateral approach. They are stabilized with internal fixation using 2–3 cannulated screws, usually without crossing the physis. After fixation, it is recommended to protect the segment with a unilateral spica cast for 3–4 weeks, in addition to avoiding weight-bearing for at least 6–8 weeks (Fig. 22.6).

In non-displaced Type IV hip fractures, in children under 3 years old, the use of a spica cast in abduction for 12 weeks is recommended. In children over 3 years old or in displaced fractures, an open reduction and internal fixation with pediatric dynamic hip screws system (DHS), or a pediatric proximal femur locking plates, through a lateral approach should be performed.

Finally, non-displaced Type V fractures can be treated with a spica cast for 4–6 weeks, if stable, with weekly radiological control. If they are displaced, this will be in flexion and abduction due to the action of the psoas and gluteus muscles. In those distal to the lesser trochanter, closed reduction and stabilization with retrograde elastic stable intramedullary nails can be obtained. In those proximal, an open reduction and osteosynthesis with pediatric DHS, or a pediatric proximal femur locking plates, through a lateral approach, are usually required (Figs. 22.7 and 22.8).

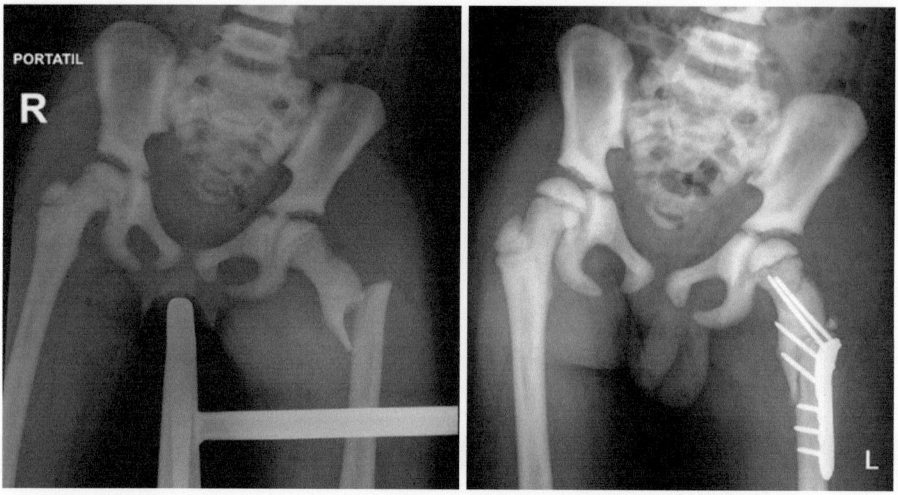

Fig. 22.7 Delbet Type V fracture in an 8-year-old child. Open reduction and internal fixation with a pediatric locking plate were performed

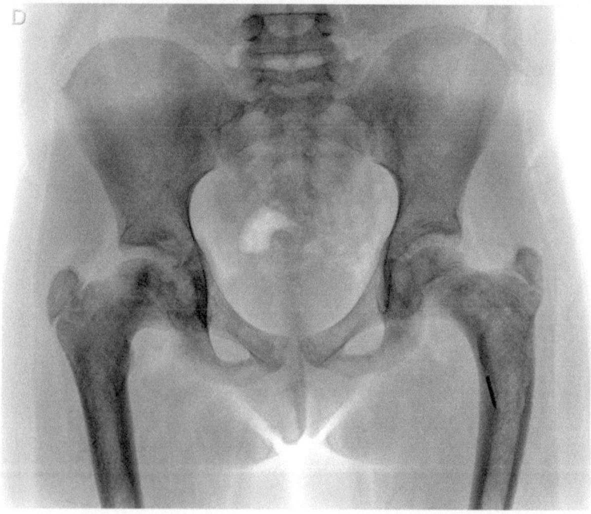

Fig. 22.8 A 10-year-old girl with sequelae of bilateral femoral fracture in pathological bone (chronic multifocal recurrent osteitis). It can be seen sequelae with Coxa brevis and coxa magna on the right hip, and coxa vara on the left hip

22.6 Complications

Avascular necrosis (AVN) is the most) frequent and most important complication, due to its poor functional outcomes. Its overall incidence is 59%. It is generally diagnosed within 2–12 months after the injury, but it may not be symptomatic until 2 years have passed. The first signs of AVN are usually pain and limitation of the range of motion.

The type of fracture and age are the best parameters for predicting AVN. Displaced Type IA fractures have an AVN incidence of 50%, Type IB of 80–100%. In Type II fractures, the overall incidence of AVN is 27%, being 50% in displaced ones. In Type III, the incidence of this complication is 27%, and in Type IV it is 14%. According to age, those over 10 years old develop AVN more frequently.

The presence of AVN seems to be related to the initial displacement of the fracture, with the failure to obtain an anatomical reduction and with the delay in definitive treatment. The evidence suggests that urgent reduction and stable fixation of the fracture, combined with capsular decompression, reduce the possibility of AVN [8].

The prognosis and treatment options vary depending on the type of AVN, the degree of deformity and collapse at the time of diagnosis, as well as the age at which the patient becomes symptomatic. The results are poor in more than 60% of patients. Ratliff [11] described three types of AVN after a hip fracture. In type I, the entire epiphysis and femoral neck are affected, from the fracture, being the worst prognosis. Type II involves only a part of the epiphysis, with a normal neck, causing minimal cephalic collapse. When necrosis goes from the fracture line to the physis, in the neck, it is described as Type III and has the best prognosis.

The consequences of AVN of the hip can be devastating. If internal fixation was installed when AVN develops, it must be removed immediately after fracture healing. Remodeling of the femoral head can occur, especially in the smaller patient, taking up to 5 years [12]. There are several treatment options depending on the age and type of AVN such as femoral osteotomies, joint distraction with external fixator, core decompression, vascularized fibula graft, and arthrodesis. All of these are salvage options, with regular results in an intermediate term. Total hip arthroplasty is the best treatment option in patients who have completed their growth.

Malunion and altered growth after a hip fracture can generate two types of deformity: coxa vara or coxa valga. Coxa vara is the second most common complication, with a global incidence of 20–30%. In Type I fractures, its incidence is 30–50%, in displaced Type II around 41%, in Type III around 11%, and approximately 10% in Type IV. It is the result of both the progressive deformity of non-displaced fractures and the loss of reduction of fractures managed with or without internal fixation.

It can also be a consequence of AVN, non-union and premature physeal closure, or even a combination of all the above factors. Anatomical reduction with stable fixation is the best method to prevent this complication. Severe coxa vara shortens the limb, causes abductor weakness, and can result in early development of hip osteoarthritis. Bone remodeling of the hip can only be expected in children under 3 years old.

In children under 8 years old, with mild coxa vara and persistent growth of the greater trochanter, epiphysiodesis of the greater trochanter is a treatment option to prevent progression of the deformity. In those over 8 years old and adolescents, remodeling cannot be expected and they are immediate candidates for surgery. If the cervico-diaphyseal angle is 110° or less, a subtrochanteric valgus osteotomy is required to recover the mechanics of the hip. Coxa valga rarely occurs for this type of fractures, with reported cases being iatrogenic [13].

Premature physeal closure has an incidence between 5% and 65%. The possible mechanisms would be physeal damage from trauma and damage to the peripheral irrigation, both from the fracture and iatrogenic. It also increases in the presence of AVN. Partial closures produce coxa vara or valga. When it is necessary to cross the physis with osteosynthesis, the use of smooth pins over cannulated screws should be preferred, and in the smallest number possible. However, Beaty [10] stated that it is more important to have stable fixation than to avoid the physis. Premature closure of the physis leads to a significant difference in lower limb length only in small children. This is because the proximal femur contributes only about 13% of the longitudinal growth of the lower limb. Contralateral epiphysiodesis may be necessary when the projected difference at skeletal maturity exceeds 2–2.5 cm.

Non-union has been reported in 6–10% of all pediatric hip fractures. The main cause is the inability to obtain or maintain an anatomical reduction. It is observed more frequently in Type II and Type III fractures that have been treated non-surgically, in fractures where an anatomical reduction is not achieved, in those with inadequate stabilization, in cases with hidden infection at the fracture site and in AVN. Non-union should be treated surgically as soon as possible, unlike AVN. Valgus osteotomy usually leads to secondary consolidation, by reducing shear forces and increasing mechanical load on the focus. Bone grafts can be used if necessary, although they are not usually necessary.

Chondrolysis is an uncommon complication; however, it generates significant sequelae. It is produced by hypoxia in the articular cartilage or associated with joint penetration of osteosynthesis. It presents with hip pain, joint blockage, and radiological reduction of the joint space. The diagnosis is usually made by MRI. The initial management is symptomatic at first, with anti-inflammatories and unloading. Some publications refer to the use of joint distraction with an external fixator to improve the joint range and reduce pain. It may require a femoral valgus osteotomy or, finally, a total hip arthroplasty.

Lastly, infection occurs in less than 1%. Given its severity and serious sequelae, early diagnosis and treatment are essential.

22.7 Final Message

Hip fractures in children and adolescents are rare injuries. Their importance lies in the fact that they present a high rate of complications. The Delbet-Colonna classification, based on the anatomical location of the fracture line, is used for their description. The treatment is very variable and is influenced by the classification, age, degree of displacement, and stability of the fracture. Despite appropriate treatment, they present a high rate of AVN, due to the vulnerability of the terminal arterial blood flow and the bone anatomy of the proximal femur in the pediatric patient.

References

1. Boardman MJ, Herman MJ, Buck B, Pizzutillo PD. Hip fractures in children. J Am Acad Orthop Surg. 2009;17(3):162–73. https://doi.org/10.5435/00124635-200903000-00005.
2. Bagatur AE, Zorer G. Complications associated with surgically treated hip fractures in children. J Pediatr Orthop B. 2002;11(3):219–28. https://doi.org/10.1097/00009957-200207000-00005.
3. Canale ST, Beaty JH. Pelvic and hip fractures. In: Rockwood CA, Wilkins KE, Beaty JH, editors. Fractures in children, ed 4. Philadelphia, PA: Lippincott-Raven; 1996. p. 1109–93.
4. Ozel BD, Ozel D, Ozkan F, Halefoglu AM. Diffusion-weighted magnetic resonance imaging of femoral head osteonecrosis in two groups of patients: Legg-Perthes-Calve and Avascular necrosis. Radiol Med. 2016 Mar;121(3):206–13.
5. Colonna PC. Fractures of the neck of the femur in children. Am J Surg. 1929;6:793–7.
6. Parker MJ. Proximal femoral fractures. In: Pynsent PB, Fairbank JCT, Carr AJ, editors. Classification of musculoskeletal trauma. Oxford: Butterworth Heinemann; 1999. p. 184–209.
7. Yeranosian M, Horneff JG, Baldwin K, Hosalkar HS. Factors affecting the outcome of fractures of the femoral neck in children and adolescents: a systematic review. Bone Joint J. 2013;95-B(1):135–42. https://doi.org/10.1302/0301-620X.95B1.30161.
8. Bukva B, Abramovic D, Vrgoc G, Marinović M, Bakota B, Dučić S, et al. Femoral neck fractures in children and the role of early hip decompression in final outcome. Injury. 2015;46(Suppl 6):S44–7. https://doi.org/10.1016/j.injury.2015.10.059.
9. Van Nortwick S, Beck N, Li M. Adolescent hip fracture-dislocation: transphyseal fracture with posterior dislocation of the proximal femoral epiphysis: a case report. JBJS Case Connect. 2016;6(3):e62. https://doi.org/10.2106/JBJS.CC.15.00271.
10. Beaty JH. Fractures of the hip in children. Orthop Clin North Am. 2006;37(2):223–vii. https://doi.org/10.1016/j.ocl.2005.11.003.
11. Ratliff AHC. Complications after fractures of the femoral neck in children and their treatment. J Bone Joint Surg. 1970;52-B:175.
12. Hughes LO, Beaty JH. Fractures of the head and neck of the femur in children. J Bone Joint Surg Am. 1994;76(2):283–92. https://doi.org/10.2106/00004623-199402000-00019.
13. Mirdad T. Fractures of the neck of femur in children: an experience at the Aseer Central Hospital, Abha, Saudi Arabia. Injury. 2002;33(9):823–7. https://doi.org/10.1016/s0020-1383(02)00013-x.

Chapter 23
Fracture of the Femoral Shaft

Javier Besomi and Eric Gordon

Femoral shaft fractures in pediatric population have a bimodal presentation, being associated, between 2 and 4 years of age, with falls, and then, during adolescence, with high-energy trauma. They represent a therapeutic challenge for the treating physician, with a wide range of therapeutic options, depending on the age and weight of the patient, the characteristics of the fracture, and its context. These options include conservative and surgical treatment, which may require the use of osteosynthesis, including an external fixator, elastic stable intramedullary nailing, rigid trochanteric lateral entry intramedullary nail, or submuscular plate.

23.1 Introduction

Femoral shaft fractures represent 1.4–1.7% of all fractures in the pediatric population [1, 2]. They are more common in men than in women, with a ratio of 2.5. The annual incidence is 16–19 per 100,000 infants [3, 4]. This incidence has a bimodal distribution, with a peak between 2 and 4 years of age, and a second peak in adolescence. Child abuse or non-accidental injuries must be ruled out in patients under 5 years old, especially when they are not yet walking. In low-energy traumas, it is important to suspect fractures in pathological bone [5].

J. Besomi (✉)
Clínica Alemana de Santiago, Universidad del Desarrollo, Santiago, Chile
e-mail: jbesomi@alemana.cl

E. Gordon
Shriners Children's St. Louis, Washington University School of Medicine,
St Louis, MO, USA
e-mail: gordone@wustl.edu

M. Sepúlveda O. (ed.), *Paediatrics Traumatology*,
https://doi.org/10.1007/978-3-031-89482-4_23

23.2 Mechanism of Injury

Femur fractures in patients between 2 and 4 years occur mainly associated with falls, either at ground level, with a torsional mechanism, or from a height. With aging, sports injuries involving high energy become relevant. In adolescence, the usual mechanism is high-energy trauma, such as car accidents or associated with extreme sports.

The iliopsoas muscle pulls the proximal fragment in flexion and external rotation, while the adductor and hamstring muscles are responsible for the shortening and varus of the distal fragment.

Femoral shaft fractures, due to the distensibility of the thigh compartments, rarely present an associated compartment syndrome or a neurovascular injury. However, it is of great relevance to perform an adequate clinical evaluation of the neurological function of the sciatic and femoral nerves, and of the femoral vessels.

23.3 Diagnosis

The anamnesis should include record of the mechanism of injury and the clinical characteristics of the patient. These include pain, functional impotence of the affected limb, with inability to weight-bearing, an increase in thigh volume, and the presence of angular and/or rotational deformity, with shortening of the limb.

The diagnosis is confirmed with femur X-rays in two planes: anteroposterior and lateral. These allow the evaluation of the location of the fracture, characterization, and degree of displacement. It is important that the radiograph includes the ipsilateral hip and knee joints, to rule out associated injuries (Fig. 23.1).

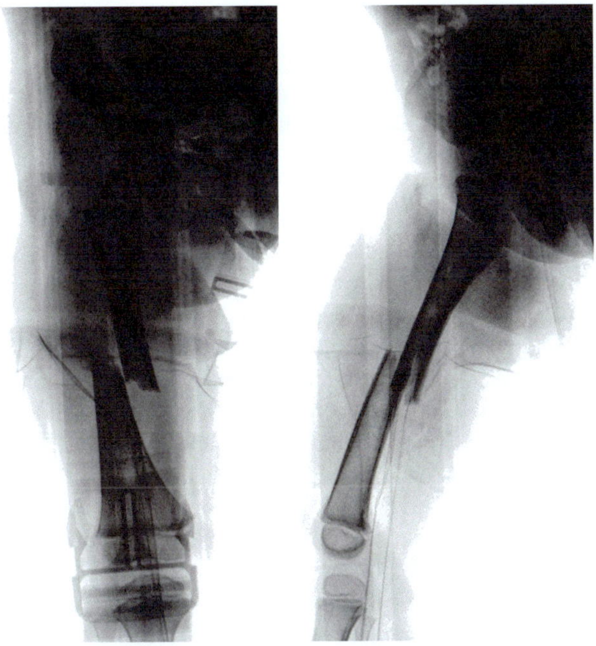

Fig. 23.1 X-ray of the right femur of a 3-year-old girl, in planes anteroposterior and lateral, including adjacent joints, hip, and knee. A diaphyseal fracture of the femur is evident

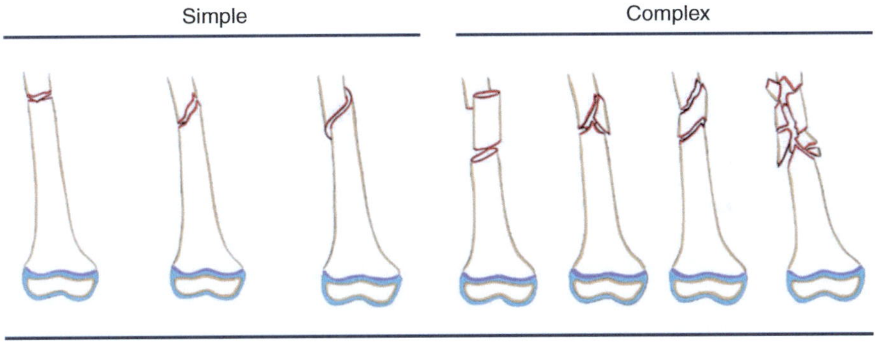

Fig. 23.2 Femur diaphyseal fracture patterns according to AO Trauma: Transverse, oblique, spiroid, segmental, butterfly wing, and comminuted

23.4 Classification

According to the AO classification of pediatric fractures in long bones, they are classified as transverse (line ≤ 30°), oblique or spiral (line ≥ 30°); simple or comminuted (Fig. 23.2).

23.5 Treatment

Broadly speaking, the treatment is divided into conservative treatment (soft tissue traction, Pavlik harnesses, and spica cast) and surgical treatment (use of external fixator, elastic stable intramedullary nailing, rigid trochanteric entry intramedullary nail, and submuscular plate). The choice will fundamentally depend on the patient's age and weight, fracture characteristics, and clinical context (of the patient, availability of instruments and osteosynthesis material, and surgeon's experience). A suggested algorithm for this decision is shown in Fig. 23.3.

In patients under 6 months old, Pavlik harnesses are a good treatment method (Fig. 23.4). The deforming forces of the abductors and psoas position the proximal fragment in flexion, abduction, and slight external rotation. The Pavlik harnesses position the distal fragment in such a way that it reduces with the proximal fragment.

Between 6 months and 2 years, the treatment of choice is closed reduction and immobilization with a spica cast (Fig. 23.5).

Between 2 and 6 years, closed reduction and immobilization with a spica cast are also suitable options and should be discussed with the parents and caregivers, because it may be poorly tolerated, requires special care, and impacts the family.

The spica cast can be bilateral or unilateral, an alternative that in this age range has shown less impact on the family. Recently, treatment with a pre-molded splint has also been reported to be effective in these patients. Elastic stable intramedullary nailing has shown less impact on the family than the spica cast, being indicated in certain circumstances.

It is recommended to explain to the parents the advantages and disadvantages of the treatment alternatives to make the best decision. In polytrauma patients, in cases of shortening greater than 2 cm, multiple fractures or open fracture, reduction and osteosynthesis with elastic stable intramedullary nailing is preferred [6, 7].

Between 6 and 11 years, reduction and fixation with elastic stable intramedullary nailing is the treatment of choice (Fig. 23.6). It is a minimally invasive technique that provides sufficient relative stability to achieve fracture healing, with good

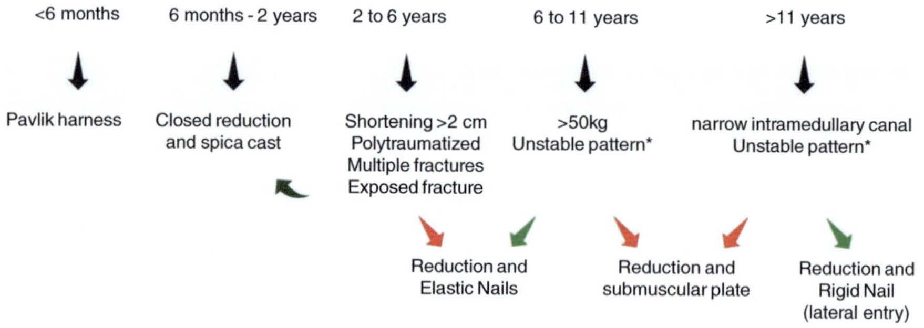

Fig. 23.3 Scheme of an algorithm for the treatment decision of a femur shaft fracture. "Unstable Pattern" is defined as a fracture line long oblique (>60°), a spiral fracture, the presence of bone comminution (>3 fragments), and those very proximal or distal

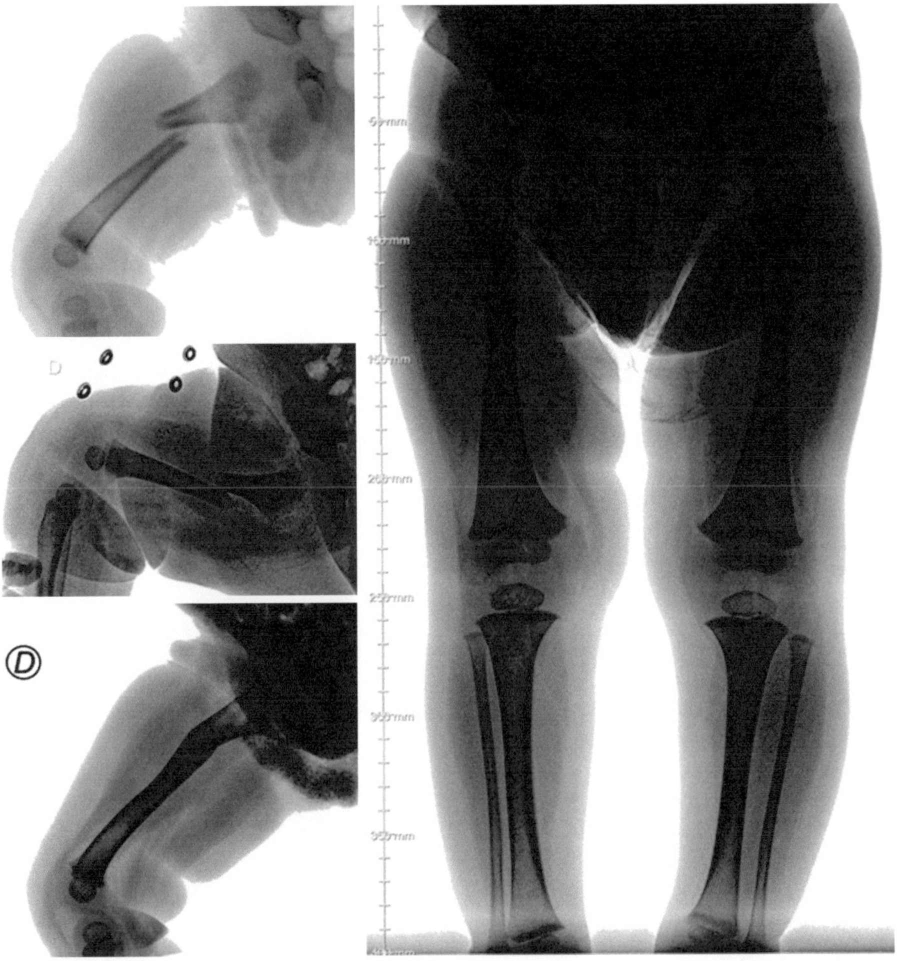

Fig. 23.4 Femur fracture in a 5-month-old child, treated with a Pavlik harness for 4 weeks. Bone healing is evident at 8 months, and without difference in limb length at 18 months after injury

clinical results. Two pre-molded nails are used, retrograde or anterograde, whose diameter is equal to 0.4 of the diameter of the isthmus of the femoral intramedullary canal. The use of endcaps, or caps, has proven useful in preventing displacement [8]. The implants can be in titanium, which offer greater elasticity, or in steel, which have shown in some studies to provide greater rigidity to the fixation and less risk of malunion [9, 10].

A multicenter study, in 230 femur fractures, showed five times more risk of complications (loss of reduction, reoperation, malunion) and worse results when using elastic stable intramedullary nailing in patients older than 11 years and/or weight greater than 50 kg [11]. On the other hand, another study showed a higher risk of shortening and complications in fractures with features with a pattern of

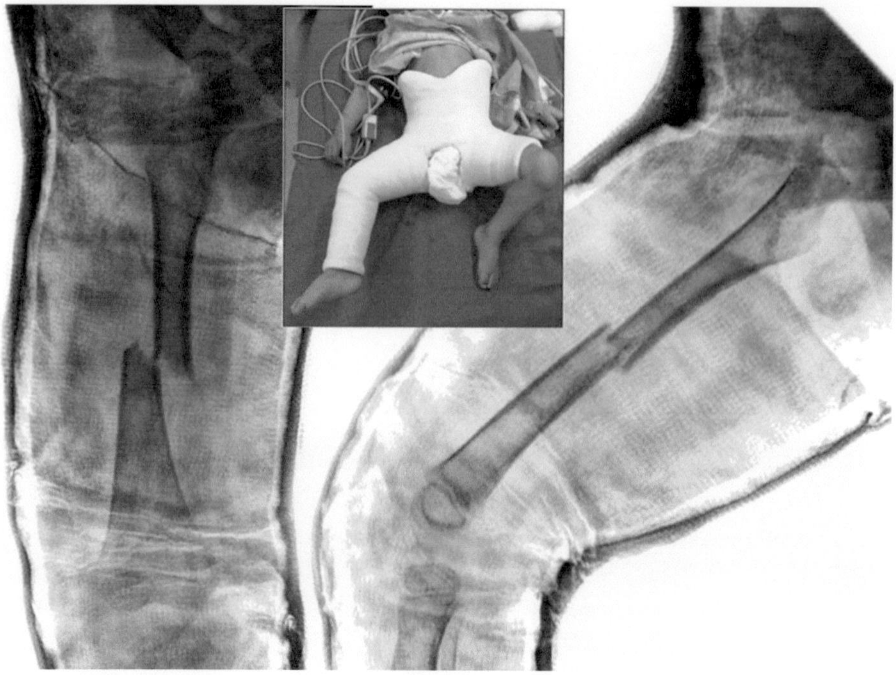

Fig. 23.5 X-rays of the right femur of a 3-year-old girl, with a diaphyseal fracture of the femur, treated with a pelvipedal cast

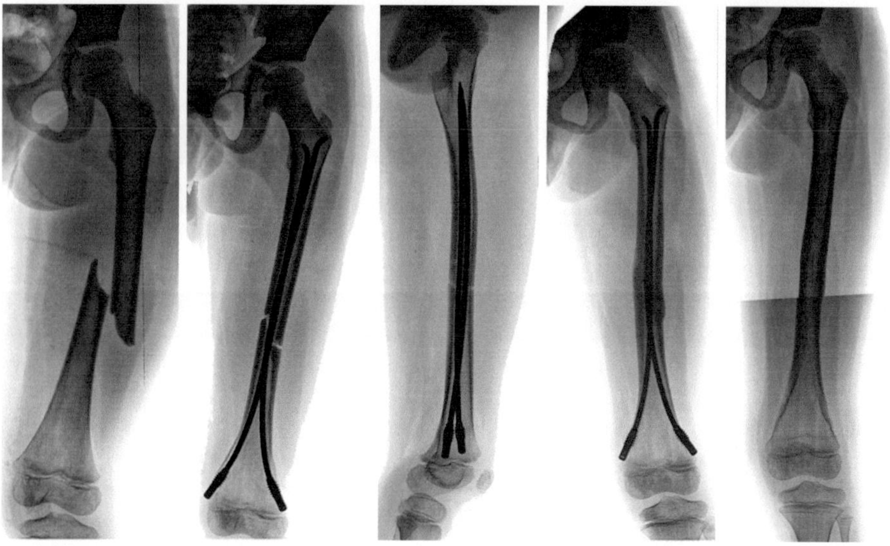

Fig. 23.6 Femur fracture in a 6-year-old child. Closed reduction and stabilization with elastic intramedullary nails, observing consolidation at 5 months. The hardware removal took place after 9 months

longitudinal instability (long oblique, spiral, comminuted) [12]. However, recent studies have shown that the use of elastic stable intramedullary nailing is a safe and effective fixation method for unstable fracture patterns, when properly performed.

Anyway, a good alternative in larger patients, who weigh more than 50 kg and have an unstable fracture pattern (long oblique feature of 0–60°, or spiral, bone comminution, or a very proximal or very distal fracture feature), is reduction and osteosynthesis with submuscular plate with minimally invasive technique (MIPO). A 4.5 mm 12–16 holes LCP plate is usually used in this technique, with 3 proximal and 3 distal screws, which is positioned between the periosteum and the vastus lateralis [13] (Fig. 23.7).

In patients over 11-years-old, the method of choice for stabilizing a femur fracture is the rigid intramedullary nail (IMN)) with a lateral trochanteric entry (Fig. 23.8). It is an osteosynthesis method that allows for early weight-bearing and has a lower risk of angular deformity. This pediatric nail should be used in a lateral entry to avoid the risk of avascular necrosis of the femoral head associated in pediatric patients with the classic entry of the IMN in the piriform fossa, or risky at the level of the apex or tip of the greater trochanter [14]. In cases with a very narrow intramedullary canal, very unstable, proximal or distal fractures, the use of the submuscular plate should be considered as a good alternative for fixation.

The use of the external fixator is useful in damage control, open and unstable fractures, both as a temporary or definitive method. However, as a definitive method, it is associated with more complications compared to other osteosynthesis methods, such as loss of reduction, poor union, new fracture, lower limb discrepancy, and

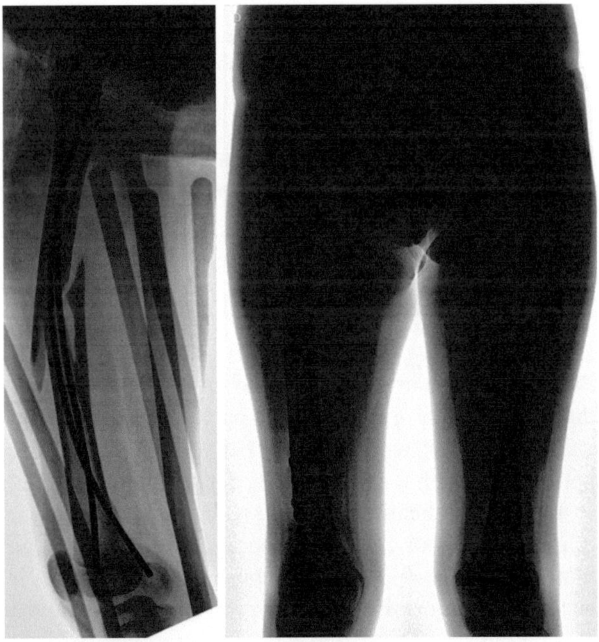

Fig. 23.7 Femur fracture in a 13-year-old girl, initially treated with elastic nails, unstable. Conversion to submuscular plate is performed

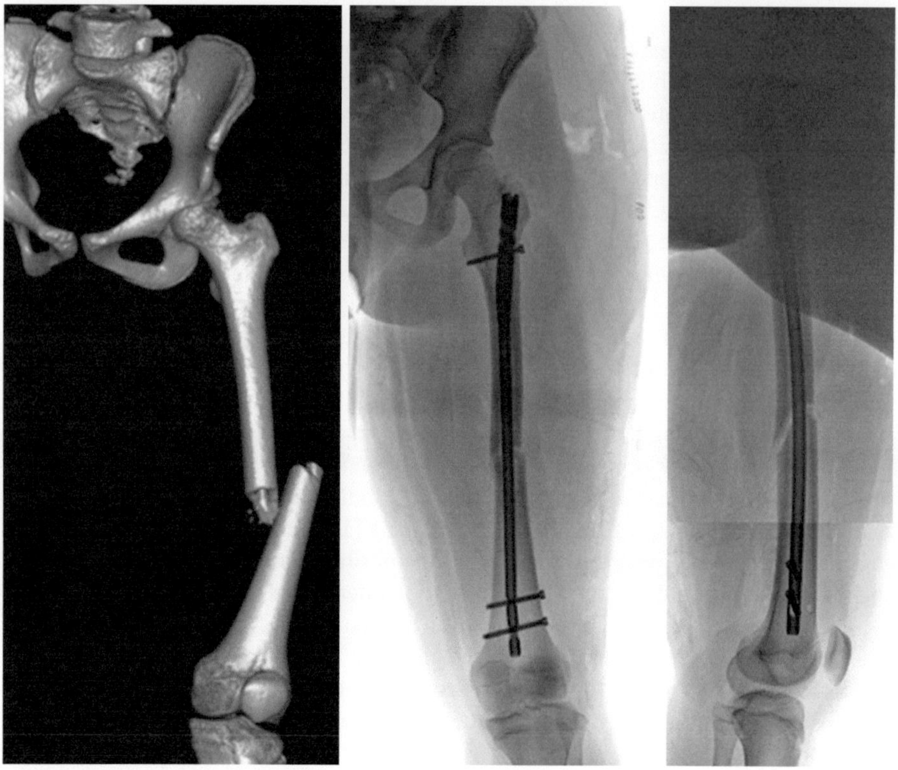

Fig. 23.8 Images of the left femur of an 11-year-old girl who presents a displaced diaphyseal fracture of the femur. Given the patient's weight (75 kg), and diameter of the intramedullary canal, it is decided to stabilize it with a rigid nail, avoiding piriformis or trochanteric entry

longer consolidation time [15, 16]. But, due to the rapid fracture healing in kids, the initial reduction with the external fixation should be as anatomically possible, since many circumstances can lead this to be the definitive treatment.

23.6 Complications

Patients with an immature skeleton may present with bone overgrowth of the femur during the repair process of a fracture, resulting in a difference in length of the lower extremities. An overgrowth of between 7 and 20 mm is described, especially in patients between 2 and 10 years, and within the first 2 years following the fracture.

Other complications include neurovascular injury, compartment syndrome, loss of reduction, poor union, shortening, non-union, discomfort from the osteosynthesis material, and re-fracture. In relation to poor union, it is classically considered as acceptable deformity values of <5–10° varus/valgus, <10–20° ante/recurvatum, <2–2.5 cm shortening, and <10° for rotational deformity.

Avascular necrosis of the femoral head, coxa valga, and narrowing of the femoral neck have been reported as complications of the use of anterograde IMN when the entry is in the piriform fossa or at the apex of the greater trochanter. Not so when using a lateral trochanteric entry [17–19].

23.7 Final Message

Femur fractures in children and adolescents are a challenge for the treating physician, both because of the pain and disability they generate for the patient, and because of the multiple treatment alternatives that exist. The patient's age and weight, the characteristics of the fracture, and the context should be considered when choosing the most appropriate treatment.

It is useful to master the different techniques in order to have a wide range of therapeutic tools, with the aim of offering the patient the best treatment, tailored to their needs. It is important to remember that, the younger the age, the greater the capacity for bone remodeling. Also, non-accidental injuries should be suspected in children under 5 years old, especially when they are not yet walking. Finally, it is important to follow up for at least 2 years from the injury, in order to timely diagnose a difference in length of the lower limbs that could occur, either due to shortening or overgrowth.

23.8 Authors' Recommendations

For the installation of a hip spica cast:

- Perform it in the operating room, using fluoroscopy.
- Position the hip at approximately 60–90° of flexion and 30° of abduction, to reduce the risk of displacement and increase comfort.
- Mold the cast with forces in recurvatum and valgus, taking care not to compress the popliteal fossa.
- Hip spica/pelvic-thigh cast, that is, hip spica on the side affected and pelvic-thigh cast on the contralateral side.

For a good elastic stable intramedullary nailing:

- Use them in the appropriate indications. Avoid using them in patients over 11years old, or over 50 kg in weight.
- Reduce with the use of traction table in older patients, and use of a roll under the thigh in younger patients.
- Follow the surgical technique precisely, with good choice of size and prior molding of the implants.

- To avoid rotational deformity, it is recommended to leave both lower limbs in the surgical field to have contralateral comparison and take a Dunn radioscopic projection at 90° comparative to evaluate [20, 21].

For the rigid CEM with lateral trochanteric entry:

- It is an effective and safe method to use from 8 years until skeletal maturity.
- Perform lateral trochanteric entry, moving away from the apex of the greater trochanter to avoid milling in the piriform fossa.
- It is not necessary to mill the canal to the endomedullary cortical bone. In children and adolescents, the fracture consolidates faster, so large diameter nails that occupy the entire endomedullary canal are not required.

References

1. Kocher MS, Sink EL, Blasier RD, Luhmann SL, Mehlman CT, Scher DM, et al. Treatment of pediatric diaphyseal femur fractures. J Am Acad Orthop Surg. 2009;17(11):718–25. https://doi.org/10.5435/00124635-200911000-00006.
2. McCartney D, Hinton A, Heinrich SD. Operative stabilization of pediatric femur fractures. Orthop Clin North Am. 1994;25(4):635–50.
3. Jv H, Svensson T, Blomqvist P, Haglund-Åkerlind Y, Janarv PM. Incidence and trends in femur shaft fractures in Swedish children between 1987 and 2005. J Pediatr Orthop. 2011;31(5):512–9. https://doi.org/10.1097/BPO.0b013e31821f9027.
4. Hinton RY, Lincoln A, Crockett MM, Sponseller P, Smith G. Fractures of the femoral shaft in children. Incidence, mechanisms, and sociodemographic risk factors. J Bone Joint Surg Am. 1999;81(4):500–9. https://doi.org/10.2106/00004623-199904000-00007.
5. Kasser JR, Beaty JM. Fractures of the diaphysis. In: Rockwood CA, Wilkins KE, editors. Rockwood and Wilkins' fractures in children. Philadelphia, PA: Lippincott-Raven; 2010. p. 797–841.
6. Gordon JE, Anderson JT, Schoenecker PL, Dobbs MB, Luhmann SJ, Hoernschemeyer DG. Treatment of femoral fractures in children aged two to six. Bone Joint J. 2020;102-B(8):1056–61. https://doi.org/10.1302/0301-620X.102B8.BJJ-2019-1060.R3.
7. Heffernan MJ, Gordon JE, Sabatini CS, Keeler KA, Lehmann CL, O'Donnell JC, et al. Treatment of femur fractures in young children: a multicenter comparison of flexible intramedullary nails to spica casting in young children aged 2 to 6 years. J Pediatr Orthop. 2015;35(2):126–9. https://doi.org/10.1097/BPO.0000000000000268.
8. Slongo T, Audigé L, Hunter JB, Berger SM. Clinical evaluation of end caps in elastic stable intramedullary nailing of femoral and tibial shaft fractures in children. Eur J Trauma Emerg Surg. 2011;37(3):305. https://doi.org/10.1007/s00068-011-0091-8.
9. Rathjen KE, Riccio AI, De La Garza D. Stainless steel flexible intramedullary fixation of unstable femoral shaft fractures in children. J Pediatr Orthop. 2007;27(4):432–41. https://doi.org/10.1097/01.bpb.0000271322.48987.46.
10. Wall EJ, Jain V, Vora V, Mehlman CT, Crawford AH. Complications of titanium and stainless steel elastic nail fixation of pediatric femoral fractures. J Bone Joint Surg Am. 2008;90(6):1305–13. https://doi.org/10.2106/JBJS.G.00328.
11. Moroz LA, Launay F, Kocher MS, Newton PO, Frick SL, Sponseller PD, et al. Titanium elastic nailing of fractures of the femur in children. Predictors of complications and poor outcome. J Bone Joint Surg Br. 2006;88(10):1361–6. https://doi.org/10.1302/0301-620X.88B10.17517.
12. Sink EL, Faro F, Polousky J, Flynn K, Gralla J. Decreased complications of pediatric femur fractures with a change in management. J Pediatr Orthop. 2010;30(7):633–7. https://doi.org/10.1097/BPO.0b013e3181efb89d.

13. Abdelgawad AA, Sieg RN, Laughlin MD, Shunia J, Kanlic EM. Submuscular bridge plating for complex pediatric femur fractures is reliable. Clin Orthop Relat Res. 2013;471(9):2797–807. https://doi.org/10.1007/s11999-013-2931-9.
14. Beaty JH, Austin SM, Warner WC, Canale ST, Nichols L. Interlocking intramedullary nailing of femoral-shaft fractures in adolescents: preliminary results and complications. J Pediatr Orthop. 1994;14(2):178–83. https://doi.org/10.1097/01241398-199403000-00009.
15. Ramseier LE, Janicki JA, Weir S, Narayanan UG. Femoral fractures in adolescents: a comparison of four methods of fixation. J Bone Joint Surg Am. 2010;92(5):1122–9. https://doi.org/10.2106/JBJS.H.01735.
16. Kocher MS, Sink EL, Blasier RD, Luhmann SJ, Mehlman CT, Scher DM, et al. American Academy of Orthopaedic Surgeons clinical practice guideline on treatment of pediatric diaphyseal femur fracture. J Bone Joint Surg Am. 2010;92(8):1790–2. https://doi.org/10.2106/JBJS.J.00137.
17. MacNeil JA, Francis A, El-Hawary R. A systematic review of rigid, locked, intramedullary nail insertion sites and avascular necrosis of the femoral head in the skeletally immature. J Pediatr Orthop. 2011;31(4):377–80. https://doi.org/10.1097/BPO.0b013e3182172613.
18. González-Herranz P, Burgos-Flores J, Rapariz JM, Lopez-Mondejar JA, Ocete JG, Amaya S. Intramedullary nailing of the femur in children. Effects on its proximal end. J Bone Joint Surg Br. 1995;77(2):262–6.
19. Raney EM, Ogden JA, Grogan DP. Premature greater trochanteric epiphysiodesis secondary to intramedullary femoral rodding. J Pediatr Orthop. 1993;13(4):516–20. https://doi.org/10.1097/01241398-199307000-00018.
20. Gwyn DT, Olney BW, Dart BR, Czuwala PJ. Rotational control of various pediatric femur fractures stabilized with titanium elastic intramedullary nails. J Pediatr Orthop. 2004;24(2):172–7. https://doi.org/10.1097/00004694-200403000-00007.
21. Frei B, Mayr J, de Bernardis G, Camathias C, Holland-Cunz S, Rutz E. Elastic stabile intramedullary nailing (ESIN) of diaphyseal femur fractures in children and adolescents: a strobe-compliant study. Medicine (Baltimore). 2019;98(14):e15085. https://doi.org/10.1097/MD.0000000000015085.

Chapter 24
Distal Femur Fractures

Claudio Meneses and Rodrigo Yáñez

Traumatic injuries at the level of the distal femur are of low frequency. However, due to the presence of one of the most active growth plates in the body, these injuries can evolve with serious alterations during the patient's growth. Therefore, their correct identification and appropriate management are relevant for the future of these patients. A large number are caused by high-energy mechanisms, so their approach is made in the context of a polytrauma, floating knee or associated neurovascular injuries, serious situations that must be identified and corrected along with the management of the fracture.

The initial radiographic study needs to be complemented with computed tomography (CT scan) if there is suspicion of articular surface involvement, or with magnetic resonance imaging (MRI) if there are doubts about a growth plate and ligamentous or meniscal injury. The therapeutic goal will be to recover the growth plate and joint anatomy and avoid causing further damage with the fracture reduction maneuvers or with the stabilization methods. The follow-up of this injury in the pediatric population should be carried out for at least 2 years, which makes these injuries be considered differently from other usual fractures in children evaluated by the orthopedic surgeon.

C. Meneses
Clínica Las Condes, Hospital Clínico San Borja Arriarán, Universidad de Chile, Santiago, Chile

R. Yáñez (✉)
Pontificia Universidad Católica de Chile, Complejo Asistencial Dr. Sótero del Río, Santiago, Chile
e-mail: rayanezp@uc.cl

M. Sepúlveda O. (ed.), *Paediatrics Traumatology*,
https://doi.org/10.1007/978-3-031-89482-4_24

24.1 Introduction

Distal femur fractures represent less than 1% of all children's fractures [1, 2]. Of femur fractures, it is the second in frequency after the fracture of the diaphysis [3]. Growth plate injuries of the distal femur represent 2% of all growth cartilage injuries [4], and 7% of those occurring in lower limbs [5]. Despite being infrequent, they are associated with a high percentage of complications, as they have a 50% incidence of growth alterations [6], which can be detected early from the first 6 months after the trauma in most cases [7], but can be evidenced up to 2 years after this.

24.2 Pathophysiology

Distal femur fractures usually occur as a result of a high-energy mechanism, either a car accident or during sports practice. The growth plate injury of the distal femur was initially called "cartwheel fracture", as it was caused by a force with the foot stuck in the spokes of a moving cartwheel [8].

The shape of the distal femur growth plate is wavy (Fig. 24.1), so the shearing forces produced by the fracture mechanism can lead to structural alterations of all the layers of the growth plate. This is associated with a high risk of growth plate bar formation [9].

At birth, the distal femur growth plate is flat. Until 2-years-old, the growth plate maintains this configuration, so a growth plate fracture will mainly damage the hypertrophic zone, causing little growth alteration (Fig. 24.2).

During growth, the growth plate develops a "W" wavy shape, with four convex quadrants of the metaphysis that fit with the concave surfaces of the epiphysis (Fig. 24.3). Therefore, after 2-years-old, due to its wavy shape, the fracture lines pass through various areas of the physis, regardless of the fracture classification, which causes a high incidence of physis growth alterations [10].

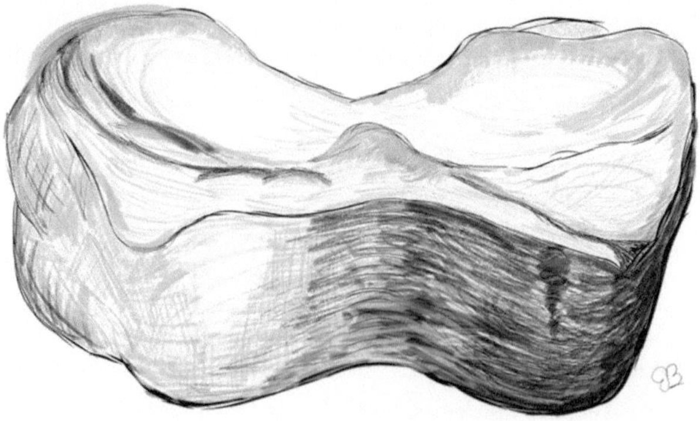

Fig. 24.1 Scheme of the undulations at the level of the physis of the distal femur

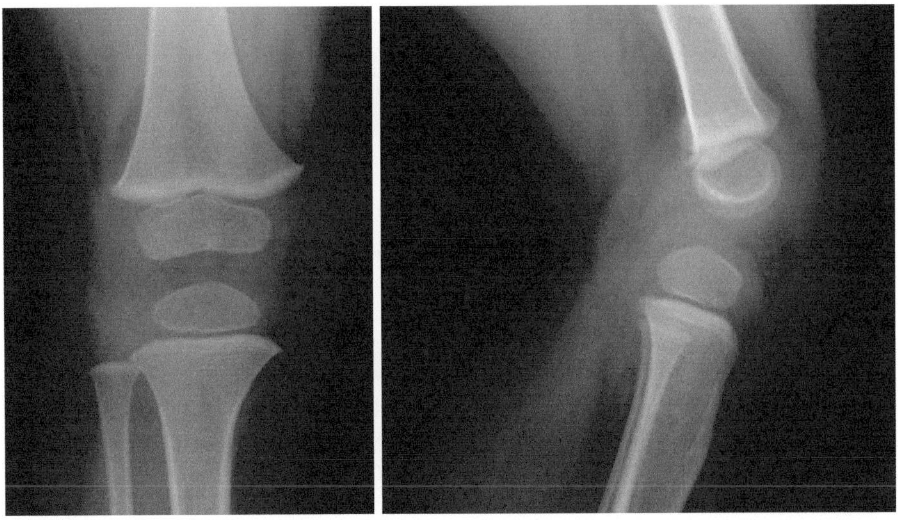

Fig. 24.2 Anteroposterior and lateral knee X-ray projections of a 3-year-old boy, where few undulations are evident, straight ossified line in the sagittal plane

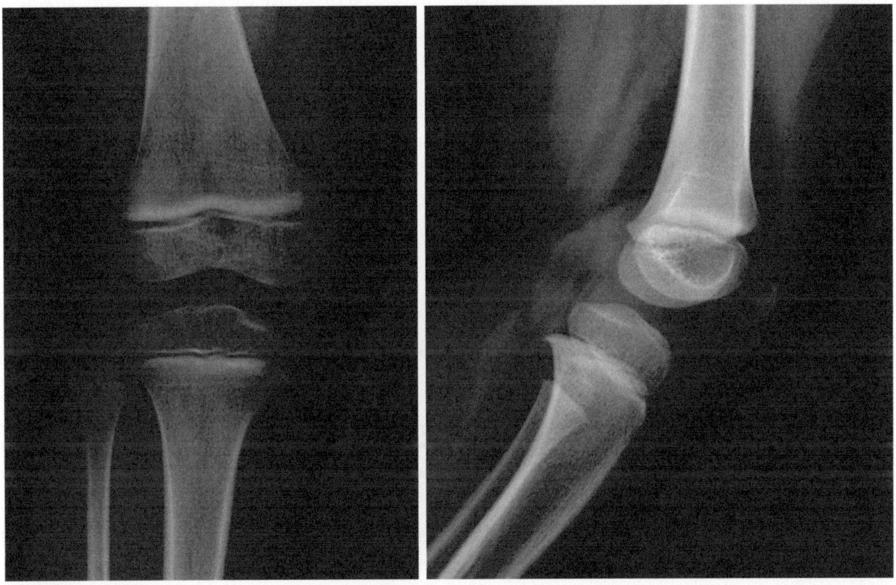

Fig. 24.3 Anteroposterior and lateral X-ray views of the right knee of a child 6 years old, with "W" shaped physis

We must also consider the high activity of this physis and its significant contribution to longitudinal growth. It gives up to 70% of the longitudinal growth of the femur and up to 35–40% of the limb [11, 12]. This segment grows in length an average of 9 mm per year, reaching during puberty 10–12 mm per year. The patient's age and the subsequent remaining growth should be considered in the potential for deformity or difference in limb length resulting from trauma [13].

24.3 Diagnosis

For the study of this injury, X-rays are taken in anteroposterior and lateral projections of the segment, which should cover the entire femur, including the hip [6]. Oblique knee projections can be helpful in identifying minimally displaced fractures [14]. Historically, X-ray on traction was requested in the face of an unclear diagnosis; however, this practice was abandoned due to the pain it caused patients [15], unnecessary given the existence of better alternative study methods.

A CT scan can be performed in case of suspicion of physeal injuries [7] and in injuries with articular involvement, which require adequately characterizing their fragments and displacement to define treatment (Fig. 24.4).

Magnetic resonance imaging (MRI) will be useful for evaluating ligamentous and intra-articular injuries, especially associated with sports-related trauma [6], which may require surgical intervention. It is also useful in patients with limited ossification of the epiphysis, in hidden fractures (Fig. 24.5) or in case of suspicion of periosteal entrapment at the fracture [15], which can complicate reduction maneuvers or cause growth alterations.

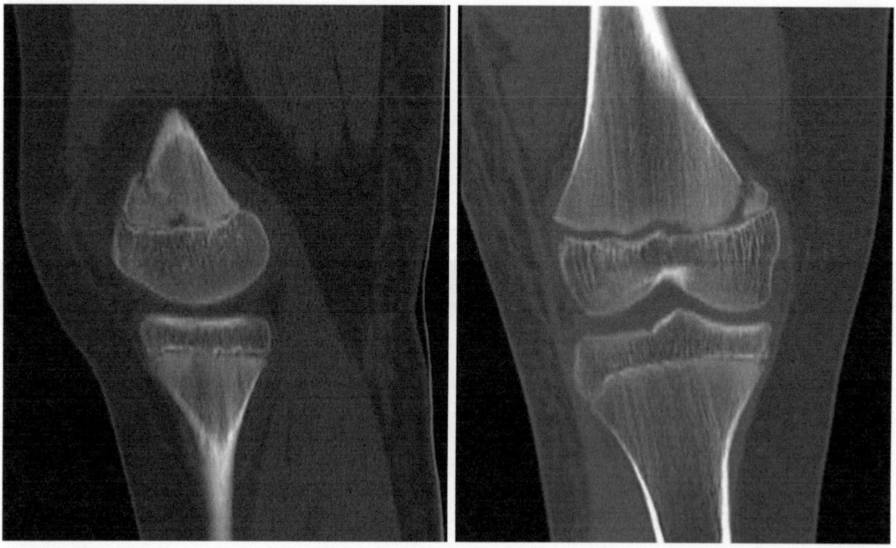

Fig. 24.4 CT scan of the knee demonstrating a Salter-Harris Type 2, non-articular fracture of the distal femur

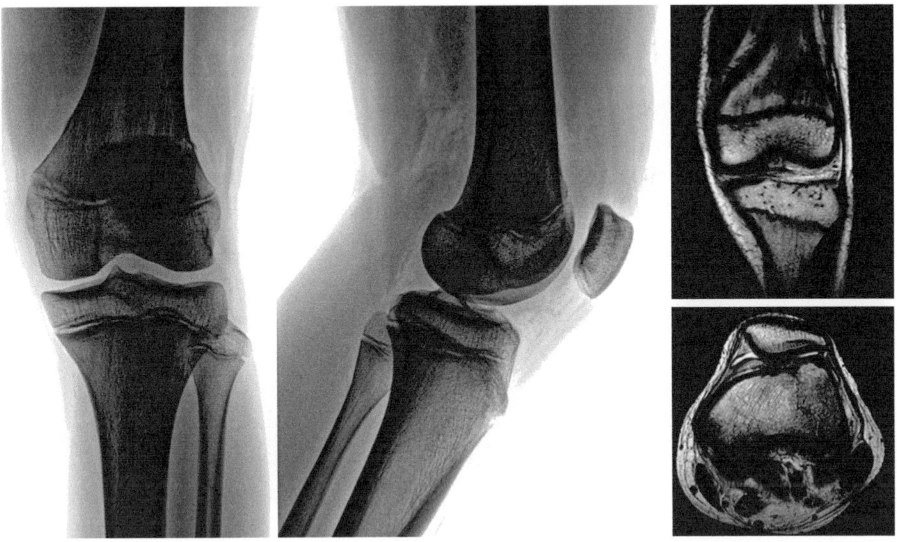

Fig. 24.5 X-ray views of a patient with suspected distal femur injury, which is demonstrated with magnetic resonance imaging

Given the association of this injury with a high-energy mechanism, other injuries must be ruled out, applying the trauma protocols of each institution, which should at least consider the radiographic study of the cervical spine, chest, and pelvis. In addition, due to the risk of vascular injury, it is important to evaluate the pulses distal to the injured segment. If there is any doubt about good irrigation, a Doppler ultrasound or a CT angiography of the limb should be requested [16].

24.4 Classification

Distal femur fractures can be divided into 3 groups: a. metaphyseal fractures; b. physeal fractures; and c. epiphyseal fractures [17].

Fractures at the level of the metaphysis represent 12% of femur fractures [18]. A non-accidental injury should be suspected when observed in children under 1 year old or who do not walk [19]. It is also common to find fractures in pathological bone in this area. They can be "buckle" or "torus" fractures, complete or multifragmentary (Fig. 24.6).

For physeal fractures, the most commonly used classification is that of Salter and Harris [20]. This divides fractures into 5 types (Fig. 24.7):

Type I: There is a separation through the physis (epiphysiolysis) without involvement of the adjacent metaphysis or epiphysis. It is the least common type and can be difficult to diagnose if there is no displacement. In such cases, suspicion

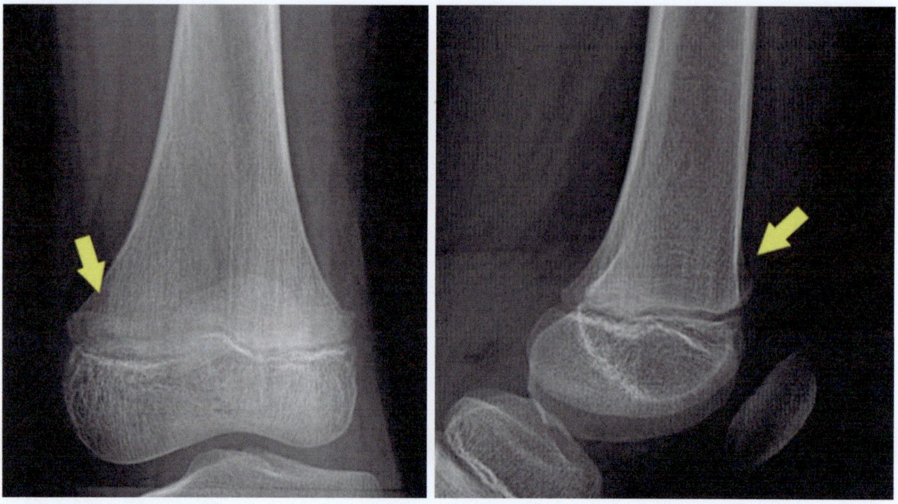

Fig. 24.6 "Labrum" or "torus" fracture of the distal femur

should be raised in patients who cannot bear their weight and have circumferential pain in the physis area [7].

Type II: This is the most common physeal fracture of the distal femur. The fracture line crosses the physis before exiting obliquely through one side of the metaphysis. Displacement usually occurs toward the side of the metaphyseal fragment. Up to about 58% of growth disturbance is described in this type of injury.

Type III: This is a fracture through the physis that exits through the epiphysis into the joint. It can be a simple or multifragmentary.

Type IV: This is an epiphyseo-metaphyseal injury. It is an intra-articular vertical fracture that passes through the metaphysis, physis, and epiphysis. Its fracture feature can be simple or complex.

Type V: This is a compressive fracture of the physis, resulting from an axial force.

Finally, intra-articular fractures are osteochondral or chondral injuries resulting from a direct blow with the knee flexed or shear forces associated with a patellar dislocation, in which case the lateral femoral condyle is affected [14].

It is important to know the term "Floating Knee," which is used to describe injuries to the ipsilateral femur and tibia, with a fracture anywhere in both bones. It is a rare injury, caused by a high-energy accident and often accompanied by injuries in other body areas. There are no studies that assess its exact incidence, but it is more common in men than in women. On physical examination, there will be an increase in volume and pain in both segments of the lower limb, shortening, and deformity. The neurovascular status may be affected, so it requires a thorough evaluation in this regard. It can be associated with ligamentous injuries of the knee, so instability of this can be found on examination [21]. The importance of this injury is given by the urgent need for stabilization, to reduce the incidence of complications.

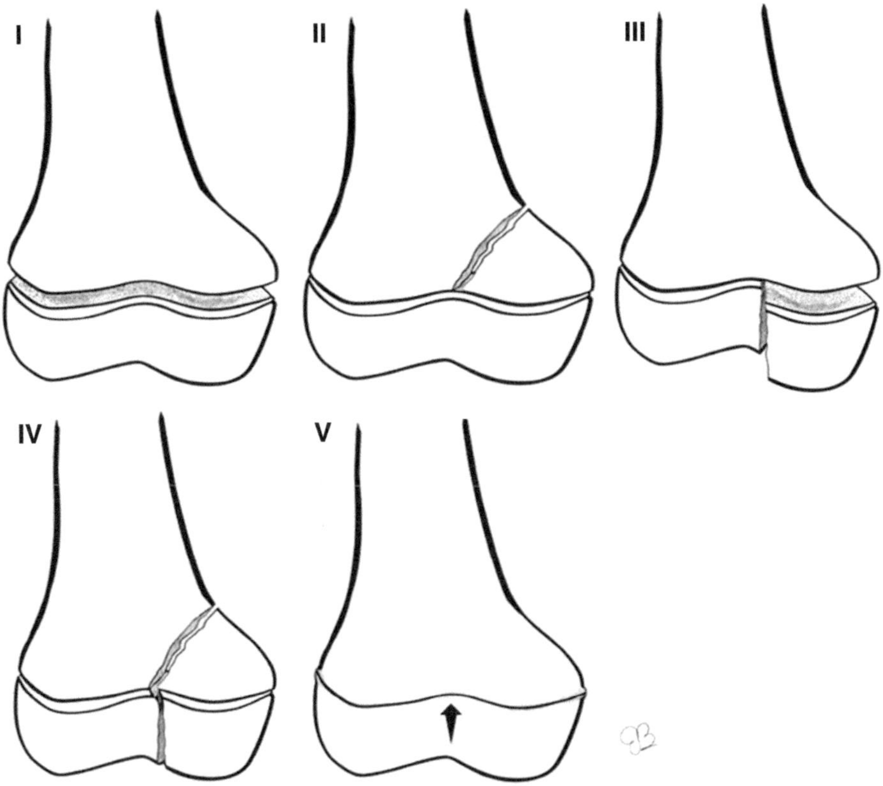

Fig. 24.7 Salter and Harris classification for distal femur fractures

24.5 Treatment

To make a decision in the management of these fractures, multiple factors must be evaluated, including the patient's age and weight, the location of the fracture (metaphyseal, physeal, or epiphyseal), its type (complete or incomplete, displaced or non-displaced), the presence of associated injuries (polytrauma, patient with neurological alterations, dysplastic bone pathology, floating knee, soft tissue injury, open fracture, vascular damage, and intra-articular injuries), the therapeutic resources available, and of course, the experience of the treating team.

There are general principles to consider for the treatment of these injuries:

The distal physis of the femur contributes with 70% of the longitudinal growth of this bone, so its damage, either by trauma or by the chosen treatment, can cause a significant sequel, such as axis alterations or difference in limb length, which should be warned to the parents or guardians of the minor immediately.

Anatomical reduction will always be better than consolidation in a bad position, but reduction maneuvers should be gentle and within the first few days. Forced or late maneuvers (more than 7 days) are associated with greater physeal damage.

Stabilization through osteosynthesis (Kirschner wires, plates with screws, cannulated screws, intramedullary nails, or external fixator) will be necessary when we face displaced fractures that require closed or open reduction, polytrauma environment that requires optimizing patient care, presence of a "Floating Knee," fracture in pathological bone, open fracture, and associated vascular injury.

The use of long leg cast, or a knee brace, is necessary in most cases, especially in those where we use nonstable methods for fixation, such as Kirschner wires. The period of immobilization varies according to age and the appearance of bone callus in radiological controls, usually between 4 and 8 weeks.

Support for rehabilitation is essential to recover joint mobility of the knee and achieve muscle strengthening and early reeducation of gait.

24.5.1 Metaphyseal Fractures

Incomplete metaphyseal fractures (a "torus" or "greenstick") and complete metaphyseal fractures without displacement (angulation less than 5°) are managed conservatively with a long leg cast for 6–8 weeks. These fractures are considered stable, but to give greater rotational control to the installed cast, it is advisable to install an anti-rotational bar under the ankle for the first 3 weeks, or a one leg spica cast.

In metaphyseal fractures with angulation of more than 5° in any plane and in displaced/overridden fractures, closed reduction should be performed, or if not achieved easily, open reduction under general anesthesia, and stabilization with a long leg cast. The exception may be a fracture angled in a minor with severe underlying neurological pathology, without walking ability, where the angulation produced does not alter his baseline situation or could even be beneficial to improve his posture. The reduction under general anesthesia should be early, and if there is a delay of more than 24 h to perform the procedure, the installation of a soft tissue traction system is recommended to manage pain and prevent further displacement, while waiting for definitive resolution. This system is installed with traction from the leg horizontally to the bed and a padded sling under the slightly flexed knee, which pulls toward the ceiling.

In the case of metaphyseal fractures that remain unstable after their closed reduction, stabilization with percutaneous Kirschner wires is recommended. If the displaced fracture is irreducible or presents an associated arterial injury that requires repair, open reduction and fixation with osteosynthesis is ideal. The recommended approach to reduce the fracture is lateral, but if it is for arterial repair, a posteromedial approach is recommended to evaluate the blood vessels in the region. After reduction, fixation can be performed using Kirschner wires 2–2.5 mm in diameter, in a crossed configuration, which is especially useful in children under 8-years-old. A long leg cast or knee brace should be added until consolidation is verified, between 6 and 8 weeks approximately, depending on the type of fracture and age of the patient.

In older or larger patients, a system of elastic stable intramedullary nails can be used, inserted anterogradely from the proximal femur (Fig. 24.8) or the use of low profile osteosynthesis plates. Among these, there are pediatric designs that allow fixing the

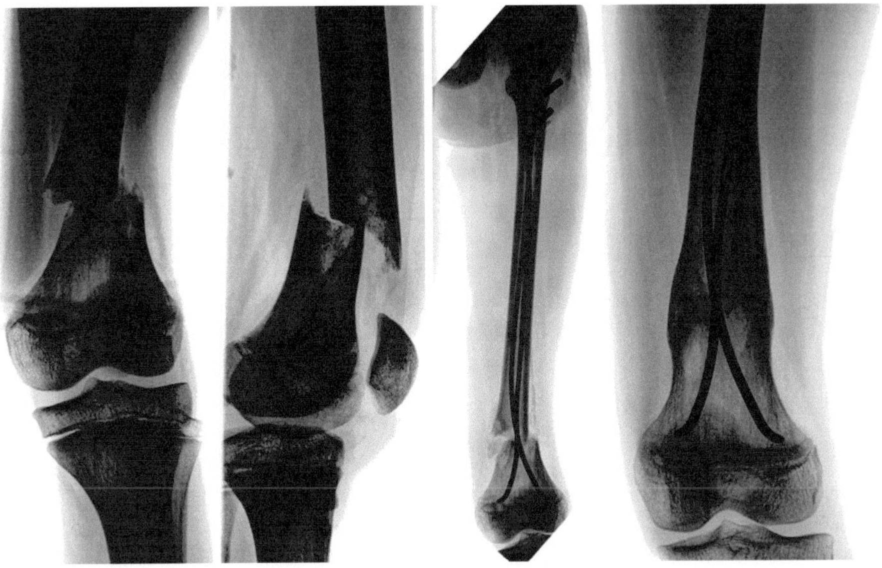

Fig. 24.8 Distal femur fracture in pathological bone (essential bone cyst), stabilized with antegrade elastic nails

distal metaphysis and the diaphysis without compromising the growth of the physis. Recently, an LCP plate for the distal femur has been developed that has a telescopic system between a portion of fixation proximal to the fracture and another portion of epiphyseal distal fixation, which allows the plate to slide along with bone growth.

Finally, there is the option of stabilization with external fixation of this type of fracture, especially useful for displaced fractures in the context of open fractures, polytrauma, or floating knee. Schanz screws of appropriate size should be used, from the lateral side, leaving 1 cm of distal metaphysis free to reduce the risk of physeal damage, and at least 2 Schanz screws should be installed in the distal fragment. A temporary fixation with a Kirschner wire in the operating room can be performed to maintain the reduction while the external fixator is installed. Fractures treated with this type of osteosynthesis can be mobilized and partial load started early according to patient tolerance. Its removal should be performed when stable consolidation is evidenced on radiographs, which time can vary depending on the type of fracture (between 6 and 8 weeks in closed fractures, and between 8 and 12 weeks in open fractures).

24.5.2 Physeal and Epiphyseal Fractures

For the treatment of fractures of the distal femoral physis, it is essential to restore the anatomy, both at the joint level and at the physis level, in order to reduce possible sequelae, both in joint function and in the growth of the affected segment. Reduction maneuvers should be performed gently and as soon as possible, under the effect of general anesthesia, as the physis damage depends both on the energy involved in the trauma, and on the forced reduction maneuvers. Follow-up checks after treatment should continue for 2 or more years, to evaluate the existence of sequelae from physis damage.

For those non-displaced physis fractures, conservative treatment is possible, by immobilizing with a long leg cast for 4–6 weeks, restricting weight-bearing on the injured limb by using crutches [14].

For displaced Salter-Harris Type I or II physis fractures, it is necessary to achieve a reduction, usually in a closed manner, and depending on the stability achieved, it will be immobilized with a long leg cast or it will be stabilized with Kirschner wires or compressive screws. The reduction maneuver consists of longitudinal traction, associating knee flexion if the epiphyseal fragment is anterior, or knee extension if the displacement is posterior. Radioscopic control should be obtained in strict anteroposterior and lateral planes of the knee. We must always confirm adequate distal perfusion after reduction, and subsequent immobilization should avoid extreme flexion or extension to reduce the risk of neurovascular damage.

If after the reduction, a stability test of the fragments is performed, and loss of reduction is observed, it should be stabilized with osteosynthesis. For Salter-Harris Type I fractures and for Type II with a small metaphyseal fragment, the use of crossed Kirschner wires is recommended (Fig. 24.9), whose distal ends are bent, and can be left under or outside the skin, as their removal will usually be along with the cast, at 6 weeks. Those Type 2 with a larger metaphyseal fragment, the recommended fixation is with 1 or 2 screws parallel to the physis, without compromising it, ideally with cannulated screw technique (Fig. 24.10).

In Salter-Harris Type III or IV physis fractures, which present articular involvement, open reduction with arthrotomy should be performed in most cases, and stabilized with internal fixation. Intraoperative arthroscopic support helps to reduce the size of the approach to be performed. After the anatomical reduction, the fracture should be fixed with 1 or 2 epiphyseal cannulated screws, parallel to the physis line.

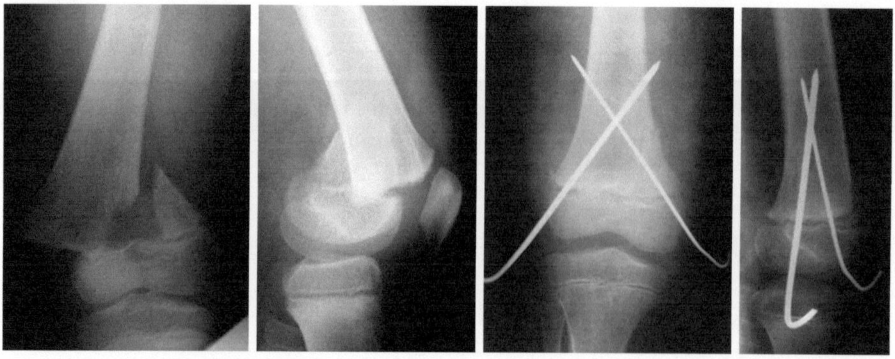

Fig. 24.9 Salter-Harris Type 2 distal femur fracture, displaced. Closed reduction and fixation with percutaneous Kirschner wires were performed

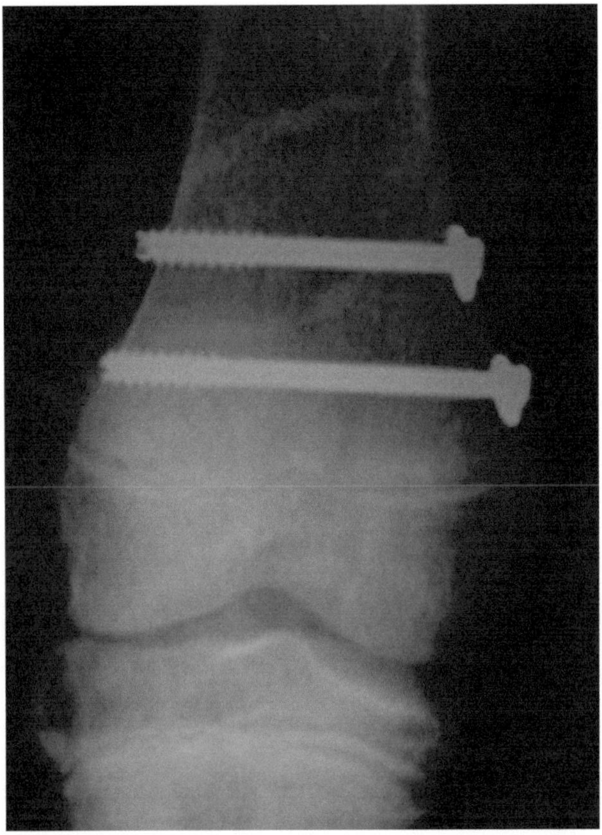

Fig. 24.10 Salter and Harris 2 type distal femur fracture, with a wide metaphyseal fragment that allows fixation with cannulated screws

The anatomical reference for the installation of screws at the level of the distal femoral epiphysis is the epiphyseal triangle in the lateral projection, which is delimited above by the physis line, posteriorly by the Blumensaat line and anteriorly by the trochlea depression (Fig. 24.11).

In those Type IV fractures with a larger metaphyseal fragment, a metaphyseal screw can be added. The screws should be installed with interfragmentary compression technique. The segment is left immobilized with a long leg cast or knee brace, avoiding weight-bearing for 4–5 weeks.

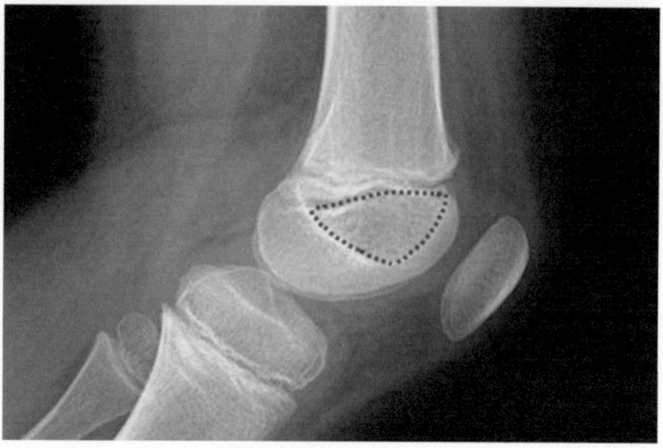

Fig. 24.11 Limits for screw insertion at the level of the distal epiphysis femoral, in the lateral plane

24.6 Complications

The alteration of growth due to damage to the distal femoral physis is a common complication, producing differences in length or axis alterations. As we previously mentioned, this physis is one of the most active in the body, contributing around 35–40% of the longitudinal growth of the lower extremity, around 9 mm of longitudinal growth per year. Therefore, the patient's age is a determining factor in the prognosis, for the projection of the growth alteration.

Fractures with Type I or II features, which in other bone segments rarely cause alterations in physis growth, are associated with 30–70% of complications in this area [22]. The physeal damage can cause an asymmetric angular deformity in the limb or a difference in limbs length, the management of which will depend on the projection made for the alteration at the end of growth. Usually, in case of a difference in length of lower limbs less than 2 cm, the management can be the use of a lift in the shoe of the affected limb. If this difference is projected between 2 and 5 cm, a physiodesis of the contralateral segment can be recommended. Finally, if a difference greater than 5 cm is projected, it is recommended to perform a bone lengthening of the segment, or a combination of procedures [14].

If a physeal bar occurs and is identified, it is recommended to perform a resection of it if it is less than 50% of the physeal area, especially in those of peripheral location, in children with more than 2 years of remaining growth. The ideal examination to study the structure of the physeal bar is the MRI, determining its size and location. For the management of an established angular deformity, the usual correction will be through a corrective osteotomy [14].

Lastly, neurovascular injury is one of the most feared complications associated with this injury and must be identified from the beginning. It requires the case to be approached in conjunction with other specialists and limits the choice of conservative management, with the external fixator being the method of choice to achieve rapid stability of the segment, with the surgical field free for secondary procedures [16].

24.7 Final Message

Distal femur fractures are low frequency injuries in the pediatric population, but in a high percentage occur in the context of polytrauma, or with associated injuries such as "floating knee" or neurovascular injury that modify their approach.

Those fractures with physeal involvement have a high percentage of a secondary growth alteration (30–70%), whose cause can be the initial trauma or iatrogenic. Patients should be monitored for at least 2 years, and in many cases, it is necessary to perform additional procedures for the correction of the sequelae.

Injuries with joint involvement (Salter-Harris Type III or IV) displaced must be reduced to recover the anatomy, both in physeal line as in the joint. Intraoperative arthroscopic support allows minimal approaches for reduction and fixation.

After reduction and stabilization, it should be maintained with an immobilization system for 4–8 weeks (except if an external fixator is used) depending on the age. Weight-bearing on the affected limb should be avoided for at least 4 weeks.

24.8 Authors' Recommendations

- For conservative treatment with long leg cast immobilization, it is recommended to install it with semi-flexion of the knee of 20–30°, for non-displaced fractures, ensuring that no weight-bearing for 4 weeks. Then, support with partial weight-bearing immobilization.
- If the fracture requires reduction, this should be done in the operating room under the effect of general anesthesia, with radiographic support. The maneuvers should be gentle and always evaluate the circulatory condition after the reduction.
- For internal fixation in patients under 8 years old or less than 30 kg in weight, it may be sufficient with 2 crossed Kirschner wires of 2–2.5 mm in diameter. In older patients, a more stable system is required, such as the use of cannulated screws, pediatric LCP plates, or external fixator.
- After 2 months, full weight-bearing and physiotherapy rehabilitation are authorized. Subsequent controls should be maintained for at least 2 years, to assess the possibility of physeal damage and growth alteration.
- For fractures with articular involvement, arthroscopic support is useful to minimize surgical approaches and perform drainage of the associated hemarthrosis.

References

1. Peterson HA, Madhok R, Benson JT, Ilstrup DM, Melton LJ 3rd. Physeal fractures: part 1. Epidemiology in Olmsted County, Minnesota, 1979-1988. J Pediatr Orthop. 1994;14(4):423–30. https://doi.org/10.1097/01241398-199407000-00002.
2. Mann DC, Rajmaira S. Distribution of physeal and nonphyseal fractures in 2,650 long-bone fractures in children aged 0-16 years. J Pediatr Orthop. 1990;10(6):713–6. https://doi.org/10.1097/01241398-199011000-00002.
3. Loder RT, O'Donnell PW, Feinberg JR. Epidemiology and mechanisms of femur fractures in children. J Pediatr Orthop. 2006;26(5):561–6. https://doi.org/10.1097/01.bpo.0000230335.19029.ab.
4. Peterson CA, Peterson HA. Analysis of the incidence of injuries to the epiphyseal growth plate. J Trauma. 1972;12(4):275–81. https://doi.org/10.1097/00005373-197204000-00002.
5. Riseborough EJ, Barrett IR, Shapiro F. Growth disturbances following distal femoral physeal fracture-separations. J Bone Joint Surg Am. 1983;65(7):885–93.
6. Young EY, Stans AA. Distal femoral Physeal fractures. J Knee Surg. 2018;31(6):486–9. https://doi.org/10.1055/s-0038-1627465.
7. Bailey MEA, Wei R, Bolton S, Richards RH. Paediatric injuries around the knee: bony injuries. Injury. 2020;51(3):611–9. https://doi.org/10.1016/j.injury.2019.12.033.
8. Hutchinson J. Lectures on injuries to the epiphyses and their results: delivered at the Royal College of surgeons. Br Med J. 1894;1:669e73.
9. Liu RW, Armstrong DG, Levine AD, Gilmore A, Thompson GH, Cooperman DR. An anatomic study of the distal femoral epiphysis. J Pediatr Orthop. 2013;33(7):743–9. https://doi.org/10.1097/BPO.0b013e31829d55bf.
10. Lippiello L, Bass R, Connolly JF. Stereological study of the developing distal femoral growth plate. J Orthop Res. 1989;7(6):868–75. https://doi.org/10.1002/jor.1100070613.
11. Pritchett JW. Longitudinal growth and growth-plate activity in the lower extremity. Clin Orthop Relat Res. 1992;275:274–9.
12. Anderson M, Messner MB, Green WT. Distribution of lengths of the normal femur and tibia in children from one to eighteen years of age. J Bone Joint Surg Am. 1964;46:1197–202.
13. Arkader A, Warner WC Jr, Horn BD, Shaw RN, Wells L. Predicting the outcome of physeal fractures of the distal femur. J Pediatr Orthop. 2007;27(6):703–8. https://doi.org/10.1097/BPO.0b013e3180dca0e5.
14. Zionts LE. Fractures around the knee in children. J Am Acad Orthop Surg. 2002;10(5):345–55. https://doi.org/10.5435/00124635-200209000-00006.
15. Little RM, Milewski MD. Physeal fractures about the knee. Curr Rev Musculoskelet Med. 2016;9(4):478–86. https://doi.org/10.1007/s12178-016-9370-7.
16. Sepúlveda M, Téllez C, Villablanca V, Birrer E. Fracturas femorales distales en niños. EFORT Open Rev. 2022;7(4):264–73. Publicado 2022 25 de abril. https://doi.org/10.1530/EOR-21-0110.
17. www.aofoundation.org
18. Smith NC, Parker D, McNicol D. Supracondylar fractures of the femur in children. J Pediatr Orthop. 2001;21(5):600–3.
19. Beals RK, Tufts E. Fractured femur in infancy: the role of child abuse. J Pediatr Orthop. 1983;3(5):583–6. https://doi.org/10.1097/01241398-198311000-00004.
20. Salter RB, Harris WR. Injuries involving the epiphyseal plate. J Bone Joint Surg Am. 1963;45:587–622.
21. Card RK, Lowe JB, Bokhari AA. Rodilla Flotante. En: StatPearls. Treasure Island, FL: StatPearls Publishing; 8 de mayo, 2022.
22. Price CTH-SJ. Lesiones extra-articulares de la rodilla. Filadelfia: Lippincott Williams & Wilkins; 2010. p. 842e85.

Chapter 25
Tibial Eminence Fracture

Florencia Espinoza, Daniel Green, and María Jesús Tuca

25.1 Introduction

Avulsion fractures of the tibial eminence (AFTE) correspond to rare injuries in children and adolescents (3/100,000 per year), representing 5% of knee joint effusions in children. The vast majority of these fractures occur in children between the ages of 8 and 14 [1, 2].

25.2 Pathophysiology

The usual mechanism of this injury is pivot-type rotation, similar to the mechanism of rupture of the anterior cruciate ligament (ACL) in adults, but AFTE can also occur as a result of direct trauma or hyperextension of the knee [3, 4].

This injury, having a mechanism similar to ACL injuries [4], involves at least elongation, or in some cases a partial injury of the ACL fibers. However, in patients with an immature skeleton, it is the chondro-epiphyseal junction that fails first, as the tibial eminence where the ACL is inserted is not yet fully ossified. Instead of suffering an intrasubstance injury of the ACL, as occurs in most adults, an avulsion fracture of the distal osteochondral insertion of the ACL occurs.

F. Espinoza
Universidad de los Andes, Santiago, Chile

D. Green
Hospital for Special Surgery, New York, USA
e-mail: GreenDW@hss.edu

M. J. Tuca (✉)
School of Medicine, Pontifical Catholic University of Chile Clinical Hospital Mutual de Seguridad, Santiago, Chile

M. Sepúlveda O. (ed.), *Paediatrics Traumatology*,
https://doi.org/10.1007/978-3-031-89482-4_25

The activity most commonly involved in these fractures is falling off a bicycle, although they can also be seen in pivot sports, such as skiing or in motor vehicle accidents [5].

25.3 Anatomy

The intercondylar eminence is the non-articular portion of the proximal tibia, between both tibial plates. It consists of a quadrilateral base and two bony prominences called tibial spines, one medial and one lateral [6].

The anterior cruciate ligament is inserted in the antero-internal part of the medial tibial spine. In its anterior portion, this ligament joins with fibers from the anterior horn of the internal and external menisci [6]. The ACL is a primary restrictor to the anterior translation of the tibia in relation to the femur, and secondarily also acts as a restrictor to the rotation and varus-valgus of the knee [7].

Most AFTE occur in skeletally immature patients, where the ACL is stronger than the eminence to which it is attached, which is partially ossified. As a result, the damage occurs in the bone insertion rather than the ligament when the knee undergoes a mechanism compatible with ACL injury [3, 8, 9]. The bone avulsion of the distal insertion of the ACL usually is limited to the intercondylar eminence, but in some cases it extends to the articular portion of the tibial plates, especially toward the medial plate.

25.4 Diagnosis

The diagnosis is given by the clinic and images. The physical examination in acute cases is characterized by the presence of a significant joint effusion, which differentiates it from intrasubstance cruciate ligament injuries or patellar dislocations, which generally have lesser effusions. Patients usually position the knee in an antalgic semi-flexion and present an inability to bear weight.

We will hardly be able to perform tests of anterior instability (Lachman Test or Anterior Drawer) or rotational instability (Pivot Shift) in acute cases, due to the pain and apprehension of the patients. In addition, we suggest avoiding them in those patient candidates for a conservative treatment, as it will not modify the initial behavior and we risk a greater displacement of the fragments.

The first imaging evaluation, to confirm the diagnosis and rule out other associated injuries, is performed using knee X-ray [1] in their anteroposterior (AP), lateral, and intercondylar tunnel projections. The most common is to observe in the lateral projection the displacement of the fragment (Fig. 25.1). In addition, the tunnel view deprojects the trochlea and the condyles to better observe the intercondylar groove, providing a better view of the fragments and their displacement.

Magnetic resonance imaging (MRI) has become the examination of choice to evaluate these injuries and define their treatment. First, because it allows obtaining

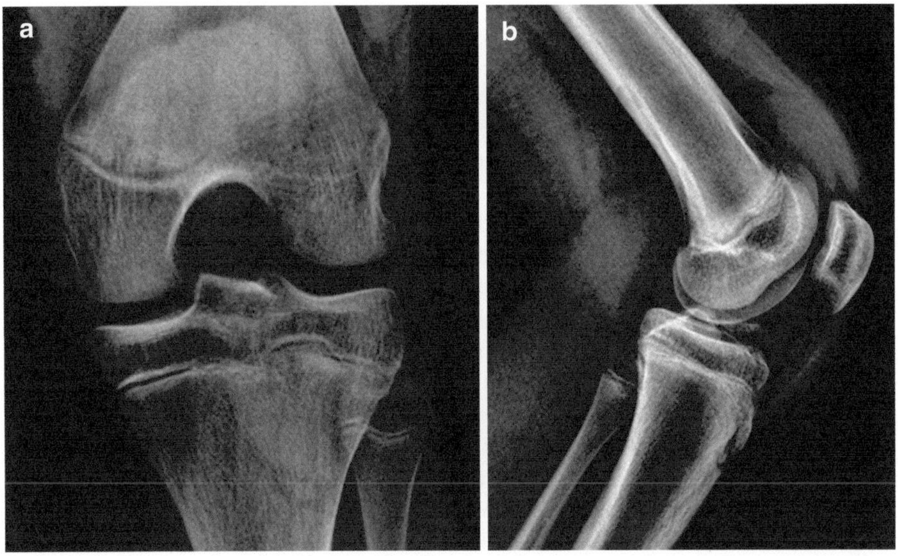

Fig. 25.1 Intercondylar tunnel and lateral radiological projections of a knee of a 13-year-old boy, showing a fracture of the tibial spine

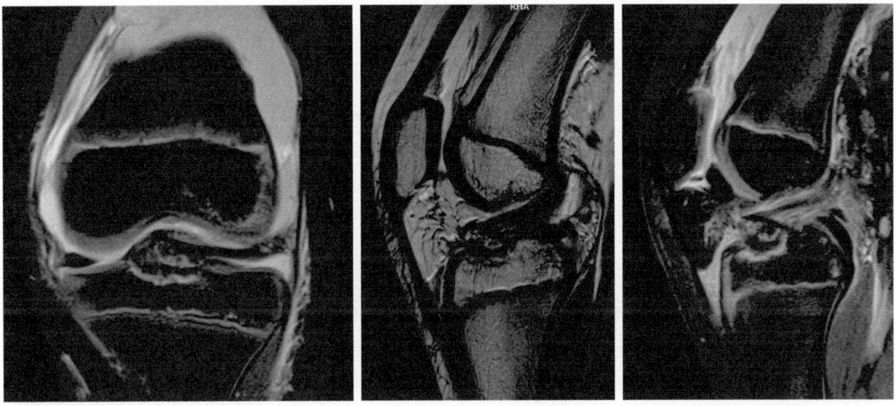

Fig. 25.2 MRI of the knee of a 9-year-old girl, with a displaced tibial spine injury

high-quality images to characterize the avulsion fragment and quantify the displacement in different planes, allowing to recognize the purely cartilaginous avulsions of the ACL, which can be invisible in simple radiographs. Secondly, the MRI helps to verify the state of the ACL fibers and rule out concomitant intrasubstance injuries, which would modify the treatment algorithm. Third, the MRI allows diagnosing associated injuries (whether meniscal tears or osteochondral fractures), which occur in 32–59% of cases [10]. Finally, it is also very useful to identify the interposition of soft tissues (menisci or intermeniscal ligament) under the fragment of the avulsion fracture, which could block the closed reduction. For all these reasons, MRI is a very useful tool in the diagnosis and therapeutic algorithm of the FAET (Fig. 25.2).

25.5 Classification

Historically, FAETs have been classified according to Meyers and McKeever (1959) [11], which grades fractures according to the displacement of the fragment using radiographs. There is consensus that Type I FAETs are for conservative treatment, and that Type III fractures require a reduction and surgical fixation. However, in Type II fractures, there is more controversy, where most surgeons agree to attempt a closed reduction and decide the treatment based on the result of this [12] (Fig. 25.3).

Even though the Meyers and McKeever classification is widely used, it is based on radiographs and does not quantify the displacement of the fragment. As we mentioned previously, today MRI is widely used in the evaluation of these patients and determines the treatment, as it allows to specify the displacement of the fracture, characterize the fragment, recognize associated injuries, and confirm the integrity of the ACL. These elements allow defining the behavior to follow and plan the surgical strategy in a better way. That is why a classification by Green & Tuca [12] based on MRI for FAETs has recently been published (Fig. 25.4).

In this classification, Grade I FAETs correspond to non-displaced or minimally displaced (<2 mm) fractures. On the radiograph, they may not be seen and are called "hidden fractures" (Fig. 25.5).

Grade II fractures are those anterior avulsions, which maintain the posterior hinge (displacement >2 mm of the anterior portion of the fracture and displacement <2 mm of the posterior portion of the fragment) (Fig. 25.6).

Grade III fractures (Fig. 25.7) are all those that meet any of the following criteria:

1. Fracture with >2 mm displacement of the posterior portion of the fragment.
2. Fracture resulting in entrapment of the meniscal ligament or intermeniscal (where the meniscus or intermeniscal ligament is inferior to a fracture fragment) blocking the reduction.

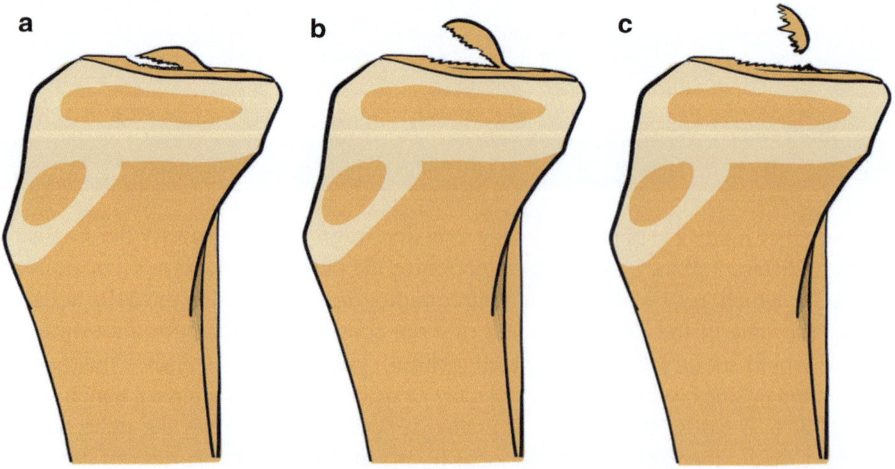

Fig. 25.3 Meyers and McKeever classification scheme. (**a**) Minimal displacement or non-displaced fragment; (**b**) anterior hinged with posterior bone contact intact; (**c**) full displacement

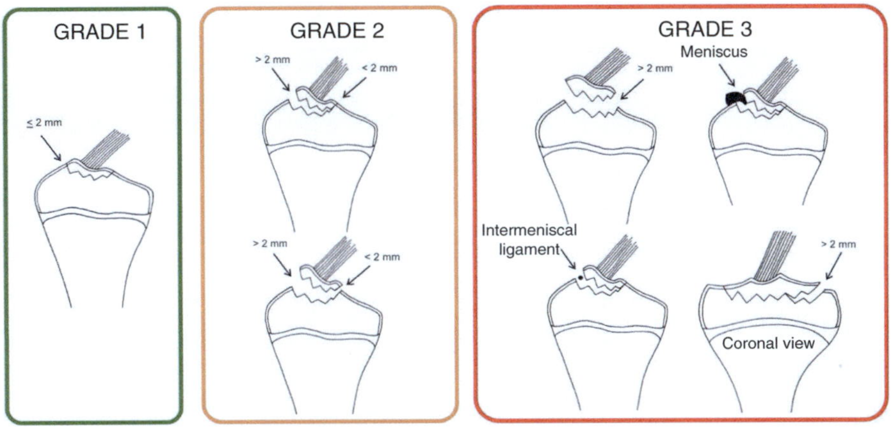

Fig. 25.4 Green and Tuca classification for tibial spine injuries, based on magnetic resonance imaging

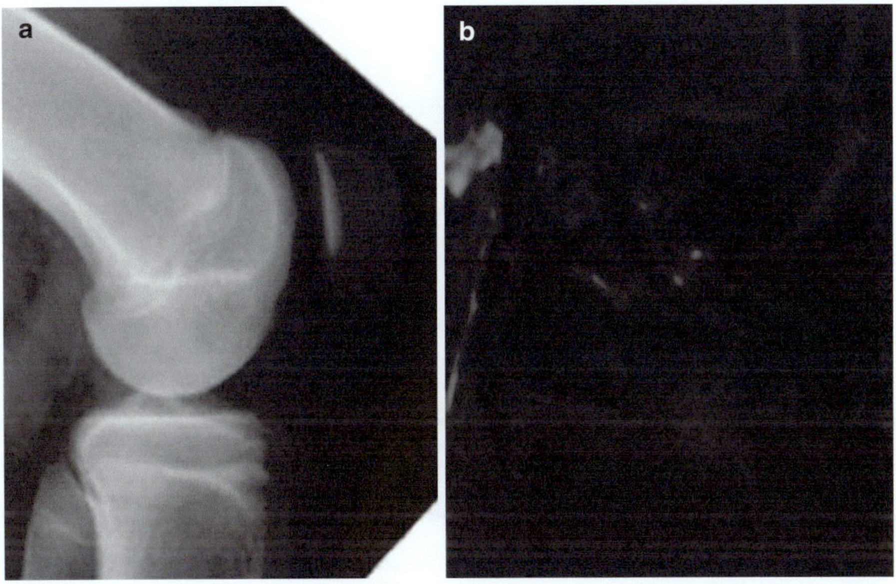

Fig. 25.5 (**a**) Lateral knee radiograph in an 11-year-old patient, where no obvious fracture is evident. (**b**) Sagittal fat-Sat MRI from the same patient showing a non-displaced avulsive fracture of tibial eminence, Green and Tuca Grade I

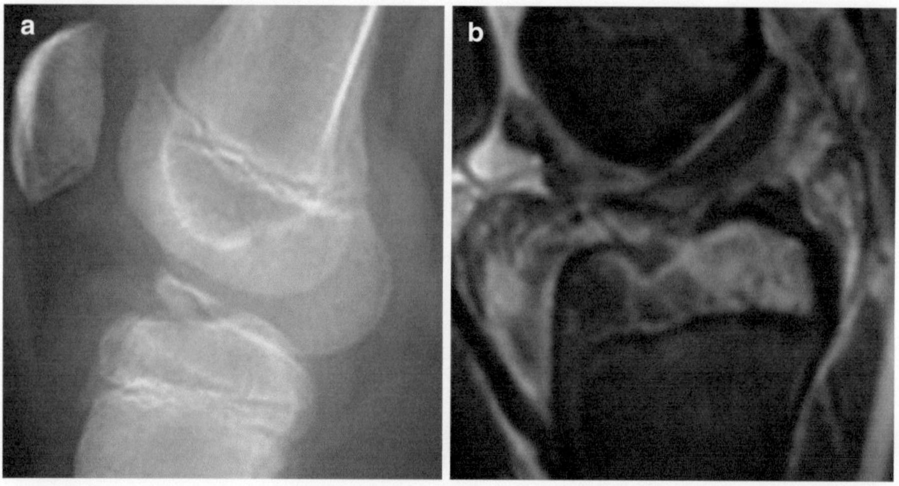

Fig. 25.6 (**a**) Lateral radiograph where AFTE is initially evident, classified as Type III according to Meyers-McKeever. (**b**) It is reclassified as Grade 2 Green and Tuca with MRI showing ≤2 mm posterior displacement and the absence of soft tissues blocking the reduction

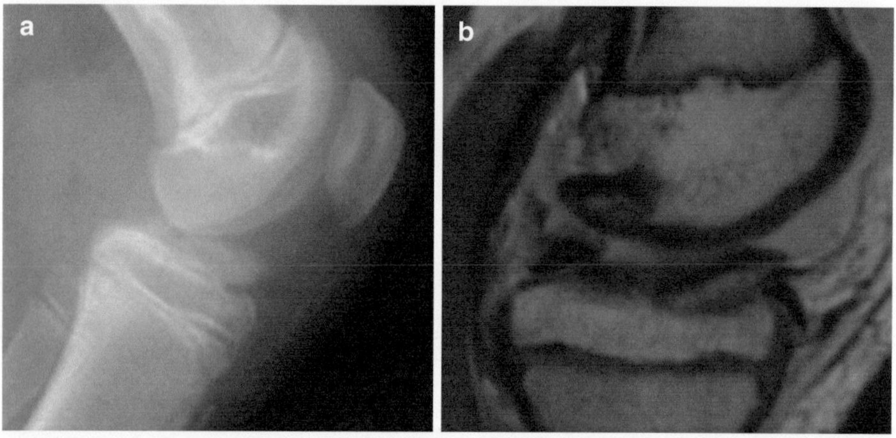

Fig. 25.7 (**a**) Lateral knee X-ray view, with AFTE classified as Type II according to Meyers-McKeever. (**b**) MRI identifying the interposition of the anterior horn of the medial meniscus, blocking the reduction of the fragment; therefore, it is reclassified as Green and Tuca Grade 3

3. Fracture that extends to the articular surface of the medial or lateral tibial plateau (most often toward the medial plateau) displaced >2 mm in the load zone.

This new classification has shown to have an inter/intraobserver performance comparable to the Meyers and Mckeever classification, but also provides a more quantitative than qualitative guide to classify fractures based on a fracture pattern, displacement of it and soft tissue involvement [12].

Using an MRI-based classification changed the therapeutic plan in 1/3 of the cases, compared to the use of simple radiographs. The recognition of the interposition of soft tissues blocking the reduction allows to redefine those FAET that have better chances of a successful closed reduction (Type II), versus those that will benefit from surgical treatment (Type III).

25.6 Treatment

Systematic reviews of pediatric patient studies, which include level III and IV studies, have categorically demonstrated that surgical treatment is superior to non-surgical treatment for displaced FAET. They report lower rates of clinical instability (14% vs 70%), subjective instability (1% vs 54%), need for future ACL reconstruction (1% vs 10%), non-union (20% vs 80%), and better functional scores [13, 14].

Faced with the question of whether closed reduction is a good option, radiographic studies have reported an average reduction of 2.45 mm [15], while MRI-based studies have reported an average reduction of only 1 mm [16]. Therefore, it can be concluded that closed reduction is unlikely in those FAET with an initial displacement >5 mm, with a higher rate of subsequent surgery for pinching or instability (17%).

25.6.1 Treatment Algorithm

Considering the mentioned evidence, most surgeons agree with the following treatment algorithm, based on the Green and Tuca classification system [12]:

- Conservative treatment (6–12 weeks with cast or knee brace 0–20°):
  - Grade 1
  - Grade 2 that achieve a successful closed reduction (<2 mm of displacement)
- Surgical reduction and fixation:
  - Grade 2 that fail in an attempt at closed reduction
  - Grade 2 with >5 mm of initial displacement
  - Grade 3
  - Associated injuries that require repair (osteochondral fracture, repairable meniscal injury)

A study [2] based on a series of 40 patients shows that, when using this treatment algorithm to face patients, there is no difference in terms of clinical or subjective outcomes between conservative treatment and surgical treatment. This study concludes that it is possible to achieve good functional results in pediatric patients who suffer from FAET, even in the Type III injuries with severe displacement have comparable outcomes to Type I injuries with minimal displacement (if they are properly managed). This demonstrates that Type I and II reducible fractures can be successfully treated with closed reduction and immobilization (conservative treatment), and that Type II and III non-reducible fractures can be satisfactorily treated with open reduction and internal fixation.

Meniscal injuries in children and adolescents undergoing surgical treatment for tibial spine fractures are found in almost 40% of cases, with a higher prevalence as age and skeletal maturity increase [17]. Thus, MRI plays a crucial role in recognizing associated injuries and anticipating the need to repair them. It also allows for the identification of soft tissue entrapment that blocks reduction, which has been described to occur in up to 30% in Type II and >50% Type III [10]. The concomitant ACL injury is more common in patients closer to skeletal maturity or adult patients. Recognizing it is relevant because the management will no longer consist of repairing or reinserting the bone avulsion, but in a probable ligament reconstruction.

Despite the lack of quality evidence, the arthroscopic approach is currently accepted as the gold standard for the reduction and fixation of displaced and irreducible FAET [18]. Compared to open surgery, arthroscopy uses a smaller incision and results in less damage to soft tissues, better pain control, and early rehabilitation. In addition, the arthroscopic approach allows for direct visualization of associated intra-articular injuries, such as meniscal tears, meniscal root injuries, loose bodies, or osteochondral lesions, and allows for simultaneous treatment of these [4, 8] (Fig. 25.8).

In response to the question of whether there is a better fixation system, there are many alternatives available, such as staples, Kirschner wires, anchors, screws, sutures, among others. Sutures and screws are the most widely used systems today and gather most of the evidence available to date.

Biomechanical studies favor the use of sutures [19–21], reporting a higher load to failure and less displacement to cyclic load. However, systematic reviews of clinical studies show no categorical differences between sutures and screws, except for the need for a second surgery for the removal of surgical materials (63–65% for screws versus 4–9% for sutures) and a difference in the rate of clinical instability (27–82% for screws versus 13–19% for sutures) [13, 14]. As for all other outcomes, such as return to sports, pivot shift, subjective instability, need for future ACL reconstruction, or arthrofibrosis, both techniques present comparable or equivalent results [13, 14, 22].

In conclusion, both screws and sutures are valid and safe fixation methods for FAET. Neither has proven to have a significant superiority over the other; however, surgeons should be aware of the advantages and disadvantages of each, and make their choice based on these (Table 25.1).

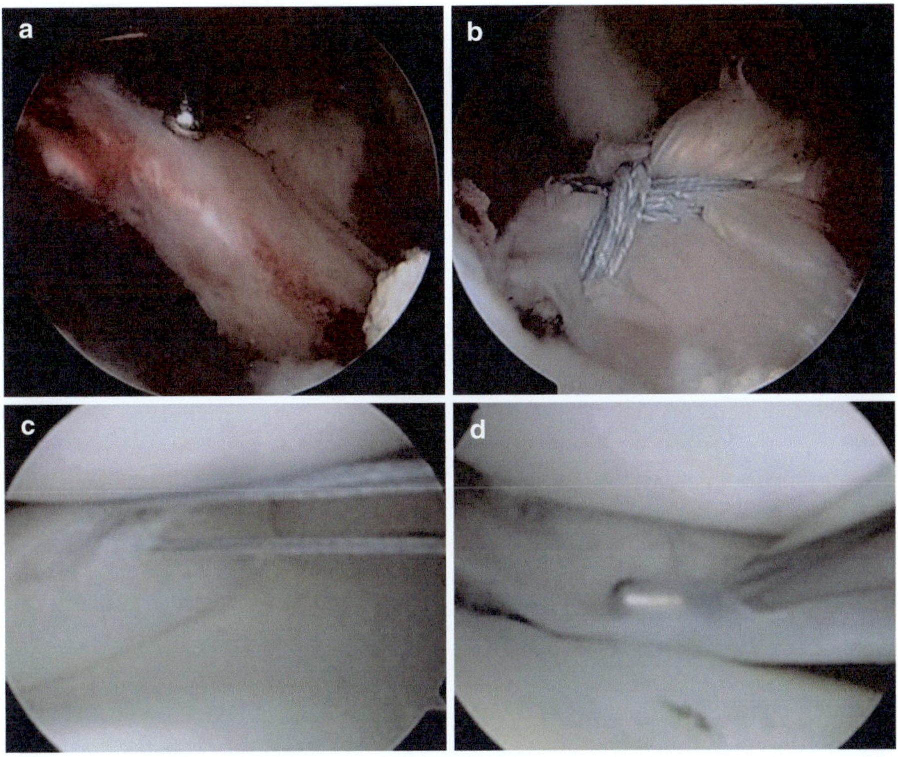

Fig. 25.8 Arthroscopic view of a knee with a diagnosis of AFTE: (**a**) anterior root of the lateral meniscus attached to the bony eminence avulsed, (**b**) arthroscopic reduction and fixation with two high resistance sutures, crosses in the anterior portion of the fragment, which were tied over a 1 cm bone bridge on the anteromedial tibia, (**c**) longitudinal tear of the posterior horn of the lateral meniscus that was repaired with two vertical sutures using an all-inside device (**d**)

Table 25.1 Comparison of advantages and disadvantages between fixation techniques with suture and with screws for AFTE

	In favor	Against
Suture	• More versatile: works for fixation of small fragments or even purely cartilaginous • Biomechanical superior in cadaveric studies • Compatible with MRI (without distortion) • Allows you to reset the ACL tension when pulling its fibers, in addition to reducing the fracture	• Technically demanding • Risk of poor reduction: top elevation of the most anterior portion of the fracture is frequent
Screw	• Technically simple • Available • Low cost	• Higher re-operation rate for hardware withdrawal (>60%) • Requires a significant bone fragment • Risk of prominence of the screws • Can lead to a greater comminution • MRI artifact

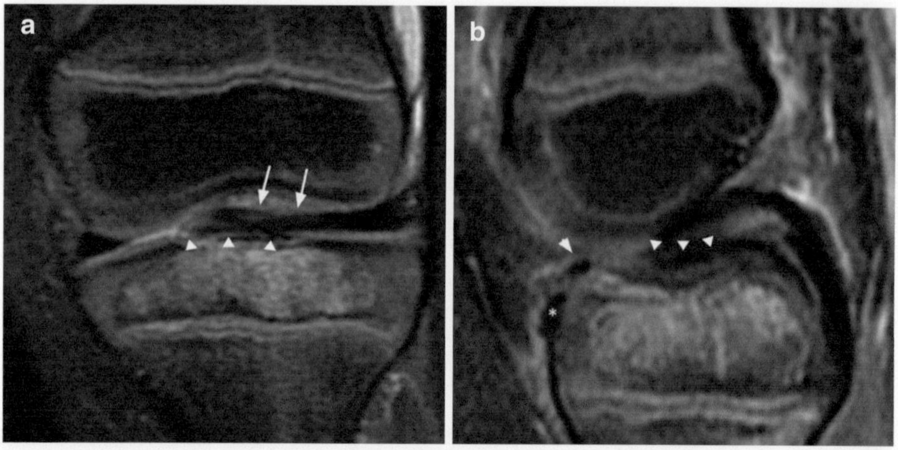

Fig. 25.9 Coronal FS MRI (**a**) showing an avulsive fragment (arrowheads) which includes the insertion of the anterior root of the lateral meniscus (long arrows). In sagittal T1 (**b**) the "double PCL" sign is evident (arrowhead), the anterior root of the medial meniscus (*) and the anterior intermeniscal ligament (short arrow)

25.7 Complications

The most common complications following the treatment of FAET are residual laxity, arthrofibrosis, non-union, malunion, and physeal arrest, although the results are generally good [1].

We must be careful with purely cartilaginous avulsions that occur in very young patients (<8 years). These are easily overlooked on plain radiographs, but magnetic resonance imaging will show a "double posterior cruciate ligament" sign [23]. It is important to suspect and look for them in a directed way in the MRI (Fig. 25.9).

Physeal arrest is very infrequent, but there are reported cases with the use of sutures and screws [24–26]. If screws are used for fixation in patients with open physes, it is recommended to perform an "all-epiphyseal" fixation or ensure early removal if it is transphyseal (once the fracture consolidation is confirmed).

In the case of performing fixation with sutures in very young patients (>4–6 years of remaining growth), performing an "all-epiphyseal" suture configuration, using absorbable sutures (Vycril), or cutting the knot through a mini-approach, the fracture consolidation is achieved.

Arthrofibrosis is the most frequent postoperative complication, present in 8–20% of cases [22, 27, 28]. The risk factors associated with the development of postoperative arthrofibrosis are preoperative stiffness, surgery >1 month after the injury, >2 h of surgery duration, malunion, prominent surgical material, and delay >4 weeks in the start of knee flexion exercises [22, 27, 29].

25.8 Authors' Recommendations

Regarding surgical treatment, our preferred technique is the use of sutures for the fixation of FAET, mainly due to its versatility and lower rate of re-operation.

Tricks for FAET suture fixation:

- Preoperative preparation:
  - 3.5 mm optics (except in very young patients <6–7 years where the use of a 2.7 mm optic is advised).
  - Supine position with the knee in 90° flexion using a lateral post and a distal foot support.
  - Padded tourniquet on the proximal part of the thigh (ensure that the width and size of the tourniquet match the patients, to avoid excessive or insufficient compression).
  - Pressure flow pump adjusted to 30–35 mmHg.
- Suggested instrumentation:
  - ACL tibial guides (compass).
  - 2.4 mm guide needle.
  - Suture retriever (wire loop or similar).
  - Suture passers: curved lasso style suture passer or arthroscopic "scorpion" style suture passer.
  - Pediatric arthroscopic cannulas.
  - Instrumentation for meniscal repair: all-inside suture device + spinal needle and PDS sutures for anterior horn tears + scorpion or lasso style suture passers in case of suspected root avulsions.
  - Cortical button for distal fixation.

ABC recommended for FAET with sutures.

A. Start with your anterolateral portal, making sure to place it just lateral to the patellar tendon and in a high position that will allow better visualization. Portals placed in a lower position will be in front of the avulsed fragment and will not allow a correct visualization of the reduction, making fixation difficult. The anteromedial portal is made under direct visualization, avoiding damaging the anterior horn of the medial meniscus and ensuring that it provides access to work on the lower surface of the fragment, but also access to the upper portion of it to achieve the reduction.

B. If your portals are insufficient or poorly positioned, do not hesitate to extend them longitudinally or add an additional portal (for example, a high patellar tendon trans portal can contribute to visualization, suture rescue, or guide passage). Remember, the key is to obtain adequate vision and good control of the fragment using two or more anterior knee portals.

C. Check the integrity of the ACL and rule out a concomitant high grade tear (this would change our plan, to perform an ACL reconstruction surgery).
D. Check the status of menisci and cartilage: before fixing the FAET, associated meniscal tears or osteochondral lesions should be treated.
E. Proceed to debride the bone bed and the lower surface of the fragment. Using the arthroscopic shaver, remove all bone clots and fibrous tissue that may be blocking the reduction. We even recommend removing more to achieve a slight over-reduction of the fragment, which will help restore the tension of the partially torn or elongated ACL fibers. This will also prevent an anterior pinching in extension, which occurs when the reduction is insufficient.
F. Protect the intermeniscal ligament: this often is located under the fragment and blocks the reduction of this. Be careful not to accidentally debride it, as while its function is controversial, it could provide stability to the anterior horns in the absence of bone insertions.
G. Anatomical reduction and temporary fixation of the fragment: use the medial and lateral bone references to ensure an anatomical reduction of the fragment. Temporarily fix it with a Kirschner wire 1.8–2.0 mm, which will facilitate the passage of sutures and the creation of tunnels.
H. If the interposition of the anterior root of the external meniscus or the intermeniscal ligament is blocking your reduction, use a PDS suture (outside-in technique) to temporarily traction them while you reduce and fix the fragment.
I. Using an arthroscopic suture passer or a curved lasso type passer, firmly transfix the ACL with at least two high strength sutures (No.2) in orthogonal configuration (one anteroinferior and the other posterosuperior). If necessary, add a third suture to confirm a secure grip of the ligament fibers.
J. Suture configuration: biomechanical studies have not shown significant differences between configurations. Our preference is to use a high strength suture plus a high strength tape, which cross over the anterior part of the fragment (forming an "x"). The tape has a wider surface area that could theoretically prevent it from tearing the ACL or the epiphyseal bone. Crossing the sutures helps to reduce the most anterior part of the fragment.
K. Arthroscopic cannulas help to rescue sutures, avoiding soft tissue bridges. They save time and simplify surgery, but they have an additional cost. If you do not have cannulas, make sure to rescue the sutures along with the wire loop to avoid soft tissue bridges.
L. Use the ACL tibial guide to direct the tibial tunnels. For fragments with an intact posterior hinge, an anteromedial and an anterolateral tunnel are sufficient to reduce and secure fixation. For those completely displaced fragments, consider adding a third central tunnel.
M. If possible, depending on the size of the fragment and the level of comminution, try to pass the tunnels through the bone fragment.
N. Hammering the drill guide against the proximal tibia will allow you to exchange the guide needle for the suture retriever (wire loop) without losing the tunnel path. Using a thin drill to cannulate the tunnel and ensure easy suture rescue is also a valid alternative.

O. Once the sutures are rescued by the anteromedial tibia, these can be knotted over a bone bridge or using a cortical button. The advantages of using a cortical button are to avoid that when knotting the sutures these can slice the soft epiphyseal bone and lose the fixation, ensuring stable fixation in cases where there is a coalition of tunnels or a bone bridge <1 cm, identifying the position of the suture knot for its future removal if necessary in a patient with high potential for remaining growth.
P. Before tying the knots, make sure there is no anterior pinching and that full extension is achieved. Be careful to avoid the superior elevation of the most anterior portion of the fragment that could block the extension. Direct arthroscopic visualization of the ROM of the knee is mandatory before securing the fixation.

25.9 Final Message

- MRI is a fundamental tool for the evaluation and therapeutic planning of patients with FAET.
- Displaced FAETs benefit from surgical treatment.
- We should choose the fixation system according to:
  - Surgeon's experience and available fixation methods.
  - Potential for remaining growth.
  - Size and comminution of the avulsed fragment.
  - That which ensures me a stable fixation to start early rehabilitation and avoid arthrofibrosis.

References

1. Tuca M, Bernal N, Luderowski E, Green DW. Tibial spine avulsion fractures: treatment update. Curr Opin Pediatr. 2019;31(1):103–11. https://doi.org/10.1097/MOP.0000000000000719.
2. Scrimshire AB, Gawad M, Davies R, George H. Management and outcomes of isolated paediatric tibial spine fractures. Injury. 2018;49(2):437–42. https://doi.org/10.1016/j.injury.2017.11.013.
3. Mitchell JJ, Sjostrom R, Mansour AA, Irion B, Hotchkiss M, Terhune EB, et al. Incidence of meniscal injury and chondral pathology in anterior tibial spine fractures of children. J Pediatr Orthop. 2015;35(2):130–5. https://doi.org/10.1097/BPO.0000000000000249.
4. Osti L, Buda M, Soldati F, Del Buono A, Osti R, Maffulli N. Arthroscopic treatment of tibial eminence fracture: a systematic review of different fixation methods. Br Med Bull. 2016;118(1):73–90. https://doi.org/10.1093/bmb/ldw018.
5. Coyle C, Jagernauth S, Ramachandran M. Tibial eminence fractures in the paediatric population: a systematic review. J Child Orthop. 2014;8(2):149–59. https://doi.org/10.1007/s11832-014-0571-6.
6. Bernasconi DJP, Campodonico M, Casanovas FJ, Cassinelli LH, Mauas D, Peirano FH, et al. Fractures of the tibial spine in children and adults. Rev Asoc Arg Ortop y Traumatol. 1996;61(1):104–8.

7. Forriol F, Maestro A, Vaquero MJ. The anterior cruciate ligament: morphology and function. Trauma Fund MAPFRE. 2008;19(1):7–18.
8. DeFroda SF, Hodax JD, Shah KN, Cruz AI. Tibial eminence fracture repair with double Hewson suture passer technique. Arthrosc Tech. 2017;6(4):e1275–9. https://doi.org/10.1016/j.eats.2017.05.005.
9. Mitchell JJ, Mayo MH, Axibal DP, Kasch AR, Fader RR, Chadayammuri V, et al. Delayed anterior cruciate ligament reconstruction in young patients with previous anterior tibial spine fractures. Am J Sports Med. 2016;44(8):2047–56. https://doi.org/10.1177/0363546516644597.
10. Edmonds EW, Fornari ED, Dashe J, Roocroft JH, King MM, Pennock AT. Results of displaced pediatric Tibial spine fractures: a comparison between open, arthroscopic, and closed management. J Pediatr Orthop. 2015;35(7):651–6. https://doi.org/10.1097/BPO.0000000000000356.
11. Meyers MH, McKeever FM. Fracture of the intercondylar eminence of the tibia. J Bone Joint Surg Am. 1959;41-A(2):209–22.
12. Green D, Tuca M, Luderowski E, Gausden E, Goodbody C, Konin G. A new, MRI-based classification system for tibial spine fractures changes clinical treatment recommendations when compared to Myers and Mckeever. Knee Surg Sports Traumatol Arthrosc. 2019;27(1):86–92. https://doi.org/10.1007/s00167-018-5039-7.
13. Gans I, Baldwin KD, Ganley TJ. Treatment and management outcomes of Tibial Eminence fractures in pediatric patients: a systematic review. Am J Sports Med. 2014;42(7):1743–50. https://doi.org/10.1177/0363546513508538.
14. Bogunovic L, Tarabichi M, Harris D, Wright R. Treatment of tibial eminence fractures: a systematic review. J Knee Surg. 2015;28(3):255–62. https://doi.org/10.1055/s-0034-1388657.
15. Janarv PM, Westblad P, Johansson C, Hirsch G. Long-term follow-up of anterior tibial spine fractures in children. J Pediatr Orthop. 1995;15(1):63–8. https://doi.org/10.1097/01241398-199501000-00014.
16. Cannamela PC, Quinlan NJ, Maak TG, Adeyemi TF, Aoki SK. Knee extension does not reliably reduce acute type II tibial spine fractures: MRI evaluation of displacement during extension versus resting flexion. Orthop J Sports Med. 2019;7(7):2325967119860066. https://doi.org/10.1177/2325967119860066.
17. Feucht MJ, Brucker PU, Camathias C, et al. Meniscal injuries in children and adolescents undergoing surgical treatment for tibial eminence fractures. Knee Surg Sports Traumatol Arthrosc. 2017;25(2):445–53. https://doi.org/10.1007/s00167-016-4184-0.
18. Doral MN, Bilge O. Editorial commentary: arthroscopic fixation of tibial eminence fractures-which technique is the best has not been defined yet! Arthroscopy. 2018;34(5):1617–20. https://doi.org/10.1016/j.arthro.2018.01.045.
19. Li J, Yu Y, Liu C, Su X, Liao W, Li Z. Arthroscopic fixation of tibial eminence fractures: a biomechanical comparative study of screw, suture, and suture anchor. Arthroscopy. 2018;34(5):1608–16. https://doi.org/10.1016/j.arthro.2017.12.018.
20. Eggers AK, Becker C, Weimann A, et al. Biomechanical evaluation of different fixation methods for tibial eminence fractures. Am J Sports Med. 2007;35(3):404–10. https://doi.org/10.1177/0363546506294677.
21. Bong MR, Romero A, Kubiak E, et al. Suture versus screw fixation of displaced tibial eminence fractures: a biomechanical comparison. Arthroscopy. 2005;21(10):1172–6. https://doi.org/10.1016/j.arthro.2005.06.019.
22. Callanan M, Allen J, Flutie B, et al. Suture versus screw fixation of tibial spine fractures in children and adolescents: a comparative study. Orthop J Sports Med. 2019;7(11):2325967119881961. https://doi.org/10.1177/2325967119881961.
23. Chotel F, Raux S, Accadbled F, et al. Cartilaginous tibial eminence fractures in children: which recommendations for management of this new entity? Knee Surg Sports Traumatol Arthrosc. 2016;24(3):688–96. https://doi.org/10.1007/s00167-015-3707-4.
24. Ahn JH, Yoo JC. Clinical outcome of arthroscopic reduction and suture for displaced acute and chronic tibial spine fractures. Knee Surg Sports Traumatol Arthrosc. 2005;13(2):116–21. https://doi.org/10.1007/s00167-004-0540-6.

25. Mylle J, Reynders P, Broos P. Transepiphysial fixation of anterior cruciate avulsion in a child. Report of a complication and review of the literature. Arch Orthop Trauma Surg. 1993;112(2):101–3. https://doi.org/10.1007/BF00420267.
26. Fabricant PD, Osbahr DC, Green DW. Management of a rare complication after screw fixation of a pediatric tibial spine avulsion fracture: a case report with follow-up to skeletal maturity. J Orthop Trauma. 2011;25(12):e115–9. https://doi.org/10.1097/BOT.0b013e3182143ef2.
27. Pandey V, Cps S, Acharya K, Rao SK. Arthroscopic suture pull-out fixation of displaced tibial spine avulsion fracture. J Knee Surg. 2017;30(1):28–35. https://doi.org/10.1055/s-0036-1579682.
28. Vander Have KL, Ganley TJ, Kocher MS, Price CT, Herrera-Soto JA. Arthrofibrosis after surgical fixation of tibial eminence fractures in children and adolescents. Am J Sports Med. 2010;38(2):298–301. https://doi.org/10.1177/0363546509348001.
29. Shin CH, Lee DJ, Choi IH, et al. Clinical and radiological outcomes of arthroscopically assisted cannulated screw fixation for tibial eminence fracture in children and adolescents. BMC Musculoskelet Disord. 2018;19:41. https://doi.org/10.1186/s12891-018-1960-7.

Chapter 26
Anterior Cruciate Ligament and Meniscal Injuries in Pediatric Patients

Julio Javier Masquijo and I. Maximiliano Espinosa

26.1 Introduction

Anterior cruciate ligament (ACL) and meniscal injuries are recognized as the most common knee injuries among pediatric athletes. These injuries have increased significantly over the past 25 years and may have severe consequences on joint function. This chapter will review the anatomy of the skeletally immature knee, clinical and imaging evaluation, and current treatment options for these conditions, along with their potential complications.

26.2 Anterior Cruciate Ligament Injuries

Anterior cruciate ligament (ACL) injuries represent a significant concern within athletic populations. Recent research indicates a notable increase in ACL injury incidence among children and adolescents, with reported rates showing a rise of 15–20% in recent years [1]. Concomitantly, the utilization of ACL reconstruction procedures in this demographic has experienced a substantial escalation, with some studies documenting an approximately 29-fold increase over the preceding decades [2]. This observed increase is considered multifactorial, attributed to factors such as enhanced recognition of the condition, improved diagnostic techniques, heightened sports participation and intensity, and the growing trend toward early athletic

J. J. Masquijo (✉)
Sanatorio Allende, Córdoba, Argentina

I. M. Espinosa
Clínica Alemana Santiago/Hospital Clínico San Borja Arriarán, Santiago, Chile
e-mail: mespinosai@alemana.cl

M. Sepúlveda O. (ed.), *Paediatrics Traumatology*,
https://doi.org/10.1007/978-3-031-89482-4_26

specialization [3]. Studies have demonstrated sex-based disparities in ACL injury incidence within the pediatric population, with females exhibiting approximately twice the risk compared to males. However, in terms of absolute numbers, the injury remains more prevalent in males [4].

Historically, the management of ACL injuries in skeletally immature patients was predominantly conservative, advocating for delayed intervention until femoral and tibial growth plate closure. However, recent evidence has indicated that this conservative approach is associated with a significantly higher incidence of secondary intra-articular injuries, including chondral and meniscal tears [5]. Consequently, many orthopedic surgeons now favor surgical intervention in the acute setting for this patient group. Reconstruction techniques employed in this population are specifically designed to restore tibiofemoral stability while simultaneously preserving the integrity of the physis (growth plate) to mitigate growth disturbances.

26.3 Mechanisms of ACL Injury

ACL injuries typically result from non-contact mechanisms, such as acute deceleration with a fixed foot and the knee near full extension, often occurring during changes of direction or landing. Contact injuries, including those resulting from a valgus collapse with 20–30° of knee flexion, can also cause ACL tears.

ACL injury is associated with several risk factors, broadly categorized as non-modifiable and modifiable. Non-modifiable factors include inherent biological and anatomical characteristics such as female sex, a history of previous ACL injury, increased Q angle or genu valgus, increased posterior tibial slope, decreased intercondylar notch width, and generalized ligamentous laxity. While primarily considered non-modifiable, certain anatomical risk factors, such as tibial slope, may potentially be addressed surgically in skeletally immature patients through techniques like guided growth.

Modifiable risk factors encompass biomechanical deficits and muscle imbalances, including decreased hip and knee flexion angles during dynamic tasks, increased internal hip rotation, dynamic knee valgus, and an imbalanced quadriceps-to-hamstring strength ratio. Identification of these modifiable risk factors is critical for the development and implementation of effective ACL injury prevention programs. These programs typically incorporate neuromuscular and proprioceptive training protocols aimed at reducing injury incidence. A recent systematic review [6] reported a significant (50%) reduction in ACL injuries among participants undergoing neuromuscular training compared to controls. This protective effect was notably more pronounced in younger populations receiving the training.

When surgical management is considered for pediatric ACL injuries, particular attention must be given to the presence of open growth plates (physes) surrounding the knee. The distal femoral physis contributes approximately 70% of femoral longitudinal growth and 37% of total lower limb length, growing at an average rate of about 1 cm/year. The proximal tibial physis contributes approximately 55% of tibial longitudinal growth and 25% of total limb length, with an average growth rate of roughly 0.64 cm/year [7]. Understanding these contributions is crucial for planning physeal-sparing surgical techniques.

To understand the surgical approaches, knowledge of the ACL's anatomy and function is essential. The ACL is classified as an intra-articular, extra-synovial ligament of the knee, forming a key component of the central pivot complex. Its primary biomechanical function is to restrain anterior tibial translation, while also contributing significantly to the knee's rotational stability. Anatomically, its proximal attachment is located on the medial wall of the lateral femoral condyle, and its distal attachment lies within the anteromedial aspect of the tibial plateau.

26.4 Diagnosis of ACL Injury

Patients presenting with suspected ACL injury typically report an acute traumatic event involving knee torsion, often accompanied by an audible "pop," immediate joint effusion, and subsequent functional impairment. Clinical examination may reveal joint effusion and pain with range of motion. Specific ligamentous laxity tests are employed to assess ACL integrity. The Anterior Drawer test is conducted with the patient supine, the hip flexed 60°, and the knee flexed 90°. The examiner stabilizes the proximal tibia and applies an anterior translational force. Excessive anterior translation relative to the contralateral limb is indicative of ACL injury. The Lachman test, another frequently utilized maneuver, is performed with the knee positioned at 30° of flexion. One hand stabilizes the distal femur while the other applies an anterior force to the proximal tibia. Similar to the Anterior Drawer test, increased anterior tibial translation, particularly when compared to the uninjured side, suggests an ACL injury. The Pivot Shift test assesses the knee's dynamic rotational stability. It involves applying a valgus force and internal rotation to the tibia while moving the knee from extension into flexion. A positive test is characterized by a sudden reduction of a subluxated tibia at approximately 30° of flexion, a phenomenon that is both palpable and visible. When evaluating knee stability, particularly in the pediatric population, specific considerations are warranted. Skeletally immature patients may exhibit inherent generalized ligamentous laxity, which necessitates careful comparison to the contralateral limb for accurate interpretation of ligamentous tests. Furthermore, when an ACL injury is suspected, it is imperative to evaluate for concomitant intra-articular and extra-articular injuries, including meniscal tears, chondral lesions, and collateral ligament damage.

Beyond clinical examination, imaging plays a crucial role in diagnosis and surgical planning. Preoperative assessment, particularly if surgical management is anticipated, should include gait analysis and comprehensive lower limb alignment evaluation. Standard radiographic evaluation of the knee should encompass anteroposterior (AP), lateral, notch, and patellar axial views (Fig. 26.1). These views are valuable for identifying associated bony injuries, such as tibial spine avulsion fractures, osseous avulsions of the collateral or posterior cruciate ligaments, and

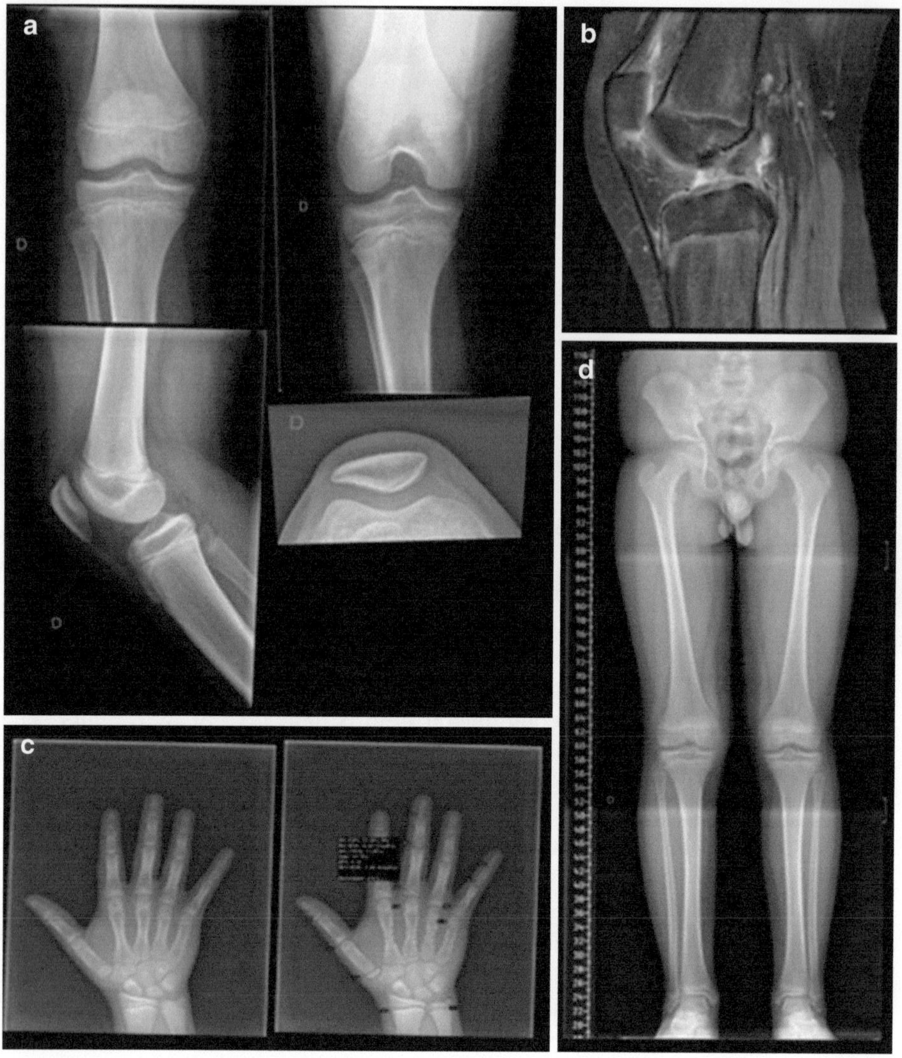

Fig. 26.1 Imaging study of the pediatric patient with an ACL injury: X-ray projections of the knee (**a**), Knee MRI (**b**), Bone age X-ray (**c**), Standing AP of lower extremities (**d**)

osteochondral fractures. They also provide initial assessment of the physeal status. A full-limb standing radiograph is recommended in all surgical candidates to accurately assess overall limb alignment and identify any pre-existing length discrepancies. Magnetic Resonance Imaging (MRI) is the preferred imaging modality for confirming a suspected ACL tear. MRI offers high diagnostic accuracy, with reported sensitivity and specificity for ACL injuries around 95% and 88%, respectively. Furthermore, it provides detailed information regarding concomitant soft tissue injuries, including meniscal and collateral ligament tears, chondral lesions, and is essential for evaluating the status of the physes.

In the skeletally immature population, accurate assessment of skeletal maturity and growth potential is imperative for guiding appropriate ACL reconstruction technique [8]. Skeletal maturity can be assessed using bone age radiographs, typically involving an anteroposterior view of the left hand and wrist, which is then compared to the standards provided in the Greulich and Pyle atlas. Alternatively, knee radiographs can be reliably used with the modified Fels Knee Skeletal Maturity System. While Tanner staging is another method described for assessing biological maturity, its reliance on secondary sexual characteristics makes it less directly indicative of skeletal growth potential in isolation, and studies have reported low reproducibility among orthopedic surgeons due to significant intra- and interobserver variability [9].

26.5 Treatment of ACL Injury

The primary treatment goals for ACL injuries in children and adolescents include pain and inflammation reduction, restoration of knee range of motion, muscle strength, and overall knee stability. Historically, conservative management was the preferred treatment approach for skeletally immature patients. This strategy typically involved activity restriction, physical therapy, and the use of a knee brace until skeletal maturity. However, recent evidence has indicated that this conservative approach is associated with suboptimal outcomes, including a higher incidence of recurrent instability episodes and an increased risk of secondary meniscal and/or chondral injuries [10].

In contrast, surgical management through ACL reconstruction is generally associated with improved functional outcomes, as evaluated by validated clinical scoring systems, and higher rates of return to sport. Nevertheless, conservative treatment remains a valid alternative for patients who do not exhibit functional instability, those with low activity demands, or in select cases of partial ACL tears.

Various surgical techniques have been developed for managing ACL injuries in skeletally immature patients, primarily categorized as physeal-sparing or transphyseal. The selection of the appropriate technique is guided by factors such as the patient's skeletal maturity, particularly the estimated remaining growth, and surgeon preference (Fig. 26.2). Generally, physeal-sparing techniques are recommended for prepubescent patients. Examples include extra-physeal methods utilizing iliotibial band autograft or all-epiphyseal reconstructions typically employing hamstring autograft (Fig. 26.3). For adolescents with approximately 2 years of anticipated growth remaining, partial or complete transphyseal techniques, often using hamstring autografts, may be considered. Patients approaching physeal closure or those who are already skeletally mature are candidates for anatomical reconstruction using techniques similar to those in adults, commonly utilizing hamstring, quadriceps tendon, or bone-patellar tendon-bone autografts. Although ACL repair techniques have been proposed as an alternative to reconstruction, current evidence does not support their routine use in skeletally immature patients. However, these methods may be considered in select cases, such as proximal ACL avulsion

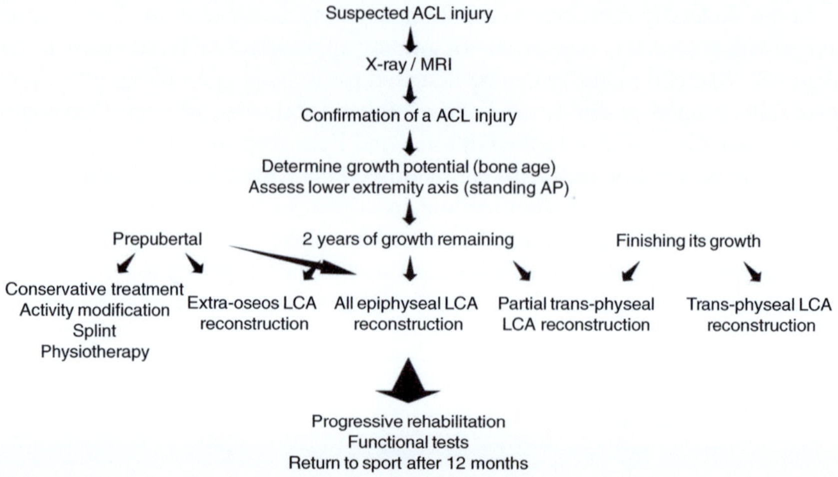

Fig. 26.2 Therapeutic algorithm for pediatric ACL injury. *Conservative management can be considered in patients who do not present functional instability, those with low demand and those with partial injuries

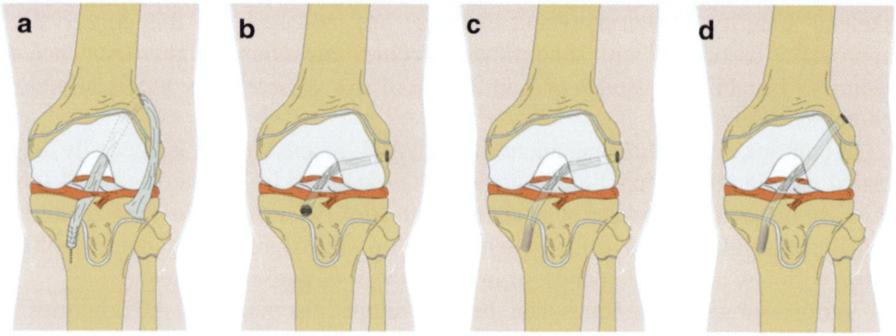

Fig. 26.3 ACL reconstruction techniques for the pediatric patient. (**a**) Extra-physeal, (**b**) all epiphyseal, (**c**) complete transphyseal, (**d**) partial transphyseal

fractures. A theoretical advantage of repair is the avoidance of bone tunnels, relying instead on anchor and suture fixation.

In skeletally immature patients requiring anterior cruciate ligament reconstruction, autograft selection is generally favored over allograft options due to evidence indicating higher failure rates associated with allograft utilization in this specific population [11].

During the preparation of bone tunnels, meticulous attention to detail is paramount to mitigate the risk of physeal injury and subsequent growth disturbances [3]. Optimal surgical technique dictates that fixation systems and bone plugs should be positioned to avoid the level of the growth plate. To further prevent the formation of physeal bone bridges, the tissue graft itself should occupy the portion of the tunnel that traverses the physis. Moreover, tunnel placement should aim for the most central location possible within the physis, and the tunnel diameter is typically restricted to less than 9 mm. This dimensional constraint is intended to maintain physeal damage below a critical threshold, estimated to be in the range of 7–9%, thereby minimizing the potential for growth arrest.

Postoperative rehabilitation protocols specifically standardized for skeletally immature patients are limited; consequently, adult rehabilitation programs are frequently adapted. These programs typically progress from an initial phase focused on pain and inflammation management to progressive neuromuscular rehabilitation, incorporating low-impact activities, jogging, cardiovascular exercises, and plyometrics in preparation for return to sport. While various criteria and protocols exist for determining readiness for return to sports, their validity in skeletally immature patients remains uncertain as they are primarily derived from adult populations. Functional testing is widely recommended, typically commencing around 6 months postoperatively, to objectively guide the rehabilitation process. These assessments aid in identifying neuromuscular and biomechanical deficits (e.g., in strength, balance, or coordination) that may represent modifiable risk factors for re-injury or graft failure. Return to sports is generally not recommended until at least 12 months post-surgery, and the decision is based on a multifactorial assessment encompassing not only biological healing but also joint stability, strength, and documented neuromuscular control.

Functional outcomes following ACL reconstruction in skeletally immature patients have been extensively evaluated across various techniques and graft types. Systematic reviews reporting outcomes using the International Knee Documentation Committee (IKDC) subjective score have demonstrated mean scores typically ranging from 81 to 100, with approximately 88% of cases achieving a grade of A or B (normal or nearly normal) [12]. Similarly, studies utilizing the Lysholm knee score have reported average scores around 94.6 (classified as good to excellent). Regarding return to sport, approximately 90% of patients successfully resume athletic activities; however, only about 80% manage to return to their pre-injury level of participation [13].

26.6 Complications of ACL Injuries

While successful outcomes are achievable with both conservative and surgical management, both approaches are associated with potential complications. Complications associated with conservative treatment may include persistent or recurrent knee instability and a heightened risk of secondary meniscal or chondral injuries. While the incidence of complications following surgical ACL reconstruction is generally low, potential risks must be considered. These risks can be minimized by accurately assessing the patient's remaining growth potential and selecting the appropriate surgical technique accordingly. Graft rupture represents one of the more common complications, with reported rates up to 19.7%. Furthermore, skeletally immature patients who sustain an ACL injury are at a considerable risk of a contralateral ACL injury, with reported rates nearing 12% [14].

Arthrofibrosis is another potential postoperative complication, with reported incidence rates up to 8.3%. Risk factors associated with arthrofibrosis include female sex, older chronological or skeletal age at surgery, use of bone-patellar tendon-bone autografts, and concurrent meniscal repair performed during ACL reconstruction.

A major concern unique to surgical ACL reconstruction in skeletally immature patients is the potential for iatrogenic physeal damage. Physeal damage resulting from bone tunnel creation can lead to angular deformities of the knee. Specifically, injury to the lateral distal femoral physis may result in genu valgum, while damage to the anterior proximal tibial physis can cause genu recurvatum. Limb length discrepancies may also occur, stemming from either premature physeal closure or accelerated growth secondary to physeal stimulation. Wong's systematic review [12] reported an incidence of angular deformities of 3.7%, primarily genu valgum, noting that 61% of these did not necessitate surgical intervention. The same review identified limb length discrepancies in 37 patients, with 51% of these cases experiencing shortening of the operated limb [12].

Less frequent, but serious, potential complications include infection and thromboembolic events. Early postoperative mobilization is strongly recommended to mitigate the risk of deep vein thrombosis (DVT). In patients with identified hypercoagulability risk factors, prophylactic anticoagulation should be considered in the postoperative period.

26.7 Meniscal Injuries: Incidence and Significance

Meniscal injuries are among the most common knee injuries in skeletally immature athletes, comparable in frequency to anterior cruciate ligament (ACL) tears. Their incidence has reportedly increased significantly in recent years. While the sequelae of meniscal tears and outcomes of meniscal repair have been extensively studied in adults, these issues have received less focus in pediatric populations, despite the high prevalence and potential for long-term negative impact on knee joint health and function.

The precise incidence and prevalence of meniscal injuries within the broader pediatric population remain challenging to ascertain. Although historically considered rare [15], more recent studies suggest the incidence is substantially higher than previously recognized [16]. For instance, the incidence of meniscal injury among US high school athletes has been reported at 40.7 per 100,000 athlete-exposures in males and 22.3 per 100,000 athlete-exposures in females [17]. Furthermore, a retrospective study of preadolescents presenting with traumatic knee hemarthrosis found that up to 45% had associated meniscal injuries [18].

26.8 Meniscal Anatomy and Biomechanics

The menisci are two asymmetrical, semicircular fibrocartilaginous structures composed of a complex network of type I collagen fibers, anchored to the tibial plateau via the meniscotibial ligaments at their anterior and posterior horns. This architecture provides structure and support, with predominant circumferential fibers resisting compressive loads and radially oriented fibers counteracting longitudinal tearing between the circumferential bundles. This unique structure develops over the first decade of life, after which pediatric menisci largely resemble those of adults in content and architecture. Meniscal vascularization undergoes significant changes postnatally. Up to approximately 9 months of age, the menisci are vascularized throughout their entire width by peripheral blood supply. Subsequently, vascularization becomes progressively limited, eventually leaving only the outer 10–30% in the "red zone" with direct blood supply [19].

26.9 Diagnosis of Meniscal Injuries

Meniscal injuries are broadly classified according to their morphologic pattern and precise anatomical location. Common tear configurations include vertical-longitudinal, oblique, radial, horizontal, and complex injuries. Vertical meniscal tears typically result from acute traumatic events and are frequently observed in conjunction with anterior cruciate ligament (ACL) injuries. In contrast, horizontal meniscal injuries are more commonly encountered in patients with discoid menisci. More recently, ramp and meniscal root injuries have been recognized and incorporated into the comprehensive classification of meniscal pathology. Ramp lesions, located at the meniscus-capsular junction of the posterior horn of the medial meniscus, are commonly identified in association with ACL tears. Anatomical and biomechanical studies have underscored the critical importance of the integrity of the posterior horn of the medial meniscus, which functions as a secondary stabilizer to anterior tibial translation. Meniscal root injuries, affecting both the medial and lateral menisci, involve tears at their respective tibial osseous insertions.

The diagnosis of meniscal injuries relies on a comprehensive approach, beginning with a detailed clinical history of the mechanism of injury and characteristic symptoms such as pain, locking, catching, or instability. Physical examination plays a crucial role, utilizing provocative maneuvers such as the McMurray test, Apley's compression, and distraction tests, along with palpation for joint line tenderness. Magnetic resonance imaging (MRI) is considered the gold standard imaging modality, offering high sensitivity and specificity for visualizing meniscal pathology. Ultimately, arthroscopy provides definitive diagnosis and allows for simultaneous surgical intervention.

26.10 Treatment of Meniscal Injuries

While small, non-displaced tears in the vascularized periphery may heal spontaneously, most symptomatic meniscal injuries in pediatric patients require surgical intervention to prevent further damage and long-term sequelae. The high healing potential observed in this age group, coupled with the poor long-term outcomes associated with subtotal and total meniscectomy, strongly support a philosophy of

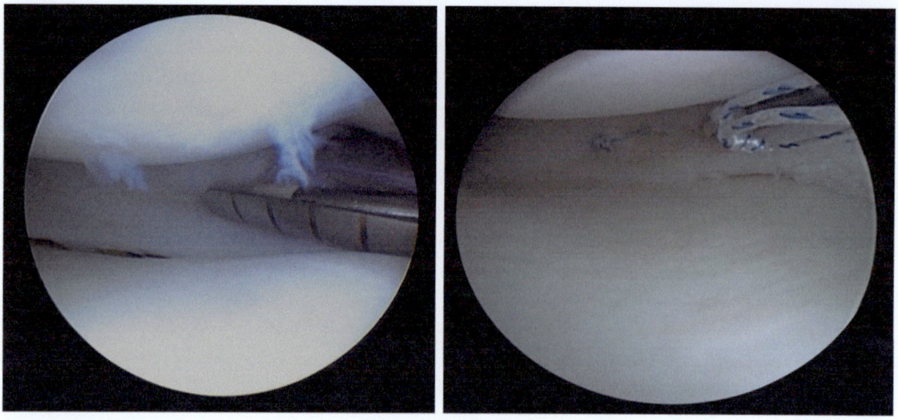

Fig. 26.4 Arthroscopic view of a meniscal repair with the "all inside" technique

meniscal preservation through surgical repair whenever feasible. Arthroscopic treatment is considered the gold standard for both diagnosis and management.

Meniscal repair can be performed using various arthroscopic techniques, including all-inside, inside-out, outside-in, or combined approaches. All-inside meniscal repair utilizes specialized devices comprising sutures attached to implants placed on both sides of the tear, which are then tensioned to reduce the tear (Fig. 26.4). Inside-out repair involves passing a double-loaded suture with flexible needles through both sides of the tear from within the joint, exiting through the capsule. The sutures are subsequently tied outside the capsule using a small open incision to mitigate the risk of entrapment of adjacent neurovascular structures. The outside-in technique is typically employed for tears located in the anterior horn.

A recent systematic review [20] reported excellent or good clinical outcomes in a high proportion of patients undergoing meniscal repair in this population. The reported failure rate requiring revision surgery was approximately 17%. Factors associated with higher meniscal healing rates include younger age, peripheral tears (specifically within the vascularized red zone, typically within 3 mm of the meniscal edge), lateral meniscus tears (compared to medial), concomitant ACL reconstruction (due to biological stimulation), surgery performed within 8 weeks of injury, and tear lengths less than 2.5 cm.

26.11 Complications of Meniscal Treatment

Complications associated with meniscal repair include failure of the tear to heal (re-tear), iatrogenic neurovascular injury, hemarthrosis, and arthrofibrosis. Minimizing complications necessitates meticulous surgical technique, thorough anatomical knowledge, appropriate patient and tear selection for the chosen repair method, and adherence to adequate postoperative rehabilitation protocols. Techniques to augment healing, such as synovial abrasion, marrow venting (creating small perforations into the bone), and fibrin clot application, have recently gained popularity.

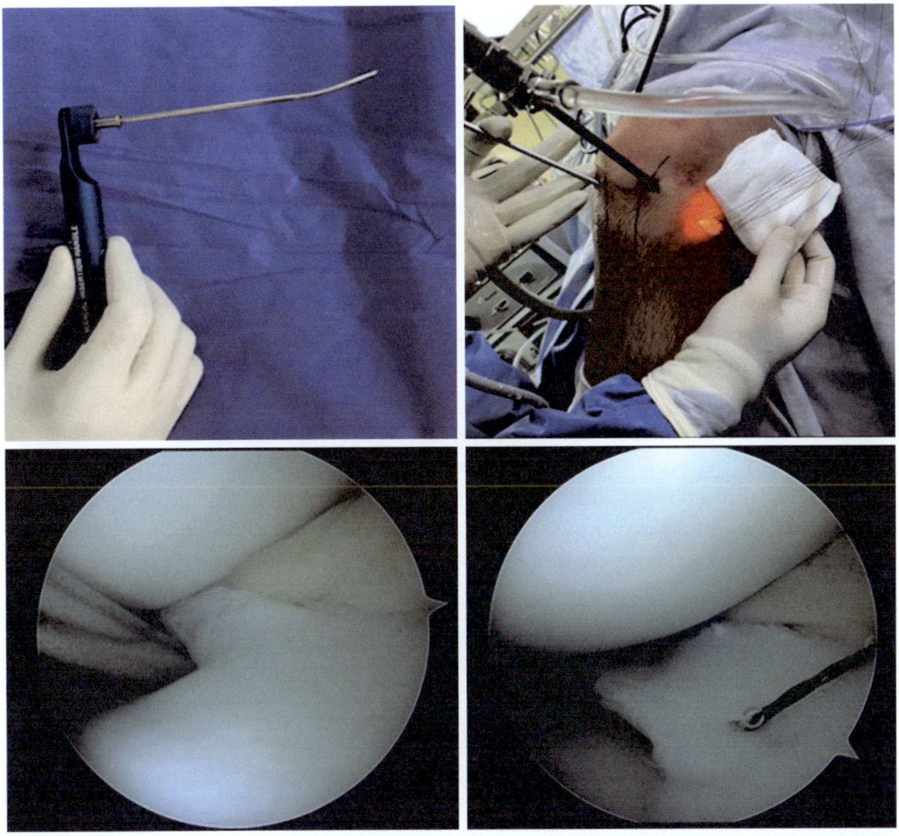

Fig. 26.5 Intraoperative and arthroscopic images of a repair meniscus with "in-side/out-side" technique

Awareness of the local anatomy is critical when performing repair. For inside-out repair, a posteromedial approach should be employed for medial meniscus repairs and a posterolateral approach for lateral meniscus repairs to safely retrieve sutures and protect adjacent neurovascular structures. Recent anatomical studies also highlight the proximity of neurovascular structures, particularly the common peroneal nerve laterally, when utilizing all-inside repair devices inserted through the anterolateral portal for lateral meniscus tears [21]. Conversely, complications following meniscectomy include the development of progressive osteoarthritis, joint pain, and instability, particularly after subtotal or total meniscectomy (Fig. 26.5).

26.12 Discoid Meniscus

Discoid meniscus (DM) is a congenital structural anomaly characterized by an enlarged, thickened meniscal body and altered collagen fiber architecture, often described as decreased and disorganized. These morphological and histological abnormalities compromise meniscal shape and stability, predisposing it to tearing and degeneration [22]. Its reported prevalence varies widely, ranging from approximately 0.4–20% depending on the population studied and diagnostic method employed [23]. DM almost exclusively affects the lateral meniscus (Fig. 26.6).

DM may be diagnosed incidentally during imaging performed for other reasons in asymptomatic individuals, or patients may present clinically with mechanical symptoms including pain, joint effusion, and audible or palpable intra-articular clicking. Magnetic Resonance Imaging (MRI) serves as a crucial diagnostic tool. When interpreted in conjunction with clinical findings, MRI confirms the diagnosis, provides detailed analysis of meniscal morphology and tear patterns, facilitates detection of associated osteochondral or ligamentous injuries, and can assess for signs of peripheral instability.

Management of discoid meniscus is primarily guided by the patient's clinical presentation and meniscal stability (Fig. 26.7). Asymptomatic DM, regardless of meniscal stability, typically requires no specific intervention; observation is indicated. For symptomatic, stable DM, the treatment of choice is arthroscopic saucerization (partial meniscectomy). This procedure aims to surgically reshape the discoid meniscus to a more functional, crescent-like morphology. Saucerization

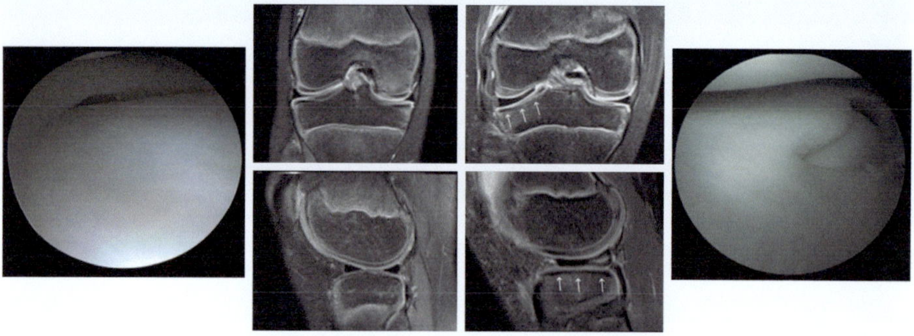

Fig. 26.6 Magnetic resonance image (in coronal/sagittal views) and arthroscopic intraoperative image where the difference between a normal meniscus and a discoid meniscus (white arrows) can be seen

Fig. 26.7 Therapeutic algorithm for the discoid meniscus

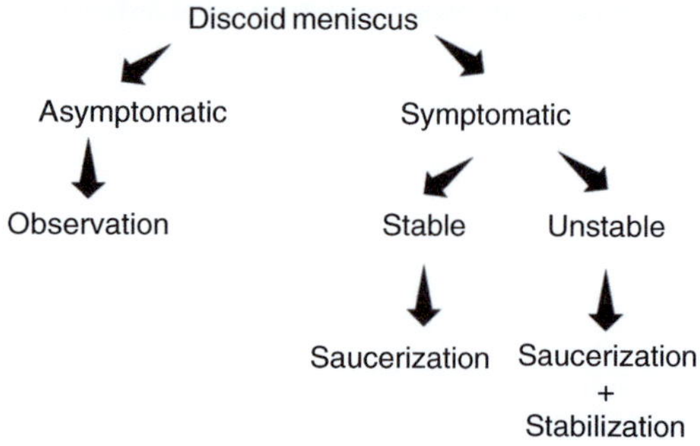

generally yields satisfactory short- and mid-term clinical outcomes [24, 25]. It is important to note that associated peripheral meniscal instability has been reported in approximately one-third of surgically treated patients [26]. In cases of symptomatic, unstable DM, the management strategy has evolved. Traditionally, these tears were treated with subtotal or total meniscectomy. However, this approach is associated with poor long-term outcomes, including persistent instability and accelerated degenerative changes in the lateral compartment of the knee [27]. Recent literature supports meniscal preservation techniques for unstable DM whenever possible. These techniques typically involve arthroscopic saucerization combined with concurrent repair of the peripheral instability. Studies reporting mid-term results of meniscal preservation techniques for unstable DM have been encouraging [28]. Evaluation of the mechanical axis of the lower limbs is an essential component in the overall management of pediatric patients with symptomatic DM, particularly those with lateral compartment pathology. Early correction of associated genu valgum deviations, potentially through guided growth techniques, may be beneficial in optimizing long-term outcomes and managing this condition.

26.13 Authors' Recommendations

- Implementation of ACL injury prevention programs is recommended for at-risk populations.
- Systematic clinical evaluation, including mandatory comparison to the contralateral limb, is essential.
- Accurate assessment of skeletal maturity is fundamental for appropriate treatment planning.
- Conservative treatment is generally reserved for patients with high adherence to rehabilitation protocols, absence of associated meniscal or chondral lesions, and partial ACL tears.
- Surgical technique selection is guided by the patient's remaining growth potential and surgeon experience and judgment.
- Technical considerations during tunnel creation are crucial for physeal preservation. Avoid placing fixation systems or bone plugs across the physis.
- To minimize physeal damage and the risk of growth arrest, bone tunnels should be positioned as centrally as possible within the physis, their diameter limited (e.g., < 9 mm), and overly oblique trajectories avoided. The tunnel segment crossing the physis should ideally be occupied by a soft tissue graft rather than left empty.
- Appropriate counseling for patients and families should include realistic expectations regarding return to sport and the potential risk of graft rupture or contralateral ACL injury.
- Meniscal tears in the pediatric population are frequently associated with other knee pathologies, such as ACL injuries, tibial spine fractures, or discoid meniscus.

- Meniscal tears in the skeletally immature knee should undergo repair whenever feasible to maximize meniscal preservation.
- Meniscal preservation surgery in pediatric and adolescent patients generally demonstrates high success rates.

26.14 Final Message

The incidence of anterior cruciate ligament (ACL) and meniscal injuries in the skeletally immature population has demonstrably risen over recent decades. Given the crucial role of these structures in knee biomechanics, timely diagnosis and appropriate management are essential for restoring joint function and safeguarding articular cartilage health. Furthermore, ACL injury prevention programs implemented in at-risk populations have demonstrated significant efficacy. While conservative management for ACL tears in this population generally yields suboptimal outcomes, it may be indicated in select cases based on specific criteria. When surgical intervention is indicated, accurate assessment of remaining growth potential is essential to guide the selection of the appropriate reconstruction technique. Advancements in meniscal repair techniques, coupled with the inherently higher healing potential observed in skeletally immature patients, strongly support the trend toward meniscal preservation surgery.

References

1. Werner BC, Yang S, Looney AM, Gwathmey FW Jr. Trends in pediatric and adolescent anterior cruciate ligament injury and reconstruction. J Pediatr Orthop. 2016;36(5):447–52. https://doi.org/10.1097/BPO.0000000000000482.
2. Nogaro MC, Abram SGF, Alvand A, Bottomley N, Jackson WFM, Price A. Paediatric and adolescent anterior cruciate ligament reconstruction surgery. Bone Joint J. 2020;102-B(2):239–45. https://doi.org/10.1302/0301-620X.102B2.BJJ-2019-0420.R2.
3. Fabricant PD, Kocher MS. Management of ACL injuries in children and adolescents. J Bone Joint Surg Am. 2017;99(7):600–12. https://doi.org/10.2106/JBJS.16.00953.
4. Beynnon BD, Vacek PM, Newell MK, Tourville TW, Smith HC, Shultz SJ, et al. The effects of level of competition, sport, and sex on the incidence of first-time noncontact anterior cruciate ligament injury. Am J Sports Med. 2014;42(8):1806–12. https://doi.org/10.1177/0363546514540862.
5. Anderson AF, Anderson CN. Correlation of meniscal and articular cartilage injuries in children and adolescents with timing of anterior cruciate ligament reconstruction. Am J Sports Med. 2015;43(2):275–81. https://doi.org/10.1177/0363546514559912.
6. Petushek EJ, Sugimoto D, Stoolmiller M, Smith G, Myer GD. Evidence-based Best-practice guidelines for preventing anterior cruciate ligament injuries in young female athletes: a systematic review and meta-analysis. Am J Sports Med. 2019;47(7):1744–53. https://doi.org/10.1177/0363546518782460.
7. Herring JA. Chapter 1. Growth and development. In: Tachdjian's pediatric orthopaedics. 6th ed. Amsterdam: Elsevier; 2020. p. 19.

8. Perkins CA, Willimon SC. Pediatric anterior cruciate ligament reconstruction. Orthop Clin North Am. 2020;51(1):55–63. https://doi.org/10.1016/j.ocl.2019.08.009.
9. Slough JM, Hennrikus W, Chang Y. Reliability of Tanner staging performed by orthopedic sports medicine surgeons. Med Sci Sports Exerc. 2013;45(7):1229–34. https://doi.org/10.1249/MSS.0b013e318285c2f7.
10. Ramski DE, Kanj WW, Franklin CC, Baldwin KD, Ganley TJ. Anterior cruciate ligament tears in children and adolescents: a meta-analysis of nonoperative versus operative treatment. Am J Sports Med. 2014;42(11):2769–76. https://doi.org/10.1177/0363546513510889.
11. Engelman GH, Carry PM, Hitt KG, Polousky JD, Vidal AF. Comparison of allograft versus autograft anterior cruciate ligament reconstruction graft survival in an active adolescent cohort. Am J Sports Med. 2014;42(10):2311–8. https://doi.org/10.1177/0363546514541935.
12. Wong SE, Feeley BT, Pandya NK. Complications after pediatric ACL reconstruction: a meta-analysis. J Pediatr Orthop. 2019;39(8):e566–71. https://doi.org/10.1097/BPO.0000000000001075.
13. Kay J, Memon M, Marx RG, Peterson D, Simunovic N, Ayeni OR. Over 90% of children and adolescents return to sport after anterior cruciate ligament reconstruction: a systematic review and meta-analysis. Knee Surg Sports Traumatol Arthrosc. 2018;26(4):1019–36. https://doi.org/10.1007/s00167-018-4830-9.
14. DeFrancesco CJ, Striano BM, Bram JT, Baldwin KD, Ganley TJ. An in-depth analysis of graft rupture and contralateral anterior cruciate ligament rupture rates after pediatric anterior cruciate ligament reconstruction. Am J Sports Med. 2020;48(10):2395–400. https://doi.org/10.1177/0363546520935437.
15. Andrish JT. Meniscal injuries in children and adolescents: diagnosis and management. J Am Acad Orthop Surg. 1996;4(5):231–7. https://doi.org/10.5435/00124635-199609000-00001.
16. Bellisari G, Samora W, Klingele K. Meniscus tears in children. Sports Med Arthrosc Rev. 2011;19(1):50–5. https://doi.org/10.1097/JSA.0b013e318204d01a.
17. Mitchell J, Graham W, Best TM, Collins C, Currie DW, Comstock RD, et al. Epidemiology of meniscal injuries in US high school athletes between 2007 and 2013. Knee Surg Sports Traumatol Arthrosc. 2016;24(3):715–22. https://doi.org/10.1007/s00167-015-3814-2.
18. Stanitski CL, Harvell JC, Fu F. Observations on acute knee hemarthrosis in children and adolescents. J Pediatr Orthop. 1993;13(4):506–10. https://doi.org/10.1097/01241398-199307000-00016.
19. Chambers HG, Chambers RC. The natural history of meniscus tears. J Pediatr Orthop. 2019;39(6 Suppl 1):S53–5. https://doi.org/10.1097/BPO.0000000000001386.
20. Liechti DJ, Constantinescu DS, Ridley TJ, Chahla J, Mitchell JJ, Vap AR. Meniscal repair in pediatric populations: a systematic review of outcomes. Orthop J Sports Med. 2019;7(5):2325967119843355. https://doi.org/10.1177/2325967119843355.
21. Shea KG, Dingel AB, Styhl A, Richmond CG, Cannamela PC, Anderson AF, et al. The position of the popliteal artery and peroneal nerve relative to the menisci in children: a cadaveric study. Orthop J Sports Med. 2019;7(6):2325967119842843. https://doi.org/10.1177/2325967119842843.
22. Kocher MS, Logan CA, Kramer DE. Discoid lateral meniscus in children: diagnosis, management, and outcomes. J Am Acad Orthop Surg. 2017;25(11):736–43. https://doi.org/10.5435/JAAOS-D-15-00491.
23. Rohren EM, Kosarek FJ, Helms CA. Discoid lateral meniscus and the frequency of meniscal tears. Skeletal Radiol. 2001;30(6):316–20. https://doi.org/10.1007/s002560100351.
24. Atay OA, Doral MN, Leblebicio lu G, Tetik O, Aydingöz U. Management of discoid lateral meniscus tears: observations in 34 knees. Arthroscopy. 2003;19(4):346–52. https://doi.org/10.1053/jars.2003.50038.
25. Ogüt T, Kesmezacar H, Akgün I, Cansü E. Arthroscopic meniscectomy for discoid lateral meniscus in children and adolescents: 4.5 year follow-up. J Pediatr Orthop B. 2003;12(6):390–7. https://doi.org/10.1097/01202412-200311000-00007.

26. Klingele KE, Kocher MS, Hresko MT, Gerbino P, Micheli LJ. Discoid lateral meniscus: prevalence of peripheral rim instability. J Pediatr Orthop. 2004;24(1):79–82. https://doi.org/10.1097/00004694-200401000-00015.
27. Lee YS, Teo SH, Ahn JH, Lee OS, Lee SH, Lee JH. Systematic review of the long-term surgical outcomes of discoid lateral meniscus. Arthroscopy. 2017;33(10):1884–95. https://doi.org/10.1016/j.arthro.2017.04.006.
28. Carabajal M, Allende GJ, Masquijo JJ. Mid-term results of arthroscopic remodeling combined with peripheral repair in children with unstable discoid meniscus. Rev Esp Cir Ortop Traumatol. 2020;64(3):206–12. https://doi.org/10.1016/j.recot.2019.10.002. English, Spanish. Epub 2019 Dec 9.

Chapter 27
Fracture of the Anterior Tuberosity of the Tibia

Gonzalo De la Fuente and Alejandro Gündel

Fractures of the tibial tuberosity are rare injuries that occur in adolescent patients, usually athletes. Their frequency is increasing due to the massive practice of sports with higher physical demand. It is important to recognize the injured structures to achieve appropriate treatment, seeking to restore the anatomy of the knee, the function of the extensor apparatus and avoid potential complications.

27.1 Introduction

Fractures of the anterior tuberosity of the tibia (ATT) are injuries that compromise the proximal apophysis of the tibia, with variable displacement, and that can be associated with intraarticular extension of the fracture and soft tissue injury. Most of these injuries occur in male athletes, with good muscular development and skeletal maturity, during sports activities that involve jumping.

The higher frequency in males is explained by their participation in sports with higher physical demand and by the later age at which the physis closure of the proximal tibial tubercle occurs.

They are rare injuries, with a reported incidence between 0.4% and 2.7%, and represent less than 1% of physeal injuries, and around 3% of all proximal tibia fractures.

G. De la Fuente
Clínica Alemana Santiago, Santiago, Chile

A. Gündel (✉)
Clínica Alemana, Hospital Militar de Santiago, Santiago, Chile

M. Sepúlveda O. (ed.), *Paediatrics Traumatology*,
https://doi.org/10.1007/978-3-031-89482-4_27

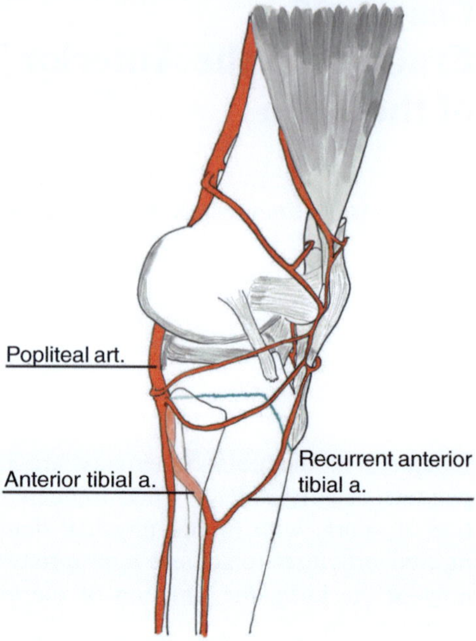

Fig. 27.1 Scheme of the relationship between the proximal tibia and the vascular structures. The popliteal artery may be trapped at the fracture site, while the recurrent anterior tibial artery is related to the incidence of compartment syndrome

27.2 Anatomy

The proximal tibia has two ossification centers, one primary, which corresponds to the proximal tibial epiphysis, and one secondary, which corresponds to the ATT, the distal insertion site of the knee extensor mechanism.

According to Ogden, the ATT initially develops as an anterior extension of the proximal tibial physis, around 12–15 weeks of gestation. During adolescence, these two ossification centers are separated by a relatively small cartilaginous bridge, which predisposes to a potential avulsive injury of the tuberosity. The physis of the ATT closes between the ages of 13 and 15 years in women and 15 and 19 years in men.

The anterior recurrent tibial artery (Fig. 27.1) is relevant in this type of injury, since, when the avulsion of the ATT occurs, some branches may retract under the fascia and muscles of the anterior compartment of the leg, which could be related to the development of a compartment syndrome.

27.3 Mechanism of Injury

These injuries usually occur in the context of sports activities, mainly basketball, and those in which competitive jumps are performed. The avulsion of the ATT occurs due to an active extension of the knee with a violent eccentric contraction of the quadriceps (more common), or by an acute passive flexion with the quadriceps in contraction (less common).

The injury pattern will depend both on the extent of skeletal maturation as well as the degree of knee flexion at the time of the injury. If the injury occurs with knee extension or with flexion less than 30°, an avulsion of the ATT usually occurs, without compromising the proximal tibial epiphysis. With flexion greater than 30°, there may be injury to the ATT, with epiphyseal or/and intraarticular involvement.

Although it is controversial, several authors suggest that Osgood Schlatter disease would be a risk factor for ATT fractures by increasing the amount of columnar cartilage in relation to the fibrocartilage in the physis, which in turn would generate greater weakness of the physis and consequent avulsion of the ATT.

27.4 Classification

There are multiple classifications for this type of fractures, mostly based on the characteristics of the fracture trait, and have been developed from the one described by Watson-Jones, who divided them into 3 types: Type 1, a small avulsion of the distal end of the ATT; Type 2, in which the entire ATT is displaced proximally, with the apex of the displacement at the level of the proximal tibial physis; and Type 3, where the fracture trait propagates through the proximal epiphysis of the tibia, toward the joint.

Ogden modifies this classification, emphasizing the intraarticular commitment and the comminution of the ATT. In Ogden Type 1, only the distal portion of the ATT is compromised; Subtype A consists of a fracture that compromises the ossification center, but without or with minimal displacement, while in Subtype B, the fragment is separated from the metaphysis. In Type 2, the ossification center is completely separated from the metaphysis; Subtype A consists of a complete ATT fragment, while in Subtype B, the ossification center is comminuted and the most distal fragment displaced toward proximal. In Type 3, the fracture trait extends toward the joint, in Subtype A, the fragment is complete, while in Subtype B, it is comminuted (Fig. 27.2).

New types of fractures have been described, either compromising the entire proximal tibial physis from anterior to posterior (Type IV), or a Type IIb associated with a Type IV (Type V).

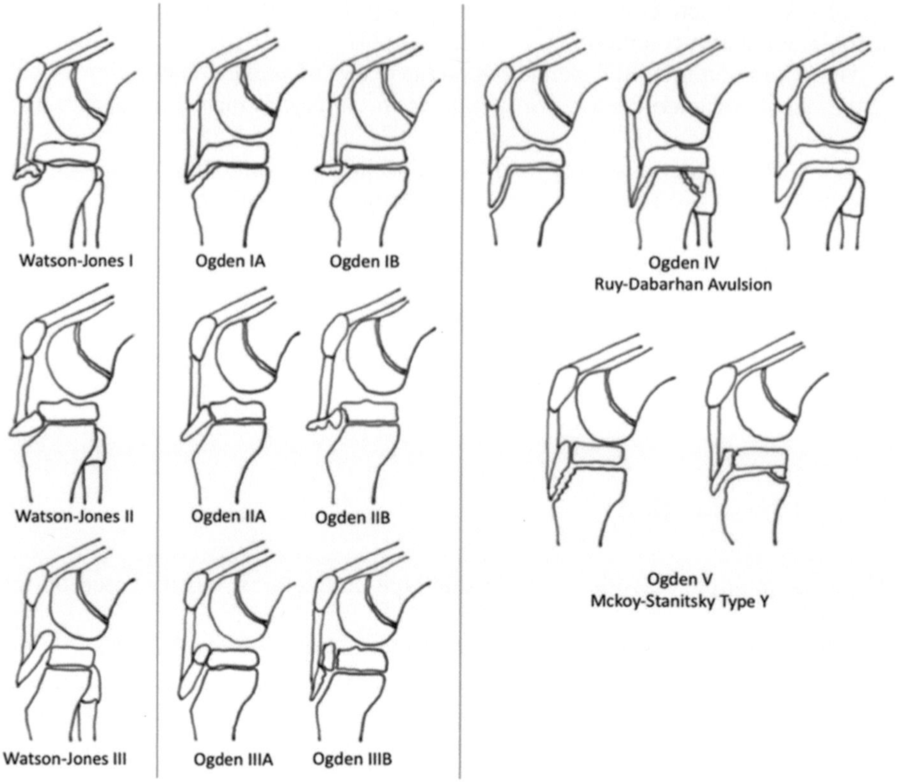

Fig. 27.2 Comparative scheme with the different classifications used to describe fractures of the anterior tuberosity of the tibia

27.5 Clinical Evaluation

Patients generally present with increased volume and pain at the level of the ATT fracture. In cases of fractures without displacement, knee extension against gravity is usually preserved and joint effusion is absent. Patients with Type 2 or Type 3 fractures cannot achieve active knee extension and most present with hemarthrosis.

The knee is usually in 20–40° flexion secondary to a hamstring contracture. In addition, they can present with a high patella depending on the degree of patellar tendon involvement. The association between ATT fractures and compartment syndrome of the leg has been described, so this should be actively sought, also the distal neurovascular evaluation of the limb is mandatory.

27.6 Imaging Study

As with all fractures, radiography is the initial study in this type of injuries. Obtaining an anteroposterior and a lateral X-ray projection of the knee is essential in the evaluation in an emergency department. Because the ATT is slightly lateral to the midline of the tibia, the lateral projection should be with a little internal rotation of the leg. Oblique projections could be useful to evaluate the intraarticular extension of the fracture; however, they are not routinely requested in all patients suspected of this injury.

In certain cases, the X-ray may be insufficient to characterize the fracture pattern, so computed tomography (CT scan) can be useful to better understand the configuration of this and assist in preoperative planning (Fig. 27.3).

Magnetic resonance imaging (MRI) is useful when there is a high index of suspicion of meniscal, ligamentous, articular cartilage, or physeal injuries (Fig. 27.4).

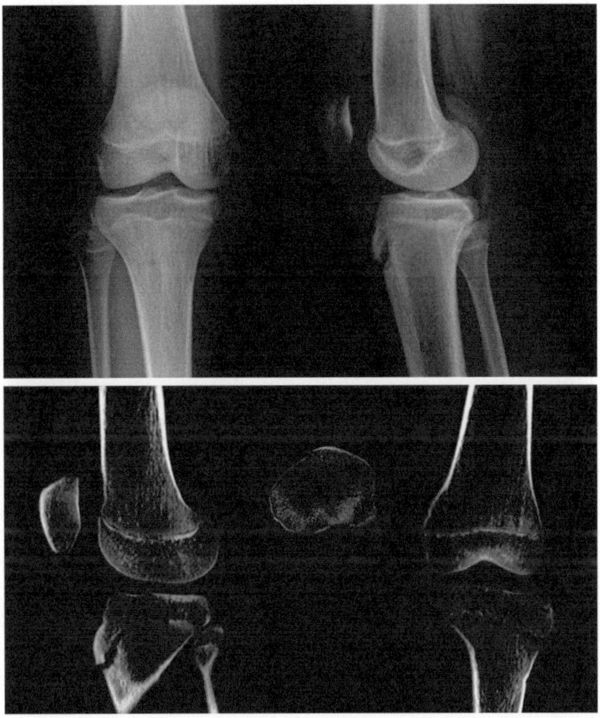

Fig. 27.3 Right knee X-rays of a 14-year-old boy with a Ogden IIIA type anterior tibial tuberosity fracture. Fracture line is evident on CT scan, where articular involvement is seen

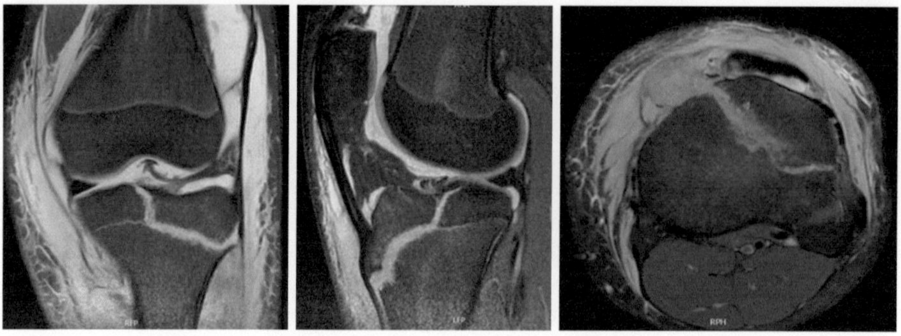

Fig. 27.4 Magnetic resonance imaging of the knee of a 14-year-old boy, where the anterior root of the lateral meniscus is trapped at the fracture feature

27.7 Treatment

The goal of treatment is to restore normal anatomy and the knee extensor mechanism. Depending on the type of fracture, the degree of displacement of the fragments, and associated injuries, they can be treated conservatively or surgically.

The treatment of Type IA fractures (non-displaced) is conservative, with a knee brace or long leg cast, with the knee in full extension, for 4–6 weeks, followed by progressive rehabilitation. In Type IB fractures, treatment can be attempted conservative, with closed reduction of the fragment and immobilization, as described for Type IA.

Type II and III fractures require surgical treatment, which usually consists of open reduction and bone fixation with a tension band or cannulated screws, from anterior to posterior (Fig. 27.5). It is recommended to use osteosynthesis with partially threaded cannulated screws to achieve better compression of the fragments. Uni or bicortical fixation has not shown a difference in functional outcomes (Fig. 27.6). It is advisable to repair and suture the periosteum and the extensor apparatus when extensive avulsion of the ATT is found.

In the postoperative period, it is recommended to protect the knee in extension for 4–6 weeks, start progressive mobilization, and resume physical and sports activities no earlier than 3 months.

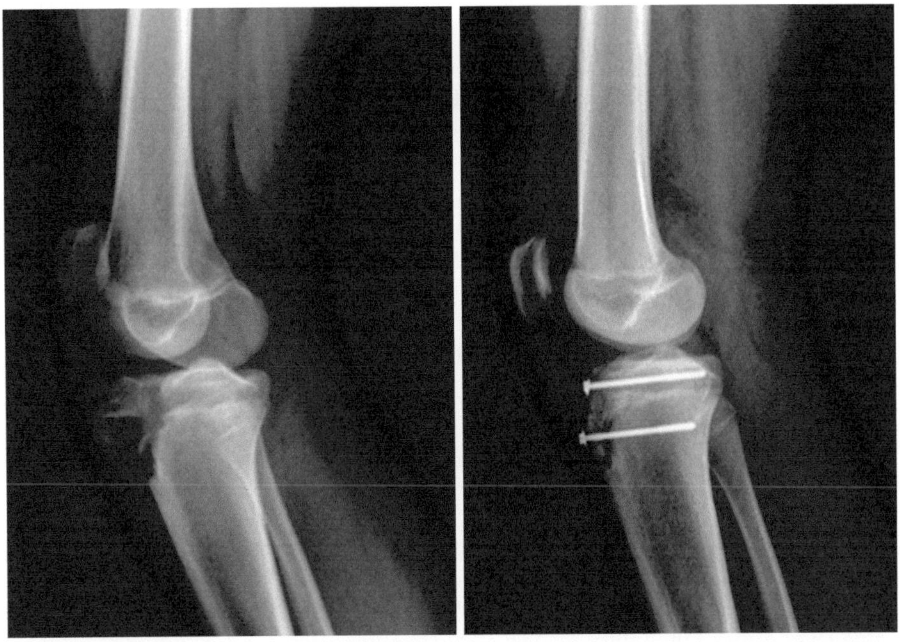

Fig. 27.5 Ogden IIIB type anterior tibial tuberosity fracture. Open reduction and osteosynthesis with screws chosen

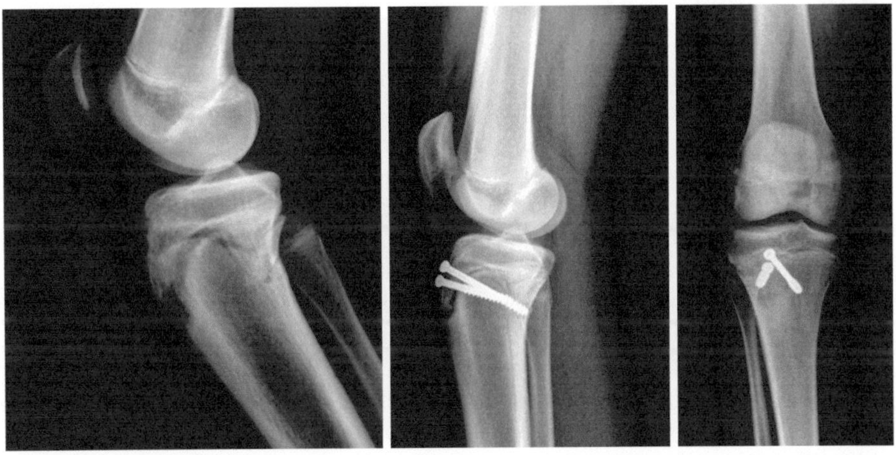

Fig. 27.6 Ogden IV type anterior tibial tuberosity fracture. Was treated with closed reduction and screws to the metaphysis

27.8 Complications

The most frequently described complication is anterior knee pain related to inflammation and bursitis caused by prominent implants (56%), but only a smaller proportion requires their removal.

Other complications described, but at a lower frequency, are new fracture, genu recurvatum, difference in length of lower limbs, and limitation of the range of knee flexion mobility.

Compartment syndrome is a serious acute complication that should always be suspected in ATT fractures, to manage it appropriately and timely. It has been described in 4–20% of cases, in different studies.

27.9 Results

Regardless of the type of fracture and the treatment performed, studies show excellent results, with bone healing close to 100%. The full range of knee mobility is achieved on average between 6 and 7 months. The return to physical activity at the same level prior to the injury reaches 98%, in approximately 7–8 months.

27.10 Authors' Advice

We request a CT scan when there is suspicion of articular extension of the fracture, which allows us to categorize and classify the injury. If possible, we complement with MRI in those fractures where joint compromise is confirmed.

In patients with Type 1A fractures, we prefer temporary immobilization for 5–7 days with a knee brace, followed by a plaster long leg brace for 4–6 weeks. Afterwards we recommend starting physiotherapy as soon as possible, focused on the recovery of the range of movement and quadriceps strengthening.

In Type IB fractures, we attempt closed reduction with knee extension; if successful, the treatment is the same as for type IA fractures. If the reduction is not satisfactory, the treatment is surgical.

In Type II, III, IV, and V fractures, the treatment of choice is surgery, with open reduction through a central longitudinal incision from the lower pole of the patella to the ATT. We perform fixation with cannulated screws. We reserve knee arthroscopy for those patients who present with an associated meniscal, ligamentous, or chondral injury. In the postoperative period, we indicate immobilization with an articulated splint, locked in extension for 4 weeks, followed by progressive physiotherapy.

Further Readings

Mosier SM, Stanitski CL. Acute tibial tubercle avulsion fractures. J Pediatr Orthop. 2004;24(2):181–4. https://doi.org/10.1097/00004694-200403000-00009.

Ogden JA, Tross RB, Murphy MJ. Fractures of the tibial tuberosity in adolescents. J Bone Joint Surg Am. 1980;62(2):205–15.

Pretell-Mazzini J, Kelly DM, Sawyer JR, Esteban EM, Spence DD, Warner WC Jr, et al. Outcomes and complications of tibial tubercle fractures in pediatric patients: a systematic review of the literature. J Pediatr Orthop. 2016;36(5):440–6. https://doi.org/10.1097/BPO.0000000000000488.

Nwachukwu BU, Rauck RC, Doyle SM. Pediatric and Adolescent Knee Surgery. Tibial tubercle avulsion fracture in children and adolescents in pediatric and adolescent knee surgery. In: Cordasco F, Green D. 1st ed. Lippincott Williams and Wilkins; N.º 1 edición (1 junio 2015) Fracture.

Rodriguez I, Sepúlveda M, Birrer E, Tuca MJ. Fracture of the anterior tibial tuberosity in children. EFORT Open Rev. 2020;5(5):260–7. Published 2020 May 5. https://doi.org/10.1302/2058-5241.5.190026.

Arkader A, Schur M, Refakis C, Capraro A, Woon R, Choi P. Unicortical fixation is sufficient for surgical treatment of tibial tubercle avulsion fractures in children. J Pediatr Orthop. 2019;39(1):e18–22. https://doi.org/10.1097/BPO.0000000000001269.

Cole WW 3rd, Brown SM, Vopat B, Heard WMR, Mulcahey MK. Epidemiology, diagnosis, and management of tibial tubercle avulsion fractures in adolescents. JBJS Rev. 2020;8(4):e0186. https://doi.org/10.2106/JBJS.RVW.19.00186.

Haber DB, Tepolt FA, McClincy MP, Hussain ZB, Kalish LA, Kocher MS. Tibial tubercle fractures in children and adolescents: a large retrospective case series. J Pediatr Orthop B. 2021;30(1):13–8. https://doi.org/10.1097/BPB.0000000000000756.

Chapter 28
Proximal Tibia Fracture

Astrid Medina and Daniel Pineda

Proximal tibia fractures in pediatric patients are relatively rare. Of the fractures of long bones at this age, they represent only 1.8%, and of all physeal fractures from 0.6–2.1%. Around 50% occur because of sports accidents, being more frequent in adolescents. Most cases correspond to Type II Salter-Harris injuries, followed in frequency by Type III injuries. Proximal tibia fractures can compromise the physis or the proximal metaphysis. Metaphyseal fractures usually occur in children between 3 and 6-years-old, and can be incomplete (in "green stick" or in "torus"), or complete. In adolescents, physeal fractures are more common, especially those that compromise the anterior tuberosity of the tibia and are associated with sports trauma.

28.1 Introduction

The ossification nucleus of the proximal tibia usually appears between the first and third month of birth.

The physis of the proximal tibia is responsible for 55% of the longitudinal growth of the tibia, and 25% of the total length of the lower limb. It grows approximately 0.6 cm per year. The closure of the proximal tibia growth cartilage is usually completed between 13 and 15 years in women, and between 15 and 18 years in men. This closure is from posterior to anterior (from posteromedial to anterolateral), which determines the fracture pattern in adolescents.

A. Medina
Fundación Cardio infantil, Clínica Reina Sofia Pediátrica y Mujer, Bogotá, Colombia

D. Pineda (✉)
Hospital Guillermo Grant Benavente de Concepción, Universidad de Concepción, Concepción, Chile

M. Sepúlveda O. (ed.), *Paediatrics Traumatology*,
https://doi.org/10.1007/978-3-031-89482-4_28

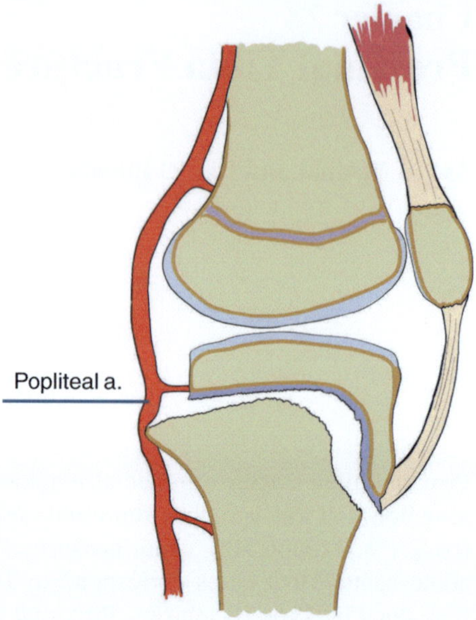

Fig. 28.1 Relationship of vascular structures, popliteal artery, with the proximal epiphysis of the tibia and its risk of injury

The proximal tibia is intrinsically stable given its anatomical relationship with some structures. In front of the metaphysis is the anterior tuberosity of the tibia, which blocks posterior displacement. The semimembranosus muscle tendon crosses medially to the physis, at the posteromedial corner. In itself, the inclined shape of the growth cartilage at this level provides greater stability. These anatomical characteristics of the area cause the epiphysis to displace anteriorly and externally in a fracture, and the metaphysis to displace posteriorly and internally.

The proximal physis of the tibia is also protected by the proximal tibioperoneal joint, while the ligamentous insertions in the area are distal to the physis, providing varus and valgus stability, as well as translational stability. It is also protected by the lateral collateral ligament, which inserts directly into the head of the fibula, and the medial collateral, which does so in the metaphysis [1].

The popliteal artery is located behind the proximal metaphysis of the tibia, separated from the bone by the popliteus muscle. Distally it is limited by the soleus arch, and its anterior tibial branch that penetrates the interosseous space. This allows little mobility, which makes it susceptible to injury in the event of a posterior displacement of the metaphysis of the proximal tibia (Fig. 28.1).

28.2 Mechanism of Injury

The intrinsic stability of the proximal tibia leads to most injuries being due to indirect mechanisms, after sudden eccentric or concentric muscle contractions. These mechanisms cause the fracture when the limb suffers a force in abduction, adduction, or hyperextension, with a knee in a fixed position, as usually occurs in landing on the limb, or takeoff when jumping [2, 3].

The direction of the fracture line will also be determined by the asymmetric physeal closure of the epiphysis with the anterior tuberosity, which occurs around 15 years. [4]. First, the posterior and medial physis closes. Then the closure continues toward the anterolateral side, until the anterior tuberosity is completely closed, which causes the metaphysis to move toward the posterior or posterolateral in relation to the epiphysis, due to the stability provided by the fibula and the presence of the anterior tuberosity of the tibia. In adolescent patients, up to 40% of associated ligament injuries can occur, with anterior cruciate ligament injuries being the most common, followed by medial collateral ligament injuries.

The presence of associated vascular injury is very low, on the order of 0.6%, and of these, 5% involve the popliteal artery. The rate of neurological or vascular injury in proximal tibial physeal fractures is on the order of 14%, with neurological injuries associated with excessive traction during reduction maneuvers. A factor to consider in these patients is that they may present spasms of the popliteal artery, up to 24 h after reduction, so they require strict monitoring. Similarly, peroneal neuropathies are usually due to traction, and recover in a period ranging from 4 to 6 months.

28.3 Classification

For classification, it is necessary to describe the location of the fracture, whether it is metaphyseal, epiphyseal, or both. The direction of displacement and associated injuries are also described. The most commonly used classification is that of Salter and Harris, with Type II being by far the most common [5]. A specific system in pediatric patients was proposed in 2009, which seeks to classify them based on the pattern of the fracture and the force that produces it [6]. This classification carries several benefits. By relating the pattern of the fracture to the mechanism that produced it, it facilitates the understanding of the pathophysiology of the fracture and the direction of the reduction. Also, being a more detailed classification, it minimizes the possibility of hidden injuries and complications (Fig. 28.2).

Hyperextension injuries carry the highest risk of vascular injury. Valgus injuries are the most common to find and are associated with a metaphyseal fragment by lateral along with proximal fibula fracture. Varus injuries are the least common. Those that occur in flexion tend to be seen more frequently in adolescents, due to the closure of the physis [7]. In younger patients, between 3 and 9 years, they occur by varus or valgus mechanism, mainly affecting the metaphysis, and usually occur from activities such as jumping on a trampoline or elastic bed.

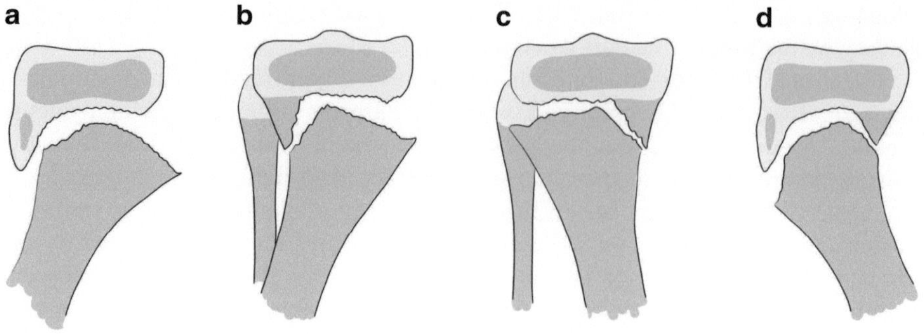

Fig. 28.2 Classification according to Salter and Harris for the most frequent proximal tibial fractures. Type 1, usually evident in the sagittal plane (**a**), and Type 2, with a lateral (**b**), medial (**c**), or posterior (**d**) metaphyseal fragment

28.4 Cozen's Phenomenon

Metaphyseal fractures of the proximal tibia are more common between the ages of 3 and 6 years, with the mechanism being a forced valgus, resulting from a fall on the lateral face of the leg, with the knee in extension [8]. In 1953, Cozen [9] described the progressive genu valgum secondary to proximal tibia fracture, with incidences reported in some series of over 90% of cases. Among the probable etiologies of this phenomenon are a lateral proximal tibia physeal arrest, inadequate fracture reduction, possible soft tissue interposition, greater growth of the proximal medial tibia physis, loss of the hamstrings in the proximal tibia, and a tensor effect of the fibula. Currently, the most accepted theory is an increase in the growth of the medial proximal tibia, due to the biological and biomechanical changes that the fracture generates [8, 10].

It is usually evident 5–6 months after the fracture, and progresses up to 2 years, presenting its greatest angulation at 1 year from the injury, with about 9.6° of metaphyseal-diaphyseal angle.

The most accepted management is observation, as the vast majority are it resolves spontaneously within a period of 2 years following the occurrence of the fracture [11, 12]. Some authors propose the clinical and radiological follow-up of patients who would have a higher risk of developing this phenomenon (with angulations greater than 4°), which are those with ipsilateral proximal fibula fracture and those with proximal metaphyseal fractures of the tibia with a medial gap (Fig. 28.3).

In those patients in whom it does not resolve spontaneously within a period of 2 years, guided growth may be a good alternative for its correction [13]. Generally, these cases present angulations greater than 15°. If a corrective osteotomy is chosen for the management of this problem, it should not be performed prematurely, as the valgus angulation has a higher probability of recurrence.

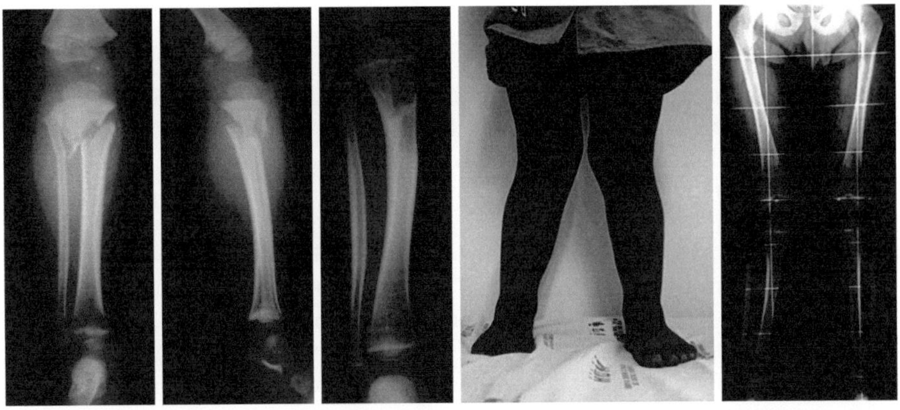

Fig. 28.3 A 3-year-old patient with a proximal tibial fracture, treated non-surgically, with casting. He developed progressive asymmetric genu valgum, secondary to Cozen's phenomenon

Fig. 28.4 "Buckle" fracture of the proximal tibial metaphysis, secondary to trampoline jumping, in a 2-year-old child

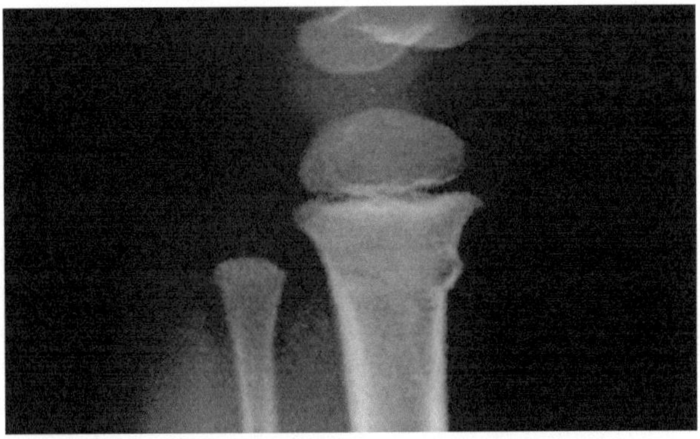

28.5 Fractures Associated with Trampoline

Fractures that occur from trampoline use, or bouncing beds, are becoming increasingly common. It is a special type of proximal metaphyseal fracture of the tibia, which occurs when children are jumping on the trampoline, usually with larger children. They can occur even without a trauma or fall mechanism [14, 15]. This fracture is linear, usually not displaced [16]. According to Kakel [17], unlike other metaphyseal fractures, it does not deform into valgus. The reason could be because it is a linear fracture or "torus," not displaced or angulated (Fig. 28.4).

Boyer describes in 1986 the mechanism of these injuries when the larger person jumps, the elastic canvas of the trampoline rebounds upwards due to inertia, so if the smaller child falls on it at that moment, they receive a significant upward impact force, applied to the child's descending leg. The force and the angle of impact at the right moment can be enough to cause a tibia fracture [18].

28.6 Diagnosis

An accurate description of the accident allows us to determine the direction of the force and suspect the injured structures. Pain, deformity, hemarthrosis, and inflammation are usually present. The patient with a non-displaced or incomplete metaphyseal fracture may only present with limping and moderate pain on knee mobilization.

In adolescent patients, fractures of the proximal tibia present more evident symptoms, with deformity and severe pain. They are usually secondary to high-energy traumas or high-impact sports injuries or jumping. In these patients, up to 40% of associated ligament injuries can occur. The injury of the anterior cruciate ligament is the most frequent, followed by the injury of the medial collateral ligament.

In hyperextension fractures, it is important to perform and document a careful examination of the neurovascular status due to the close relationship of the popliteal artery with the proximal end of the tibia. The examination of distal pulses, pedis, and posterior tibial, along with the examination of the peroneal and tibial nerves, is mandatory.

It should be considered that these patients may present a spasm of the popliteal artery due to the trauma, which can appear up to 24 h after the reduction, so monitoring should be strict.

Similarly, neurological injuries can occur due to traction of the peroneal nerve, which usually recover in a period ranging from 4 to 6 months.

Regarding imaging studies, knee X-ray in anteroposterior and lateral projections is usually sufficient for diagnosis. In addition to the fracture line, an increase in the space between the patella and the femur, suggestive of hemarthrosis, may be noticed.

In adolescent patients, in addition to X-rays, a computed tomography (CT scan) should be taken to assess possible joint extension, and magnetic resonance imaging (MRI) should be used in cases where associated soft tissue injuries are suspected.

28.7 Treatment

Non-displaced fractures of the proximal tibial metaphysis are immobilized using a long leg cast molded to the limb, keeping the knee at 30° of flexion, for 4–6 weeks.

If the fracture is displaced, a closed reduction under anesthesia is advised, with the support of fluoroscopy to visualize an anatomical reduction.

If the angulation is in valgus, the limb is generally reduced by adducting it with the knee extended. This manipulation should be gentle, in order not to injure the peroneal nerve. After the reduction, a long leg cast is applied, molded in varus, and keeping the knee at 30° of flexion. A radiographic check is necessary after a week, to rule out fracture displacement. If the reduction is not achieved, a small approach is recommended to evaluate the fracture site, and to remove the tissues that usually interpose in there. Stabilization of the fracture with osteosynthesis is usually not necessary, so stability is achieved applying a cast in a similar way to conservative treatment.

After 4–6 weeks, thc immobilization is removed, and a rehabilitation plan is initiated until the recovery of the knee and ankle mobility ranges is achieved, improving the muscular balance of the limb. It is important to warn the family about the need for strict follow-up for the next 18 months, due to the described risk of a Cozen phenomenon [19].

Non-displaced physeal fractures are immobilized in a long leg cast, with the knee in extension for 4–6 weeks.

Fractures through the physis, displaced, imply a higher energy mechanism, and are usually unstable. Extra-articular fractures that compromise the physis are treated with closed or open reduction, and osteosynthesis in unstable ones. To reduce the fracture in these cases, it is necessary to flex the knee, seeking to relax the posterior muscles. Fixation of these fractures with 2 crossed Kirschner wires, transphyseal, of 2.0 mm is recommended.

In the case of injuries through the physis with a displaced lateral metaphyseal fragment, the reduction is performed by adducting the limb, with the knee extended, and correcting the valgus. The metaphyseal fragment can be stabilized with a cannulated screw.

If the displacement is posterior, the close vascular relationship must be remembered, so the reduction is performed by gentle traction, correcting the deformity, and then stabilization is performed, if necessary. These fractures can also present periosteal interposition in the facture site, which can prevent closed reduction.

The treatment of intra-articular fractures follows the same principles as for most of this type in pediatric patients. If the fracture is displaced intra-articular and associated injuries are suspected, depending on the age and degree of displacement, arthroscopic assistance can be used for a closed reduction, or an open reduction, with the use of stable osteosynthesis for fixation [20]. Epiphyseal or metaphyseal screws can be used. It is necessary to check ligament stability, which may also require surgical intervention, either at the same time or deferred.

After the fracture has healed, it is important to carry out clinical and radiographic follow-up to assess the possibility of secondary deformities, asymmetries, or limb length differences, as a sequel to early closures of the proximal tibial physis [21].

In the rehabilitation of these injuries, it is important to bear in mind that they are associated with sports injuries and high-impact trauma. Therefore, adolescent athletes should complete their rehabilitation process with specific vertical jump training, in order to improve coordination and mitigate traction forces during the landing phase. Proprioceptive training, in combination with strength training, prevents injuries from uncoordinated movements. Coaches should be advised not to push athletes beyond their physical capacity, as it is established that muscle fatigue is a risk factor for knee injuries.

28.8 Complications

The proximal tibial physis is responsible for 55% of the longitudinal growth of the tibia, and 25% of the total length of the limb. It grows approximately 0.6 cm per year. Injuries that compromise the physis, especially in young children, have a high risk of resulting in a clinically significant limb length discrepancy. Depending on the magnitude, it may be necessary to perform a physiodesis of the unaffected limb, for which the prediction of the timing of the correction is extremely useful. This can be done by multiple methods (Multiplier, Dimeglio, etc.).

Angular deformities occur due to early and asymmetrical closure of the physis. The magnitude is directly related to the age of the patient at which the fracture occurred.

It is important to follow up the fracture with both leg standing radiographs of the limbs (scanograms), which allow the evaluation of the anatomical and mechanical axes, the comparative length of the limbs, to establish a correct treatment plan.

Another less frequent, but devastating complication is vascular injury. This can be secondary to an arterial tear due to the posterior displacement of the proximal tibial metaphysis. Given its close anatomical relationship, it should be considered in fractures due to hyperextension with posterior displacement of the proximal tibia. In the literature, the presence of associated vascular injury is low, around 0.6% and of these, 5% involve the popliteal artery. In the case of a vascular injury that requires surgical exploration, the reduction and stabilization of the fracture should be performed first [22]. Vascular injury can also be a consequence of compartment syndrome, due to the increase in pressures of the leg muscle compartments resulting from the trauma, even more so if the treatment is with a closed cast that can further increase the pressure. The patient and their family should be warned of the clinical signs of alarm, and strict directed observation by the treating physician is required.

28.9 Associated Injuries

The incidence of knee instability, in adolescents with complex fractures of the proximal tibia, can reach up to 53%. Injuries to the medial collateral ligament and the anterior cruciate ligament are common. These ligaments are likely injured first, before the forces are transmitted to the epiphysis. A directed search for these injuries should be carried out, to achieve appropriate management.

28.10 Final Message

Proximal tibia fractures are relatively rare in the pediatric population, due to their anatomical characteristics that protect them and make them intrinsically stable. However, when they occur they can have serious complications.

The mechanism of injury has an important relationship with age, and it is fundamental to understand it in order to carry out an appropriate therapeutic approach. In adolescents, fractures generally involve the physis and are secondary to high-impact sports traumas that generate traction forces. In high-energy fractures, with posterior displacements or that compromise the stability of the knee, the close relationship with the popliteal vessels that can generate acute or late vascular alterations should be remembered.

In pediatric patients, the Cozen's phenomenon can occur after a metaphyseal fracture of the tibia and requires strict observation of its evolution to determine the treatment, being the great majority of spontaneous resolution.

References

1. Saade-Lemus S, Nguyen JC, Francavilla ML, Martin-Saavedra JS, Ho-Fung VM, Kaplan SL. Buckle fracture of the proximal tibia in children and frequency of association with trampoline and inflatable bouncer use. Pediatr Radiol. 2019;49(10):1327–34. https://doi.org/10.1007/s00247-019-04450-0.
2. Steiger CN, Ceroni D. Mechanism and predisposing factors for proximal tibial epiphysiolysis in adolescents during sports activities. Int Orthop. 2019;43(6):1395–403. https://doi.org/10.1007/s00264-018-4168-4.
3. Omar M, Petri M, Ettinger M, Decker S, Krettek C, Gaulke R. Simultaneous bilateral transitional fractures of the proximal tibia after minor sports trauma. Case Rep Orthop. 2013;2013:724802. https://doi.org/10.1155/2013/724802.
4. Aymen F, Youcef O, Aymen S, Issam A, Abderrazek A. Triplane fracture of the proximal tibia: a case report and literature review. Pan Afr Med J. 2019;33:40. Published 2019 May 21. https://doi.org/10.11604/pamj.2019.33.40.17953.
5. Watanabe H, Majima T, Takahashi K, Iizawa N, Oshima Y, Takai S. Posterior tibial slope angle is associated with flexion-type Salter-Harris II and Watson-Jones type IV fractures of the proximal tibia. Knee Surg Sports Traumatol Arthrosc. 2019;27(9):2994–3000. https://doi.org/10.1007/s00167-018-5319-2.
6. Mubarak SJ, Kim JR, Edmonds EW, Pring ME, Bastrom TP. Classification of proximal tibial fractures in children. J Child Orthop. 2009;3(3):191–7. https://doi.org/10.1007/s11832-009-0167-8.
7. Israni P, Panat M. Proximal tibial epiphysis injury (flexion type, salter-Harris type 1). J Orthop Case Rep. 2016;6(4):62–5. https://doi.org/10.13107/jocr.2250-0685.572.
8. Yang BW, Shore BJ, Rademacher E, May C, Watkins CJ, Glotzbecker MP. Prevalence of Cozen's phenomenon of the proximal tibia. J Pediatr Orthop. 2019;39(6):e417–21. https://doi.org/10.1097/BPO.0000000000001354.
9. Cozen L. Fracture of the proximal portion of the tibia in children followed by valgus deformity. Surg Gynecol Obstet. 1953;97(2):183–8.
10. Dorman S, Jariwala A, Campbell D. Cozen's phenomenon: a reminder. Scott Med J. 2013;58(3):e10–3. https://doi.org/10.1177/0036933013496922.
11. Bae K, Jeon JY, Park SS, Park J, Kang MS. Initial angular deformity and its recovery of the proximal tibial metaphyseal fracture according to the cause: trampoline-related injury versus other injuries. J Child Orthop. 2020;14(4):304–11. https://doi.org/10.1302/1863-2548.14.200072.
12. Vrettakos AN, Evaggelidis DC, Kyrkos MJ, Tsatsos AV, Nenopoulos A, Beslikas T. Lower limb deformity following proximal tibia physeal injury: long-term follow-up. J Orthop Traumatol. 2012;13(1):7–11. https://doi.org/10.1007/s10195-012-0179-x.

13. Morin M, Klatt J, Stevens PM. Cozen's deformity: resolved by guided growth. Strategies Trauma Limb Reconstr. 2018;13(2):87–93. https://doi.org/10.1007/s11751-018-0309-y.
14. Jääskelä M, Kuivalainen L, Victorzon S, Serlo W, Lempainen L, Sinikumpu JJ. Trampoline-related proximal tibia impaction fractures in children: a population-based approach to epidemiology and radiographic findings between 2006 and 2017. J Child Orthop. 2020;14(2):125–31. https://doi.org/10.1302/1863-2548.14.190177.
15. Stranzinger E, Leidolt L, Eich G, Klimek PM. The anterior tilt angle of the proximal tibia epiphyseal plate: a significant radiological finding in young children with trampoline fractures. Eur J Radiol. 2014;83(8):1433–6. https://doi.org/10.1016/j.ejrad.2014.05.013.
16. Muljadi JA, Chaijenkij K, Arirachakaran A, Kongtharvonskul J. Comparative surgical risk between type of trampoline (size and place) and type of patients (age and sex) in trampoline related injury: a systematic review and indirect meta-analysis. BMC Sports Sci Med Rehabil. 2020;12:37. https://doi.org/10.1186/s13102-020-00185-w.
17. Kakel R. Trampoline fracture of the proximal tibial metaphysis in children may not progress into valgus: a report of seven cases and a brief review. Orthop Traumatol Surg Res. 2012;98(4):446–9. https://doi.org/10.1016/j.otsr.2012.02.007.
18. Boyer RS, Jaffe RB, Nixon GW, Condon VR. Trampoline fractures of the proximal tibia in children. Am J Roentgenol. 1986;146:83–5.
19. Papamerkouriou YM, Tsoumpos P, Tagaris G, Christodoulou G. Does Cozen's phenomenon warrant surgical intervention? J Child Orthop. 2020;14(3):213–20. https://doi.org/10.1302/1863-2548.14.190147.
20. Pace JL, McCulloch PC, Momoh EO, Nasreddine AY, Kocher MS. Operatively treated type IV tibial tubercle apophyseal fractures. J Pediatr Orthop. 2013;33(8):791–6. https://doi.org/10.1097/BPO.0b013e3182968984.
21. Yoo MJ, Yoo JI, Lee JY, Park YJ, Kang-Heo. Treatment of typical trampoline fracture of the proximal tibia in children: results of minimum 1 year follow-up. Eur J Trauma Emerg Surg. 2021;47(3):811–6. https://doi.org/10.1007/s00068-019-01266-3.
22. Shinomiya R, Sunagawa T, Nakashima Y, Nakabayashi A, Makitsubo M, Adachi N. Slow progressive popliteal artery insufficiency after neglected proximal tibial physeal fracture: a case report. J Pediatr Orthop B. 2018;27(1):35–9. https://doi.org/10.1097/BPB.0000000000000379.

Chapter 29
Tibial Shaft Fracture

Hernán Guzmán and Constanza Ramírez

Tibial shaft fractures are common injuries in the child population. Their presentation varies according to the age of the patient and the mechanism of injury. They present peculiarities related to their management, their prognosis, associated injuries and even potential medical-legal repercussions in children exposed to non-accidental trauma.

For their treatment, a good prognosis is recognized through conservative treatment, but also that residual deformities of the axes are poorly tolerated over time. Therapeutic options range from immobilization with a cast, to a reduction and surgical fixation. The choice of treatment should be based on objective criteria that allow obtaining the best results, with the least impact on the child and his family.

29.1 Introduction

Few fractures in pediatric patients have a range of presentation patterns and therapeutic options as varied as the diaphyseal fracture of the tibia. It has been expressed that, in the tibia, each fracture has its own "personality." In this chapter, we will analyze the different variables that influence the form of presentation and evolution of tibial shaft fractures in the pediatric patient.

We will describe the mechanical, biological, anatomical, and clinical factors that influence the "personality" and behavior of these fractures. The criteria for

H. Guzmán
Clínica Las Condes, Santiago, Chile

C. Ramírez (✉)
Clínica MEDS, Hospital Sotero del Río, Santiago, Chile
e-mail: constanza.ramirez@meds.cl

M. Sepúlveda O. (ed.), *Paediatrics Traumatology*,
https://doi.org/10.1007/978-3-031-89482-4_29

considering an adequate reduction and the therapeutic means available, their indications and complications will be defined.

29.2 Epidemiology

The fracture of the tibia is the third most frequent fracture in the long bones of the pediatric population and can represent 15% of all fractures in pediatric age [1]. It occurs throughout childhood, and the average age of presentation is 8 years, affecting men in a proportion of 2:1, with respect to women; 70% of them present as an isolated fracture of the tibia and the fibula fracture is associated with the remaining 30% [2].

29.3 Pathophysiology

Isolated tibia fractures are usually associated with low-energy traumas. The most common presentations are oblique or spiral fractures, located in the middle and distal third. These fractures are produced by torsional or rotational mechanisms, usually by falls with the foot fixed on the ground, with the body in motion.

In patients under 3 years, this rotational mechanism is characteristic and is usually responsible for a special form of injury, known as "Toddler fracture" or "first steps fracture," as it is common in young children who are starting to walk. It should be noted that the tibia is the third most affected bone in non-accidental trauma; even some series report that 16% of children affected by physical abuse present a tibia fracture [3].

Spiral or short oblique fractures usually respect the fibula, presenting as isolated fractures of the tibia. In cases of higher energy rotational mechanism, as occurs in sports activities in older patients, an associated fracture of the fibula with an oblique or spiral line, at a different level than in the tibia, may occur.

Higher energy traumas, and direct impacts on the leg, are associated with transverse or comminuted fractures, which can produce a fibula fracture of the same type of pattern and at the same level. This fibular involvement at the same level as the tibia gives this injury a high degree of instability. These fractures are associated with traffic accidents, falls from heights, and high-impact or physical contact sports.

29.4 Anatomy

The tibia and fibula make up the skeleton of the leg, providing insertion to the muscles destined for the foot, and being responsible for the load of the limb.

The fibula supports between 6% and 17% of body weight, and its main function is to provide insertion points for the anterolateral muscles of the leg and lateral stability to the ankle. The tibia is the main responsible for the load-bearing weight, and in its proximal third, it provides insertion to the anterolateral and posterior muscles of the leg.

In its distal half, the tibia has no muscle insertions, which can be a factor that hinders the bone healing at that level. The musculature of the leg is organized into four compartments, which partially surround the tibia, as its anteromedial side is totally subcutaneous, without muscle coverage.

The anterolateral musculature of the leg (specifically the anterior tibial muscles, long extensor of the toes, and long extensor of the hallux) influences the displacements of the fragments of a tibial shaft fracture. In a mid-third fracture of the tibia with associated fibula fracture, the anterolateral musculature pulls the distal segment into valgus, as there is no sufficient medial musculature to prevent it.

When the fibula is intact, there is less tendency to shortening, but greater tendency to varus deviation. In this case, the fibula acts as a pivot against the action of the musculature. When the anterolateral musculature contracts, the tibia tends to shorten, but the fibula prevents it by deviating the distal segment toward the varus [4] (Fig. 29.1).

An important point to consider among the anatomical characteristics of the leg that influence the management of tibial fractures is the absence of muscle coverage on its anteromedial aspect. Thus, one of the treatment techniques for unstable fractures, stable elastic intramedullary nailing, which requires muscle function to

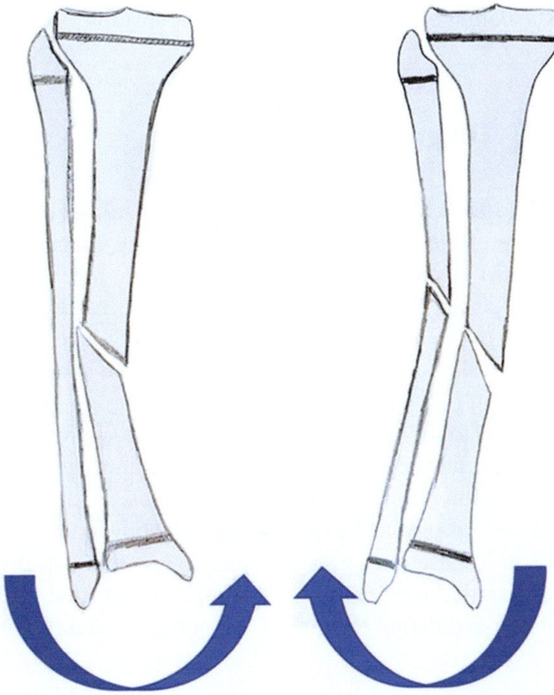

Fig. 29.1 In an isolated tibial fracture, the fibula acts as a pivot against the anterolateral musculature, deviating the distal segment in varus. When there is a fracture of the tibia and fibula, there is no resistance to the anterolateral muscular action, resulting in a distal valgus angulation

transform traction forces into compression forces, achieves less stability in this segment due to the lack of muscle activity on the anteromedial aspect, which must be considered during the therapeutic decision.

The perfusion of the leg and foot are the responsibility of the anterior tibial and posterior tibial arteries. The first of these is located in the anterolateral compartment, and the second in the deep posterior compartment. The posterior tibial artery branches into the nutrient artery of the tibia, in the proximal third. This artery gives rise to an endosteal circulation network that communicates with branches coming from both tibial arteries, and that reach the periosteum, through muscle insertions. The lack of muscle insertions in the distal third of the tibia, and throughout its anteromedial face, limits the circulatory supply of this bone [4]. This anatomical condition influences the ability to heal fractures and defend against infections.

The existence of four inextensible muscle compartments, in conjunction with the vascularity of the leg, results in high-energy traumas with severe soft tissue damage with a high risk of direct vascular damage or damage to the vessels responsible for muscle perfusion. In addition, the increase in pressure in these compartments due to trauma and secondary edema can lead to the development of a compartment syndrome, which is less common than in the adult population due to the tissue elasticity of the pediatric population, but can be associated with high-energy traumas, with catastrophic consequences, so it should always be investigated [5].

The consolidation of fractures in the tibia in growing patients usually does not present problems, and it takes between 8 and 12 weeks, depending on the patient's age. The non-union rate is very low, but delays in consolidation associated with soft tissue damage, lower perfusion, and/or instability of the fracture are not uncommon.

29.5 Diagnosis

In children who can communicate and adolescents, the trauma history is evident, and the clinical suspicion in the presence of pain, functional impotence, and/or deformity of the affected limb is clear. The mechanism of injury, type of accident, and the energy of the trauma should be thoroughly investigated, assessing possible injuries to other systems and fractures in other segments. The physical examination should evaluate the soft tissues condition, the neurovascular status, and the presence of signs of compartment syndrome.

In the smaller patients, especially at the age of onset of walking or prior to this, there may not be evidence of an acute traumatic episode, and both pain and functional impotence may be less noticeable.

A careful physical examination will show pain when palpating the subcutaneous tibia, and sometimes a slight increase in volume at that level.

A detailed medical history should be recorded, especially investigating a possible non-accidental origin of the tibia fracture. Cases in which the traumatic mechanism described does not match the type of fracture that occurs in patients who do not yet walk, that the story of the history is contradictory or inconsistent, when there is a delay in consulting, or when there are records of previous care for traumatic injuries, are more suspicious.

It is important to record a detailed examination of the patient, their skin, and other skeletal segments, looking for signs of other traumatic injuries.

In most fractures of the tibial shaft, the imaging diagnosis is based on X-rays, in anteroposterior and lateral projections, which should include the knee and the ankle. Special attention should be paid to the search for transitional type fractures in the ankle in older patients, given their association.

We recommend complementing the study with radiological study of the ankle with anteroposterior, lateral, and mortise X-ray projections, and even consider the use of computed tomography (CT scan) of the ankle in the suspicion of articular involvement.

In children under 3 years old with a high suspicion of fracture, but without evidence in the usual projections, the study can be complemented with oblique projections. Despite this, there is a group of patients in which the presence of the fracture will not be objectified after the radiological study.

The possibility of performing a study with scintigraphy, and even with magnetic resonance imaging (MRI) to demonstrate the existence of the fracture is described, but usually with the clinical history and the findings of the physical examination, the initial treatment can be defined in the suspicion of the injury, and repeat radiographic study at 10–15 days, where the existence of initial consolidation phenomena confirms the diagnosis.

In the suspicion of a non-accidental trauma injury, the study protocol of the care center should be activated, which should include X-rays of the entire skeleton and systematized evaluation of other systems, in addition to the social and legal study (see Chap. 3).

29.6 Classification

Leg fractures in pediatric patients are classified based on their location (metaphyseal, epiphyseal, or diaphyseal). In addition, the presence of physeal involvement, the fracture line (transverse, oblique, spiral, butterfly wing, comminuted), the state of the fibula (intact or fractured), the degree of displacement, and whether it is an open fracture are recorded in its description. In the case of this last group, the Gustilo and Anderson classification is used.

There is also the AO classification specific for fractures in long bones in pediatric age, which allows the characterization of the lesion in a specific way, useful in scientific analysis.

29.7 Treatment

The treatment of diaphyseal fractures of the tibia in children and adolescents depends on the fracture pattern, mechanism, skeletal maturity, soft tissue status, and the existence of other concomitant injuries. In most cases, these fractures can be managed non-surgically, performing their reduction when necessary, and stabilizing them with a well-molded cast.

29.7.1 Conservative Treatment

The goal of treating a fracture of the diaphysis of the tibia is to achieve its consolidation while maintaining the functional anatomical axes, so the initial or post-reduction alignment must comply with the parameters considered acceptable.

Although the emphasis should be placed on obtaining reductions as close to the anatomical in the coronal plane, without rotational malalignment, an acceptable angulation is considered one that does not exceed 5–10° in any plane (Table 29.1) [6, 7].

In the case of displaced fractures, it must be verified that there is at least a 50% of contact between the fragments, and a maximum of 1 cm of shortening.

The cast for the conservative treatment of these fractures is a long leg cast. It is installed starting with a short leg cast, below the knee, performing a 3-point support to maintain the proper reduction, seeking to prevent varus deformity when the fibula is intact, and valgus when it is fractured.

The long leg cast is completed once a reduction in the appropriate axis of the fracture is verified, adding the upper segment, with the knee at 20–40° of flexion. This position is useful for fracture rotational control, relaxing the gastrocnemius muscles and preventing the patient from weight bearing on the limb [8]. The risk of posterior angulation is decreased by leaving the ankle in a position of 15–20° of plantar flexion (Fig. 29.2).

If the cast is installed in the acute period of the trauma, it is important to leave an anterior opening to decrease the risk of compartment syndrome, caused by an increase in volume of the soft tissues. In the case of patients with an increased risk of presenting this complication, hospitalization for observation is suggested, with the limb elevated and neurovascular monitoring, even possibly deferring the installation of the definitive immobilization 1 or 2 days.

Table 29.1 Recommended limits of residual deformity for conservative treatment

Age	<8 years	>8 years
Varus	10°	5°
Valgus	5°	5°
Sagittal angulation	10°	5°
Shortening	10 mm	5 mm
Rotation	5°	5°

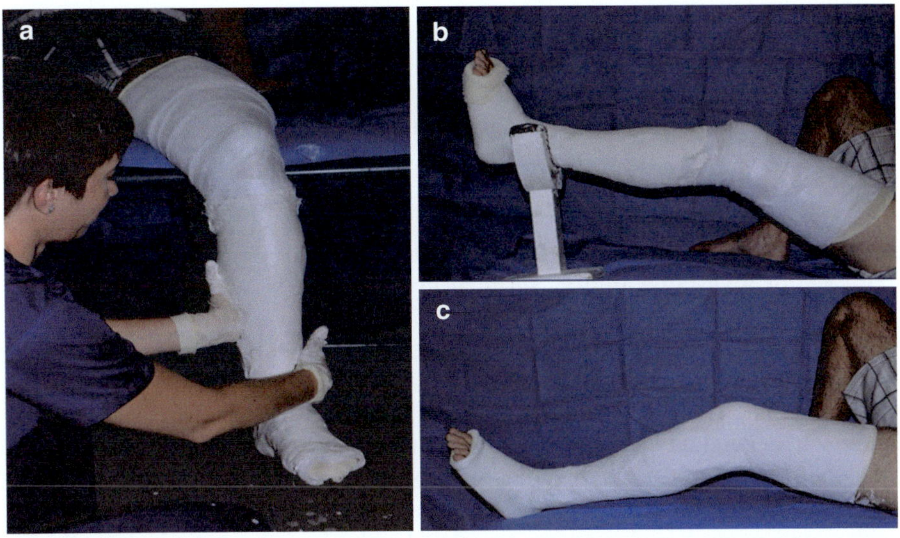

Fig. 29.2 Installation of a long leg cast. (**a**) Molding of a short leg cast to maintain fracture reduction. (**b**) Once the short leg is positioned, the cast is completed up to the thigh. (**c**) Long leg cast with knee flexion 20–40° and slight plantar flexion of the ankle

If the displacement exceeds the acceptable parameters, a closed reduction under anesthesia or sedation is performed, with a maneuver opposite to that which caused the fracture. It should be evaluated under fluoroscopy, seeking to determine an adequate position of the fragments prior to the installation of the long leg cast. It should be considered that in high-energy trauma, with involvement of the tibia and fibula, the tibia fracture tends to be very unstable and difficult to reduce, with a tendency to posterior angulation (anterior apex) in the sagittal plane.

With the long leg cast, the patient is instructed to avoid weight bearing for 3–4 weeks, after which the change to a walking boot is made, depending on the patient's age and with the presence of radiological signs of bone healing. Once there is a bone callus, it is recommended to start bearing weight progressively, since there is evidence that the time of consolidation for tibia fractures is shortened with early weight bearing [7–9].

It is recommended to perform weekly radiological control during the first 2–3 weeks after the reduction, to evaluate that there has not been displacement or unacceptable angulation. If there is an angulation greater than 5° in the control, it is recommended to perform a new reduction of the fracture or a cast wedging. The latter can be performed during the first 2 weeks of treatment, with an opening or closing wedge, the size of which will be determined according to the angulation to correct.

29.7.2 Surgical Treatment

Although its indication is less frequent, it is the treatment of choice for unstable fractures, whose reduction cannot be maintained with cast immobilization, or when there is a loss of reduction that cannot be corrected non-invasively. This treatment is also recommended for comminuted fractures, those with significant shortening, and those that do not allow for conservative treatment, in the context of polytrauma, with a high risk of compartment syndrome, a floating knee or a vascular injury. Surgical management is also indicated in open fractures.

The available osteosynthesis techniques and methods are multiple, including percutaneous fixation with Kirschner wires, elastic stable intramedullary nailing, the use of external fixation, and internal fixation with plates. The choice of technique will depend on the fracture pattern, patient's age, skeletal maturity, existence of associated injuries, and the surgeon's experience. In younger patients, and with special consideration in fractures of the distal third of the tibial diaphysis, fixation with percutaneous Kirschner wires associated with a long leg cast with knee flexion can be used (Fig. 29.3).

Intramedullary nailing with elastic titanium or steel nails is the most commonly used technique in diaphyseal tibia fractures in children and adolescents. It is a minimally invasive technique, which avoids damaging the physis and allows for early mobilization and weight bearing, making it an option with excellent results. An important point to consider is the risk of coronal angulation when the entry of both

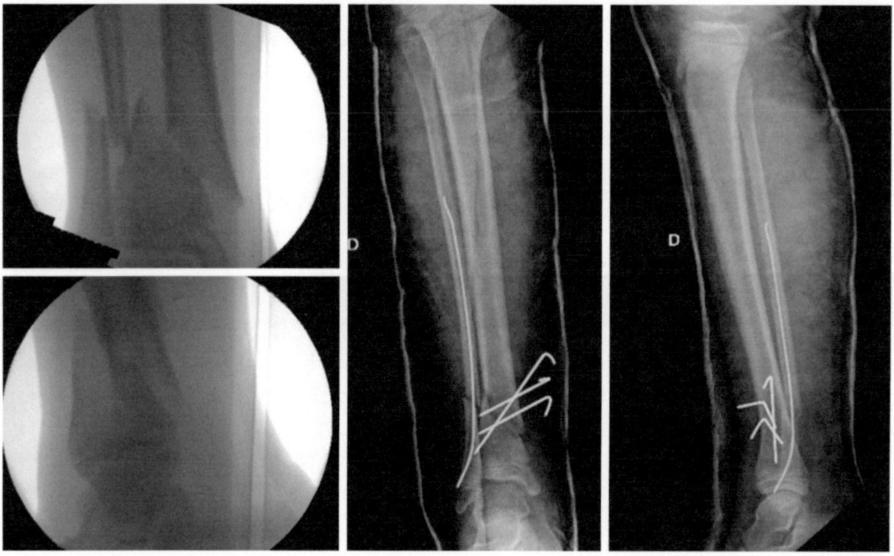

Fig. 29.3 Short oblique fracture of the distal third of the tibia. The tibial fracture was stabilized with 3 percutaneous Kirschner wires and protected with a long leg cast

nails is made on the same side, so it is recommended to make a lateral and medial entry (Fig. 29.4).

The entry of the nails should avoid damaging the proximal physis and the apophysis of the anterior tuberosity of the tibia, due to the risk of secondary growth alterations. In some cases, patients treated with this technique require some additional immobilization with a short leg cast, to support the stability of the reduction in the initial period.

Among the complications of the elastic stable intramedullary nailing technique, the migration of the nails is described, and few cases of infection associated with open fractures, as well as the complications inherent to these fractures, such as residual angular deformities and union delays [10]. Complications are more frequent in older patients and adolescents (Fig. 29.5).

The stabilization of the tibia fracture with external fixators has its main indication in the treatment of open fractures at this level, allowing the management of adjacent soft tissues. However, they can be an option in high-energy closed fractures, especially comminuted or segmentary, which compromise the length of the tibia, and can associate a significant compromise of soft tissues.

The external fixator, in monoplanar or multiplanar configuration, can be used as definitive fixation or as initial stabilization that can then be converted to another

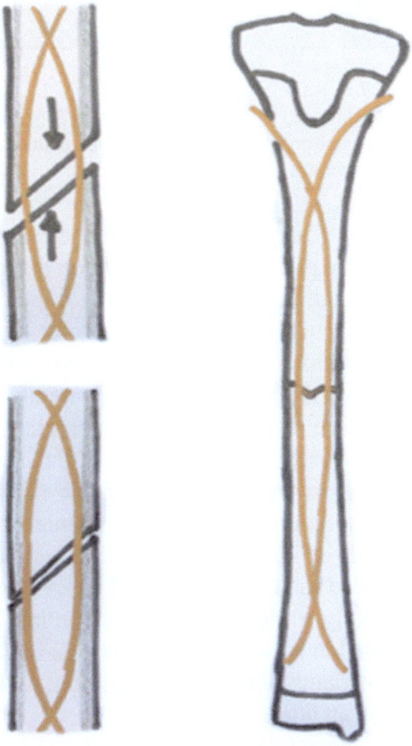

Fig. 29.4 Recommended configuration for the use of elastic stable intramedullary nails in tibial fractures. A "double C" configuration is used for the anterograde technique. The entry is made in the anterior-medial and anterior-lateral part of the proximal metaphyseal cortex, 2 cm distal to the proximal epiphysis, next to the tibial tuberosity. The nails must be shaped prior to insertion, to allow the apex of the curve to be at the fracture site, since greater contact with the internal cortex allows for improved axial and translational stability

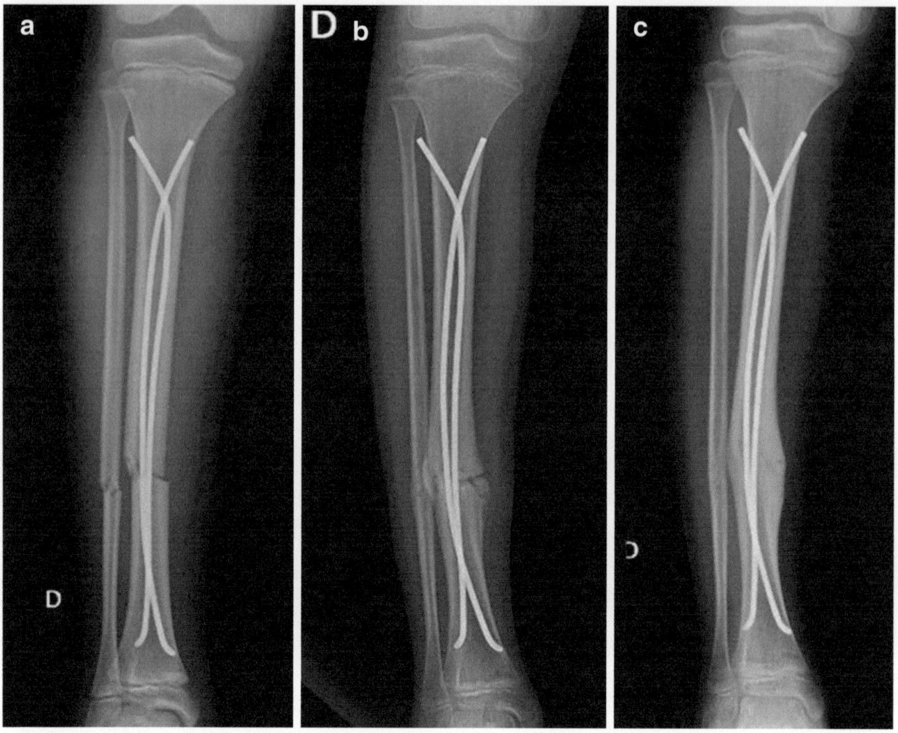

Fig. 29.5 Radiographs of unstable leg fracture treated with closed reduction and stable elastic intramedullary nails. (**a**) Immediate postoperative outcome. (**b**) Signs of delayed consolidation at 14 weeks of progression, using a removable short boot. (**c**) Consolidated fracture after 4 weeks of use of a weight bearing walking boot

technique, usually elastic stable intramedullary nailing. Depending on the size and age of the patient, external fixation can be stable enough to allow early weight bearing, in addition to restoring length in complex fractures. Some systems even allow the gradual correction of bone defects and residual deformities. The most frequent complication of this technique is infection at the pin entry point, but malunion, consolidation delay, and re-fracture are also described.

The use of osteosynthesis with plates in the tibial diaphysis in children is infrequent because the exposure of the fracture site and the surgical approach can decrease irrigation, increasing the risk of healing delay and non-union. They are useful in comminuted and segmental fractures of difficult containment with other methods (Fig. 29.6). The development of minimally invasive techniques has expanded their use for special cases.

Finally, rigid locked intramedullary nails have limited use, as they cannot be installed in a tibia with open physis in the entry area. Their use is restricted to pediatric patients with mature skeleton, without major difference in their management than in an adult patient.

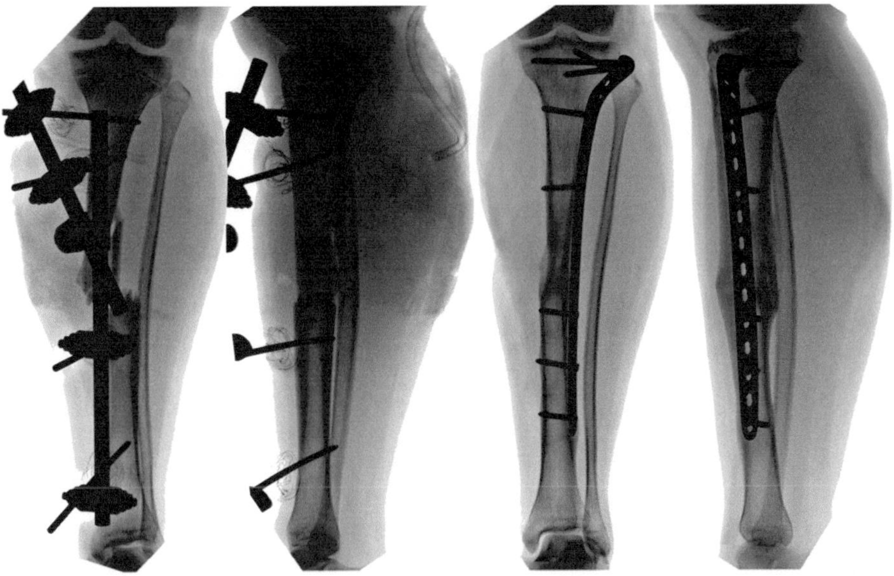

Fig. 29.6 Exposed, segmental, diaphyseal, and proximal physeal fracture of the left tibia in a 14-year-old patient. Initially, the patient was stabilized with an external fixator for soft tissue management, followed by definitive fixation with a plate using the MIPO technique

29.8 Open Fracture of the Leg

Generally, open fractures of the leg are more complex than closed fractures, with a worse prognosis. The risk of infection for these injuries varies between 5% and 15%. The healing time is longer than for closed fractures and depends on the involvement of the soft tissues, the patient's age, the fracture line, bone loss, and the presence of infection. The management of the soft tissues may require flaps or grafts, depending on the severity of the injuries.

All require surgical treatment, regardless of the patient's age. This consists of surgical debridement, with adequate removal of necrotic tissue. In addition, prophylactic antibiotic treatment and tetanus prophylaxis should be indicated, if necessary, in accordance with local regulations.

After completing the surgical debridement, achieving a clean field, the fracture reduction is performed (closed or open, as necessary) and fixation with the chosen surgical technique. External fixation is the most used in fractures with great involvement of soft tissues (Fig. 29.7), while elastic stable intramedullary nailing is recommended in those with adequate coverage of soft tissues. In selected cases, it is possible to manage these fractures with a cast, making a "window" in the plaster that allows the management of the involved soft tissues.

Current evidence establishes that the timely administration of antibiotics in these fractures is the most significant factor in preventing infection associated with an

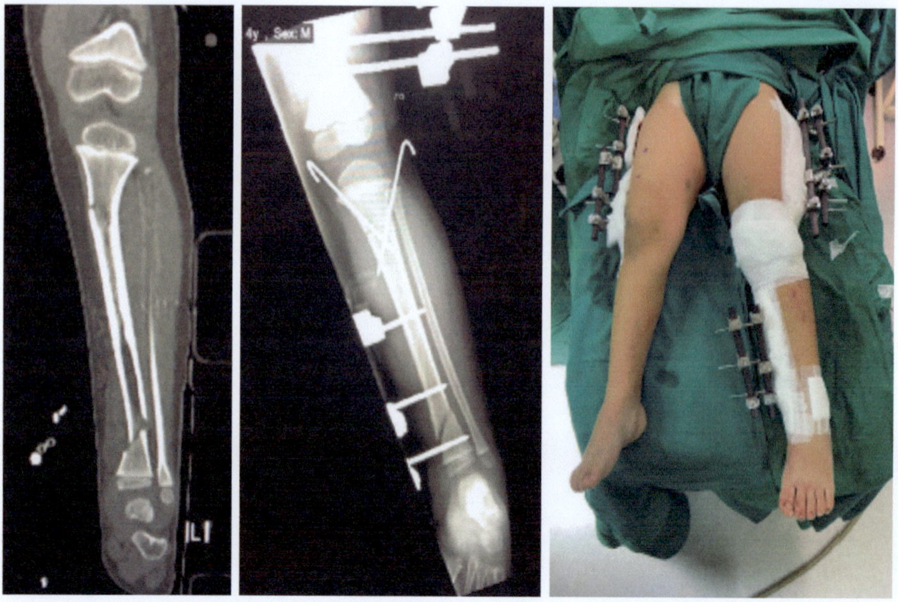

Fig. 29.7 Leg fracture in a 4-year-old patient, due to a traffic accident. An external fixator was used to manage the fracture in the context of a patient with multiple trauma (pelvic fracture, fracture of both femurs and TBI, in addition to the leg fracture), as damage control

open fracture, even more than the time elapsed to surgical cleaning, so its administration should not be delayed [11].

29.9 Complications

Compartment syndrome in leg fractures in the pediatric population is less prevalent than in adults, however, an incidence of up to 4% of fractures is reported, which will depend on the patient's age, type of fracture, and mechanism of injury. It is even reported that up to 10% of patients would have alterations when measuring intracompartmental pressure [12].

The diagnosis can be difficult to make, so its suspicion is fundamental and patients must be strictly monitored to detect signs early. The presence of anxiety, agitation, and an increase in analgesic requirements (known as the 3 "A's") can be indicators of the presence of compartment syndrome in children, with better sensitivity than the signs used in adult patients (pallor, disproportionate pain, or passive mobilization of the toes, paresthesia, paresis, absence of pulses, and poikilothermia, known as the 6 "P's") [13].

If suspicion arises, it should be treated immediately, with fasciotomies of the anterior, lateral, superficial, and deep compartments, since the ischemia produced can lead to muscle and nerve injuries, with serious functional sequelae.

Delayed union is an infrequent complication in low-energy fractures, which consolidate within a period of 8–12 weeks. However, it can occur in high-energy fractures, open, displaced, with bone loss, that have become infected, or that required an external fixator. In the case of delayed union of a tibia fracture without a fibula fracture, a fibula osteotomy can be performed, distal to the fracture, to allow compression of the tibial fracture site.

Another alternative is the use of bone graft in case of atrophic non-unions, which require cellularity input, or stabilization with a plate or intramedullary nail in case of needing to improve stability.

Angular deformities secondary to malunion are usually secondary to inadequate reduction and/or stabilization. Although, there is angular remodeling in the tibia, its potential is less than in the femur or forearm. Angulations close to the physis or those with anterior apex, in varus and in a single plane, have a better ability to remodel than those with posterior apex, in valgus or multiplanar. Patients under 8 years can remodel angulations of up to 10° in the coronal or sagittal plane, and those older than that age remodel only up to 5°. It is considered that rotational deformities do not remodel.

Differences in length of lower limbs occur due to increased growth of the fractured extremity, and it is more common in patients under 10 years old with comminuted or open fractures. For this reason, it is recommended to follow these fractures for at least 2 years to reveal alterations in axes or length, even though their incidence is lower than in fractures of the femoral diaphysis.

29.10 Final Message

The confrontation and management of diaphyseal fractures of the tibia in pediatric patients are a challenge for the specialist. It is imperative to have knowledge of all the factors that influence the evolution and prognosis of these injuries, as well as the different treatment alternatives, their advantages, limitations, and possible complications. It should not be forgotten that the mere healing of the fracture is not the only objective of treatment, but it must be ensured that the axis and length of the skeleton are restored, as well as the integrity and function of the soft tissues of the affected limb.

29.11 Authors' Advice

Conservative treatment, long leg cast procedure:

- Preferably use plaster of Paris, as it allows better molding, and open linearly to reduce the risk of compression against edema, and allows the performance of wedging later, if necessary.

- If possible, the patient should be seated on the stretcher with the limb hanging, and good analgesia, to relax the musculature around the fracture.
- Both malleoli should be carefully padded, reinforcing the distal and proximal ends, in addition to the anterior and posterior region of the knee, to avoid areas of injury by compression.
- In the first stage, the installation of the distal end of the plaster is performed, which helps to align and reduce the fracture by the effect of weight, performing the molding at the level of the malleoli.
- During the installation of the short leg cast, second stage, the definitive reduction of the fracture is performed, so the molding is fundamental and the support in 3 points should be considered to counteract the displacement of the fracture. Remember that the tibia is triangular, so the molding should have this shape on its anterior side of the cast.
- The position of the reduction must be maintained until the setting of the short leg cast.
- It is important to make cuts in the proximal border of the plaster, to avoid circular compressions when continuing with the plaster toward proximal.
- The third stage, completing the long leg cast, can be performed in decubitus since the fracture is already reduced.
- If considered necessary, the resistance can be increased by the posterior side with the use of a cast valve at that level.
- It is essential to complete the long leg cast with the knee flexed between 20 and 40°, to relax the calf and hamstring muscles. Care must be taken when holding the popliteal region to avoid a deformation of the plaster that can generate a posterior compression.

Conservative treatment, axis correction with cast wedging:

- Useful in angulations in a single plane (especially varus-valgus), allowing to correct angulations between 10° and 15°.
- The opening wedge has better result and predictability (Fig. 29.8).
- It is performed in plaster of Paris, closed and dry.
- Its highest performance is when it is carried out between 7 and 10 days from the fracture, due to the presence of soft callus.
- The fracture is located, and a semi-circumferential cut is made with a saw in the middle of the perimeter opposite to the apex of the angulation. The cut is then separated with a plaster spreader. A wooden or plastic wedge is installed to maintain separation, ensuring that they remain fixed and do not migrate into the plaster. Cotton can be installed inside the plaster to reduce the possibility of this happening. Close the wedge with plaster of Paris after satisfactory immediate radiological control.
- The magnitude of the opening depends on the angulation of the fracture, but it is recommended not to exceed 2 cm.
- Ensure that there is no compression on the skin in the area of the fulcrum of the wedge (side opposite to the opening). Special care in the corrections of valgus angulations, as the fulcrum is on subcutaneous tibia. For this, a "window" can be

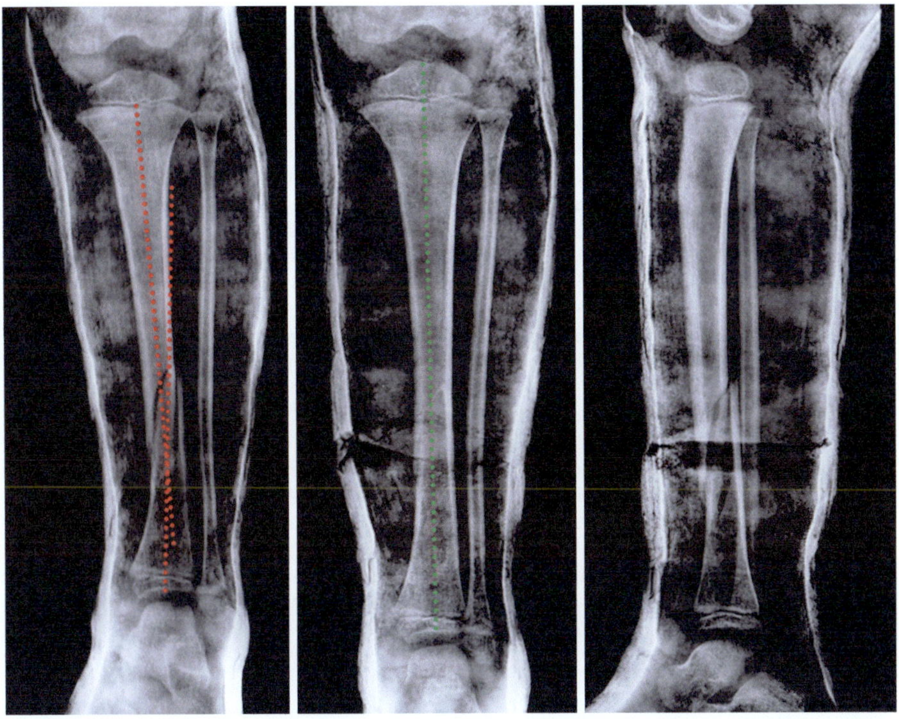

Fig. 29.8 X-rays of the left leg of a 5-year-old child, in whom a varus deviation is verified, which is corrected by means of an opening casting wedge at the level of the fracture site

made to the plaster in the area of the fulcrum, the next day, to ensure that there is no plaster compression.

– Finally, this plaster must be replaced with a new one between 7 and 10 days.

References

1. Patel NK, Horstman J, Kuester V, Sambandam S, Mounasamy V. Pediatric tibial shaft fractures. Indian J Orthop. 2018;52(5):522–8. https://doi.org/10.4103/ortho.IJOrtho_486_17.
2. Mashru RP, Herman MJ, Pizzutillo PD. Tibial shaft fractures in children and adolescents. J Am Acad Orthop Surg. 2005;13(5):345–52. https://doi.org/10.5435/00124635-200509000-00008.
3. Berthold O, Frericks B, John T, Clemens V, Fegert JM, Moers AV. Abuse as a cause of childhood fractures. Dtsch Arztebl Int. 2018;115(46):769–75. https://doi.org/10.3238/arztebl.2018.0769.
4. Mooney J, Hennrikus W. Fractures of the shaft of the tibia and fibula. In: Flynn JM, Skaggs DL, Waters PM, editors. Rockwood and Wilkins fractures in children. 8th ed. Philadelphia, PA: Wolters Kluwer Health; 2014. p. 1874–932.
5. Raducha JE, Swarup I, Schachne JM, Cruz AI Jr, Fabricant PD. Tibial shaft fractures in children and adolescents. JBJS Rev. 2019;7(2):e4. https://doi.org/10.2106/JBJS.RVW.18.00047.

6. Ho CA. Tibia shaft fractures in adolescents: how and when can they be managed successfully with cast treatment? J Pediatr Orthop. 2016;36(Suppl 1):S15–8. https://doi.org/10.1097/BPO.0000000000000762.
7. Hogue GD, Wilkins KE, Kim IS. Management of pediatric tibial shaft fractures. J Am Acad Orthop Surg. 2019;27(20):769–78. https://doi.org/10.5435/JAAOS-D-17-00819.
8. Herman MJ, Martinek MA, Abzug JM. Complications of tibial eminence and diaphyseal fractures in children: prevention and treatment. J Am Acad Orthop Surg. 2014;22(11):730–41. https://doi.org/10.5435/JAAOS-22-11-730.
9. Silva M, Eagan MJ, Wong MA, Dichter DH, Ebramzadeh E, Zionts LE. A comparison of two approaches for the closed treatment of low-energy tibial fractures in children. J Bone Joint Surg Am. 2012;94(20):1853–60. https://doi.org/10.2106/JBJS.J.01728.
10. Kinney MC, Nagle D, Bastrom T, Linn MS, Schwartz AK, Pennock AT. Operative versus conservative management of displaced tibial shaft fracture in adolescents. J Pediatr Orthop. 2016;36(7):661–6. https://doi.org/10.1097/BPO.0000000000000532.
11. Ibrahim T, Riaz M, Hegazy A, Erwin PJ, Tleyjeh IM. Delayed surgical debridement in pediatric open fractures: a systematic review and meta-analysis. J Child Orthop. 2014;8(2):135–41. https://doi.org/10.1007/s11832-014-0567-2.
12. Shore BJ, Glotzbecker MP, Zurakowski D, Gelbard E, Hedequist DJ, Matheney TH. Acute compartment syndrome in children and teenagers with tibial shaft fractures: incidence and multivariable risk factors. J Orthop Trauma. 2013;27(11):616–21. https://doi.org/10.1097/BOT.0b013e31828f949c.
13. Livingston KS, Glotzbecker MP, Shore BJ. Pediatric acute compartment syndrome. J Am Acad Orthop Surg. 2017;25(5):358–64. https://doi.org/10.5435/JAAOS-D-15-00655.

Chapter 30
Ankle Fracture

Cristian Olmedo and Rodrigo Zuñiga

Physeal ankle injuries are the second most common in the child population. Injuries due to direct or indirect mechanisms, associated with sports practice and the misuse of trampolines. In adolescents, we can find injuries similar to adults or the presence of syndesmotic injuries, where clinical suspicion is of utmost importance. Most injuries are managed conservatively, leaving surgical treatment for specific situations. If these injuries are managed properly, medium and long-term complications (arthritis, misalignments) are avoided, with acute complications being rare.

30.1 Introduction

Ankle fractures in the pediatric population represent 5% of all fractures in this age-group. Physeal injuries of the distal tibia and fibula account for between 25% and 38% of all physeal fractures and are the third most common in childhood, after those of the phalanges and distal radius [1–3].

In general, in childhood, distal physeal injuries are more common than leg fractures in their middle third, and a high percentage occur in sports activity [2, 3], falls from heights, or domestic injuries [3, 4]. A 58% of physeal ankle injuries occur during sports practice.

Metaphyseal fractures of the distal tibia are scarcely described in epidemiology, and there are only English series, by Domzalski [4], which describes that they would be between 0.35% and 0.45% of the total fractures. In our clinical practice, 9% of

---

C. Olmedo
Clínica Alemana, Universidad del Desarrollo, Santiago, Chile

R. Zuñiga (✉)
Hospital San Borja Arriarán, Universidad de Chile, Santiago, Chile

M. Sepúlveda O. (ed.), *Paediatrics Traumatology*,
https://doi.org/10.1007/978-3-031-89482-4_30

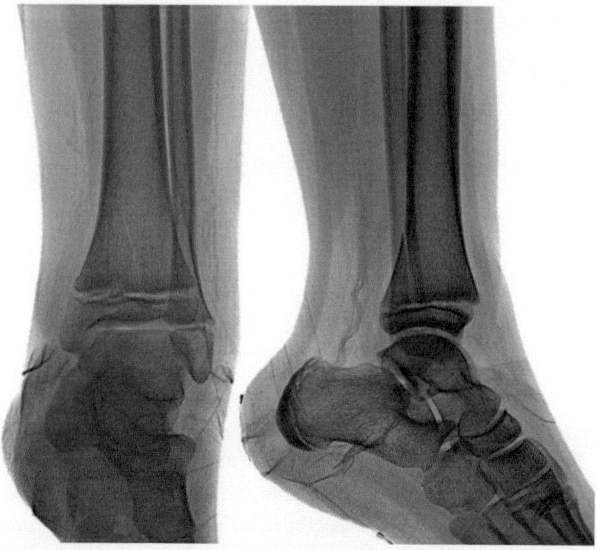

Fig. 30.1 Left ankle X-ray of a 13-year-old boy with a Salter and Harris type 2 physeal injury of the distal tibia

consultations were due to bicycle accidents, and 38% due to direct or indirect trauma to the lower limb. Currently, there is an increasing trend of injuries in ankles in the pediatric population associated with the use of trampoline or elastic bed, injuries that can be bony or ligamentous.

Physeal fractures are more common in men than in women (Fig. 30.1). The distribution is similar by age segments, being more frequent between 8 and 15 years [1].

Distal closure of the distal tibial physis occurs asymmetrically, from the anteromedial area, then posterior and ending its closure in the anterolateral area. The complete closure of this physis is described at 16–17 years in men and 14–15 years in women. This physeal cartilage contributes between 30% and 40% of the longitudinal growth of the tibia, on average 3–5 mm per year [5], so an adequate control must be carried out in the face of significant remaining growth after a trauma injury.

Syndesmotic ankle injuries are associated with adolescent population who practice impact sports and/or with torsional mechanisms during sports, such as football, or in those with a fixed ankle, such as snowboarding and skiing [2]. These injuries are described in up to 1% of pediatric ankle injuries [6].

Most fractures of the distal tibia and leg are managed conservatively [7, 8]. However, under special conditions, surgical treatment may be required, such as in cases of open fractures, associated with polytrauma, neurovascular injury, compartment syndrome, severe soft tissue injury, metaphyseal comminution adjacent to the physis, among other causes [8–10].

30.2 Injury Mechanism

The injury mechanism can be found in the Dias-Tachdjian classification, which describes different types of tears and the forces involved in them [1, 11]. It provides important information about the deforming forces, and consequently how to reduce the fracture.

The first part of each type includes the position of the foot at the time of injury, while the second part corresponds to the injury mechanism itself. It describes four types: Type A. Supination—external rotation, Type B. Pronation—- eversion - external rotation, Type C. Supination—plantar flexion, and Type D. Supination—inversion (Fig. 30.2).

There are also transitional injuries, given the closure process of the distal tibial physis, which will be treated in another chapter (Chap. 31).

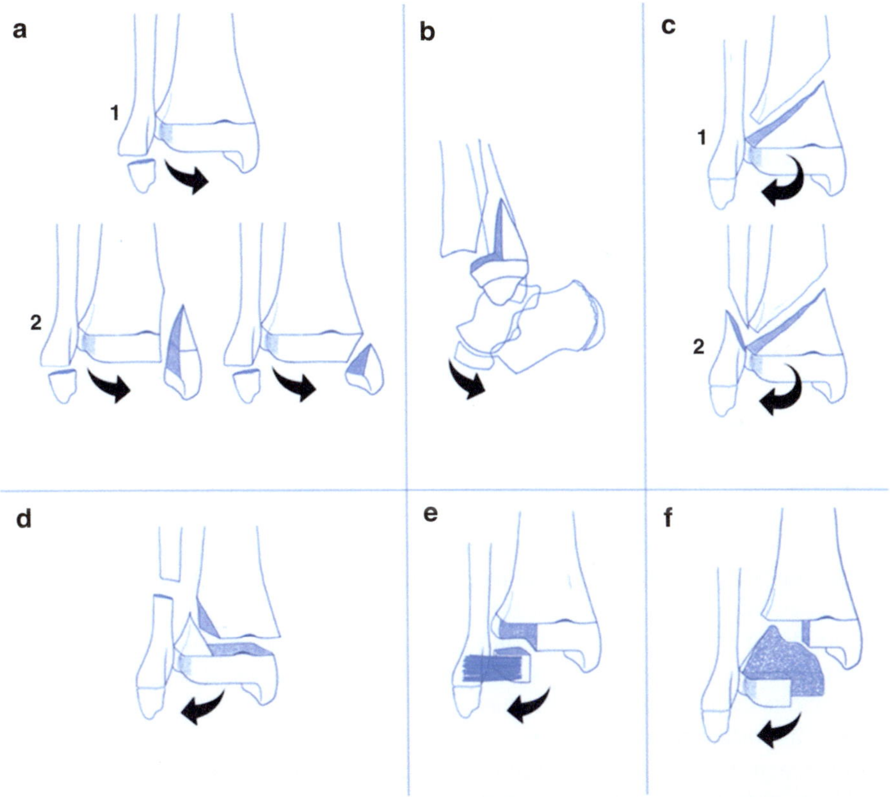

Fig. 30.2 Días-Tachdjian classification, with its 6 types, by injury mechanism: Type A, supination—inversion, Type B, supination—plantar flexion, Type C, supination—external rotation, and Type D, pronation—eversion. Also included are transitional fractures, Type E, Salter-Harris III of the distal tibial epiphysis, and Type F, triplanar fracture

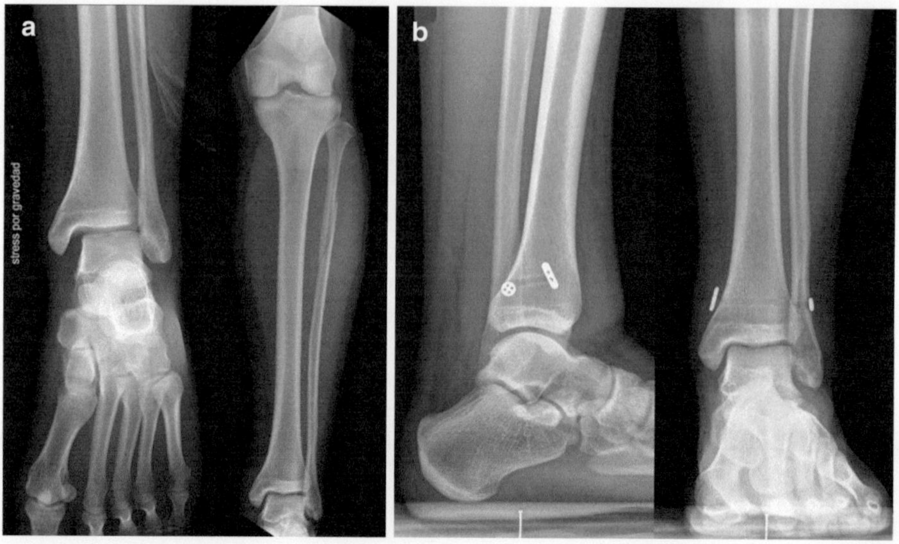

Fig. 30.3 Proximal fibula fracture (Maisonneuve) in a 14-year-old adolescent, with a syndesmosis injury evident on gravity stress X-ray (**a**). The syndesmosis was stabilized with a system of buttons and sutures (**b**)

Approaching adolescence, we find fractures with behavior similar to that of adults, with variable malleolar involvement. We will also find syndesmotic injuries in the juvenile population [2, 6], where the vast majority are stable, with specific injury mechanisms, that should alert us, requiring a high index of suspicion for their study and treatment (Fig. 30.3).

30.3 Anatomy

The distal tibia has a triangular configuration, with its medial face in direct relation to the teguments, its convex lateral face with a notch for the fibula through which it articulates with it, and a posterior face.

The distal fibula, lateral malleolus or fibula, is elongated and flattened transversely. Its anterior part is convex, smooth, and subcutaneous. It is longer and more voluminous than the medial malleolus.

It is important to always remember the scarce cover of the soft tissues in the distal area of the leg, for the coverture of osteosynthesis [12].

The load forces are mainly supported by the tibia, as the fibula contributes with approximately 1/6 of this resistance [13–15].

The ossification nucleus of the distal tibia appears between 6 and 24 months. The physis begins to close around 15 years, in a process that lasts approximately 18 months. The distal fibula presents an ossification nucleus that appears between 9 and 24 months, locating the physis at the level of the joint, and its closure usually precedes that of the tibia by 12–24 months [1].

The tibio-fibular-talar joint is a synovial trochlea type, allowing plantar and dorsal flexion movements of the talus, between the two malleoli. The distal physis of the tibia is extraarticular. In addition, it has a syndesmosis or tibio-fibular joint, held transversely by the anteroinferior tibio-fibular ligaments (which play an important role in transitional fractures), posteroinferior, by the interosseous membrane, the interosseous ligament, and the transverse tibio-fibular ligament, which together provide stability.

The syndesmosis continues proximally with the interosseous membrane [13–16]. This presents an elastic union between the tibia and the fibula and provides a place for the insertion of the long muscles of the foot. There are multiple studies that show that the post-traumatic increase in the syndesmal space leads to worse results, as well as that the increase of 1 mm of this space leads to an increase in the joint contact pressure of 50% [13].

The articular cartilage is relatively thin, so defects and articular steps can produce post-traumatic osteoarthritis in the medium and long term [14].

The articular facet of the distal tibia (Plafond) has approximately 3° of valgus. The mortise presents 20°–30° of external rotation with respect to the knee [13].

The anterior talofibular ligament is the most frequently injured and plays a fundamental role in limiting the anterior displacement of the talus and the plantar flexion of the ankle. The calcaneofibular is the only ligament that bridges between the talocrural and subtalar joints. It has insertions in the axis of rotation which allows flexion-extension movements of the talocrural joint. Since it connects two joints, this ligament allows movements of the subtalar joint. The posterior talofibular ligament is relaxed in plantar flexion and in neutral, and it tightens in dorsiflexion. The posterior intermalleolar ligament tightens during dorsiflexion and relaxes during plantar flexion. This means that excessive dorsiflexion forces can cause its rupture, or osteochondral injuries by avulsion. In the case of plantar flexion, a pinching between the talus and the tibia could be observed, due to the relaxed position of this. Finally, the medial complex or "spring-deltoid" is composed of superficial and deep fibers, 6 bands, 3 constant (spring ligament, tibionavicular, and deep tibiotalar), and 3 variable (superficial posterior tibiotalar, tibiocalcaneal, and deep anterior tibiotalar) [16].

30.4 Diagnosis

The diagnosis of most injuries is clinical and radiological. We can find variable forms of presentation [3], including functional impotence (the patient who limps or does not support), local volume increase, pain, deformity, bone exposure, joint effusion, feeling of instability, soft tissue injury, and even neurovascular compromise.

It is always important to evaluate the distal pulses (posterior tibial and dorsalis pedis), record their presence, and observe the perfusion of the toes (should be <2 s the fill after compression), the sensitivity of the distal territories, and the mobility of the toes.

Syndesmotic injuries may be accompanied by localized pain in the syndesmosis, pain with active and passive external rotation of the foot, and pain with forced dorsiflexion. The special tests for its evaluation are the "squeeze-test," the external rotation test, the fibular ballottement test (or translation), the Cotton test, and the cross leg test. Around 20% of syndesmotic injuries are not detected in the clinical examination [2].

The Ottawa criteria for the indication of a radiological study in emergencies, with high sensitivity in the adult population, cannot be applied with the same sensitivity in the pediatric population [16–18], so if there is suspicion of injury, it is advisable to request a basic radiographic set, especially in children below 10 years.

The anteroposterior (AP), lateral, and tibiofibular mortise ankle X-ray projections (Fig. 30.4) will help us to assess the location of the fracture (metaphyseal, physeal, and epiphyseal), the type of fracture pattern (complete or incomplete), the characteristic of the fracture line (oblique, transverse, spiral, and comminuted), the presence of intra-articular involvement, and bone avulsions [3]. It is important to evaluate the opening of the medial clear space, and the tibiofibular overlap (decrease or diastasis as such).

A comparative AP X-ray, under load or stress, is reserved for those patients in whom a ligamentous compromise is suspected, mainly syndesmal, remembering that the clear medial space and the tibia fibula overlap vary with age, being equal to the adult over 14 years old. Keep in mind that the stress X-ray due to gravity allows us to evaluate the integrity of the medial ligamentous complex of the ankle [3].

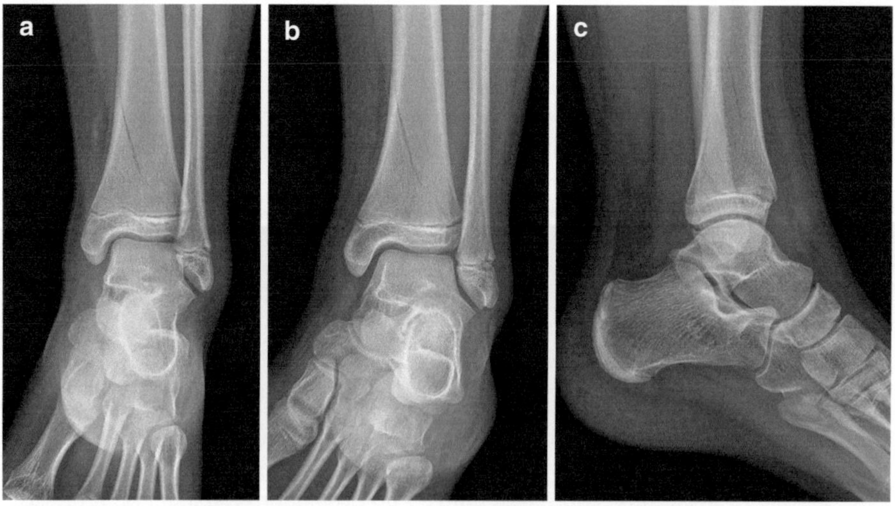

Fig. 30.4 Anteroposterior (**a**), mortise (**b**), and lateral (**c**) X-ray projections of the left ankle of a 10-year-old girl with a Dias-Tachdjian B type fracture

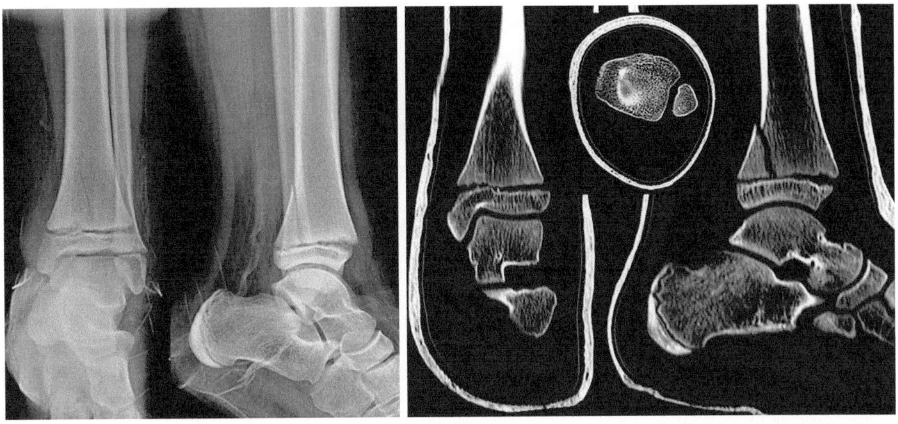

Fig. 30.5 X-ray of the left ankle of a 13-year-old boy (**a**), with a fracture in which joint involvement was suspected), which was ruled out with a CT scan (**b**), that shows a Dias-Tachdjian B fracture

Computed axial tomography (CT scan) is recommended when there is articular involvement (Fig. 30.5), or when the fracture line is complex (e.g., extraarticular triplanar or metaphyseal comminution). It allows for better preoperative planning [3, 19]. The loaded CT scan, a recently available exam, would allow for better evaluation of syndesmal instabilities, misalignments, and asymmetric joint compromises.

The contribution of magnetic resonance imaging (MRI) in the initial study is not very relevant, except for academic purposes. It does become essential in the evaluation after the fracture consolidation, for the differential diagnosis in a persistently painful ankle, when we suspect the presence of a physeal bar, or for the definitive diagnosis of syndesmal injuries.

30.5 Classification

The classifications of distal leg and ankle fractures classically are divided by anatomical segment or by injury mechanism.

The anatomical classification will be the initial one and will allow us to understand and then subdivide it going forward. We can subdivide the metaphyseal area according to the type of fracture line, and the epiphyseal area according to Salter-Harris (Scheme 30.1).

Metaphyseal injuries are considered, defined by the AO, as the square formed by the lines of equal measures based on the width of the distal tibia and fibula physis [4, 20]. The relevance of this location is the type of fracture, given the implications in its stability.

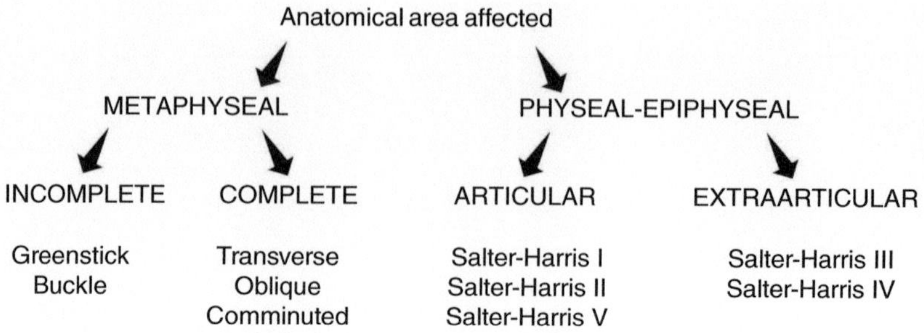

Scheme 30.1 Anatomical classification of ankle fractures

Table 30.1 Prevalence of ankle injuries by patient age

Age	Types of fracture
<1 year	Metaphyseal injuries suspected of abuse
<5 years	Incomplete, isolated fibula fracture, complete metaphyseal, Gillespie
>5 years	Complete, medial ossification nucleus injury or fibular
Adolescent	Transitional, avulsive, malleolar, syndesmal injuries

Physeal injuries are classified according to Salter and Harris (SH), being the most prevalent the SH Type II fracture [11, 21]. The avulsion of the perichondral ring of the distal tibia, or SH Type IV, should not be forgotten [22].

Also, epiphyseal injuries can be due to avulsive fractures of the fibula and/or medial malleolus in pediatric patients.

It should be noted that a metaphyseal corner fracture should make us suspect of non-accidental injuries (NAI) [23–25], being its classic presentation in the medial metaphyseal area of the tibia.

As we have seen, the injury mechanism is recorded in the Dias-Tachdjian classification. The AO trauma pediatric fracture classification attempts to describe by segment and group the previous ones.

In the adolescent age they approach the adult classifications, being able to find unimalleolar fractures (medial or lateral), bimalleolar, trimalleolar, and with syndesmal injury. We can also divide ankle fractures according to the age of prevalence, which helps to guide the diagnosis (Table 30.1).

30.6 Treatment

Distal metaphyseal fractures are usually associated with two patterns described in the literature: recurvatum combined with valgus, and procurvatum associated with varus [4]. In these fractures is found the Gillespie fracture, which corresponds to a greenstick fracture of the tibia with the complete posterior cortex that must be immobilized in equinus to avoid the increase of the angulation.

Conservative management with immobilization is indicated for fractures not displaced in the initial evaluation, and in the short-term follow-up (first 2 weeks). This can be done indifferently with removable immobilizations or short leg casts, depending on the adherence of the patient and/or their family.

Treatment can be performed with a closed reduction and initial long leg cast in unstable displaced fractures that maintain the reduction within the cast. Here, weekly control for the first 2 weeks is important to evaluate its adequate containment. In stable fractures after their reduction, a short leg cast can be used, contraindicating the load for 3 weeks, so as not to lose the reduction.

The closed reduction can be performed in the emergency room under sedation, or in the operating room, according to the preference of the treating physician. It is relevant to obtain an immediate X-ray control to ensure that the cast was installed with a good technique, and that the fracture is well reduced and contained (Fig. 30.6). If it is not possible to achieve a stable closed reduction, it should be considered that there is trapped periosteum, especially in metaphyseal lesions.

Physeal displacements >3 mm (especially if there is a growth remnant greater than 3 years), articular defects >2 mm, and any articular step require surgical treatment through closed and/or open reduction of these, to thus ensure adequate medium and long-term results [5, 11].

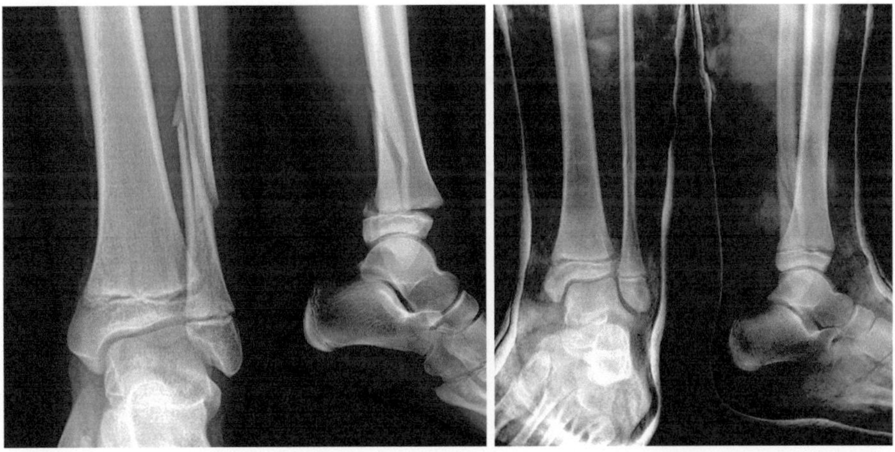

Fig. 30.6 X-ray of the ankle of a 10-year-old girl, with a fracture reduced under sedation. Its stable reduction is subsequently verified, well contained in a short leg cast

Articular epiphyseal lesions require an anatomical articular line reduction, without steps (for example, medial physeal lesions of the tibia SH Type II or Type IV). For fixation, we consider the use of cannulated screws or Kirschner wires. We use screws when we have a significant Thurstan Holland fragment to hold. When this is small, we use crossed Kirschner wires. In relation to fractures with an epiphyseal component (SH Type III and Type IV), we use screws that respect the physis and ideally go parallel to it.

In general, the reduction of the fibula is achieved with the reduction of the tibia, in distal tibial physeal lesions. It is very unusual to have to use osteosynthesis in the fibula, for which usually an elastic nail is sufficient in most cases.

Different is the case when managing fractures with a closed physis, or almost closed in adolescents, where the fibular length and the articular congruence are relevant. The concept of stability is important in this age group, which can be demonstrated with load/stress radiographs in unimalleolar fractures (Fig. 30.7). Bimalleolar or trimalleolar fractures or with syndesmal involvement are considered unstable and of surgical resolution with open reduction and internal fixation.

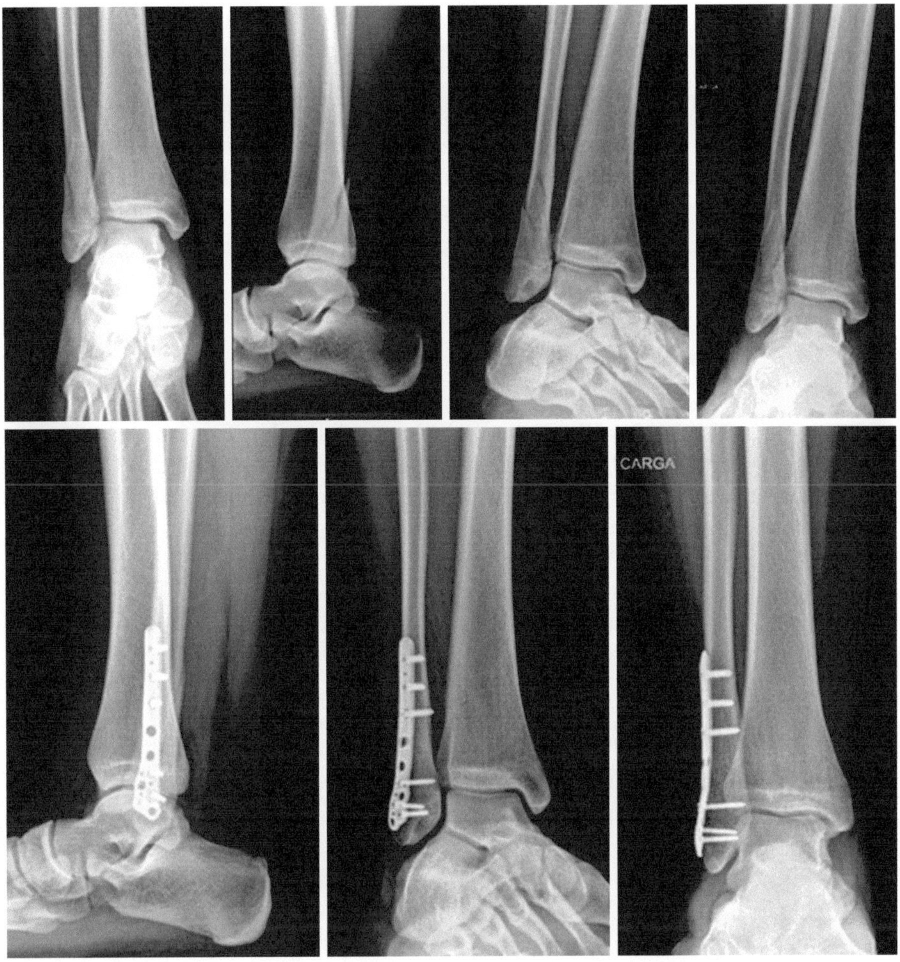

Fig. 30.7 Ankle X-rays of a 14-year-old adolescent with a unimaleolar fracture of the fibula, where a gravity stress X-ray (**a**) shows instability, for which surgical treatment is performed (**b**)

30.7 Complications

In relation to ankle physeal fractures, premature closure of the physis is reported in about 12.6%, according to a recent meta-analysis [5]. In other studies, the incidence is variable, from 17% to 60% [11, 21].

Other complications that are described are secondary deformity post-fracture or malunion [3, 21], the formation of a distal tibio-fibular synostosis [4, 26], the complication of superficial wounds, even with secondary deep infection [3], the non-union [3], and the post-traumatic arthritis [3]. All these are mainly associated with the persistence of articular steps or untreated malunion, which determine alterations of the ankle axis.

It is important to determine the associated syndesmal or ligamentary instabilities, or the presence of osteochondral lesions, as the untimely diagnosis is related to the development of post-traumatic arthritis.

Compartment syndrome is a rare entity in ankle fractures, but it should be taken into account [3]. It is important to recognize the "Extensor Retinaculum Syndrome," with the clinical presentation of significant pain on the top of the foot, hypoesthesia of the first interdigital space, and pain on extension of the hallux and/or lesser toes [27].

30.8 Final Message

Children and adolescents will eventually become adults; therefore, they need a congruent ankle joint to avoid degeneration in the medium and long term. For this reason, it is the responsibility of the treating physician to perform a correct evaluation and treatment of injuries in these patients, having a high index of suspicion in unstable syndesmotic injuries, achieving joint congruence in all ankle fractures, and understanding the basics for the proper management of physeal injuries, with the aim of not having future misalignments when there is still remaining growth.

30.9 Authors' Advice

- Ankle fractures are common in the pediatric population, most of them are treated conservatively.
- Determine surgical management by conducting a thorough study. Articular steps should not be tolerated.
- In adolescents, there should be a high suspicion of syndesmotic injuries.
- Remember that joint congruence and mortise are key for a good outcome.

References

1. Flynn JM, Skaggs DL, Waters PM. Rockwood & Wilkins fractures in children. 8th ed. Philadelphia, PA: Wolters Kluwer; 2014.
2. Shore BJ, Kramer DE. Management of syndesmotic ankle injuries in children and adolescents. J Pediatr Orthop. 2016;36(Suppl 1):S11–4. https://doi.org/10.1097/BPO.0000000000000767.
3. Olgun ZD, Maestre S. Management of pediatric ankle fractures. Curr Rev Musculoskelet Med. 2018;11(3):475–84. https://doi.org/10.1007/s12178-018-9510-3.
4. Domzalski ME, Lipton GE, Lee D, Guille JT. Fractures of the distal tibial metaphysis in children: patterns of injury and results of treatment. J Pediatr Orthop. 2006;26(2):171–6. https://doi.org/10.1097/01.bpo.0000218523.82996.76.

5. Jalkanen J, Sinikumpu JJ, Puhakka J, Laaksonen T, Nietosvaara Y, Kosola J, et al. Physeal fractures of distal tibia: a systematic review and meta-analysis [published online ahead of print, 2021 Apr 12]. J Pediatr Orthop. 2021;41 https://doi.org/10.1097/BPO.0000000000001833.
6. Kramer DE, Cleary MX, Miller PE, Yen YM, Shore BJ. Syndesmosis injuries in the pediatric and adolescent athlete: an analysis of risk factors related to operative intervention. J Child Orthop. 2017;11(1):57–63. https://doi.org/10.1302/1863-2548.11.160180.
7. Bauer J, Hirzinger C, Metzger R. Quadruple ESIN (elastic stable intramedullary nailing): modified treatment in pediatric distal tibial fractures. J Pediatr Orthop. 2017;37(2):e100–3. https://doi.org/10.1097/BPO.0000000000000705.
8. Özkul E, Gem M, Arslan H, Alemdar C, Azboy ASG. Minimally invasive plate osteosynthesis in open pediatric Tibial fractures. J Pediatr Orthop. 2016;36(4):416–22. https://doi.org/10.1097/BPO.0000000000000451.
9. Iobst CA. Hexapod external fixation of tibia fractures in children. J Pediatr Orthop. 2016;36(Suppl 1):S24–8. https://doi.org/10.1097/BPO.0000000000000764.
10. Rogers GP, Tan HB, Foster P, Harwood P. Complex tibial shaft fractures in children involving the distal Physis managed with the Ilizarov method. Strategies Trauma Limb Reconstr. 2019;14(1):20–4. https://doi.org/10.5005/jp-journals-10080-1421.
11. Wuerz TH, Gurd DP. Pediatric physeal ankle fracture. J Am Acad Orthop Surg. 2013;21(4):234–44. https://doi.org/10.5435/JAAOS-21-04-234.
12. Rouvière H. Human anatomy volume III limbs. J Chem Inf Model. 2013;53:1689–99.
13. DiGiovanni C, Greisberg J. Core knowledge in orthopedics: foot and ankle. 1st ed. Amsterdam: Elsevier; 2007. https://doi.org/10.1177/1938640008324663.
14. Gau CC, Yao TC, Gan ST, Lin SJ, Yeh KW, Chen LC, et al. Age, gender, height and weight in relation to joint cartilage thickness among school-aged children from ultrasonographic measurement. Pediatr Rheumatol Online J. 2021;19(1):71. https://doi.org/10.1186/s12969-021-00554-w.
15. Lippert H. Anatomy. In: In: Structure and morphology of the human body. 4th ed. Madrid: Marbán; 2002.
16. Golanó P, Vega J, de Leeuw PA, Malagelada F, Manzanares MC, Götzens V, et al. Anatomy of the ankle ligaments: a pictorial essay. Knee Surg Sports Traumatol Arthrosc. 2010;18(5):557–69. https://doi.org/10.1007/s00167-010-1100-x.
17. Ellenbogen AL, Rice AL, Vyas P. Retrospective comparison of the low risk ankle rules and the Ottawa ankle rules in a pediatric population. Am J Emerg Med. 2017;35(9):1262–5. https://doi.org/10.1016/j.ajem.2017.03.058.
18. Clark KD, Tanner S. Evaluation of the Ottawa ankle rules in children. Pediatr Emerg Care. 2003;19(2):73–8. https://doi.org/10.1097/00006565-200304000-00003.
19. Thawrani D, Kuester V, Gabos PG, Kruse RW, Littleton AG, Rogers KJ, et al. Reliability and necessity of computerized tomography in distal tibial physeal injuries. J Pediatr Orthop. 2011;31(7):745–50. https://doi.org/10.1097/BPO.0b013e31822d385f.
20. Audigé L, Slongo T, Lutz N, Blumenthal A, Joeris A. The AO pediatric comprehensive classification of long bone fractures (PCCF). Acta Orthop. 2017;88(2):133–9. https://doi.org/10.1080/17453674.2016.1258534.
21. Cai H, Wang Z, Cai H. Surgical indications for distal tibial epiphyseal fractures in children. Orthopedics. 2015;38(3):e189–95. https://doi.org/10.3928/01477447-20150305-55.
22. Masquijo JJ, Lanfranchi L, Allende V. Salter-Harris VI physeal fractures of the ankle and foot. Rev Asoc Argent Ortop Traumatol [Internet]. 2015;80(2):104–12. Available from: http://www.scielo.org.ar/scielo.php?script=sci_arttext&pid=S1852-74342015000200006&lng=es&nrm=iso
23. Adamsbaum C, De Boissieu P, Teglas JP, Rey-Salmon C. Classic metaphyseal lesions among victims of abuse. J Pediatr. 2019;209:154–159.e2. https://doi.org/10.1016/j.jpeds.2019.02.013.
24. Tsai A, Johnston PR, Perez-Rossello JM, Breen MA, Kleinman PK. The distal tibial classic metaphyseal lesion: medial versus lateral cortical injury. Pediatr Radiol. 2018;48(7):973–8. https://doi.org/10.1007/s00247-018-4103-2.

25. Chaturvedi A, Mann L, Cain U, Chaturvedi A, Klionsky NB. Acute fractures and dislocations of the ankle and foot in children. Radiographics. 2020;40(3):754–74. https://doi.org/10.1148/rg.2020190154.
26. Jung ST, Wang SI, Moon YJ, Mubarak SJ, Kim JR. Posttraumatic tibiofibular synostosis after treatment of distal tibiofibular fractures in children. J Pediatr Orthop. 2017;37(8):532–6. https://doi.org/10.1097/BPO.0000000000000708.
27. Mubarak SJ. Extensor retinaculum syndrome of the ankle after injury to the distal tibial physis. J Bone Joint Surg Br. 2002;84(1):11–4. https://doi.org/10.1302/0301-620x.84b1.11800.

Chapter 31
Transitional Ankle Fractures

Pablo Echenique and Pablo Wagner

Transitional ankle fractures are injuries to the distal physis of the tibia that occur in children and adolescents aged between 10 and 17 years-old, in whom physeal closure has begun. During this period, the physis ossifies in a predictable order, causing fractures with special characteristics, attributable to incomplete physeal closure.

31.1 Epidemiology

Traumatic ankle injuries are common in pediatric patients (1/1000 per year) and are second only to hand and wrist injuries in patients aged 10–15 years old. Ankle fractures occur twice as often in males and represent 5% of all pediatric fractures, and 9–18% of all physeal injuries. Specifically, triplane fractures represent 5–15% of pediatric ankle fractures and occur in adolescents with an average age of 13 years old and a range of 10–17 years old [1]. Tillaux fractures represent 2.9% of distal tibial physeal fractures.

P. Echenique
Clínica Alemana de Valdivia, Mutual de Seguridad C.Ch.C, Hospital Base Valdivia, Universidad Austral de Chile, Valdivia, Chile

P. Wagner (✉)
Clinica Alemana de Santiago-Universidad del desarrollo, Hospital Militar de Santiago-Universidad de los Andes, Santiago, Chile

M. Sepúlveda O. (ed.), *Paediatrics Traumatology*,
https://doi.org/10.1007/978-3-031-89482-4_31

31.2 Pathophysiology

Skeletal growth of the distal tibia continues until the age of 16 years old in males and 14 years old in females. The closure of the distal tibial physis occurs in a pattern, widely described in the literature, starting in the center of the physis and progressing towards anteromedial, then posteromedial, and finally lateral (Fig. 31.1).

Once the closure of the distal tibial physis begins, there is a transition period of 18–20 months in which it is incomplete. The unfused portions of the ankle physis have a higher risk of fracture during this period of incomplete growth plate closure, giving rise to the so-called transitional fractures. Triplane fractures occur at the beginning of this period, while juvenile Tillaux fractures occur closer to the end of physeal closure [2].

Triplane ankle fractures are complex traumatic injuries, involving the metaphysis, physis, and epiphysis. The term "triplane" refers to the three-dimensional orientation of the fracture lines in the distal tibia and represents a diagnostic challenge [3]. The fracture at the level of the epiphysis is in the sagittal plane and is radiographically visible in the anteroposterior x-ray projection of the ankle (AP). The fracture at the level of the metaphysis is in the coronal plane, in its posterior area, and is observed in the lateral x-ray projection of the ankle (Fig. 31.2). The fracture compromises a portion of the physis in the axial plane, providing the third plane.

Juvenile Tillaux fractures only involve the lateral epiphysis of the distal tibia. These occur when the medial physis is already closed, following a forced mechanism of external rotation of the foot, with or without associated abduction. As a result of this movement, the tibiofibular syndesmotic ligaments (in their anterior distal segment) cause the avulsion of this epiphyseal segment, generating a Salter-Harris Type IV fracture (Fig. 31.3).

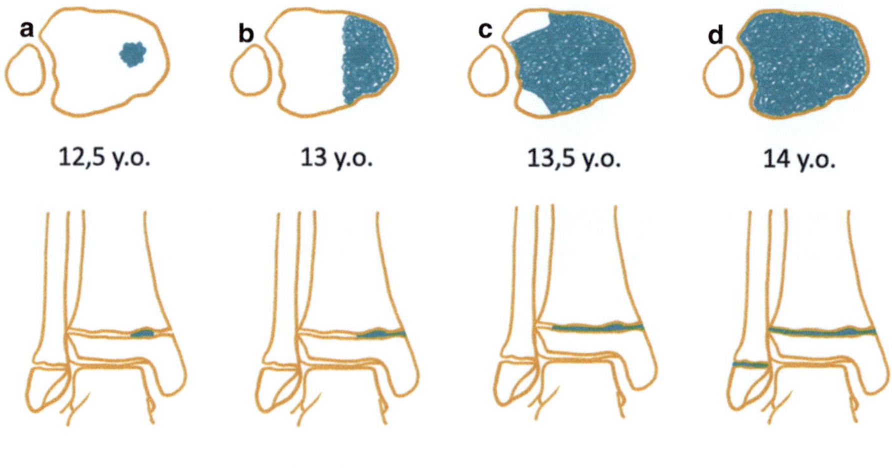

Fig. 31.1 Closure pattern of the distal tibial physis. Closure begins in the central medial zone (**a**), continuing towards medial closure (**b**), later advancing to lateral (**c**), and ending in the anterolateral and anteromedial zones, (**d**) complete physis closure

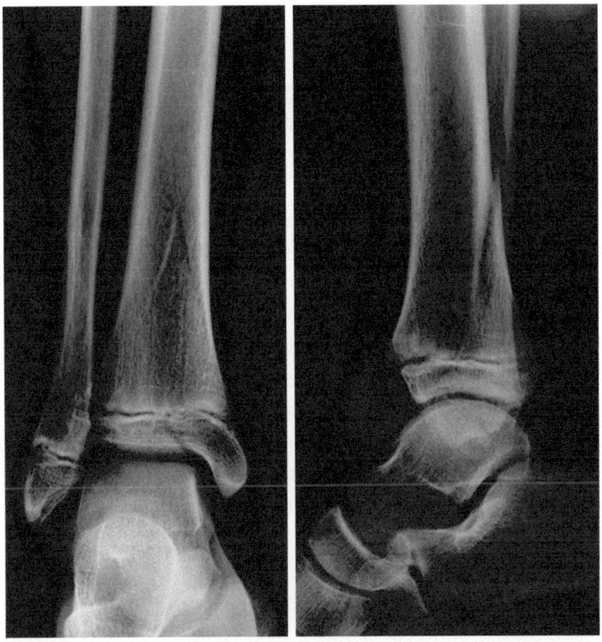

Fig. 31.2 X-ray showing triplanar ankle fracture. In the anteroposterior projection, the sagittal epiphyseal fracture line can be seen, and in the lateral projection, the coronal metaphyseal fracture line

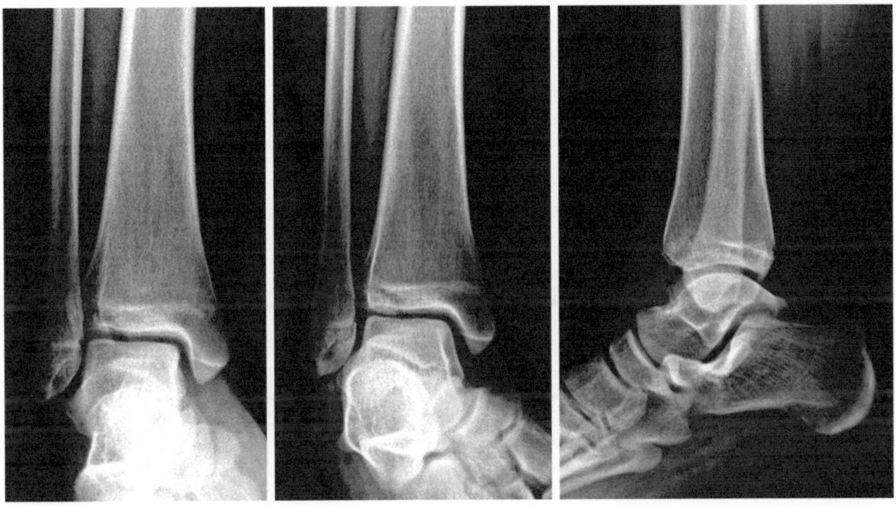

Fig. 31.3 Juvenile Tillaux fracture. In the anteroposterior and oblique (mortise) x-ray projections, the sagittal epiphyseal fracture line can be seen, with a joint step

31.3 Diagnosis

Adolescent patients generally report a twist of the ankle, which can be due to low or high-energy mechanisms during a sports activity, falls from heights, and traffic accidents. It presents with pain in the ankle and inability to weight bear.

The reported mechanism is usually a force of supination and external rotation, associated or not with axial compression, which explains the triplane fractures and the juvenile Tillaux type, which are the most common of the transitional fractures, since the lateral physis is the weakest area of the segment, the last to complete its closure, and the insertion point of the resistant anteroinferior tibiofibular ligament (AITFL). Medial triplane fractures are rare and occur as a result of an adduction and/or internal rotation force.

Upon clinical examination, swelling and/or bruising are observed. Patients present pain on direct palpation of the physis, circumferentially. Joint instability or obvious deformity is rarely appreciated, but it can occur in severe injuries. A complete neurovascular examination should be performed and documented to rule out associated injuries [4].

Ankle triplane fractures are often underestimated with the sole analysis of x-rays, as each projection only reveals a single fracture line. The combined set of x-ray projections (anteroposterior -AP-, mortise and lateral ankle) are essential in its diagnosis.

The AP projection of the ankle, and even better, the mortise projection of the ankle, reveal the sagittal fracture line in the epiphysis (Salter-Harris Type III) and is the key to confirming the diagnostic suspicion.

The lateral projection of the ankle shows the coronal fracture line at the level of the metaphysis in its posterior portion (Salter-Harris Type II). The fracture that passes through the physis in the axial plane (Salter-Harris Type I) will be more evident in radiographs with a higher degree of displacement. Due to the involvement of metaphysis, physis, and epiphysis, they could be classified as a variant of Salter-Harris Type IV injuries; however, due to their complicated and varied configuration, it is better to treat them as a different clinical entity [5]. It is noteworthy that the rare medial triplane fracture differs from the lateral injury, in that the metaphyseal fracture occurs in the sagittal plane and the epiphyseal injury is more medial and of coronal orientation, possibly or not compromising the articular cartilage in the medial malleolus (Fig. 31.4) [6].

Juvenile Tillaux type fractures are usually seen on x-rays, with the oblique projection of the ankle being the most useful [7], but it is recommended to evaluate with computed tomography (CT-scan) the displacement at the articular level (Fig. 31.5) [8].

While CT-scan is not essential for all cases of triplane fractures, it is a great tool for evaluating the exact fracture pattern, allowing for improved classification according to the number of parts or fragments. It also allows determining the degree of articular line displacement, which can support the need for surgical resolution. It can also change the therapeutic approach, both prior to or after a closed reduction,

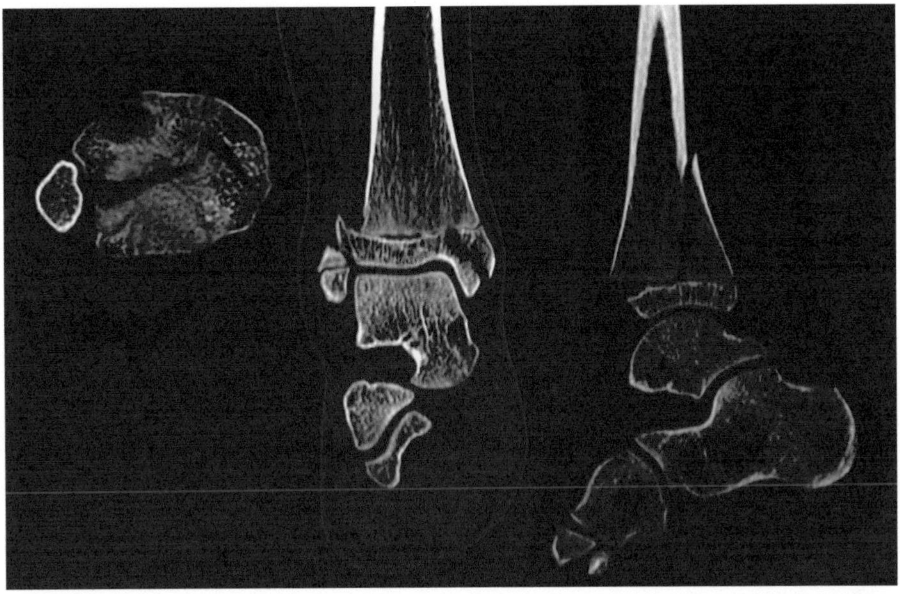

Fig. 31.4 CT-scan of a right ankle showing a medial triplanar fracture, with no joint involvement in the sagittal plane

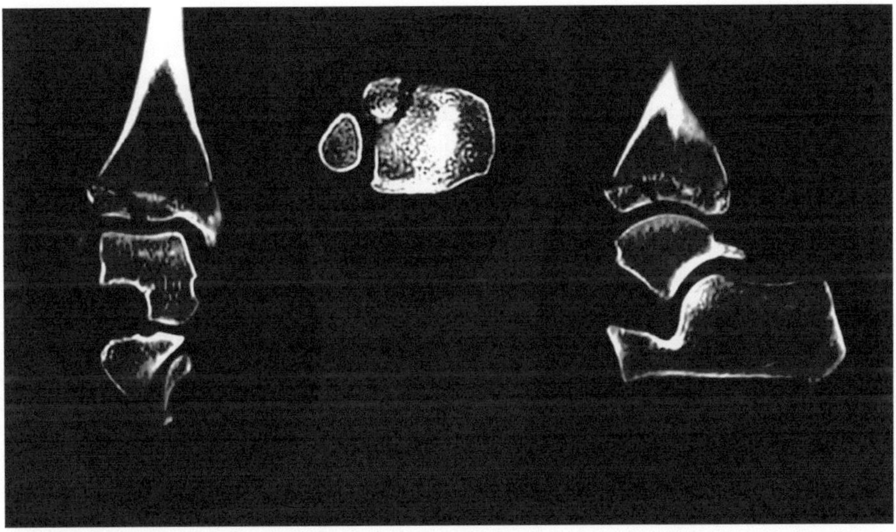

Fig. 31.5 CT-scan of the right ankle of a 14-year-old girl, showing intra-articular displacement of a juvenile Tillaux type fracture, with significant joint gap

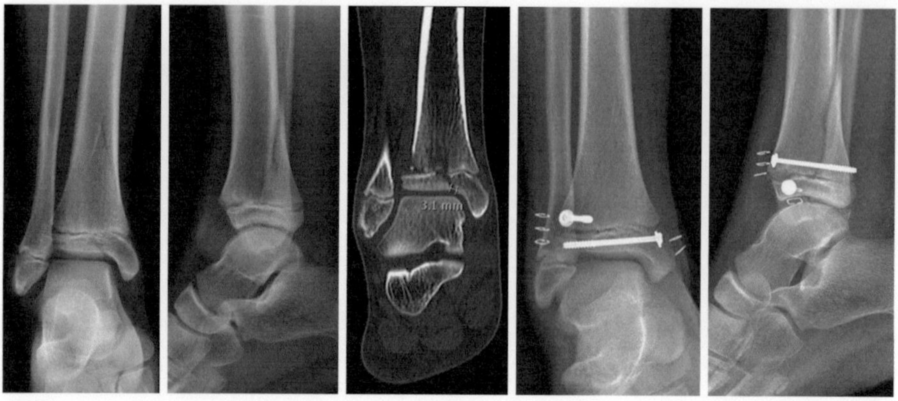

Fig. 31.6 Right ankle x-rays showing triplanar fracture. The preoperative study with CT-scan allows locating the ideal position of osteosynthesis to close the fracture lines

helping to accurately determine the insertion point and trajectory of the screws, according to the three-dimensional configuration of the injury (Fig. 31.6) [9, 10].

31.4 Classification

Ankle triplane fractures are classified according to the number of fragments and to the pattern of the injury.

According to the number of parts or fragments we can have: two parts (anterolateral and posterior epiphysis, anteromedial epiphysis), three parts (anterolateral epiphysis, posterior epiphysis, anteromedial epiphysis), and four parts (comminuted) (Fig. 31.7).

According to the pattern of the fracture line, they are divided into: lateral, middle, and intramalleolar. The lateral pattern is the most common, with an epiphyseal fracture line in the sagittal plane, physeal in the axial plane, and metaphyseal in the coronal plane. The middle pattern presents a feature epiphyseal in the coronal plane, physis in the axial plane, and metaphyseal in the sagittal plane. Finally, the intramalleolar pattern can have three types: Type I, intra-articular affecting the load-bearing surface; Type II intra-articular not affecting the load-bearing surface; and Type III, extra-articular.

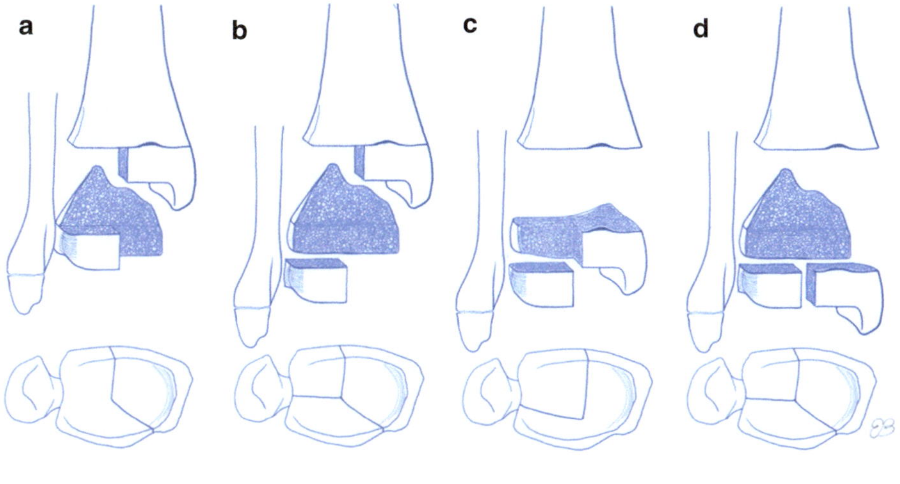

Fig. 31.7 Types of triplanar fracture based on the number of fragments: two parts (**a**), three parts (**b** and **c**), four parts (**d**) [18]

31.5 Treatment

The treatment of triplane ankle fractures depends on the degree of displacement of the fracture fragments, especially the articular displacement visualized on the CT-scan.

Non-displaced or minimally displaced injuries (less than 2 mm) can be effectively treated with a long leg cast, while those with more than 2 mm of displacement are recommended for surgical treatment, with closed or open reduction, and internal fixation [3].

The reduction maneuver for the classic pattern of triplane ankle fracture is by internal rotation of the ankle. It is recommended to control with CT-scan after closed reduction to evaluate residual displacement and joint separation and define if this is tolerable.

Surgical treatment is reserved for those triplane fractures with more than 2 mm of intra-articular displacement, or injuries that lost adequate reduction after the attempt at conservative management. Stable fixation is achieved with one or two screws placed parallel to the physis. The placement of the screws can be done in the metaphysis, in the epiphysis, or in both, depending on the fracture pattern.

There is no evidence to suggest the superiority of fixation with cannulated screws compared to non-cannulated, or fully threaded compared to partially threaded for triplane ankle fractures.

The goal of surgery is to restore the congruence of the articular surface to optimize results. Care must be taken to place the screws as perpendicular as possible to the fracture lines, maximizing compression and maintaining reduction. Both closed reduction techniques and open reduction have been equally effective in achieving correction, as long as they are performed at the right time.

The authors' preference in the case of indicating conservative treatment of a triplane ankle fracture is the use of a long leg cast with knee flexion to control rotation. This is used for 3 weeks, without allowing weight bearing. After this, it is changed to a short cast boot or cam walker, with partial weight bearing, for 3 weeks.

For surgical treatment, we recommend percutaneous reduction with a malleolar forceps through small incisions, and fixation with one or two 3.5 mm screws, cannulated, partially threaded, placed in parallel orientation to the physis. The exact orientation of the screws perpendicular to the fracture line is planned with the preoperative CT-scan, so we perform this study in all surgical cases [11].

Lateral triplane fractures, with lateral epiphyseal injury, are fixed with a screw placed from anterolateral to posteromedial, while the metaphyseal fragment is fixed with screws from anterior to posterior. Usually one or two screws are sufficient to maintain stable reduction, ensuring that all the threads of the screws pass the fracture line if using partially threaded screws, and that they do not remain prominent at their ends (Fig. 31.8).

Both when performing minimal approaches and when inserting screws, extreme care must be taken not to injure the neurovascular and tendinous structures at risk. Special care must be taken with the superficial peroneal nerve, often visible in the anterolateral area of the ankle, and with the anterior tibial neurovascular bundle, the deep peroneal nerve and the artery, which run posterior to the extensor hallucis longus. In the anteromedial area, we must be careful to avoid damaging the internal

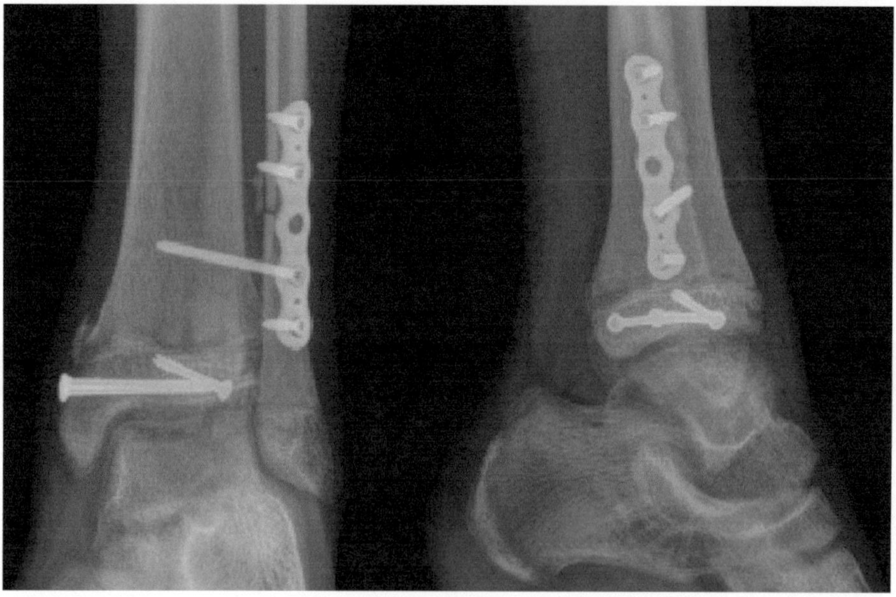

Fig. 31.8 Patient with triplanar fracture and syndesmoid injury. Closed reduction and fixation with epiphyseal screws, fibula plating, and syndesmoid screw to stabilize the mortise was performed

saphenous vein and the saphenous nerve, which are located approximately 1 cm medial to the anterior tibial tendon (between this and the medial malleolus) [12].

We recommend the usc of arthroscopy to visualize the reduction of the articular fracture line, especially if there is suspicion of interposition of soft tissues or free articular fragments that prevent closed reduction and must be resected (Fig. 31.9).

The treatment of juvenile Tillaux type fractures will be determined by the degree of displacement at the articular level. If the displacement is less than 2 mm, the treatment can be conservative. The use of a short leg cast for 1 month, without load, followed by load to tolerance with a cam walker for 2 weeks is recommended. At the time of cast removal, it is suggested to support with physiotherapy for gait rehabilitation.

If the displacement at the joint level is 2 mm or more, surgical treatment is recommended [13], as this is associated with the appearance of degenerative radiological signs in 6–9 years after injury, generally asymptomatic at that time, but with an uncertain long-term prognosis [14].

Surgical treatment consists of performing a reduction of the fracture by internal rotation of the foot, so that the fracture line should not be evident in the radioscopic view in the anteroposterior and mortise projections. It proceeds to stabilize with a compressive screw (cannulated or not cannulated) of diameter 3.0–4.0 mm, usually percutaneously.

If the fracture line persists after closed reduction, a minimal lateral ankle approach should be performed, or use arthroscopic support, to obtain an anatomical reduction of the fracture. Once achieved, it is fixed with a screw from anterolateral to posteromedial, in the distal tibial epiphysis, which can cross the physis given the scarce remaining growth in this lesion [15] (Fig. 31.10).

It should be noted, in the context of triplanar ankle fractures, that the presence of diaphyseal fractures of the tibia, distal fractures of the fibula and multifragmentary

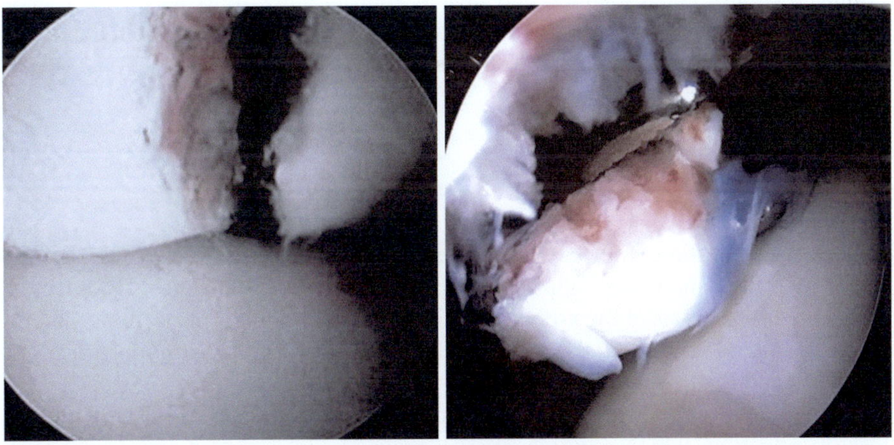

Fig. 31.9 Arthroscopic evaluation of joint injury in a triplanar fracture. Loose intra-articular fragments may be present in high-energy injuries and must be removed to achieve reduction

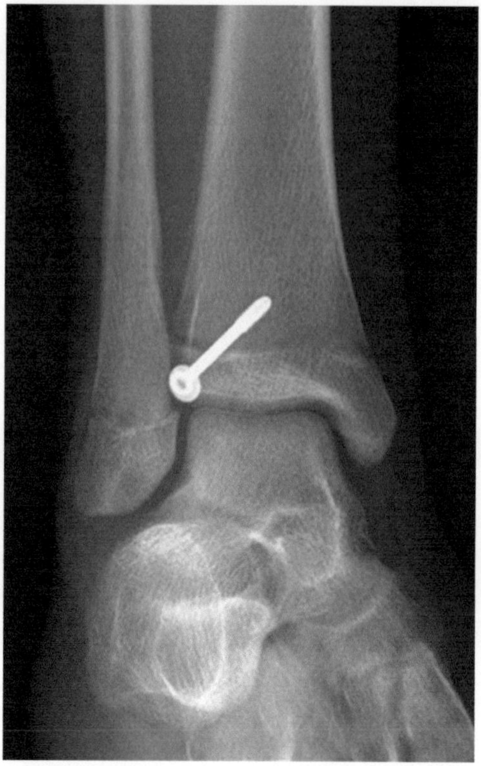

Fig. 31.10 Juvenile Tillaux type fracture, treated with closed reduction and screw fixation, which may pass through the physis

fractures of the tibial epiphysis, indicate a higher degree of energy of the injury [16]. This should alert about the possibility of associated injuries at the level of the syndesmosis and the deltoid ligament (although less frequent). These injuries should be evaluated in a directed manner, and treated appropriately, to avoid residual ankle instability. If the fracture of the tibia and/or fibula are displaced, their fixation is recommended along with the syndesmosis [17].

31.6 Prognosis

The prognosis of these injuries is usually excellent when the transitional ankle fracture is identified and treated appropriately. Therefore, timely diagnosis is essential, with a precise analysis of the x-rays of the injured ankle in all its projections (anteroposterior, lateral, and mortise), and complement with CT-scan for a more accurate diagnosis and treatment.

Complications of conservative treatment of these injuries are rare. These include loss of reduction, which requires surgical management to avoid major problems. Also described are non-union of the fracture, malunion, persistent pain, and early degenerative changes, especially in those cases where there is persistent displacement or joint incongruity greater than 2 mm.

Adverse events from surgical treatment are rare and include hemarthrosis, infection, non-union, transient neuropathy, symptomatic osteosynthesis (subchondral screws in the epiphyseal area increase the pressure of joint contact, and it is recommended to remove them within a period of 1 year).

Damage to the physis, with the formation of a physeal bar, is described in 7–21% of cases. The importance has been questioned not to pass through the physis with osteosynthesis, given the proximity of the time of physeal closure. In the case of juvenile Tillaux fractures, this is not relevant, as the end of the physeal closure is in process. However, for patients with triplane ankle fractures, who may have more than 2 years of remaining growth, the risk of damage and secondary complications is present, so it is appropriate to avoid damaging the physis as much as possible, and we must carry out a prolonged clinical and radiological follow-up in these cases.

31.7 Final Message

Transitional ankle fractures occur in adolescents between the ages of 12 and 17-years-old. The type of fracture will mainly depend on the degree of closure of the distal tibial physis. Treatment is conservative if there is no significant displacement of the fracture line, and surgical if this is 2 mm or more. An anatomical reduction is required to obtain good long-term results.

References

1. Shamrock AG, Varacallo M. Triplane ankle fracture. In: StatPearls. Treasure Island, FL: StatPearls Publishing; 2022.
2. Olgun ZD, Maestre S. Management of pediatric ankle fractures. Curr Rev Musculoskelet Med. 2018;11(3):475–84. https://doi.org/10.1007/s12178-018-9510-3.
3. Rosenbaum A, DiPreta JA, Uhl RL. Review of distal tibial epiphyseal transitional fractures. Orthopedics. 2012;35(12):1046–9. https://doi.org/10.3928/01477447-20121120-07.
4. Su AW, Larson AN. Pediatric ankle fractures: concepts and treatment principles. Foot Ankle Clin. 2015;20(4):705–19. https://doi.org/10.1016/j.fcl.2015.07.004.
5. Thawrani D, Kuester V, Gabos PG, et al. Reliability and necessity of computerized tomography in distal tibial physeal injuries. J Pediatr Orthop. 2011;31(7):745–50. https://doi.org/10.1097/BPO.0b013e31822d385f.
6. Yung CS, Kuong EE, Chow W. A previously unreported type of extra-articular triplane fracture: a revised classification system. J Orthop Surg (Hong Kong). 2019;27(1):2309499019828500. https://doi.org/10.1177/2309499019828500.
7. Mosca VS. Techniques of operative reduction and fixation of triplane and juvenile Tillaux fractures in adolescents. Oper Tech Orthop. 1995;5:171–7. https://doi.org/10.1016/S1048-6666(95)80010-7.
8. Horn BD, Crisci K, Krug M, Pizzutillo PD, MacEwen GD. Radiologic evaluation of juvenile tillaux fractures of the distal tibia. J Pediatr Orthop. 2001;21(2):162–4.

9. Hirsch M, Flores F, Ardiles O, Rios D. Understanding triplane fractures of the distal tibia. Chil J Radiol. 2016;22(3):114–20. https://doi.org/10.1016/j.rchira.2016.09.002.
10. Eismann EA, Stephan ZA, Mehlman CT, et al. Pediatric triplane ankle fractures: impact of radiographs and computed tomography on fracture classification and treatment planning. J Bone Joint Surg Am. 2015;97(12):995–1002. https://doi.org/10.2106/JBJS.N.01208.
11. Hadad MJ, Sullivan BT, Sponseller PD. Surgically relevant patterns in triplane fractures: a mapping study. J Bone Joint Surg Am. 2018;100(12):1039–46. https://doi.org/10.2106/JBJS.17.01279.
12. Frank RM, Hsu AR, Gross CE, Walton DM, Lee S. Open and arthroscopic surgical anatomy of the ankle. Anat Res Int. 2013;2013:1–9. https://doi.org/10.1155/2013/182650.
13. Rapariz JM, Ocete G, González-Herranz P, et al. Distal tibial triplane fractures: long-term follow-up. J Pediatr Orthop. 1996;16(1):113–8. https://doi.org/10.1097/00004694-199601000-00023.
14. Crawford AH. Triplane and Tillaux fractures: is a 2 mm residual gap acceptable? J Pediatr Orthop. 2012;32(Suppl 1):S69–73. https://doi.org/10.1097/BPO.0b013e31824b25a1.
15. McGillion S, Jackson M, Lahoti O. Arthroscopically assisted percutaneous fixation of triplane fracture of the distal tibia. J Pediatr Orthop B. 2007;16(5):313–6. https://doi.org/10.1097/BPB.0b013e3281568bab.
16. D'Angelo F, Solarino G, Tanas D, Zani A, Cherubino P, Moretti B. Outcome of distal tibia physeal fractures: a review of cases as related to risk factors. Injury. 2017;48(Suppl 3):S7–S11. https://doi.org/10.1016/S0020-1383(17)30650-2.
17. Cuzmar-Grimalt D, Escudero-Heldt M, Aldunate-González JT, Plaza-Guzmán N. Ankle fracture in adolescents: triplanar ankle fracture associated with leg fracture. Acta Ortop Mex. 2016;30(3):144–6. Spanish
18. Cancino B, Sepúlveda M, Birrer E. Ankle fractures in children. EFORT Open Rev. 2021;6(7):593–606. https://doi.org/10.1302/2058-5241.6.200042.

Chapter 32
Traumatic Injuries of the Pediatric Foot

Natalia Cifuentes and Consuelo Peirano

Traumatic foot injuries account for about 10% of fractures in pediatric age. Most pediatric foot fractures are conservatively treated, but special attention should be taken to fractures with articular compromise, those involving high-energy mechanisms, and the proper management of soft tissues.

While the prognosis is favorable, with good functional results, it is necessary to identify those fractures that inherently have a higher risk of developing complications, such as phalangeal fractures with joint component, hallux phalangeal fractures, distal phalangeal physeal fractures that extend to the nail matrix, Jones fracture of the fifth metatarsal, Lisfranc injury, talus and calcaneus fractures.

32.1 Introduction

Fractures and dislocations of the pediatric foot are common injuries, accounting for about 10% of fractures in this age range [1, 2]. Phalangeal and metatarsal fractures account for almost 90% of fractures at this level [3].

They pose a diagnostic challenge because the mechanism of injury is not always known, as very young patients do not always provide information, and often anxiety, fear, and pain hinder the physical examination. To this we must add the complexity of pediatric foot radiology due to its large cartilaginous component in the tarsal bones, presence of ossification nuclei, apophyses, and accessory bones.

N. Cifuentes
Hospital Clínico Herminda Martín, Chillán, Chile

C. Peirano (✉)
Hospital Clínico Regional, Concepción, Chile

M. Sepúlveda O. (ed.), *Paediatrics Traumatology*,
https://doi.org/10.1007/978-3-031-89482-4_32

There is a concept that the bones of the infant foot, being predominantly cartilaginous, have a great potential for remodeling, and therefore fractures have traditionally been treated conservatively. However, there are few studies that follow up in the long term to determine the real implications in adulthood [4].

The increase in competitive sports activity and higher energy injuries in adolescents have determined the need to choose for surgical management in some cases to avoid possible complications. Among them, compartment syndrome, extensor retinaculum syndrome, complex regional pain syndrome, infections, neurovascular injuries, complications related to the cast, undiagnosed injuries in polytrauma patients, osteonecrosis, premature physeal closure, malunion, non-union, arthrofibrosis, and post-traumatic arthritis are described.

It is important to analyze the kinematics of the trauma, the mechanism of injury. It is also essential to properly evaluate the involved area, the soft tissues, and the correct management of these, as they can be as or more important than bone injuries.

32.2 Pathophysiology

Children and adolescents are increasingly involved in activities and sports that involve high energy, in turn determining more complex traumatic injuries [5]. In the initial evaluation of the pediatric foot, Ogden [6] showed that cartilaginous bone has great elasticity, absorbing and dissipating the energy of trauma differently than in adults, resulting in different fracture patterns. Therefore, the management of injuries differs in childhood and adolescence. The tolerance ranges for angulations and displacements vary according to age, and in some fractures there are no agreed values.

A thorough understanding of the growing foot, from the point of view of bone, ligament, apophyseal, and physis anatomy, is fundamental for an adequate clinical evaluation of the area to be examined and recognition of acute traumatic injuries [7].

32.3 Anatomy

The foot is divided into three anatomical zones: forefoot, midfoot, and hindfoot.

The distal third, which corresponds to the forefoot, includes the phalanges, metatarsals, and metatarsophalangeal joints.

The midfoot includes the three cuneiforms, the navicular, and the cuboid, with the tarsometatarsal joints marking the boundary between the forefoot and the midfoot. At this level, we have the plantar ligaments, which are stronger than the dorsal stabilizers. Among them, the Lisfranc ligament is of vital importance in the biomechanics of the foot, considering that there is no intermetatarsal ligament between the first and second metatarsal.

The hindfoot is made up of the calcaneus and the talus. The Chopart joint separates the midfoot from the hindfoot. The hindfoot has a large joint called the subtalar joint, which is composed of three articular facets [8].

It is especially important to know the presence of secondary ossification centers (Fig. 32.1), supernumerary bones (Fig. 32.2), and growth plates to make a correct diagnosis, as they can be confused with traumatic injuries, despite having a distinctive location and radiological characteristics (regular edges, peripheral sclerosis). The calcaneus and the talus have the primary ossification center present at birth, while that of the cuboid becomes evident a few months after birth and the primary ossification nucleus of the navicular appears around 3 years old.

Given the same trauma, the foot of a child, adolescent, and adult dissipate energy in different directions, generating different fracture patterns. Sometimes these features are difficult to identify on x-rays, making magnetic resonance imaging (MRI) and computed tomography (CT-scan) fundamental tools for an adequate diagnosis [7].

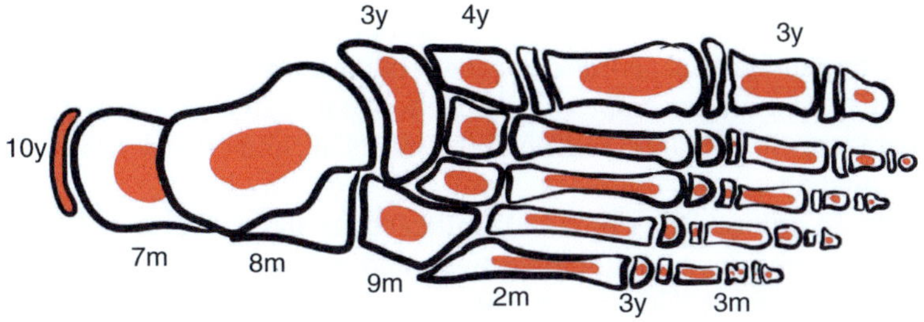

Fig. 32.1 Secondary ossification centers at the foot level (y = years; m = months in utero)

Fig. 32.2 Normal location of supernumerary bones in the foot

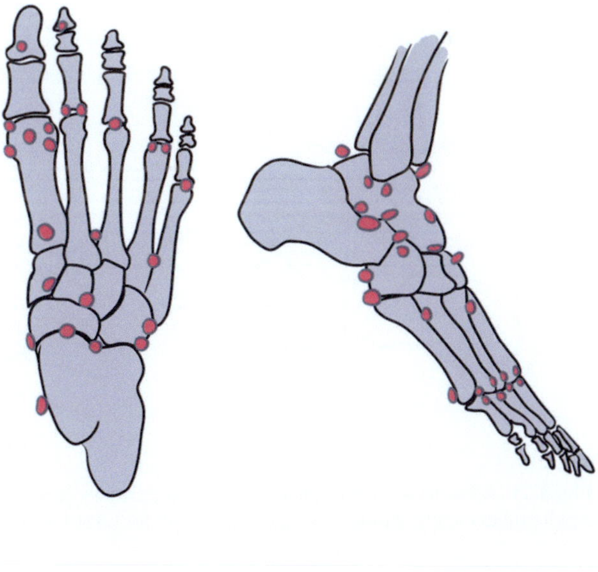

32.4 Diagnosis

In pediatric fractures, it is common not to have a report of the injury mechanism from the patient, or a witness to the accident. Factors such as the energy and speed involved, the position of the foot at the time of the accident, and the actual height of the fall, are difficult to obtain reliably, despite being fundamental to predict possible injuries.

The general evaluation of the patient, as with all musculoskeletal injuries, should be performed with the patient undressed. If possible, gait should be evaluated, determining if there is refusal to load on any limb or painful limping. It is important to objectify antialgic positions and the presence of associated injuries, which are of vital importance in the polytrauma patient.

One should observe standing, the alignment of the limb (varus, valgus), the presence of previous conditions (flat foot, high arch, congenital malformations), skin involvement and evaluate the ranges of motion compared with the healthy limb, the exact location of pain, both spontaneous and on palpation. This last point is difficult to objectify in the vast majority of cases, so it is recommended to perform a systematic palpation of the foot, in addition to identifying increases in volume and/or bruising. The neurological and vascular status of the limb should always be recorded.

There may be a subtle compromise of the foot's irrigation in a closed trauma due to the characteristic tolerance of the compartments in children and the abundant collateral circulation.

The Ottawa criteria [9] (Fig. 32.3), validated for the pediatric population, help determine the need for a radiological study and guide to the likely compromised segment (ankle or foot). The presence of pain on palpation in the lateral and medial malleolus, at the level of the navicular, at the base of the fifth metatarsal and the inability to take four steps on the limb, is indicative of the need for an x-ray study.

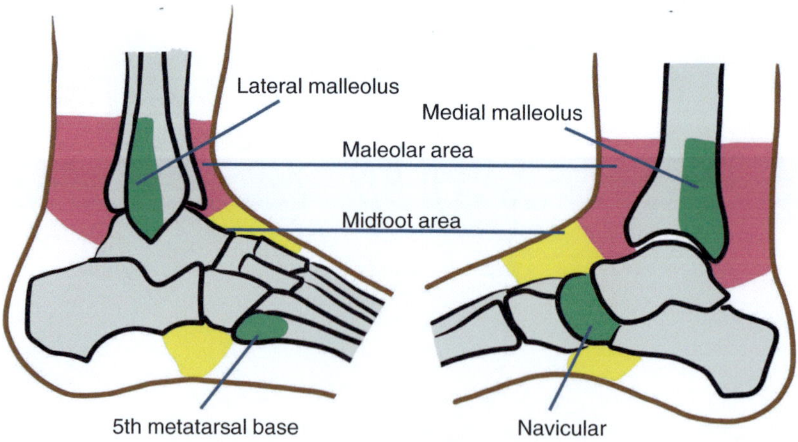

Fig. 32.3 Areas to be evaluated according to the Ottawa criteria. If pain is present in any of them, a radiological study should be requested to look for bone lesions

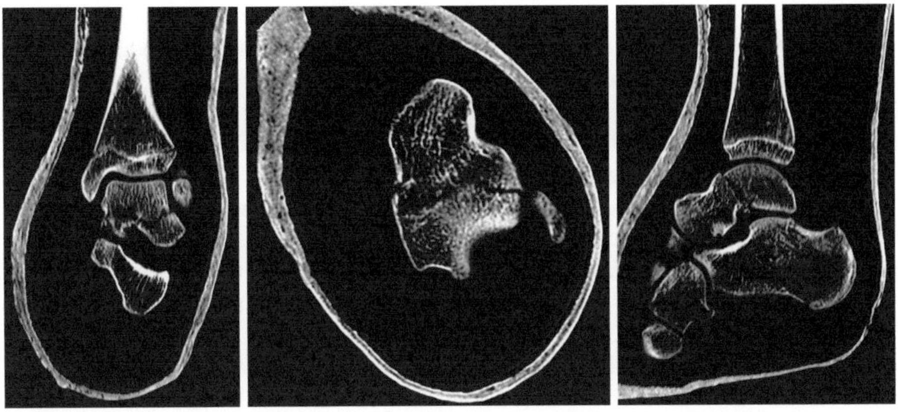

Fig. 32.4 CT-scan of the ankle of a 10-year-old girl, showing fracture of the talar neck

The anteroposterior (AP), lateral and mortise ankle x-ray projections, in addition to the oblique projection of the foot, can be complemented with radiographs for specific injuries, according to examination findings (sesamoids, axial of calcaneus, subtalar facet).

It is suggested to perform joint stability tests, both of the ankle and foot (anterior drawer, talar tilt, "Squeeze test," Lisfranc), but always taking into account the patient's age, the degree of anxiety and the presence of pain, due to the elastic nature of the tissues in prepubertal age may not provide more information and only increase discomfort, decreasing the possibility of achieving cooperation from the patient.

In some cases, it will be necessary to request a CT-scan to improve the definition of the fracture, allowing a three-dimensional evaluation of the compromised structures (Fig. 32.4). MRI is the ideal imaging exam for the evaluation of soft tissues, including tendons and ligaments, as well as cartilage and the presence of bone edema.

Finally, the use of bone scintigraphy allows identifying areas of bone tissue turnover, such as in stress fractures, tumoral lesions, or infectious ones.

32.5 Talus Fractures

This is an infrequent injury in children, with a prevalence of 0.008% of all pediatric fractures [10] reported in the literature.

They are the result of high-energy trauma involving axial load with the ankle in dorsiflexion (traffic accidents, fall from height). They are also described in low-energy traumas, associated with sports activities, where they present as avulsion fractures, with a good prognosis.

On clinical examination, we will find edema and pain on the anterolateral side of the ankle, associated with functional impotence, refusal to weight bearing, and even deformity in case of displacement. The radiological study should include AP, lateral, and oblique foot x-ray projections. It is also recommended to complement the study with the Canale and Kelly x-ray projection, with the beam pointing to the center of the foot, at 75° of inclination, and the foot positioned at 15° of elevated inclination from the side. This projection allows evaluating the neck of the talus, unprojecting from the navicular. In case of diagnostic suspicion, it may be necessary to complement the study with a CT-scan.

The most frequently compromised anatomical site is the neck of the talus, which can be associated with fractures of the malleoli, compression injury of the calcaneo-cuboid joint, and Salter-Harris Type III or Type IV fractures of the distal tibia.

In 1970, Hawkins [11] classified these fractures into three types, which was modified by Canale and Kelly [12], who added a fourth type (Fig. 32.5).

The higher the degree of the classification, the greater the energy involved, and therefore, the greater the risk of soft tissue injury, neurovascular and tendon involvement (Table 32.1). Kızılay and Aytan [13] reports a case of a Hawkins Type III talus fracture in a 9-year-old child, with interposition of the posterior tibial artery, the tibial nerve, and the posterior tibial tendon and the long flexor digitorum, associated with a fracture of the medial malleolus.

Fractures of the head of the talus are very infrequent, usually secondary to mid-tarsal dislocations (Chopart).

The fracture of the lateral process is frequently misdiagnosed, as it is interpreted as a lateral ankle sprain because it presents with external perimaleolar edema, external inframaleolar pain, and refusal to the load. It is associated with a dorsiflexion and inversion mechanism of the ankle, combined with axial load, with the transmission of shearing forces from the calcaneus to the lateral process. It was initially described associated with snowboarding, but cases are also reported from skateboarding accidents. The study should be completed with CT-scan to define the presence of articular involvement, the size of the fragment, and its real displacement.

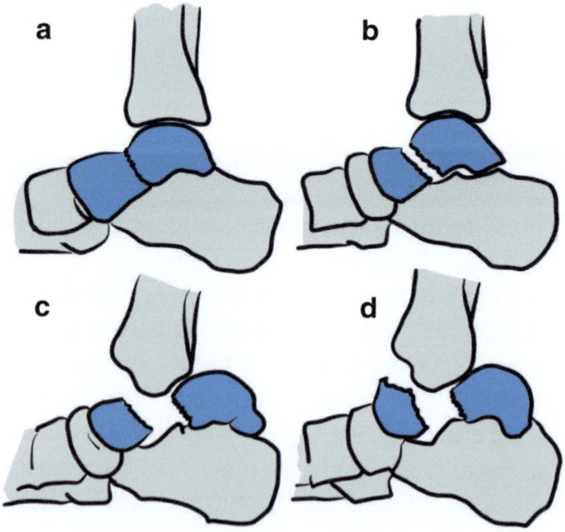

Fig. 32.5 Diagram of the modified Hawkins classification for talus fractures. (**a**) type I; (**b**) type II; (**c**) type III; (**d**) type IV

Table 32.1 Description of the Hawkins classification, modified by Canale and Kelly [12], and its relationship with the risk of avascular necrosis (AVN)

Type	Security	Subtalar	Ankle	Talonavicular	NAV risk
I	Not displaced		–	–	Low
II	Displaced	Subluxated/ dislocated	–	–	42%
III	Displaced	Subluxated/ dislocated	Subluxed/ dislocated	–	91%
IV	Displaced	Subluxated/ dislocated	Subluxed/ dislocated	Subluxed/ dislocated	>95%

The fracture of the posterior process is rare and must be differentiated from the Stieda process and the os trigonum.

Finally, it is important to remember the existence of osteochondral lesions of the talar dome. Up to 45% of them are associated with ligament injury or ankle fracture, located anterolaterally. These lesions are of traumatic etiology in virtually all cases, unlike those located medially, which are more posterior, non-traumatic, with up to 25% bilateral presentation. The study for these lesions includes AP, lateral, and mortise ankle x-ray projections, adding the projections in plantar flexion and oblique. Their classification requires a study with CT-scan and/or MRI to determine the treatment.

In general terms, for the pediatric patient, conservative treatment is preferred. Avulsive lesions are managed symptomatically, with a short leg cast or a Cam Walker being sufficient, with unloading for 1–2 weeks, and then protected loading for 1–2 more weeks.

The treatment of non-displaced lateral process fractures and without involvement of articular facets is conservative, with a short boot cast and unloading for 4 weeks. In cases with displacement and/or joint involvement, it is necessary to perform reduction and osteosynthesis being able to fix the fracture with smooth Kirschner wires or with screws.

Type I neck fractures are managed conservatively, with a short leg cast and unloading for 4–8 weeks, depending on the age of the patient.

The displaced talus fracture corresponds to a surgical emergency due to its high rate of avascular necrosis [13]. In the cases with displacement >5 mm or angulation >5° in the anteroposterior plane, a reduction, closed or open, must be performed. In case of requiring stabilization with osteosynthesis, the choice is cannulated screws from posterior to anterior, thus preserving the articular cartilage and with better biomechanical resistance. While there are no consensus values for acceptable alignment in children, the goal should be an articular step less than 2 mm. It is immobilized with a short leg cast and is kept unloaded for a period of 4–8 weeks, then allowing protected loading as tolerated (Fig. 32.6).

The most feared complication of a talus fracture is avascular necrosis, more common in neck fractures, and directly related to the severity of the initial injury. It can

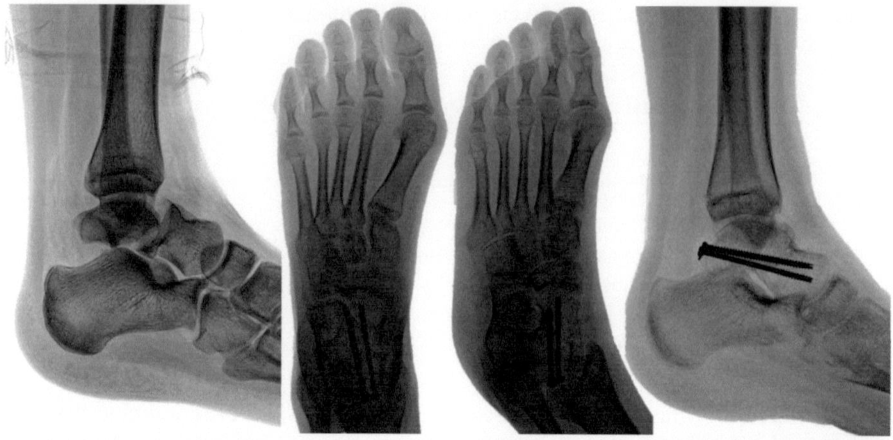

Fig. 32.6 X-ray of an 11-year-old girl with a Hawkins type III talus fracture, treated by reduction and stabilization with cannulated screws

develop up to 6 months after the trauma, so radiological follow-up is recommended for at least 18 months. The Hawkins sign, which is the subchondral radiolucency in the dome of the talus, is an indicator of revascularization that becomes evident between 6 and 8 weeks. This is a good prognosis marker, but inconsistent in pediatric patients [6].

The diagnosis of osteonecrosis prior to radiological collapse can be made with MRI, with the presence of the "double ring" sign, which corresponds to an image of a hyperintense area (inner ring) surrounded by a hypointense halo (outer ring) in T2 [14].

Malunion, either due to underestimating the initial displacement, incomplete reduction or postoperative loss of it, produces a varus hindfoot, with a forefoot in adduction and supination, due to shortening of the medial column. Incongruity of the subtalar joint can also be observed, due to the fact that the remodeling potential of the talus is not unlimited [15].

Other rarer complications to see are non-union, delayed consolidation, post-traumatic arthritis, and local complications (soft tissue or infection).

32.6 Calcaneus Fractures

These are low-frequency injuries, representing between 0.05% and 0.15% of all pediatric fractures. They have a higher incidence between the ages of 8 and 12 years old. These injuries are associated with high-energy mechanisms, such as falls from height, traffic accidents.

They are usually extra-articular fractures (65% of calcaneus fractures), with little displacement, and with adequate results with conservative management. During adolescence, the incidence of articular fractures increases, with patterns like adults, that require surgical management.

A high index of suspicion should be maintained, as the findings on x-rays can be subtle due to not presenting a large displacement, resulting in a delay in diagnosis that reaches up to 40% of cases. It is important to note that one third of calcaneus fractures are associated with other injuries, such as ankle, leg, and vertebral fractures, so the study should cover these areas.

The initial radiological study should include x-rays in AP, lateral, oblique, and axial projections of the calcaneus (Harris Projection). Regarding radiological measurements, the Böhler and Gissane angles do not have standardized values for the pediatric population, and the partial ossification of the calcaneus makes these measurements complex. However, in 2011, Boyle et al. [16] published the first study on the measurement of these angles in pediatric patients aged 0–14 years old, obtaining an average value of 35.2° for the Böhler angle and 111.3° for the Gissane angle, which could be used as a reference. To complement the imaging study and define articular involvement, CT-scan evaluation is essential.

For these injuries, the Essex-Lopresti classification is used, which identifies "tongue" type injuries and those with articular depression (Fig. 32.7), in addition to defining extra-articular or intra-articular involvement with the Wiley classification (Fig. 32.8).

Stress fractures of the calcaneal tuberosity in preschool patients are described, which present with heel pain associated with claudication without known trauma, with an initial radiograph without findings, which when repeated after 2 weeks shows marked sclerosis in the tuberosity area. They do not require specific treatment, only observation.

In adolescent athletes, the avulsion fracture of the posterior tuberosity can occur, which when it involves a large fragment and significant displacement ("beak sign"), corresponds to an emergency due to the risk of imminent exposure.

In cases of extra-articular or articular fractures without depression, conservative management consists of a short leg cast, with non-weight bearing for 4–6 weeks, depending on age, followed by protected load to tolerance.

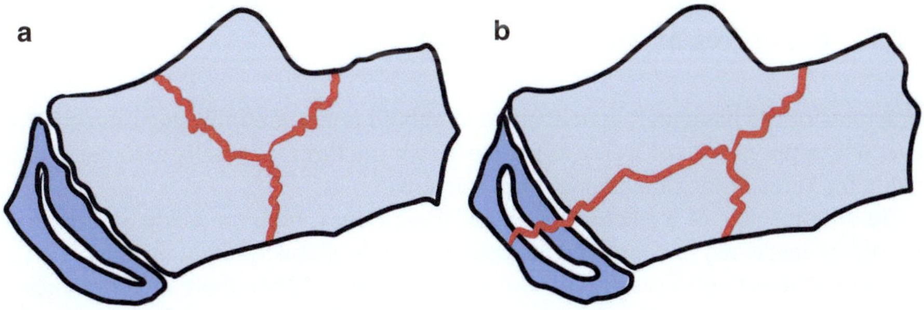

Fig. 32.7 Essex-Lopresti classification scheme. (**a**) central depression type; (**b**) "tongue" type

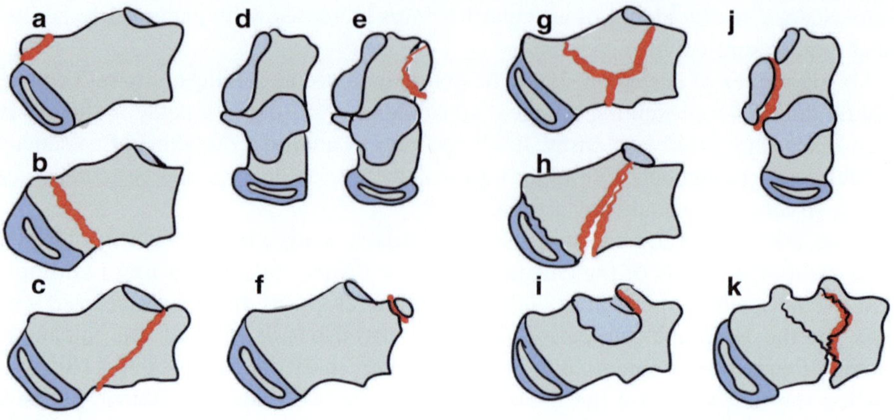

Fig. 32.8 Wiley classification of calcaneal fractures. (**a**) tuberosity avulsion; (**b**) vertical of the body; (**c**) horizontal of the body; (**d**) medial process avulsion; (**e, f**) anterior process avulsion; (**g**) non-displaced; (**h**) tongue-type; (**i**) centrolateral fracture; (**j**) sustentaculum fracture; (**k**) displaced multifragmentary

Fractures with an articular compromise, associated with depression of the posterior facet, have an indication for surgical treatment, with an approach through the sinus of the tarsus, with direct visualization of the fragment for its reduction, without yet consensus on the choice of the most suitable osteosynthesis material, which can be Kirschner wires or screws, depending on the patient's age. There are case reports of articular fractures managed conservatively in patients under 8 years old, with satisfactory short-term functional results, without evidence yet to recommend this behavior.

The results of the treatment of pediatric calcaneus fracture show a low incidence of complications, without compromise of gait or residual pain, even in articular fractures with minimal displacement treated conservatively. There are no long-term follow-up reports of displaced articular fractures, which allow determining the incidence of post-traumatic subtalar arthritis.

32.7 Fractures at the Tarsal Level

Fractures of the navicular, cuneiform, and cuboid bones are infrequent in pediatric age, with a prevalence of 2–7% of pediatric foot fractures, generally associated with ankle fractures or tarsometatarsal joint fractures.

In the presence of a fracture in any of these bones, both the ankle and the foot should be inspected in a targeted manner, in search of concomitant injuries.

Most of these injuries are avulsive or stress-related. When there are high-energy mechanisms, displaced fractures or "explosion type" comminuted fractures can be identified, associated with Lisfranc type tarsometatarsal injuries and others.

Avulsive or stress fractures can be managed with a short leg cast off-load for 3–4 weeks, followed by protected load bearing for 2 weeks; they have a good prognosis, without functional sequelae or residual pain. In the case of displaced fractures, as they are bones that are part of joint complexes, reduction and osteosynthesis should be prioritized if necessary, to restore the biomechanics of the midfoot. Complications are given by the high-energy mechanism and associated injuries.

32.8 Lisfranc Injury

Lisfranc luxofracture is infrequent in pediatric age and difficult to diagnose due to the radiological characteristics of the pediatric foot. The joint involvement can be only ligamentous, so a high index of suspicion must be maintained.

This injury can occur due to high-energy traumas (traffic accidents, falls from height) or low energy. Three different mechanisms are described (Fig. 32.9):

- Jumping and landing on tiptoe, which produces axial load with metatarsophalangeal flexion.
- Falling backwards with the forefoot fixed on the ground.
- Compression force on the heel, when kneeling, which generates dorsiflexion and plantar flexion forces.

In the pediatric population, low-energy mechanisms, related to sports activities, cause exclusively ligamentous injuries that can be managed conservatively.

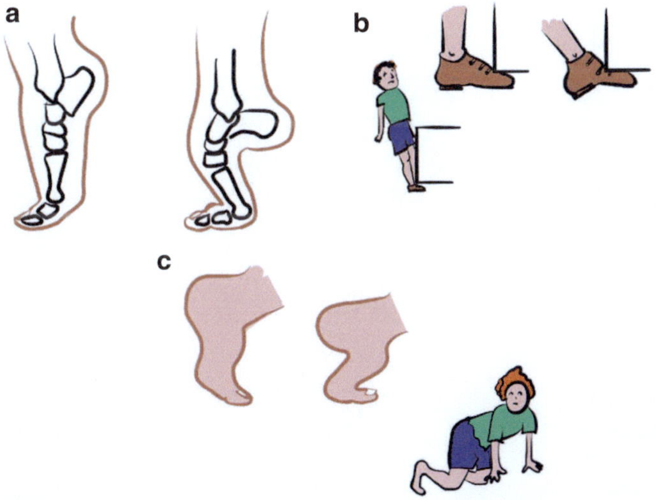

Fig. 32.9 Mechanisms of Lisfranc injury in pediatric patients: (**a**) jump and support on tiptoe; (**b**) fall on back with fixed foot; (**c**) dorsiflexion of forefoot with plantar flexion of midfoot, on knees

In the infant foot, the distance between the bases of the first and second metatarsals is constant at all ages (<3 mm), unlike the distance between the base of the second metatarsal and the medial cuneiform, which gradually decreases until the age of 7 years old, when it reaches the adult value (<2 mm) [17].

On physical examination, swelling of the dorsal side of the foot, functional impotence with refusal to load, pain in the midfoot is observed. The characteristic plantar bruising in adults is inconsistent in children.

The radiological study begins with comparative weight-bearing AP, lateral and oblique foot x-rays. In the AP radiograph, the lateral edge of the first metatarsal is in line with the lateral edge of the medial cuneiform, and the medial edge of the second metatarsal in line with the medial edge of the second cuneiform. In the oblique x-ray projection, the medial edge of the fourth metatarsal is in line with the medial edge of the cuboid. The radiological sign that corresponds to a small avulsive fracture of the medial base of the second metatarsal ("fleck sign"), which corresponds to the Lisfranc ligament, is infrequent in children.

In cases where radiology is not conclusive, it can be supplemented with CT-scan or MRI.

For these injuries, the Hardcastle classification is used (Fig. 32.10):

Type A: total incongruity of the entire tarsometatarsal joint in one direction, sagittal, coronal, or combined.
Type B: partial incongruity, medial displacement of the first metatarsal or lateral displacement of the second-third-fourth-fifth. More common in patients pediatric.
Type C: divergent pattern, medial displacement of the first metatarsal and lateral of second-third-fourth-fifth.

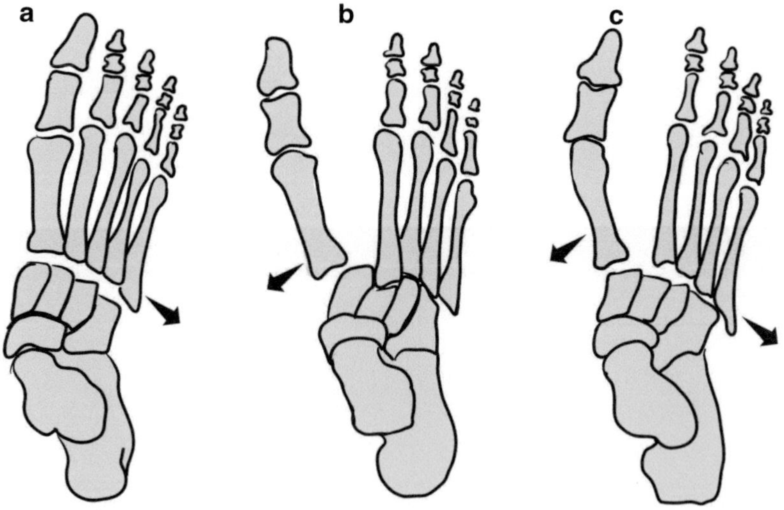

Fig. 32.10 Hardcastle classification. (**a**) Total unidirectional incongruence; (**b**) partial incongruence; (**c**) divergent pattern

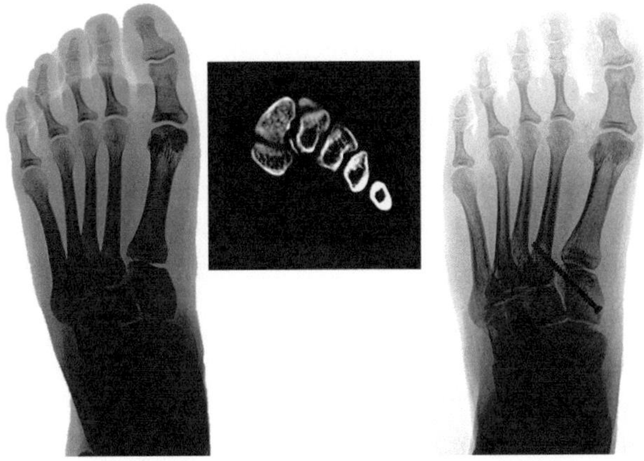

Fig. 32.11 Lisfranc injury in a 13-year-old girl. The CT-scan showed the "fleck" sign, confirming avulsion of the Lisfranc ligament. She was treated with stabilization with a cannulated screw

The treatment of non-displaced fractures or with minimal displacement (<2–3 mm), should consider the condition of the soft tissues. The application of a cast should be deferred due to the risk of compartment syndrome.

The short leg cast is used for 3–4 weeks, non-weight bearing, then protected load for 2–3 weeks. In patients close to adolescence, the need for physiotherapy should be evaluated.

For those displaced fractures, reduction should be performed, closed and/or open, with osteosynthesis (Fig. 32.11), which can be with Kirschner wires, screws, or plates, depending on the characteristics of the fracture and associated injuries, in addition to the age of the patient. After this, it should be immobilized for 3–4 weeks.

As low-energy injuries are more frequent in this age group, complications associated with soft tissues are of low frequency, and the prognosis tends to be with full recovery of the function and low incidence of chronic pain associated with instability [18].

There are some midfoot fractures encompassed in the term "bunk-bed fracture," with a mechanism like Lisfranc's, but in a pediatric population under 6 years old:

1. Incomplete fracture of the base first metatarsal, torus, or Salter-Harris Type I.
2. Compression fracture of the cuboid, which on the radiograph is seen as an area of greater sclerosis towards proximal.

Both fractures are managed conservatively, with a short leg cast for 3–4 weeks.

32.9 Metatarsal Fractures

They correspond to the most frequent fractures of the pediatric foot (60%). In general terms, subcapital and diaphyseal fractures present little displacement and angulation, with wide tolerance ranges for the central metatarsals.

If reduction is required, it is achieved with closed maneuvers, and in the face of instability, percutaneous osteosynthesis with smooth Kirschner wires is sufficient, associated with a short leg cast, for 3–4 weeks in the case of subcapitals, and 4–6 weeks in the diaphyseal; the first half of the immobilization time off-load and then protected load. In children under 5 years old, the isolated fracture of the first metatarsal is more frequent and over that age, the isolated fracture of the fifth. The fractures of the second-third-fourth metatarsal do not occur in isolation, so all metatarsals should be evaluated in search of more subtle concomitant injuries (Fig. 32.12).

The injuries can be by direct mechanism: contusion by fall of blunt object or crushing, with features usually in the middle third of the diaphyses; or indirect: by axial loads or torsional forces, which generate spiral features at the level of the proximal third of the diaphysis or subcapitals.

On examination, we will find pain, bruising and swelling in the midfoot. A high index of suspicion should be maintained due to the risk of compartment syndrome. In indirect mechanisms, the involvement of soft parts is more subtle and may only manifest as refusal to load.

The initial study is performed with AP, lateral, and oblique foot x-rays. It is important to define the treatment, evaluate angulations and displacements both in the anteroposterior and sagittal plane. There is no specific classification for these fractures. In case of patients under 5 years old with initial negative findings on x-rays, but with a high clinical suspicious, it is suggested to temporarily immobilize with short leg splint and re-evaluate with x-ray in 10–14 days, in search for bone repair signs.

The absolute indications for surgical management are an open fracture, articular involvement, compartment syndrome, and non-union. Acceptable values of angulation and shortening in children are not clearly defined, but reduction should be considered in the following cases: dorsal angulation >20°, shortening >5 mm, risk of

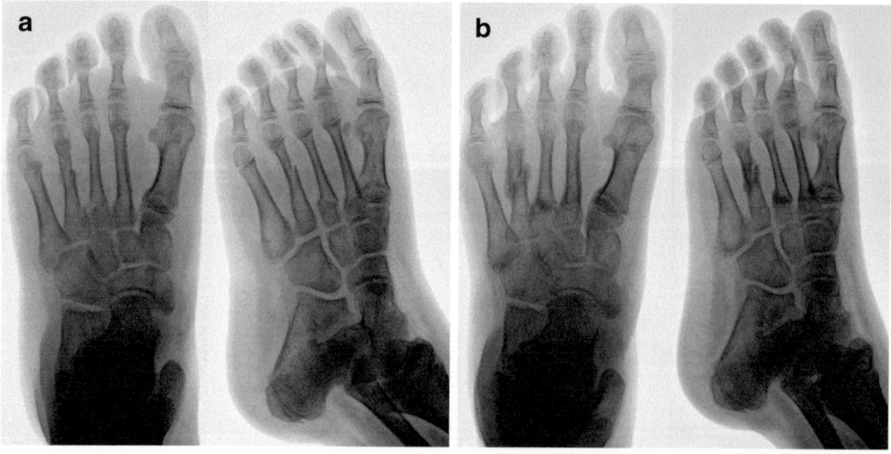

Fig. 32.12 Foot x-rays of a 9-year-old boy with fractures of the 2nd, 3rd, and 4th metatarsals (**a**). He was treated conservatively, with evidence of consolidation after 4 weeks of evolution (**b**)

exposure. In relation to the first metatarsal, it is advisable to perform reduction with dorsal angulation >10° and shortening of any magnitude. In the adolescent population, a displacement greater than 75% of the diaphyseal width is added as a relative indication for reduction [19].

The complications of these injuries are more related to the involvement of soft tissues. In the specific case of the fracture, the risk of delay in consolidation could occur in open fractures or loss of reductions in up to 15% [20].

32.10 Fracture of the Base of the Fifth Metatarsal

Fractures of the base of the fifth metatarsal account for 40% of all metatarsal fractures, and 90% of them are concentrated in those >10 years old. It is associated with a forced inversion or adduction of the foot resting on the ground.

Clinically, it presents with pain on load on the lateral edge of the foot, localized edema at the base of the fifth metatarsal of variable amount, with bruising being infrequent. The initial study is with AP, lateral and oblique foot x-rays, which are sufficient to make a diagnosis and define the therapeutic approach.

The fracture line is usually perpendicular to the diaphyseal axis, which allows differential diagnosis with the apophyseal ossification nucleus and accessory nuclei (os vesalianum and os peroneum). Remember that the ossification center appears at 8 years old and fuses around 12 years old in women and 15 years old in men. The axis of the accessory nucleus is parallel to that of the diaphysis, and in the case of avulsion of this, a minimum displacement is appreciated [21].

The avulsive fracture of the tuberosity is produced by the action of the peroneus brevis tendon, but could involve the origin of the abductor digiti minimi muscle.

Classification

- Avulsive fracture of the tuberosity.
- Ossification nucleus fracture.
- Jones fracture.

Avulsive fractures, proximal to the metaphysio-diaphyseal junction, and non-displaced, are conservatively treated, with short leg cast and unloading for 3–4 weeks, followed by protected load for 2 weeks, with good results.

Fractures located distal to the metaphysio-diaphyseal junction require strict clinical and radiological follow-up. In case of an initial non-significant displacement, unloading is indicated for 4–6 weeks with a short leg cast and then protected load for 3 weeks (Fig. 32.13).

Distal fractures have a higher risk of delayed consolidation and non-union, which increases with late diagnosis, presenting with persistent pain and functional impotence. The Jones fracture in patients under 13 years old has the highest risk of non-union, as well as a history of pain prior to trauma (stress fracture). In case any of these complications are identified, surgical reduction, fracture focus reactivation, bone graft in case of pseudoarthrosis, and osteosynthesis with compressive

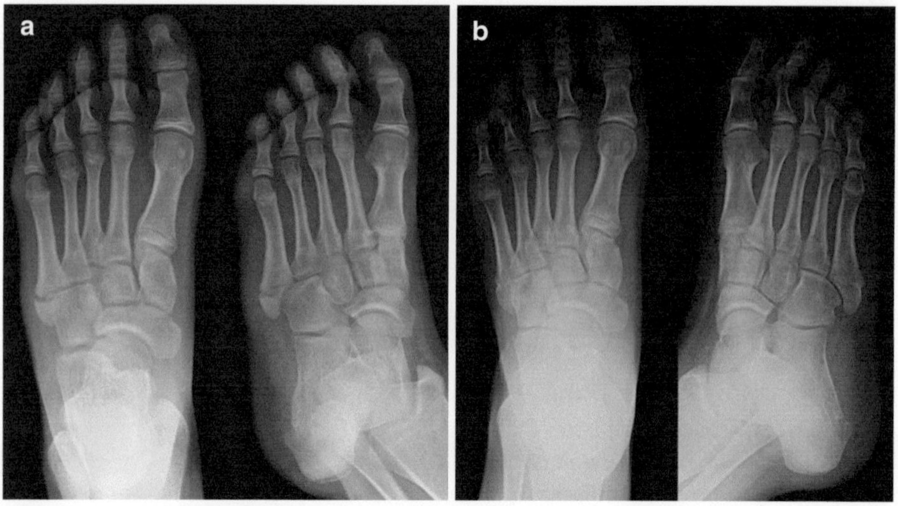

Fig. 32.13 Adolescent with a Jones fracture of the 5th metatarsal (**a**). Consolidation is evident after 6 weeks of conservative treatment (**b**)

technique (4.0–4.5 mm screws) are indicated, although the use of smooth Kirschner wires in the acute period is described, the last associated with immobilization and unloading.

32.11 Toe Fractures

These are common injuries, accounting for 18% of fractures of the pediatric foot. These occur due to heavy objects falling on the foot, or direct contusion when walking barefoot. In addition to evaluating the state of the soft tissues, it is necessary to identify any compromise of the nail bed, as if present, it corresponds to an open fracture, often being Salter and Harris type I or II injuries, displaced.

For diagnosis and to determine the need for reduction, a study with AP, lateral, and oblique foot x-rays is usually sufficient. The proximal phalanx is usually the one involved.

In the case of a displaced Salter-Harris Type I or Type II fracture in only one plane (Fig. 32.14), a reduction with local anesthesia (traction and correction of the deformity in the opposite direction to the deformity), radiological control, and immobilization with a bandage to the adjacent toe (barreling) is sufficient.

If the angulation is in two planes or an unstable subcapital feature, reduction in the operating room is indicated. Generally, closed reduction is enough, osteosynthesis with a Kirschner wire using a percutaneous technique and, depending on the patient's age, immobilization with barreling or a short leg cast and off-load for 2–3 weeks, after which the immobilization and wire are removed.

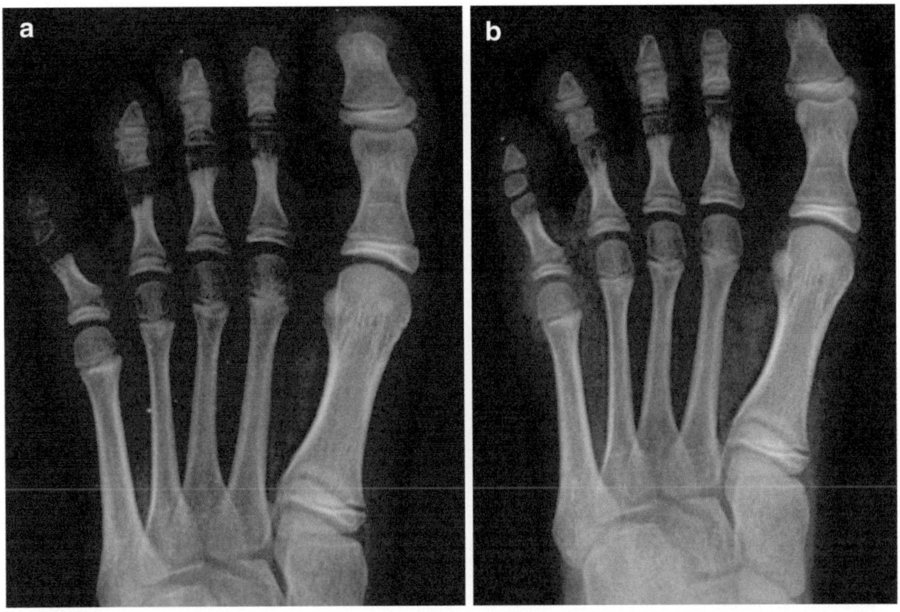

Fig. 32.14 (**a**) Displaced Salter and Harris II type fracture of the proximal phalanx of the 5th toe. (**b**) Post-reduction control under local anesthesia

A specific classification is not applied in phalange fractures, but it is relevant to determine the involvement of the nail bed, as the presence of peri-ungual blood, eponychium injury or subungual hematoma makes it necessary to rule out an open fracture Salter-Harris Type I or Type II, with dorsal displacement. It is recommended to drain the subungual hematoma when it covers >50% of the nail. In the hallux, the displaced physis fracture of the distal phalanx associated with exposure through the nail bed with matrix damage, is called a Pinckney fracture, and is generally secondary to sports injuries [22].

Most of these injuries have a good prognosis, with non-surgical treatment. In general terms, from the second to the fifth toes, immobilization through barreling bandage results in sufficient stability and analgesia, allowing heel loading as tolerated. The bone healing time fluctuates between 3 and 4 weeks, and a short leg cast can be added for protected walking, if necessary (multiple fractures).

Open fractures should be managed according to general principles: cleaning, suturing, stabilization (if necessary), and repair of the nail bed and matrix to avoid alteration of the morphology of the nail.

Hallux fractures that compromise the physis and epiphysis can involve the articular surface (Fig. 32.15). When the joint extension exceeds 25% of the surface, or the displacement is greater than 2–3 mm, closed or open reduction and osteosynthesis with smooth Kirschner wires or mini screws according to age are indicated [23, 24].

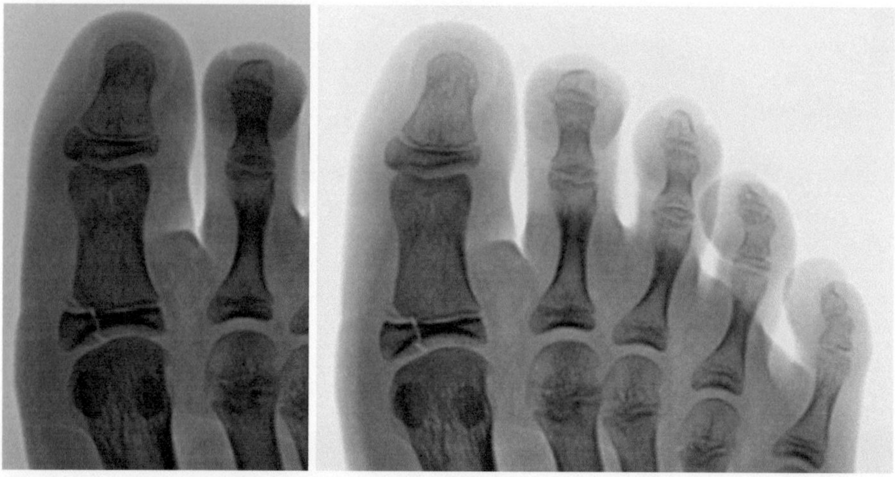

Fig. 32.15 Fracture of the proximal phalanx epiphysis of the hallux in a 9-year-old girl. She was treated non-surgically due to minimal initial displacement of the injury

32.12 Stress Fractures

Repetitive activities that exceed the regeneration capacity of bone tissue cause stress fractures. In athletes with an immature skeleton, the accelerated increase in muscle mass, the presence of still developing bones with thinner cortices, lower proportional bone mineral density and hormonal factors, predispose to this type of injuries.

The foot occupies the second place in frequency of these injuries, with the metatarsals and tarsal bones, respectively, being the tibia the bone with the highest incidence. The sports that are most related to stress fractures of the metatarsals are ballet, athletics and gymnastics.

We will find localized pain in the plantar or dorsum of the foot, of long duration. The x-ray study has low sensitivity (15%), may show periosteal reaction, cortical thickening and sclerosis. Three-phase bone scintigraphy has better sensitivity, but low specificity. MRI is the choice in these injuries [25].

The treatment will depend on the location, complication with acute fracture, age, and activity level of the patient; generally, they are managed conservatively with unloading and modification of predisposing factors (see Chap. 5).

32.13 Wheel Spoke Injuries

Wheel spoke injuries are a common reason for consultation in pediatric emergency services, with a higher incidence between the ages of 2 and 8 years old, related to the improper transportation of children as passengers on bicycles that do not have protective measures or seats intended for this purpose [26].

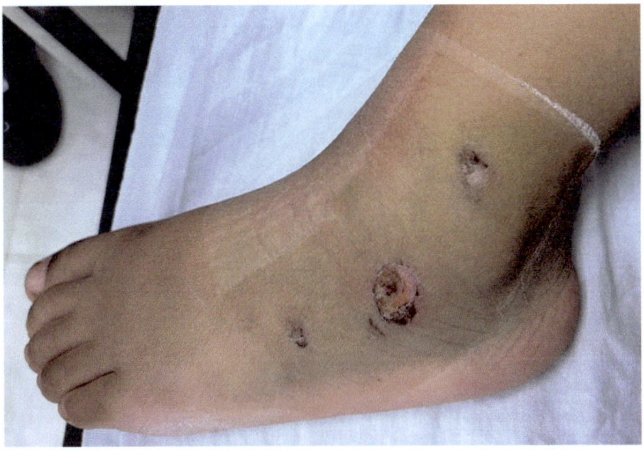

Fig. 32.16 Soft tissue injuries, caused by erosion with bicycle wheel spokes, at the ankle and foot level, in an 8-year-old child

The injury occurs through three mechanisms:

- Tissue laceration due to the "knife" effect of the spoke
- Crushing from the impact between the wheel and arch
- Damage from the shear vector resulting from these two forces

Given the above, the final magnitude of the soft tissue injury will be evident within 48–72 h, due to the effect on the local microvasculature.

The initial evaluation is of vital importance, where the state of the soft tissues, neurovascular and osteoarticular involvement should be included. X-rays must be requested, from the ankle and foot, and can show incomplete metaphyseal fractures of the distal tibia/fibula, with physeal involvement.

In this type of injury, the serial evaluation through time of the state of the soft tissues is fundamental, considering its evolutionary nature, since in general if associated fractures are found, they are managed non-surgically, requiring only immobilization (Fig. 32.16).

32.14 Foot Compartment Syndrome

The tissues of the pediatric foot have greater elasticity than those of the adult, mainly due to their cartilaginous bone composition and higher water content, but in the face of high-energy traumas, the risk of compartment syndrome should always be considered. Open fractures do not decrease the potential risk of occurrence.

The sustained increase in pressure in the nine compartments of the foot decreases perfusion, causing muscle necrosis and nerve ischemia; prolonged ischemia can result in irreversible damage to the muscles, nerves, and skin. The importance of early identification and timely treatment lies in the severity of the functional sequelae it entails, constituting one of the surgical emergencies in traumatology.

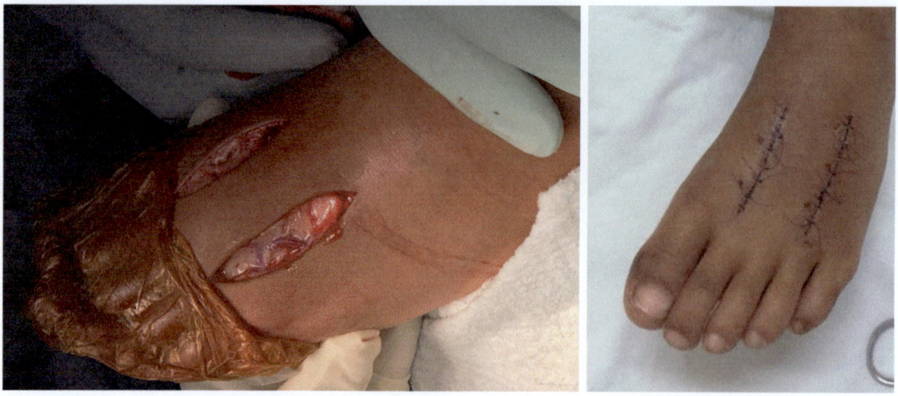

Fig. 32.17 Foot fasciotomy in a 7-year-old child due to high-energy trauma and secondary compartment syndrome. Closure of the fasciotomies is observed at 3 weeks, with complete coverage

Normal pressure values in the compartments of infants are higher than in adults, and it has not yet been possible to standardize cut-off values according to age, so pressure measurement as the only diagnostic tool is not validated.

The diagnosis continues to be clinical. The "5P's", described to identify a compartment syndrome, do not present early in children, demonstrating little utility in timely diagnosis. In pediatric age, the "3A's" should be identified: Anxiety, increase in Analgesic needs, Agitation; with the increase in analgesic requirements being the earliest of them. The presence of any of these signs in a patient who has suffered a severe foot injury should raise suspicion of an imminent compartment syndrome and the need for an emergency fasciotomy.

Generally, after 48–72 h, if there is not associated extensive soft tissue injury or coverage deficit, primary skin closure is feasible, obtaining good functional results (Fig. 32.17).

The prevalence of pediatric foot compartment syndrome is unknown. Wallin [29] presents a systematic review of the available literature from 1990 to 2012, with studies that support the good results after fasciotomy in pediatric patients, with medium-term follow-ups. Among the complications are chronic pain, claw toes, cavus foot, and paresthesias.

32.15 Final Message

Foot fractures are among the most common injuries in pediatric age. Although most of them are amenable to conservative management due to their great potential for healing and remodeling, this is not infinite, and this premise does not apply to all the bones of the foot, not across all ages.

The radiology of the pediatric foot is complex, so the application of a systematized radiological evaluation, knowledge of standardized measurements and their proper application and interpretation for the choice of the correct treatment in each case, is of vital importance.

32.16 Authors' Recommendations

- The talus fracture, with a high-energy mechanism, is generally associated with ankle fractures, so an imaging study of the ankle and foot should be requested in the initial evaluation.
- Always consider within the differential diagnosis of lateral ankle sprain due to a fall on a skateboard, the fracture of the lateral process of the talus.
- Any contusion of the hallux with evidence of peri-ungual bleeding at the base should be evaluated to rule out an open physeal fracture of the distal phalanx.
- Subcapital and diaphyseal fractures of the central metatarsals have a great potential for consolidation and remodeling, so it is recommended to consider the patient's age, taking into account the premise "treat the child, not the x-ray.".
- Maintain a high index of suspicion in causal mechanisms of Lisfranc Injury, evaluate the x-rays systematically, and request specialized imaging studies in cases that warrant it.
- Open foot fractures do not decrease the risk of compartment syndrome, remember the "3A's", and maintain a high index of suspicion.

References

1. Landin LA. Epidemiology of children's fractures. J Pediatr Orthop B. 1997;6(2):79–83. https://doi.org/10.1097/01202412-199704000-00002.
2. Denning JR, Mehlman CT. The community Orthopaedic surgeon taking trauma call: pediatric foot fracture pearls and pitfalls. J Orthop Trauma. 2019;33(Suppl 8):S27–32. https://doi.org/10.1097/BOT.0000000000001547.
3. Cooper C, Dennison EM, Leufkens HG, Bishop N, van Staa TP. Epidemiology of childhood fractures in Britain: a study using the general practice research database. J Bone Miner Res. 2004;19(12):1976–81. https://doi.org/10.1359/JBMR.040902.
4. Blount W. Injuries of the foot. In: Beaty JH, Kasser JR, editors. Fractures in children. Philadelphia, PA: Williams and Wilkins; 1955. p. 195–6.
5. Adirim TA, Cheng TL. Overview of injuries in the young athlete. Sports Med. 2003;33(1):75–81. https://doi.org/10.2165/00007256-200333010-00006.
6. Ogden J. The foot. In: Ogden J, editor. Skeletal injury in the child. New York: Springer; 2000. p. 626–7.
7. Rockwood and Wilkins. Fractures in children. 9th ed; 2020; vol. 30. pp. 1883–964.
8. Green A. The pediatric foot and ankle. Pediatr Clin N Am. 2020;67(1):169–83. https://doi.org/10.1016/j.pcl.2019.09.007.
9. Stiell I. Ottawa ankle rules. Can Fam Physician. 1996;42:478–80.
10. Thermann H, Schratt HE, Hüfner T, Tscherne H. Die Frakturen des kindlichen fusses [Fractures of the pediatric foot]. Unfallchirurg. 1998;101(1):2–11. https://doi.org/10.1007/s001130050225.

11. Hawkins LG. Fractures of the neck of the talus. J Bone Joint Surg Am. 1970;52(5):991–1002.
12. Canale ST, Kelly FB Jr. Fractures of the neck of the talus. Long-term evaluation of seventy-one cases. J Bone Joint Surg Am. 1978;60(2):143–56.
13. Kızılay YO, Aytan O. Low-energy Hawkins type III Talar neck fracture-dislocation with neurovascular and tendon entrapment in a pediatric patient. J Foot Ankle Surg. 2017;56(6):1288–91. https://doi.org/10.1053/j.jfas.2017.05.007.
14. Reginelli A, Russo A, Turrizziani F, Picascia R, Micheletti E, Galeazzi V, et al. Imaging of pediatric foot disorders. Acta Biomed. 2018;89(1-S):34–47. https://doi.org/10.23750/abm.v89i1-S.7009.
15. Denning JR. Complications of pediatric foot and ankle fractures. Orthop Clin North Am. 2017;48(1):59–70. https://doi.org/10.1016/j.ocl.2016.08.010.
16. Boyle MJ, Walker CG, Crawford HA. The pediatric Bohler's angle and crucial angle of Gissane: a case series. J Orthop Surg Res. 2011;6:2. https://doi.org/10.1186/1749-799X-6-2.
17. Knijnenberg LM, Dingemans SA, Terra MP, Struijs PAA, Schep NWL, Schepers T. Radiographic anatomy of the pediatric Lisfranc joint. J Pediatr Orthop. 2018;38(10):510–3. https://doi.org/10.1097/BPO.0000000000000864.
18. Mahan ST, Lierhaus AM, Spencer SA, Kasser JR. Treatment dilemma in multiple metatarsal fractures: when to operate? J Pediatr Orthop B. 2016;25(4):354–60. https://doi.org/10.1097/BPB.0000000000000311.
19. Robertson NB, Roocroft JH, Edmonds EW. Childhood metatarsal shaft fractures: treatment outcomes and relative indications for surgical intervention. J Child Orthop. 2012;6(2):125–9. https://doi.org/10.1007/s11832-012-0403-5.
20. Pinckney LE, Currarino G, Kennedy LA. The stubbed great toe: a cause of occult compound fracture and infection. Radiology. 1981;138(2):375–7. https://doi.org/10.1148/radiology.138.2.7455117.
21. Crawford AH, Mehlman CT, Parikh SN. Fractures and dislocations of the foot and ankle. In: Mencio GA, Swiontkowski MF, editors. Green's skeletal trauma in children. 5th ed. Philadelphia, PA: Elsevier Saunders; 2015. p. 473–542.
22. Crawford H. Fractures and dislocations of the foot. In: Flynn JM, Skaggs DL, Waters PM, editors. Rockwood and Wilkins' fracture in children. 8th ed. Philadelphia, PA: Wolters Kluwer; 2015. p. 1225–70.
23. Park DY, Han KJ, Han SH, Cho JH. Barefoot stubbing injuries to the great toe in children: a new classification by injury mechanism. J Orthop Trauma. 2013;27(11):651–5. https://doi.org/10.1097/BOT.0b013e31828e5d39.
24. Jaimes C, Khwaja A, Chauvin N. Ankle and foot injuries in the young athlete. Semin Musculoskelet Radiol. 2018;22(01):104–17. https://doi.org/10.1055/s-0037-1609012.
25. Noonan KJ, McCarthy JJ. Compartment syndrome in the pediatric patient. J Pediatr Orthop. 2010;30(2 Supplement):96–101.
26. Wallin K, Nguyen H, Russell L, Lee DK. Acute traumatic compartment syndrome in pediatric foot: a systematic review and case report. J Foot Ankle Surg. 2016;55(4):817–20. https://doi.org/10.1053/j.jfas.2016.02.010.

Index

A
Acromioclavicular disjunction, 129
Advanced Trauma Life Support (ATLS), 52
Amputation, 117
Ankle fractures, 425
  anatomy, 428, 429
  classification, 426, 431, 432
  complications, 435
  diagnosis, 429–431
  incidence, 425, 426
  injury mechanism, 427, 428
  recommendations, 436
  syndesmotic injuries, 426
  treatment, 433, 434
Anterior cruciate ligament (ACL), 373, 374
  AFTE, 357–360, 363, 364
  complications, 379, 380
  diagnosis, 375, 376
  injury mechanism, 374
  recommendations, 384
  treatment, 377–379
Anterior tuberosity of the tibia (ATT), 389
  anatomy, 390
  classifications, 391
  clinical evaluation, 392
  complications, 396
  imaging, 393, 394
  incidence, 389
  knee mobility, 396
  mechanism of injury, 390, 391
  recommendation, 396
  treatment, 394
Antibiotic prophylaxis, 111, 112
Anxiety, 470
Arthrofibrosis, 366
Avascular necrosis (AVN), 171, 326, 327
Avulsion fractures of the tibial eminence (AFTE)
  anatomy, 358
  classification, 360, 362, 363
  complications, 366
  diagnosis, 358, 359, 365
  pathophysiology, 357
  recommendations, 367–369
  treatment, 363, 364
Avulsion injury, 179
Avulsive fracture, 465

B
Bado classification, 233, 234
Baumann angle, 197
Bone fragility, 99, 100
Bone repair
  characteristics, 3
  conservative treatment, 76–78
  growth factors
    bone grafts, 12, 13
    cell therapy, 12
    distraction osteogenesis, 12
    micromobility, 11
  growth plate, 8, 9
  inflammatory phase, 10
  ossification process, 7, 8
  remodeling phase, 11
  reparative phase, 10, 11
  secondary repair, 9
  tissue structure, 3–7

M. Sepúlveda O. (ed.), *Paediatrics Traumatology*,
https://doi.org/10.1007/978-3-031-89482-4

C

Calcaneus fractures, 458–460
Cast index, 267
Cervical spine injury, 50
Child abuse, 35
Chondrogenesis, 10
Chondrolysis, 328
Clavicle fracture
  anatomy, 124, 125
  classification, 127
  definition, 123
  diagnosis, 125–127
  epidemiology, 123
  mechanism of injury, 124
  recommandation, 134
  treatment, 128–134
Clavicle fractures, 81
Clinodactyly deformity, 276
Collagen proteins, 6
Conservative treatment
  bone repair, 76–78
  characteristics, 75, 76
  complications, 84
  diagnosis, 79, 81
  humeral condyle fractures, 163
  indications, 81
  options for, 82, 83
  recommendations, 85, 86
Consolidation, 255
Coxa vara, 327
Cubitus Varus, 204

D

Damage Control Orthopedic Surgery, 50
Deltopectoral approach, 144
Diaphyseal fracture, radius and ulna
  anatomy, 248
  classification, 249, 250
  complications, 255–257
  diagnosis, 249
  incidence, 245
  mechanisms of injury, 246–248
  recommendations, 257, 258
  treatment, 250–255
Diaphyseal fractures, 91
Discoid meniscus (DM), 383, 384
Distal femur fractures
  classification, 347–349
  complications, 354, 357
  diagnosis, 346, 347
  incidence, 344
  pathophysiology, 344, 345
  radiographic study, 343
  recommendations, 355
  treatment
    metaphyseal fractures, 350, 351
    physeal and epiphyseal fractures, 351–353
    principles, 349
    stabilization, 350
Distal radius fracture, 262
  classification, 263
  complications, 270, 272
  diagnosis, 262, 263
  epidemiology, 261
  incidence, 261
  mechanism of injury, 262
  recommendations, 272
  treatment, 264–267, 269, 270
Distraction osteogenesis, 12

E

Early Total Care (ETC), 50
Elastic intramedullary nailing (ESIN)
  anteroposterior and lateral projection, 93
  diameter of, 95
  indications, 95–97
  materials, 94
  planes, 92
  radial neck fractures, 209, 214, 221–225
  rotational movements, 92
  T-handle, 93
Elbow, 159, 161–165, 167, 169, 170
Elbow dislocation, 177, 179, 180, 183, 184, 188
Epiphyseal fractures, 351–353
Epiphyseal vessels, 18
Essex-Lopresti classification, 459
External fixation (EF), 98, 99

F

Fassier-Duval type telescopic nails, 100
Femoral epiphysis, 318
Femoral metaphysis, 318
Femoral shaft fractures, 331
  classification, 333
  complications, 338, 339
  diagnosis, 332, 333
  incidence, 331
  mechanism of injury, 332
  recommendations, 339, 340
  treatment, 334, 335, 337
Femur fractures, *see* Femoral shaft fractures

Fingertip injuries, 289
  anatomy
    distal phalanx, 292
    nail complex, 291
    pulp, 292
  classification, 293
  definition, 289
  diagnosis, 293
  epidemiology, 290
  pathophysiology, 290
  treatment
    amputation, conservative treatment, 298
    distal phalanx fracture, repair and fixation, 297, 298
    local flaps, 298–301
    nail bed avulsions, 297
    nail bed injury, suture or adhesives, 296
    subungual hematoma, trephine and drain, 294
    traumatic onysectomy, 295, 296
Fish tail deformity, 170
Floating knee, 348
Foot injury
  anatomy, 452, 453
  calcaneus fractures, 458–460
  compartment syndrome, 469, 470
  diagnosis, 454, 455
  incidence, 451
  lisfranc injury, 461–463
  metatarsal fractures, 463–466
  pathophysiology, 452
  prognosis, 451
  recommendations, 471
  sports activity, 452
  stress fractures, 468
  talus fractures, 455–458
  tarsal level, 460, 461
  toe fractures, 466–468
  wheel spoke injuries, 468, 469
Forearm fractures, *see* Diaphyseal fracture, radius and ulna

G

Gartland classification, 199
Growth plate
  anatomy, 16–18
  bone repair, 8, 9
  classification, 22–25
  complications, 29–31
  definition, 15
  diagnosis, 20
  incidence, 25, 26
  mechanism of injury, 26
  regulation, 18, 19
  trauma, 20
  treatment, 26–29
Gustilo and Anderson (GA) classification, 111
Gustilo-Anderson classification, 55

H

Hallux fractures, 467
Hand fractures, 275
  anatomy, 277, 278
  clinodactyly deformity, 276
  diagnosis, 279, 280
  incidence, 275
  mechanism of injury, 278, 279
  surgical indications, 276
  treatment
    bicondylar fractures, 283
    comminuted fractures, 284
    complications, 287
    diaphyseal fractures, 284, 285
    middle and proximal phalanges, 286, 287
    subcapital fractures, 282, 283
    unicondylar phalangeal fractures, 281, 282
Hardcastle classification, 462
Havers Systems, 4
Hawkins classification, 457
Hedgehog pathway, 4
Hemodynamic instability, 313
Hip fractures, in children and adolescents
  classification, 320–322
  complications, 326–328
  diagnosis, 319, 320
  incidence, 317
  pathophysiology, 318, 319
  treatment, 323–326
Holstein-Lewis fracture, 154
Humeral condyle fractures
  classification, 159–161
  complications, 168–172
  conservative treatment, 163
  definition, 159
  diagnosis, 161–163
  post-operative management, 167
  surgical treatment, 163–166
  treatment outcomes, 167, 168
Humeral shaft fractures
  classification, 150
  complications, 154
  diagnosis, 149

Humeral shaft fractures (*cont.*)
  epidemiology, 147
  mechanism of injury, 148, 149
  recommendations, 155, 156
  treatment, 152, 153
Hypertrophic zone, 16

I
Injury Severity Score (ISS), 53
Insulin-Like Growth Factor I (IGF-I), 18
Intramedullary nail (IMN), 337

J
Juvenile Tillaux fracture, 440–442

K
Kirschner wires, 101, 102, 130, 133, 143, 152, 163, 164, 185, 187, 200, 204–206, 282, 416, 417, 434, 466
Knee injury, *see* Distal femur fractures

L
Legg-Calvé-Perthes disease, 319
Letts classification, 234, 235
Lisfranc injury, 461–463
Locked compression plate (LCP), 97, 98
Lower limb injuries, 65

M
Malunion, 188, 204, 327, 458
Mangled Extremity Severity Score (MESS), 117
Medial epicondyle fractures
  anatomy, 177, 178
  avulsion injury, 179
  classification, 183, 184
  complications, 188
  diagnosis, 179, 180, 182
  direct trauma, 179
  incidence, 177
  recommendations, 186, 187
  treatment, 184–186
Meniscal injuries
  complications, 383
  diagnosis of, 381
  discoid meniscus, 383, 384
  mechanism of, 380
  prevalence, 380
  recommendations, 384
  treatment, 381, 383
Metaphyseal corner fractures, 40
Metaphyseal fractures, 350, 351
Metaphyseal vessels, 18
Metatarsal fractures, 463–466
Monteggia fracture-dislocation
  classification, 234, 235
  complications, 238, 239
  diagnosis, 236, 237
  history, 233
  mechanism of injury, 235, 236
  recommendation, 239–241
  treatment, 237, 238

N
Nail bed avulsions, 297
Nail bed injury, 296
Neer-Horwitz classification, 142
Niche Cells, 10
Non-accidental injuries (NAI)
  definitions, 35
  diagnosis, 36–38, 40, 41
  prevalence, 35
  risk factors, 36
  treatment, 43
Non-collagen proteins, 6
Non-union, 169, 170, 255, 327, 328

O
Open fractures
  amputation, 117
  antibiotic prophylaxis, 111, 112
  classification, 111
  complications, 117
  debridement and irrigation, 112
  incidence, 109
  stabilization, 114, 116
  treatment, 110, 111
Orthopedic management, 54, 55
Ossification process, 7
  endochondral, 8
  intramembranous, 8
Ossification zone, 17
Osteoblasts, 5, 6
Osteocalcin (OCN), 6
Osteochondrosis, 62
Osteoclasts, 5
Osteocytes, 6
Osteogenesis imperfecta, 6, 100
Osteopontin, 4

Osteoprotegerin (OPG), 5
Osteosynthesis, 89, 90, 104–106, 153, 254, 313, 331, 416, 418
Overuse musculoskeletal injuries
anatomy, 60
classification, 62
epidemiology, 60
lower limbs, 65
morbidity, 59
pathophysiology, 61, 62
pelvis, 67
prevention, 71
recommendations, 72
spine, 69
stress fractures, 69, 70
treatment, 63, 64, 70
upper limbs, 64, 65

P
Parathyroid hormone (PTH), 12
Pavlik harnesses, 334
Pediatric Trauma Score (PTS), 53
Pelvic injuries, 67
anatomical factors, 306
characteristics, 305
classification, 307, 308
diagnosis, 308–310
epidemiology, 306
etiology, 306
traumatic brain injury, 307
treatment, 311, 313, 314
Pelvis fractures, 51
Perichondral complex, 17
Physis, 101, 102, *see* Growth plate
Pinckney fracture, 467
Polytrauma patient
abdominal injuries, 54
cause of death, 48
characteristics, 48
evaluation and treatment, 50–52
history, 47
imaging, 52, 53
implementation, 47
orthopedic management, 54, 55
scoring systems, 53
systemic response, 49, 50
thoracic trauma, 54
traumatic brain injury, 54
Proximal humerus fractures
anatomy, 138, 139
classification, 141
complications, 145
cysts, 145
definition, 137
diagnosis, 140, 141
external rotation, 145
incidence, 137
injury mechanism, 139
shoulder dislocation, 145
treatment, 142–145
Proximal tibial fractures
classification, 401, 402
complications, 406
Cozen's phenomenon, 402
diagnosis, 404
incidence, 399
knee instability, 406
mechanism of injury, 400, 401
physis, 400
popliteal artery, 400
trampoline, 403
treatment, 404, 405
Pseudoparalysis, 140

R
Radial neck fractures
clinical evaluation and radiology, 211, 212
conservative/non-operative decision analysis, 215–221
X-ray, 215
dislocation, 226–228
ESIN, 209, 221–225
injury mechanism, 210, 211
non-operative and operative treatment, 212–214
postoperative management and outcome, 225
principles, 228–230
treatment strategy, 214
Rang and Smith classification, 183
Ranvier zone, 17
Rib fractures, 40
Runx2 transcription factor, 6

S
Salter and Harris (SH) classification, 23–25
Screw fixation, 103
Seymour fractures, 297
Skeletal Survey, 40
Sonic Hedgehog (Shh), 5
Spica cast, 334, 339
Spine injuries, 69
Spondylolysis, 69

Sternoclavicular joint, 133
Stress fractures, 69, 70, 461, 468
Subungual hematomas, 294
Supracondylar fractures, 191
  classification, 199, 200
  complications, 204–206
  diagnosis, 194–197, 199
  incidence, 192
  mechanism of injury, 192, 194
  treatment, 200, 201, 203, 204
Surgical treatment
  bone fragility, 99, 100
  characteristics, 90
  diaphyseal fractures, 91
  elastic intramedullary nailing
    anteroposterior and lateral projection, 93
    diameter of, 95
    indications, 95–97
    materials, 94
    planes, 92
    rotational movements, 92
    T-handle, 93
  external fixation, 98, 99
  humeral condyle fractures, 163–166
  LCP, 97, 98
  osteosynthesis, 89, 90, 104–106
  pathophysiology, 90
  periosteum, 92
  physis, 101, 102
  role of fixation, 91, 92
  screws, 103
Syndesmosis, 429

T
Talus fractures, 455–458
Technetium (Tc99), 320
Thoracic trauma, 54
Tibial fractures, 95
Tibial shaft fractures
  anatomy, 410–412
  classification, 413
  clinical presentation, 409
  complications, 420, 421
  conservative treatment, 414, 415
  diagnosis, 412, 413
  epidemiology, 410
  open fractures, 419
  pathophysiology, 410
  personality, 409
  recommendation, 421, 422
  surgical treatment, 416–419
Tibial tuberosity, *see* Anterior tuberosity of the tibia (ATT)
Titanium elastic nails (TEN), 252
Toe fractures, 466–468
Transitional ankle fractures
  classification, 444, 445
  diagnosis, 442–444
  epidemiology, 439
  pathophysiology, 440, 441
  prognosis, 448, 449
  treatment, 445–448
Traumatic Brain Injury (TBI), 54
Triplane fractures, *see* Transitional ankle fractures

U
Ulnar nerve injury, 188
Unicondylar phalangeal fractures, 281, 282
Upper limb injuries, 64, 65

V
Vacuum assisted closure (VAC) device, 117

W
Wheel spoke injuries, 468, 469
Wiley classification, 460

Z
Zanca projection, 130

MIX
Papier aus verantwortungsvollen Quellen
Paper from responsible sources
FSC® C105338

If you have any concerns about our products,
you can contact us on
ProductSafety@springernature.com

In case Publisher is established outside the EU,
the EU authorized representative is:
Springer Nature Customer Service Center GmbH
Europaplatz 3, 69115 Heidelberg, Germany

Printed by Libri Plureos GmbH
in Hamburg, Germany